Nutrition Education
Linking Research, Theory, and Practice

Isobel R. Contento, PhD
Mary Swartz Rose Professor of Nutrition Education
Teachers College Columbia University

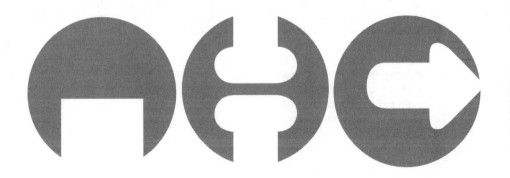

JONES AND BARTLETT PUBLISHERS
Sudbury, Massachusetts
BOSTON   TORONTO   LONDON   SINGAPORE

World Headquarters

Jones and Bartlett Publishers
40 Tall Pine Drive
Sudbury, MA 01776
978-443-5000
info@jbpub.com
www.jbpub.com

Jones and Bartlett Publishers Canada
6339 Ormindale Way
Mississauga, Ontario L5V 1J2
CANADA

Jones and Bartlett Publishers International
Barb House, Barb Mews
London W6 7PA
UK

Production Credits
Acquisitions Editor: Jacqueline Mark-Geraci
Senior Production Editor: Julie Champagne Bolduc
Associate Editor: Patrice M. Andrews
Editorial Assistant: Amy L. Flagg
Production Assistant: Jennifer M. Ryan
Marketing Manager: Wendy Thayer
Manufacturing Buyer: Therese Connell
Composition: Shawn Girsberger
Cover Design: Anne Spencer
Senior Photo Researcher and Photographer: Kimberly Potvin
Cover Image: © Mark B. Bauschke/ShutterStock, Inc.
Printing and Binding: Malloy, Inc.
Cover Printing: Malloy, Inc.

Library of Congress Cataloging-in-Publication Data
Contento, Isobel.
  Nutrition education : linking research, theory, and practice / Isobel Contento.
     p. ; cm.
  Includes bibliographical references.
  ISBN-13: 978-0-7637-3806-8 (alk. paper)
  ISBN-10: 0-7637-3806-9
 1. Nutrition. 2. Health education. 3. Food habits. I. Title.
  [DNLM: 1. Health Education--methods. 2. Nutrition Therapy--methods. 3. Food Habits. WB 18 C759n 2006]
  RA784.C596 2006
  613.2--dc22
                              2006101796
6048

Printed in the United States of America
12 11 10 09 08 10 9 8 7 6 5 4 3

Brief Contents

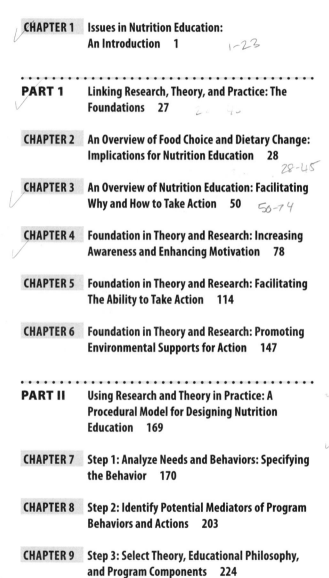

Contents

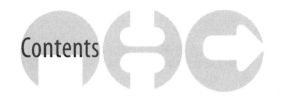

Preface

The importance of nutrition education has become increasingly recognized now that there is consensus that people's food choices, dietary practices, and physical activity behaviors influence health. The public's increased risk of chronic disease and the concern about the high rate of overweight have added urgency to the need for nutrition education. Nutrition education can be delivered through multiple venues and its scope is very broad. Consequently, this text focuses on how to design, deliver, and evaluate the types of educational interventions and programs that the vast majority of nutrition educators conduct on an ongoing basis in their places of work.

During the past decade there has been considerable research in the behavioral aspects of nutrition and in nutrition education. Nutrition educators have gained a better understanding of why people eat what they do and how they make change. New research is available regarding how nutrition education can increase the motivation, skills, and opportunities for people to engage in health-promoting actions. There is also increased appreciation that our food choices are embedded in social and environmental contexts that have considerable influence on these choices. The role of nutrition education is thus to address the numerous personal and environmental influences on food choices and dietary behaviors—potential mediators of action and behavior change—so as to assist individuals in practicing healthy behaviors.

Enriched by teamwork among nutrition educators and other professionals, such as health educators, psychologists, and physicians, this research has generated theoretical frameworks that can guide nutrition education. From such research we know that nutrition education is more likely to be effective when it clearly identifies the behaviors or practices of a given group that can contribute to improved health, then uses theory and evidence to identify the motivations of people to engage in these behaviors and practices, help them to overcome barriers, and promote environments that are supportive. Nutrition education thus needs to be action- or issue-focused, evidence-based, and framed by theory.

Helping students make the transition from knowing about some of the key theories of motivation and behavior change and applying them is a challenge. This book is based on my experience, nutrition education research, and participation in nutrition education in a variety of settings. In particular, this text is based on the experience of teaching nutrition students in their first course on nutrition education. I have found that most nutrition students who have learned a considerable body of knowledge about food and nutrition are not able to link research and behavior theory with practice effectively.

I have devised a procedural model to make it easier for students to design effective nutrition education. Using a six-step process, this procedural model shows how *behavioral theory* is translated into *theory-based strategies*, and then into *practical ways* to implement these strategies. It integrates theory, research, and practice, providing advice on designing, implementing, and evaluating theory-based nutrition education. Over the years, this procedural model has been refined and streamlined as students (and practitioners) have used it to design their sessions and we have observed how well this system works in practice.

This book is divided into three parts. Part I, "Linking Research, Theory, and Practice: The Foundations" provides a background in useful theories for nutrition education and the research evidence for effective practice. Part II, "Using Research and Theory in Practice: A Procedural Model for Designing Nutrition Education" describes the six-step process for translating theory and evidence into theory-based educational strategies. It also offers specific practical activities that we can conduct as nutrition educators. Part III, "Research and Theory in Action: Implementing Nutrition Education" describes the nuts and bolts of implementing nutrition education to various audiences through a variety of venues.

This book includes a variety of features to prepare students to provide effective nutrition education to specific groups.

- "Nutrition Education in Action" boxes in each chapter highlight concepts discussed in the chapter through an example of best practice or research.
- The Case Study introduced in Chapter 7 and followed throughout Chapters 8–14 illustrates each step of the procedural model for designing nutrition education.
- Worksheets are provided in Chapters 7–14 for students to develop their own sessions or program using the design system.
- Learning objectives at the beginning of each chapter improve retention of the material presented.
- Review questions at the end of each chapter reinforce key concepts.
- References at the end of each chapter provide an opportunity for further study.

The reading of this book should be accompanied, where there is time, by reading about additional, contemporary examples of research and best practices in journals, professional association newsletters, or government nutrition and health websites, and attending professional meetings. It is also important to keep up with the concerns of the public by following newspaper and television stories about food and nutrition. The public needs and wants what nutrition educators can offer. This book is designed to help students gain the knowledge and skills to provide such nutrition education.

Issues in Nutrition Education:
An Introduction

OVERVIEW   This chapter introduces the reader to the field of nutrition education, its history and its aims. It provides a definition of nutrition education that will be used in this book, and an overview of the book.

OBJECTIVES   At the end of the chapter, you will be able to

- State why nutrition education is both important and difficult to do
- State whether nutrition education is effective
- Understand differing points of view about the purposes and scope of nutrition education
- Define nutrition education
- Describe what nutrition educators do

SCENARIO

Before you begin, reflect on what you think about nutrition education Why is nutrition education necessary, given that so much food and nutrition information is available to the public in the media? Define *nutrition education*. What do you think its goals should be? What kinds of content do you think are appropriate for nutrition education? Write a short paragraph on your prior experience and expectations. After you have read the book or at the end of the semester, you can come back and review what you wrote here and reflect on any changes in your thinking.

Introduction

This is an exciting time for the field of nutrition education. Everyone seems to be interested in food. Most newspapers have weekly sections on food. Restaurant guides have proliferated, and chefs are now celebrities. Cooking shows are popular on television, and in some areas entire television channels are devoted to food. The cookbook and food sections of bookstores have grown, and diet books abound. Food is also an important topic of conversation. As you have probably experienced, mentioning that you are in the field of nutrition means that people immediately have questions for you. Clearly, food is not just a necessity but also one of life's great pleasures. Almost two hundred years ago, Brillat-Savarin pointed out in a book on the physiology of taste that "the pleasure of eating . . . occurs necessarily at least once a day, and may be repeated without inconvenience two or three times in this space of time; . . . it can be combined with all our other pleasures, and even console us for their absence" (Brillat-Savarin, 1825).

At the same time, current eating patterns are associated with 4 of the 10 leading causes of death in developed countries such as the United States: coronary heart disease, some types of cancer, stroke, and type 2 diabetes (Frazão, 1999; National Center for Health Statistics [NCHS], 2003). Dietary factors also are associated with osteoporosis, a major underlying cause of bone fractures in older persons (Frazão, 1996). Obesity is on the rise, carrying with it an increased risk of various chronic diseases. From the late 1970s to the 1990s, the prevalence of overweight among many age groups doubled, so that between 10% and 15% of young people aged 6 to 17 years are now considered overweight, and about half the adult population of the United States is considered either overweight or obese (Flegal et al., 2002; Hill et al., 2003; Hedley et al., 2004). The rate of obesity has jumped in every state. In 1990, obesity rates in most states were below 14%; now most states have an obesity rate of 20% or more (Figure 1-1). Consequently, excesses and imbalances of some food components in the diet have replaced once commonplace nutrient deficiencies as a source of concern (U.S. Department of Health and Human Services [DHHS], 1988; Food and Nutrition Board, 1989; DHHS, 2000).

It is becoming clear that many of today's health conditions are influenced, at least in part, by people's behaviors and are related to lifestyle (DHHS, 2001). Indeed, it has been estimated that diet and other social and behavioral factors such as smoking, sedentary lifestyles, alcohol use, and accidents account for about half of all the causes of death in the United States (Institute of Medicine [IOM], 2000).

The fact that many chronic diseases are to some extent the result of individual and social patterns of behavior (DHHS, 1988; Food and Nutrition Board, 1989; IOM, 2000; DHHS, 2000) means that positive changes in individual dietary behaviors, community conditions of living, social structures, and food-related policies may lead to reduction in risk of disease. Prevention becomes a possibility. In addition, people

are becoming increasingly interested not just in preventing disease but also in enhancing their health. Better health provides people a better quality of life and enhanced functioning so that they are able to do the many things in life they value. By exercising control over modifiable behavioral and socioenvironmental factors that affect health, people can live more healthfully as well as longer. Consequently, recommendations have been made for implementing national strategies to improve health and reduce disease risk (DHHS, 2000; IOM, 2000).

Interest in food and health issues is also high among consumers. Annual surveys of supermarket shoppers show that nutrition is increasingly important as a factor in people's shopping decisions (Food Marketing Institute, 2004). Food companies and food service providers, recognizing that "nutrition" is a buzzword that sells products, are also getting in on the act. They have created fat-free baked goods, low-fat yogurt, and a host of other products to satisfy one set of enthusiasms, as well as low-carbohydrate products in response to another set of enthusiasms. Reduced-sodium products sit side by side with their original, higher-salt versions. The fruit and vegetables sections of many supermarkets have doubled and tripled in size. Some fast food chains are broiling instead of frying and are offering salads and other items perceived to be "healthy."

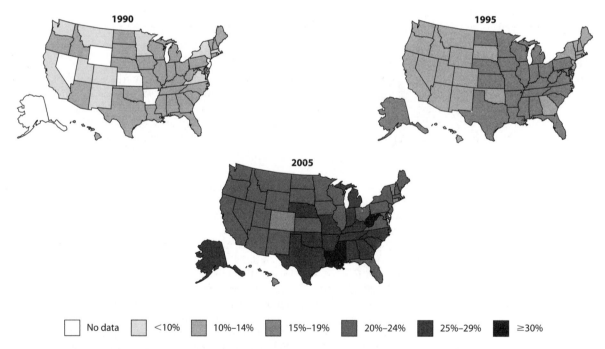

FIGURE 1-1 Obesity trends* among U.S. adults: 1990, 1995, 2005.

* BMI≥30, or about 30 pounds overweight for 5'4" person.
Source: Centers for Disease Control and Prevention. Behavioral Risk Factor Surveillance Systems (BRFSS). www.cdc.gov.bfrss.

Is Nutrition Education Needed?

It would appear, then, that eating well should be getting easier for everyone. If the news media are providing information, and healthful foods abound in food supermarkets, is nutrition education needed? The answer is a definite "yes" for several reasons.

But first, a clarification about the term *nutrition education. Nutrition* is the word we use to talk about the way in which food nourishes people. Good nutrition is essential for growth and development in children, and for health and well-being in people of all ages, as we have discussed, and the relationship between nutrition and health involves many dietary components. Nutrition education is thus education about nutrition. However, people eat foods, not nutrients, so that what is generally referred to as "nutrition education" is education about foods as well as about nutrition.

Dietary Patterns Are Not Optimal

Despite the abundance of food and food products, dietary intakes for many are not optimal. Survey trends show that the average per person intakes of various foods and food products in the United States over the years have improved in some categories but are not as healthful as they could be in others. For example, Americans today consume a little less fresh fruit than 100 years ago and a lot more processed fruit, particularly orange juice; vegetable consumption has increased in the past 25 years, but it is about the same as it was 100 years ago when home-produced vegetables were the major source. Moreover, about 50% of vegetable consumption is white potatoes, much of which are in the form of french fries or potato chips. And while average milk intakes have declined in the past 50 years, intakes of soda have increased over the same period, from 10 gallons per person per year to about 55 gallons. Meat consumption is high, as is the quantity of total added fats and sugars. Finally, survey data show that about 74% of American adults have eating patterns that "need improvement" and another 16% have diets that are "poor" as measured by the Healthy Eating Index (Center for Nutrition Policy and Promotion [CNPP], 2004). Young children start out well, with one third having "good" diets, but by age 9, only 12% have good diets, nearly the same as for adults (CNPP, 2001).

These eating patterns can be compared to the U.S. government's dietary guidance graphic, MyPyramid, which depicts a healthful eating pattern based on scientific evidence. This graphic, shown in Figure 1-2, indicates the amount that people should eat, on average, from each of several basic food groups. The width of each group in the graphic represents how much individuals should eat from each group: more from grains and vegetables, for example, than from milk or meat. The food groups are presented in the shape of a pyramid to convey the concept that *within* each group, individuals should eat *more* lower-fat or higher-fiber foods in that group, which are shown in the bottom of the figure, and *fewer* highly processed, higher-fat, or lower-fiber foods within that group, which are in the tip of the pyramid and are not shown.

National data show that Americans are not eating in the way recommended by this pyramid (CNPP, 2004; Cook & Friday, 2004). They are eating on average 6.8 servings of grain, of which only 0.8 are whole grains, and 4.5 servings of fruit and vegetables, when 5 to 9 are recommended. Although about 50% of Americans meet the recommended daily amounts of 6 to 11 servings or ounces of grains, only 34% do so when caloric intake is taken into consideration. Likewise, only about a quarter of the population meets the recommended 5 or more servings a day of fruits and vegetables for their caloric intake. These data are shown in Table 1-1. Indeed, only about 1 of 10 Americans meets all the recommended intakes from all the basic food groups. These consumption data are depicted graphically in Figure 1-3, which shows that American eating patterns are like an inverted pyramid: narrower at the base and broader at the top. We are eating more from the highly processed, higher-fat, or lower-fiber foods within each group than from the lower-fat, higher-fiber foods within each group. At the same time, we as a nation eat on average 43% of our daily calories from the "other foods" category.

Complex Food Choice Environment

Another reason why people need help making dietary choices is that the food environment has become increasingly complex. People in previous centuries lived on several hundred different foods, mostly locally grown. In 1928, large supermarkets in the United States stocked about 900 items. By the

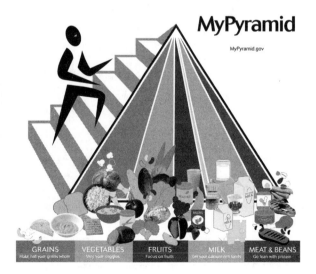

FIGURE 1-2 MyPyramid.

Source: www.MyPyramid.gov.

TABLE 1-1 We Are Not Watching What We Eat

Americans are doing fairly well at watching cholesterol intake. But we're not eating nearly enough fruit and vegetables, and only about 40% are taking it easy on the fat, and about one third on the salt.

	Daily Recommended Amounts	Percentages of People Meeting Daily Recommendations
Grains	6–11 servings	51% (34% for calories)
Vegetables	3–5 servings	42% (34% for calories)
Fruits	2–4 servings	30% (24% for calories)
Milk	2–3 servings	33% (26% for age)
Meat	2–3 servings	44% (38% for calories)
Total fat	30% of calories	38%
Saturated fat	Less than 10% of calories	41%
Cholesterol	300 milligrams or less	69%
Sodium	2,400 milligrams or less	32%
Variety	Eight or more different items in a day	55%

Sources: Cook, A.J., and J.E. Friday. 2004. *Pyramid servings intakes in the United States 1999–2002, 1 day* (CNRG Table Set 3.0). Beltsville, MD: USDA, Agricultural Research Service, Community Nutrition Research Group. http://www.ba.ars.usda.gov/cnrg; and Basiotis, P.P., A. Carlson, S.A. Gerrior, W.Y. Juan, and M. Lino. 2004. The Healthy Eating Index 1999–2000: Charting dietary patterns of Americans. *Family Economics and Nutrition Review* 16(1):39–48.

1980s, a typical supermarket stocked approximately 12,000 food items, taken from an available supply of 60,000 items (Molitor, 1980). Even more dramatic increases have occurred during the past two decades as a growing food industry converts basic foods into an ever-expanding array of food products through increasingly complex technologies. Some 50,000 different brand-name processed food items now perch on many supermarket shelves, from an available supply of 320,000 in the marketplace (Lipton, Edmondson, & Manchester, 1998; Gallo, 1998). In addition, the food preparation that was once done by a family member is now frequently in the hands of a stranger, since 40% of all foods consumed are eaten away from home. Even food that is eaten in the home often has been prepared, purchased, and brought in from elsewhere. Consumers must make choices among these options.

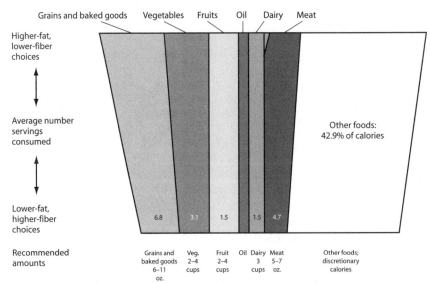

FIGURE 1-3 Food consumption pyramid: Average servings consumed by the U.S. population compared with MyPyramid recommendations.

Source: Community Nutrition Research Group, Agriculture Research Service. 2000, October. *Pyramid servings intakes by U.S. children and adults 1994-1996, 1998.* Beltsville, MD: U.S. Department of Agriculture.

The criteria for food choice have also expanded. Many consumers make choices on the basis of environmental concerns as well as health. For example, most food items come highly packaged, and many have traveled long distances. Many consumers and professionals note that the way food is grown, processed, packaged, distributed, and consumed has serious consequences for the sustainability of our food systems, and believe that it is important to consider these consequences in making food choices (Gussow & Clancy, 1986; Gussow, 1999; Clancy, 1999; Gussow, 2006). Others are interested in social justice concerns and want to choose foods that were produced using fair labor practices. For all these reasons, individual and community food choices have become very complex.

Complex Information Environment

The complexity of the foods available in the marketplace makes wise selection even harder. Our ancestors readily knew the foods they were eating just by looking at them, or could learn about them from family or cultural traditions. Most of the 50,000 items in today's supermarket bear little resemblance to the simple foodstuffs previously eaten by humans. Foods with artificial sweeteners in them are being joined by foods made with artificial fats. Some 10,000 "new" food-related items are being introduced by food processors in the United States every year (or about 30 a day). Knowledge about these items cannot possibly be derived from simply looking at them, nor can their composition and effects on the body be learned by stories and attitudes passed down through the generations. People must learn about foods through other means.

The increasing complexity of this food environment demands consumers who are nutritionally literate. Yet nutritional literacy does not come easily. For packaged foods, nutritional labels are very important. Although 80% of consumers report that they attempt to read food labels, most admit that they don't always understand what they mean (Levy, Patterson, & Kristal, 2000). Some labels on products are actually misleading—lean frozen dinners labeled as "95% fat free" can contain 30% of calories as fat; 2% "low fat" milk also has 30% of its calories as fat. We ask people to "eat no more than 30% to 35% of calories from fat," yet it is almost impossible for consumers to know what that means in terms of food. Moreover, diet books highlight low-fat diets as the ideal one year and low-carbohydrate diets the next year.

Consumer Bewilderment and Concern

No wonder, then, that consumers are bewildered. Although many Americans are concerned about their health and are indeed eating more healthful foods than they were a decade or so ago, the average person's diet is getting better and worse at the same time. For instance, mothers may buy skim milk for their families along with high-fat premium "home-style"

ice cream, the latter because of its perceived superior quality. One national poll indicated that consumers who decrease their intake of fat by eating smaller servings of a fatty food, such as a fatty cut of meat, might nevertheless add 5 to 6 tablespoons of dressing to the salad they have chosen to eat instead. The net result is that they are getting more fat and possibly fewer nutrients from their diet.

These contradictory behaviors often derive from genuine confusion about what is good to eat. Although food manufacturers have responded to consumer concern about healthful food, they have introduced at least as many less healthful items as they have more healthful ones. There is considerable confusion in developing countries as well: many people exchange locally grown whole foods for imported, processed items, believing the latter to be better for health. Well-off people in such countries are thus developing the same chronic diseases as more affluent countries and are experiencing increased obesity rates at the same time that those who are poor are suffering from malnutrition (Monteiro, Conde, & Popkin, 2004).

All these facts suggest that people need education about food and nutrition.

The Challenge of Educating People About Eating Well: Why Do We Need This Book?

Our analysis so far would suggest that what consumers need is information on food composition, label reading skills, and skills in preparing foods in a healthy fashion. However, if practical information of this sort is all people need to eat more healthfully, then a book such as this one would not be needed. If nutrition education were simply *telling* people a variety of needed information, then what we would need is a book devoted to describing interesting ways to translate the findings of nutrition science for different audiences.

However, research provides evidence that even if everyone became more knowledgeable about food and nutrition, and food companies produced more healthful food products, consumers would still need help making nutritious food choices. There is more to good nutrition than knowing which foods to eat and having those foods available. Information is not enough. The potent influences of biological factors, cultural and social preferences, and emotional and psychological factors make the job of assisting people to eat well demanding. Understanding these and addressing them are the major tasks of nutrition education.

Biological Influences

Some have argued that people have an innate "body wisdom" that will guide them to naturally select healthful foods, thus implying that nutrition education is not needed. Much of this line of thought grew out of the work of Clara Davis, who studied the spontaneous food choices of infants (Davis, 1928). The infants, aged 6 to 11 months, were weaned by allowing them to self-select their entire diets from a total of 34 foods, without added salt or sugar, which were rotated—a few at a time—at each meal. Davis reported that after several months of such "spontaneous" food selection, the children's nutritional status and health were excellent. However, one should note that the 34 foods were all simply prepared, minimally processed, and nutritious whole foods, such as steamed vegetables, fruit juice, milk, meat, and oatmeal. There were no poisons, and nothing was allowed to influence the children's food choices except their own appetites: the food items were offered by caretakers who were trained to provide no encouragements or discouragements while the children ate. It comes as no surprise that the infants' health was superb. Whether infants would demonstrate a similar "instinct" if they were offered tasty, energy-dense, low-nutrient food items has not been examined, but such an outcome seems unlikely given experiments in which rats exposed to such diets became obese. Nor do conditions of freedom from all outside influences exist in real-world settings.

We have no evidence that any sort of innate "body wisdom" could function in an environment in which exposure to negative influences of all kinds seems almost inescapable. However, we do seem to possess biological mechanisms that in a less complex world would have helped us select a varied and adequate diet. Yudkin (1978) has argued that in the past, people could get what they *needed* simply by eating what they *wanted*. This is probably because through the centuries people obtained their needed nutrients mostly by getting enough calories. It has been shown, for example, that there is a direct correspondence between the number of calories supplied in a mixed diet of whole, minimally processed foods and the many nutrients it contains, such as protein, calcium, vitamin A, thiamin, and iron (Astrand, 1982). The key is in getting a varied diet. Humans appear to have a built-in mechanism that helps ensure that we eat a variety of foods. As people eat more of a particular food in the course of a short time period such as a meal, they come to like its taste less, but the desire for other foods offered remains relatively unchanged (Rolls, 2000). We all know this phenomenon: when we are so full as not to be able to eat another mouthful of the entree, we find ourselves quite able to eat dessert! Although the experience of hunger ensures that we will eat, our enjoyment of tasty foods combined with this sensory-specific satiety mechanism, as it is called, would have ensured —in a "primitive' environment—that we move from one food to another and thus select a balanced diet over the long term. Interestingly, a varied diet also appears to make us eat more, a fact that may have helped our ancestors but which, in a food-rich environment, may now work against us.

Biological mechanisms important to the survival of the human race may therefore contribute to many of our current health problems. Technology has made it possible to manipulate foods' sensory properties to make them sweeter or saltier or richer tasting or more colorful at will (Gussow & Contento, 1984). Thus, technology has fully separated the tastiness of foods from their nutritional worth. In addition, current technology creates notorious hazards for energy perception. The fat content of many processed foods is not clearly evident from either the appearance of the food, its feel and taste, or from the packaging and shape of the item. The energy content of a variety of similar-tasting foods can vary considerably. And the array of such processed food products, made tasty by the addition of fat, sugar, and salt, is vast. This means that by following their food preferences—eating a variety of tasty foods—people are no longer assured that they will get a nutritionally adequate diet. Indeed, such behavior increases the likelihood of overconsumption of high-fat, low-fiber diets that may place people at greater risk for a number of chronic diseases. There appears to be no set point for the amount of fat or sugar people will eat. At the same time, most studies and surveys show that taste is the major determinant of people's choices in foods. Taken together, people's desire to eat foods that are tasty and marketers' desire to put into the marketplace foods that cater to people's biological attraction to sugar, fat, and salt make the task of educating for a healthful diet a difficult one.

Cultural and Social Preferences

Whatever biological predispositions humans possess operate in the context of food availability, and as Rozin (1982) has noted, what is available to eat is determined not only by what is available geographically and economically but also by what a culture dictates is appropriate to eat. Although humans as a worldwide group eat just about everything edible, any particular group of people uses only a small proportion of the possible sources of nutrients around them. Consequently, Rozin says that "the best predictor of the food preferences, habits and attitudes of any particular human would be information about his/her ethnic group (and hence, native cuisine) rather than any biological measure one might imagine" (Rozin, 1982).

Indeed, anthropologist Margaret Mead years ago argued that traditionally, in all known societies, it was not biological mechanisms but transmission of culturally imposed eating patterns that kept humans alive. Each such eating pattern was derived from the group's experience with foods, and this experience was transmitted through the culture. These traditional food patterns were not necessarily optimal but were nutritionally viable and enabled people to survive at least through the reproductive years (Gussow & Contento, 1984). Biological preference and cultural influences are thus intertwined. What is made available by a culture comes to taste good: we may eat what we like, but we also come to like what we eat.

Today, what is available to eat in the United States is determined largely by what is mass produced by food companies and available in the supermarket. These products are highly promoted by the communication instruments of mass culture (television, advertising, and so forth), leading to consumer demand. Because so many of today's food products are neither biologically or culturally familiar, culturally transmitted traditional "craft skills" are most often no longer useful (Leiss, 1976; Gussow & Contento, 1984).

Studies show that taste and availability are closely followed by convenience in influencing food selection. Modern culture emphasizes convenience or quickness in preparing or obtaining foods, to fit in with today's hectic lifestyles. Many people today think of a food as available only if it can be purchased already prepared or can be prepared quickly without much effort. For example, more and more people are eating out or buying carry-out foods from full-service and fast-food restaurants. Away-from-home foods account for 32% of calories (up from 18% in the 1970s) and about half of total food expenditures (Stewart, Blisard, & Jolliffe, 2006). Yet quick and convenient foods that are readily available commercially are not always the most healthful, nor are they produced, transported, or packaged in the most ecologically sound manner. All these cultural and social influences can make educating about foods, nutrition, and dietary change difficult.

Family and Psychological Factors

People have many expectations about the food they eat: it should taste good, it should look good, it should impress friends when they serve it to them, it should be healthful, it should help them stay thin, and it should remind them of the warmth of family. They have many beliefs and attitudes relating to food in general and to specific foods in particular. The opinions of family or important others as well as moral and religious values also influence food choices.

Within the constraints of biology and culture, people as they grow up also develop individual food preferences and patterns of eating because any given individual amasses a unique set of experiences with respect to food (Rozin, 1982). This uniqueness stems partly from the fact that an individual's exposure to the culture is filtered through the family's interpretation of culture. For example, there is evidence that one of the major influences on the acquisition of eating patterns by children is familiarity with given foods (Birch, 1999). Such familiarity is determined by what the family serves, which in turn reflects the family's cultural and other beliefs about food. Unique individual eating patterns also arise because individuals have particular food experiences during their lifetime.

Thus, eating patterns and dietary behaviors are influenced by many familial and psychological factors, as well as by cultural and social ones. People learn very early that the foods they eat or don't eat will elicit reactions from parents, teachers, and friends ("If we push away our vegetables, Mommy may get cross at us"). During adolescence, peer pressure dominates what people choose to eat. Even as adults, few business lunches pass without a few mental nutritional notes ("Joe Davis was the only one who ordered red meat during lunch").

Eating is clearly deeply embedded in the early development of individuals and continues to be tied in with many other aspects of life. Consequently, any changes in eating behaviors may involve many other changes as well, such as family traditions, social and professional occasions that involve food, making time in busy schedules for eating well, or changing how one handles stress (for example, by exercising instead of eating). A person must be motivated to make changes and to maintain them. Sometimes we mistake people's demonstrated interest in what they eat for a commitment to eat well. Interest is shown by attendance at workshops and requests for recipes. Commitment or motivation is shown by actually preparing—and eating—the recipes requested.

Sense of Empowerment

Even if a person is motivated, the sheer number of food products available makes decision making a daunting task for the consumer. It is also a daunting task for the nutrition educator because the consumer needs a great deal of complex information, yet in an information-overloaded society, the consumer wants or can handle only simple messages. So the challenge to the nutrition educator is how to convert complex information into simple but accurate messages that consumers will attend to and act on.

At the same time, to understand some of the choices they have to make, people will need to be able to analyze and evaluate complex information in the midst of conflicting claims. For example, Are calories the most important item on a food label? Is a breakfast cereal that is high in sugar but low in fat a better choice for children? Which food preservation methods are safe? Does it make a difference whether one chooses organically produced foods or foods produced by more conventional agriculture? And differences in terms of what—impact of food on personal health, or impact of food production methods on the long-term sustainability of the food system? What about genetically engineered foods—should they be labeled? Thus, eaters need critical thinking skills. In addition, they need affective skills such as assertiveness, self-management, and negotiation skills that enhance their sense of competence and control over their own food choices. People also need skills in preparing healthful foods quickly and conveniently. Finally, for community as well as personal empowerment, people need to have the skills and opportunity to identify food- and nutrition-related issues facing their communities and work with others to address these issues appropriately.

Material Resources and the Environmental Context

No amount of motivation and skills, however, will put healthful food on the table if material resources are inadequate for people to purchase (or grow) and prepare the food. Material resources include not only money but also time, labor, and fuel. Affordability of healthful food, as well as food availability, is crucial, particularly for low-resources audiences in low-income neighborhoods. Having in one's neighborhood only convenience stores that charge high prices and carry limited supplies of healthful foods makes eating well extremely difficult. Whole-grain products and fruits and vegetables are not as available in fast food outlets, workplace cafeterias, or other places convenient to people's out-of-home activities as are more highly processed food items, and they often cost more (Drewnowski, Darmn, & Briend, 2004).

Nor can the best of intentions be implemented and behaviors maintained if social structures, food marketing practices, food policies, and other aspects of the food environment are not conducive to health. Fast foods that tend to be higher in fat, sugar, and salt are everywhere—convenient, tasty, and inexpensive—and their portion sizes are often large. Surveys have found that almost 60% of Americans eat away from home on any given day and are thus exposed to such foods (Agricultural Research Service, 2000).

In addition, the dietary pattern emphasized by marketers, shown in Figure 1-4, is very different from the dietary pattern recommended by the U.S. MyPyramid (see Figure 1-2) as likely to enhance nutritional health—one high in whole grains, fruits, and vegetables; adequate in dairy and meat; and sparing in foods that are high in fat and sugar. More marketing and advertising dollars are spent promoting food products in the "other foods/discretionary calories" category than are spent on foods in the basic food groups, as we have seen, resulting in increased consumption and demand. Finally, people of all ages, particularly children, have become

more sedentary in the last 30 years. We use more labor-saving devices and cars, and spend more time watching TV and using computers. People have hectic jobs and work long hours, leaving less time for physical activity. Thus people cannot eat as many calories as they once could in order to meet their other nutrient needs. The issues that demand attention from nutrition educators, then, are not only individual food-related behaviors and personal choice but also external environmental factors such as material resources, social structures, food policies, and marketing practices.

Defining Nutrition Education

We have seen that nutrition education is both necessary and challenging to do. But what exactly is nutrition education and what should it seek to accomplish?

Brief History of Nutrition Education

Although families and cultures have been educating about food since the dawn of human history, the formal field of nutrition education can be considered to have had its start when governments began publishing dietary guidance recommendations for the public based on the findings of nutrition science and taking into account cultural eating patterns. In the United States, the first food guide was published by the U.S. Department of Agriculture in 1917 as a teaching tool with the goal of improving the health of the nation's people. A basic understanding of the need for carbohydrates, proteins, and fats had emerged in the late 1800s. The need for other "protective substances" for human health became apparent with the discovery and characterization of the first

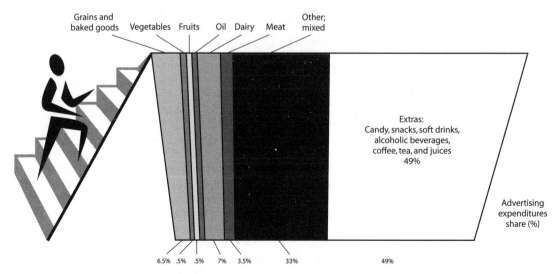

FIGURE 1-4　Food marketing pyramid: Advertising expenditures by food manufacturers.

Source: Gallo, A. 1999. Food advertising in the United States. In *America's eating habits: Changes and consequences* (Agricultural Information Bulletin No. 750), edited by E. Frazão. Washington, DC: U.S. Department of Agriculture.

vitamins in the early 1900s. The importance of minerals in food for human health also became known—for example, the importance of milk as a source of calcium for bone health. With continuing research and identification of vitamins and minerals needed for good health, sufficient information had emerged by 1917 to provide guidance to the public. In this first food guide, foods were placed into groups based on their nutrient composition, and people were provided with recommendations as to how many foods to eat from each group to be healthy. The concern was for nutritional adequacy—that is, the purpose of the food guides was to ensure that people ate the right foods in sufficient amounts to provide all the nutrients that they needed for growth and health. The early guides were directed at entire families, as shown in Figure 1-5. Later food guides were directed at individuals.

The number of groups, as well as which foods were categorized into which groups, has changed from time to time over the past century in these teaching tools, based on the findings of nutrition science, cultural food patterns, the interests of food producers, and other factors. Different graphics have been used over the decades to communicate this dietary guidance and make the message understandable and useful to consumers. Figure 1-6 shows a graphic in which recommended foods were placed into seven food groups, used in the 1930s, and Figure 1-7 shows what was commonly called "the Basic Four," in use in the 1950s and 1960s.

By the early 1970s there was increasing recognition that the major dietary concerns for a majority of Americans were no longer related to nutrient-deficiency diseases but to the risk of chronic diseases such as heart disease, diabetes, cancer, and overweight. Consequently the nature of the dietary advice changed. As nutrition researcher Hegsted (1979) noted at the time, "In the past, the message was, in essence, to eat more of everything. Now we are faced with the more difficult problem of teaching the public to be more discriminating. Increasingly, the message will be to eat less." After considerable discussion and debate among health professionals, the U.S. Congress, federal government agencies, and the food industry, a set of dietary guidelines, called the *Dietary Guidelines for Americans*, was adopted in 1980. The dietary guidelines were published jointly by the U.S. Department of Agriculture (USDA) and the Department of Health and Human Services (DHHS). They were designed to assist the public in making food choices that would provide for sufficient amounts of all the essential nutrients as well as reduce the risk of chronic disease and maintain a healthy weight, although they did not specifically recommend that people eat less. These guidelines are revised every five years to ensure that they incorporate the latest nutrition science research findings and food policy considerations (see www.health.gov/dietaryguidelines/).

About the same time, the graphic for the food guide as an educational tool itself was also changed dramatically. After

careful work on the part of nutritionists working in government, considerable debate by nutrition professionals, lobbying by the food industry, and extensive consumer research, the graphic in the United States was changed from a series of equal-sized boxes representing each of the food groups, as in the Basic Four, to a pyramid shape and was called the Food Guide Pyramid (Figure 1-8). The pyramid shape was intended to better convey to the public the fact that the number of servings from each of the food groups differs according to group; that is, it emphasized the notion of proportionality. For example, the largest number of daily servings should come from the grain group (the bottom of the pyramid). The next largest number of daily servings should come from the fruits and vegetables groups, followed by the dairy and meat groups. The quantities shown for each of the pyramid groups were the basics recommended for good health. Foods high in sugar and fat were placed in the tip of the pyramid and were to be eaten sparingly.

The Food Guide Pyramid was modified in 2005 and is now called MyPyramid (see Figure 1-2). MyPyramid is a graphic that is linked to information on the Web (www.MyPyramid.gov), where people can download the graphic as well as information on how to personalize the recommendations for their own needs. The information is also linked to the *Dietary Guidelines* document, which provides the basis of the pyramid recommendations. Foods higher in fiber and lower in fat and sugar within each food group should be eaten more often. Foods high in fats and sugars that were predominant in an "others" group that was at the tip of the Food Guide Pyramid and labeled "Eat sparingly" are no longer shown in the MyPyramid graphic. Instead, people who have "discretionary calories" (between 100 and 300 calories for most people) can spend them on "other foods" or additional foods from the "basic five" food groups. However, as noted before, in actuality foods from this "discretionary calories" group contribute substantially to individuals' intakes (Figure 1-3) and account for about half the advertising expenditures by food companies for food items (Figure 1-4).

It should be noted, however, that the nation's goal for nutrition education has remained unchanged from the initial food guide in 1917 to the latest government recommendations embodied in the dietary guidance documents just described: to improve the health of the nation's people.

What Is Nutrition Education?

What, then, is nutrition education? There are many definitions of nutrition education, based on different views about its purpose. These differing views are explored in this section. After that, we will arrive at a definition to be used in this book.

One view may be called the *information dissemination approach*, which sees nutrition education as limited to the dissemination of nutrition science–based information only. In

FIGURE 1-5 Example of the USDA's family-oriented food guidelines, 1921.

Source: U.S. Department of Agriculture. www.nal.usda.gov/fnic/history/early.htm.

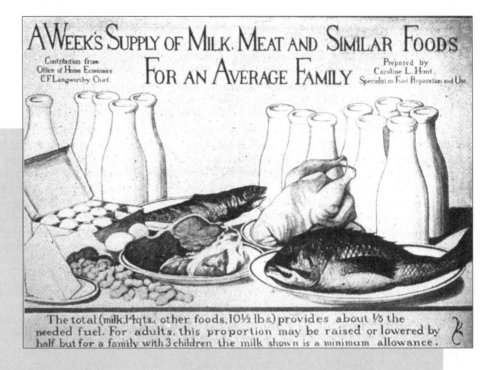

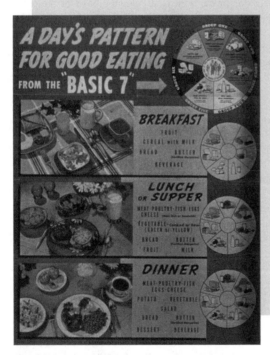

FIGURE 1-6 Food guide, 1944: The Wheel of Good Eating.

Source: U.S. Department of Agriculture. www.nal.usda.gov/fnic/history/early.htm.

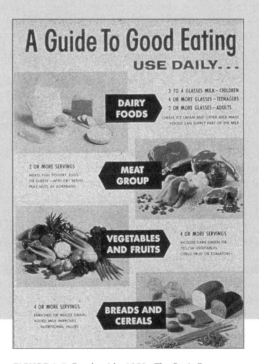

FIGURE 1-7 Food guide, 1950s: The Basic Four.

Source: U.S. Department of Agriculture. www.nal.usda.gov/fnic/history/early.htm.

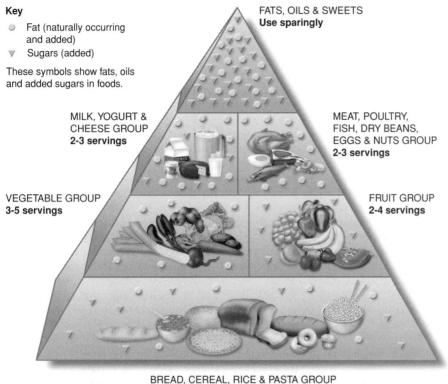

Key

- ⬤ Fat (naturally occurring and added)
- ▽ Sugars (added)

These symbols show fats, oils and added sugars in foods.

FATS, OILS & SWEETS
Use sparingly

MILK, YOGURT & CHEESE GROUP
2-3 servings

MEAT, POULTRY, FISH, DRY BEANS, EGGS & NUTS GROUP
2-3 servings

VEGETABLE GROUP
3-5 servings

FRUIT GROUP
2-4 servings

BREAD, CEREAL, RICE & PASTA GROUP
6-11 servings

FIGURE 1-8 The Food Guide Pyramid, 1990s.

Source: U.S. Department of Agriculture. The Food Guide Pyramid. *Home and Garden Bulletin*, No. 252; August 1992, revised October 1996.

this approach the goal of nutrition education is simply—and only—to provide consumers with the information about food and nutrients needed to make decisions about what to eat, rejecting the notion that nutrition professionals should also *actively promote* healthful choices. Consumers are viewed as being savvy and not liking to be told what to do. They will eat healthfully if only they have the information they need. Indeed, when the *Dietary Guidelines for Americans* was first published in 1980, there was considerable criticism of it. Newspapers carried headlines such as "Government Now Reaches Into Your Home to Tell You What to Eat!"

As if to reassure the public, the *Surgeon General's Report on Health Promotion and Disease Prevention*, published soon thereafter, stated that "One of the fears associated with health education, especially government-sponsored efforts, is that it interferes with individual freedom, by attempting to modify individual lifestyles. Actually, the goal of health education is just the opposite—to guarantee the individual's freedom of choice regarding his own health by giving him the reliable information he needs to make decisions about how he wants to live" (DHHS, 1979).

Nutrition education in this approach is viewed as limited to the process of translating the findings of nutrition science to various audiences using methods from the fields of educa-

tion and communication. Nutrition educators are seen only as information dispatchers. Messages to be communicated are derived from the findings of nutrition science research, and the methods of communicating the messages are derived from the principles of education. The goal of nutrition education is thus to provide "accurate, reliable and science-based information consumers need to make informed choices" (Dietary Guidelines Alliance, 1996). Effectiveness can be gauged by the extent to which consumers know the needed information.

Certainly freedom of choice is a major value in this society, and information about foods and nutrition is a central element of nutrition education. It is also essential that this information be evidence based and accurate. In addition, because the food and nutrition science content is complex, and because ongoing research studies and controversial issues need to be correctly interpreted, nutrition educators must be sufficiently and appropriately trained in the science of nutrition (American Dietetic Association [ADA], 1990).

However, there are criticisms of this approach that limits nutrition education to information dissemination only. First, surveys consistently show that most Americans believe that they are well informed about nutrition (Balzer, 1997; IFIC Foundation, 1999). The finding that they are also not eating according to recommendations argues that information alone is clearly not enough.

Given the nature, volume, and complexity of the information necessary for true informed choice, an approach limited to information dissemination is not really possible in practice (Contento, 1980; Gussow & Contento, 1984). That is, all nutrition education programs will inevitably have to make choices about what information and skills to address in any given situation. For example, no usable food product label can carry information on all 60 or so nutrients essential for good health. Just leaving out data on some nutrients and including others biases the information. Nor can a single educational session or even a several-session program provide all the needed information for true informed choice on all nutritional matters. In making a choice of which issues to emphasize and what content to cover, the nutrition educator must make a judgment because there is not enough time to give "all the facts" about everything. Even in group settings involving open-ended discussion and mutual dialogue, only certain issues can be explored at any given time. Choices regarding program content always have to be made. Thus, it is impossible for nutrition education to be value free even if it wanted to be.

When definitions that embody the information dissemination-only approach are examined carefully, one finds that they do not really mean information dissemination in any neutral sense. For example, the American Dietetic Association has described nutrition education as the "process that assists the public in applying nutrition knowledge," but adds that it is also "the deliberate effort to improve the nutritional well-being of people" (ADA, 1990). Similarly, the government document noted earlier that argues for a freedom-of-choice approach adds that "choices are genuinely free only when the individual has effectively been given full information about the decision and the risks attendant to it, as well as the necessary decision-making skills to avoid or manage those risks; and the opportunities for individual action [are] facilitated and barriers to action lessened" (DHHS, 1979). These definitions either imply that nutrition education does have a particular value (e.g., "encouraging good nutritional practices") or that nutrition education involves many other activities besides giving information to assist people in making changes in their behavior (e.g., it includes activities to "facilitate" individual action or to "lessen" barriers).

Finally, some critics point out that nutrition education should not be value free even if it could be. For example, nutritionist Jean Mayer (1986) noted that "Nutritionists, unlike biochemists and physiologists, but like cardiologists and pediatricians, have to see their science as one whose goal is to benefit people."

The second approach to nutrition education, *facilitating behaviors conducive to health,* is based on the premise that given that a major goal of nutrition education is to improve the health of the nation's people and that people's health conditions are to some extent the result of individual and social patterns of behavior, it is appropriate for nutrition education to facilitate the adoption or maintenance of individual behaviors and community practices that are conducive to long-term health. As we have noted, consumers believe they are well informed. In addition, research evidence suggests that knowledge may be a necessary, but not a sufficient, condition for reaching the goal of improved health. Knowledge of nutrition information by itself does not usually lead to desirable food choices and other nutrition-positive food practices. As discussed earlier, food behaviors and eating practices are influenced by many powerful psychosocial and other factors in addition to knowledge.

In this view, then, nutrition education involves much more than simply imparting food and nutrition information in the most attractive and effective way. Nutrition education facilitates behaviors that are conducive to health by focusing on the personal motivations and competence, interpersonal interactions, and environmental factors that influence individual and community patterns of behavior. In this approach, nutrition education is seen as a "form of planned change that involves the deliberate effort to improve nutritional well-being by providing information or other types of educational/behavioral interventions" (Sims, 1987). The term *educational intervention* is often used, and in this approach the role of the nutrition educator moves from that of an "information dispatcher" to a "facilitator of behavior change" of individuals and communities.

A specific example can illustrate this point. A nutrition educator was interested in increasing the rate of breastfeeding, as recommended by health professionals, among a group of low-income women in a food assistance program. As is typical of most nutritionists, she had planned to discuss the nutritional benefits of breastfeeding and teach the women how to do it successfully. However, when she went to talk with the women ahead of the scheduled time, she found that the women knew all about breastfeeding and its numerous benefits, and many had attempted it before, but that they were embarrassed to do it. That is, they had the knowledge and skills, but the difficulty lay in the emotional and cultural barriers to breastfeeding. So she changed her session to discuss the barriers to breastfeeding, including embarrassment, and potential ways to overcome these barriers. That is, her goal was to facilitate the adoption of a *behavior*—breastfeeding—that was judged by the pediatric nutrition community as desirable based on scientific evidence. To achieve this goal, she addressed personal, interpersonal, and cultural factors that would facilitate the adoption of this behavior rather than focusing on nutrition science content alone.

Programs may thus involve strategies specifically designed to facilitate change in behaviors and practices identified by current scientific knowledge as health risks or capable of having an impact on food system sustainability. This "communication/behavior change" approach has formed the basis of most nutrition research studies and community projects in the food and nutrition arena in the past two decades. These have included mass media campaigns, community-based projects, and school curricula to increase fruit and vegetable consumption (e.g., Campbell et al., 1999; Potter et al., 2000; Ammerman et al., 2002; Blanchette & Brug, 2005), calcium intake (Reed et al., 2002), and physical activity (McKenzie et al.,1996) and to reduce fat intake (Luepker et al., 1996). Evaluation in this approach is measured by improvements in the food and nutrition behaviors of individuals and communities.

The approach of focusing on facilitating behavior change has also been criticized. What if some years from now researchers discover that the recommendations we are urging on the public today were not beneficial or, worse yet, were harmful? In addition, it has been argued that by exhorting the public to adopt certain behaviors and forgo others, "we are bothering and frightening people about too many things" for which we as professionals do not have definitive answers, and we are seen as advocating a "denial of pleasure" (Becker, 1986). Also, if we employ persuasive communication techniques, are we not being manipulative and therefore stretching what is appropriate in terms of our role as educators? Taken to an extreme, preventive approaches can be seen as paternalistic and coercive, where educational interventions are for people's "own good" or for the benefit of society in terms of reduced medical costs or a better-fed workforce and the like.

The facilitating behavior change approach is based on the assumption that individuals have a great deal of influence over their personal decisions and actions and that changes in these personal behaviors can significantly change health outcomes. These assumptions arose from the discovery of physiological risk factors for chronic diseases, such as serum cholesterol, and the realization that lifestyle behavioral factors such as poor diet and lack of exercise can contribute to these risk factors. Thus, unhealthy behaviors themselves can be viewed as behavioral risk factors. Consequently, health promotion and nutrition education often consist of intervention strategies designed to alter these behavioral risk factors.

However, precisely because the individual behavior change approach helps people to acquire the motivation and competence to take increased control over their own food choices and health, people are held personally accountable for the state of their health. It can be a quick step from this personal responsibility approach to blaming the victim when individuals become ill (Allegrante & Green, 1981; Green & Kreuter, 1999). That is, this approach can result in "person blame" rather than "system blame." It becomes easy to ignore the fact that there are genetic factors affecting health, as well as powerful institutional and social conditions that shape and reinforce behavior.

Furthermore, in this approach the behavior or practices to be addressed are most often identified as needs or problems not by the groups or communities themselves but by governmental or professional groups familiar with scientific evidence. It has been argued that an active, participatory approach in which people are actively involved in all stages of nutrition education is more likely to be effective in the long run. Participants can then identify issues of interest to them, which may not always involve behavioral changes but rather a variety of other issues, such as food accessibility, family cohesiveness, or other values in life (Arnold et al., 2001; Buchanan, 2004; Kent, 1988; Rody, 1988). In this approach, self-reliance and empowerment are the outcomes, not necessarily dietary behavior change.

The third approach to nutrition education is to *focus on environmental change*. It has become increasingly clear that environmental factors are a major influence on food choices and nutrition-related practices. Indeed, behavior and environment have a reciprocal relationship with each other (Bandura, 1986). Dietary change is more likely when the physical environmental is health promoting, so that personal decisions and motivations are supported and reinforced—that is, when healthful foods are available and accessible in the workplace, in schools, and in communities. Consequently, many nutrition education interventions now also address the environmental context. The environmental component can involve altering the physical food choice environment by such means as making changes in the foods offered in school meal programs and in workplace cafeterias, or increasing the availability of neighborhood farmers' markets. The environmental component can include changes in the social environment, such as providing social support for healthful eating.

Some health professionals have gone so far as to argue that many of our behaviors are due in part to economic, organizational, and political factors in society that actually *encourage* at-risk behaviors (McKinley, 1974). A story, attributed to sociologist Irving Zola, tells of a physician trying to explain the dilemmas of the modern practice of medicine: "You know," he said, "sometimes it feels like this. There I am standing by the shore of a swiftly flowing river and I hear the cry of a drowning man. So I jump into the river, put my arms around him, pull him to shore and apply artificial respiration. Just when he begins to breathe, there is another cry for help. So I jump into the river, reach him, pull him to shore, apply artificial respiration, and just as he begins to breathe, another cry for help. So back in the river again, reaching, pulling; applying artificial respiration and then another yell. Again and again without end goes the sequence. You know, I am so busy jumping in, pulling them to shore, applying artificial respiration, that I have no time to see who the hell is upstream pushing all of them in." Some thus contend that health professionals devote too many resources and attention to "downstream activities" that are short term and ultimately futile (McKinley, 1974). We should instead be devoting more attention "upstream" to the "manufacturers of illness," whose activities "foster and habituate certain at-risk behaviors."

These considerations have led to some debate in the health promotion field about the relative importance of facilitating individual behavior change versus broader institutional and social approaches to health, behavioral versus environmental strategies, and blaming the victim versus blaming the manufacturers of illness (Green & Kreuter, 1999). Ultimately, all agree that attention to both individual and environmental factors is important.

In the health promotion field, the work of health education, which focuses on education of the public, is distinguished from the larger, more comprehensive and multifaceted enterprise of health promotion. *Health education* has been described as any combination of learning experiences designed to facilitate voluntary actions conducive to health. *Health promotion* takes into consideration the environment as well, and is thus defined as the combination of educational and ecological supports for actions and conditions of living conducive to health (Green & Kreuter, 1999). In practice, there is obviously a continuum between health education and health promotion.

What Can We Conclude?

Clearly, enhancement of knowledge and decision-making skills for informed choice is vital in nutrition education. The public needs accurate science-based information on foods and on the relationships among food, nutrition, and health. Given that there are some 50,000 food items in the average U.S supermarket, consumers also need to know how to select foods for optimal health from the vast array of available products. Indeed, they will need to know more than just which nutrients are present in which of today's food products. The public will also need to know "how to be discriminating about dietary advice that comes, sought and unsought, from a variety of unequally reliable sources such as popular books, advertising, packaging labels, newspapers, and materials from food industry sources or 'health' food stores" (Contento, 1980).

Finally, people make choices in light of their life situations and values. For example, for a mother of young children, eating together as a family may be more important than the quality of what they eat. Balancing these myriad food choice criteria will require considerable analytical and evaluative skills on the part of consumers as well as the ability to construct conceptual frameworks and develop "personal food policies." Therefore nutrition education needs also to enhance people's critical thinking skills.

Although we acknowledge that eating behavior—healthful or otherwise—is voluntarily chosen by people in light of their own life situations, we also recognize that implicit in the national goal to improve the health of the nation's people is the value-laden goal of enhancing the nutritional well-being of individuals and populations. This means that nutrition education also involves promoting health, helping people to see the value of health for themselves, and facilitating people's attempts to eat healthfully. For example, the U.S. government has at times embarked on national campaigns to improve the nation's health. One such attempt, conducted in collaboration with the Produce for Better Health Foundation, was to encourage people to eat more fruits and vegetables. Mass media campaigns were conducted, and grocery store bags were used to carry the message "Five a Day for Better Health!" or "Eat your colors."

Many nutrition professionals are concerned that using health-promoting activities or persuasive communications as part of nutrition education may be coercive. Yet, the food industry (manufacturers, the food service sector, and retailers) spent $26 billion in 2000 on advertising and promotions (Elitzak, 2001). Advertising and marketing to children was $15 billion in 2002 (double of that in 1992) (McNeal, 1992; Center for Science in the Public Interest [CSPI], 2003). About $150 million a year is spent on advertising for candy bars, $580 million for soft drinks, and more than $1.5 billion for fast food (Leading advertisers, Ad Age, 2001).People are exposed to 3 hours of food advertising every week, all year, whereas government health-related campaigns may amount to only a few million dollars a year (e.g., $4 million for the National Cancer Institute's 5 A Day program, $34 million for the Centers for Disease Control's Division of Nutrition and Physical Activity, $10 million for USDA's Team Nutrition), and people may never attend a nutrition education program or see a nutritionist during their entire lives. Such a situation cannot result in genuinely free, informed choice. Thus nutrition educators have an obligation to bring health concerns to the attention of individuals to promote health and to guarantee fully free choices. Indeed, as Gillespie (1987) pointed out, "persuasive communication is consistent with our democratic educational values if the attempts to change attitudes or behavior explain the reasons why recommended behaviors are desirable and indicate the strength of scientific evidence supporting such recommendations. Participants should be involved in decisions to change their food behavior not only as an ingredient in program success but also to guard against manipulation."

The 5 A Day campaign mentioned earlier illustrates these considerations. The message was based on extensive research that shows that eating five or more fruits and vegetables a day has many health benefits and carries no known risks. Considerable consumer behavior research was also conducted to understand the consumers' point of view. From these activities a campaign was developed in which consumers were told of the benefits to them of eating fruits and vegetables ("for better health"), given the research evidence provided by a credible source (the National Cancer Institute), and then urged to eat fruits and vegetables. Some strategies went further: for example, fruit and vegetable bags in grocery stores for consumers provided a listing of the nutrient composition of several dozen fruits and vegetables so as to facilitate food choices. Messages directed at individuals were accompanied by changes in the environmental context as well, such as billboards placed in prominent places and increased availability of fruits and vegetables in many grocery stores.

Defining Nutrition Education

Taking into account these considerations and various definitions of nutrition education and health education, we define *nutrition education* for the purposes of this book as any combination of educational strategies, accompanied by environmental supports, designed to facilitate voluntary adoption of food choices and other food- and nutrition-related behaviors conducive to health and well-being; nutrition education is delivered through multiple venues and involves activities at the individual, community, and policy levels (Contento et al., 1995; Society for Nutrition Education [SNE], 1995, 2006; American Dietetic Association, 2003).

The phrase "combination of educational strategies" emphasizes that because many factors influence behavior, nutrition education needs to employ a variety of educational strategies and learning experiences that are appropriately directed at these multiple influences on, or determinants of, food choice and dietary behavior in order to facilitate dietary change. Nutrition education focuses on enhancing health and facilitating solutions. Education is *not* synonymous with information dissemination, although the public and many in the nutrition science, biomedical, public health, and policy fields think it is. The word comes from the Latin *educare*, meaning to bring up or lead out, and can be seen as a process that not only provides knowledge, information, and skills but also fosters development, growth, and change. These educational strategies are at the heart of this book and are described in great detail in the remaining chapters. They are content-free processes that can be used to address the many issues that are of concern or of interest to the public, to professionals, or to the nation at large.

Use of the word *designed* means that nutrition education is a systematically planned set of activities. Such systematically planned nutrition education can occur through multiple venues, such as schools, communities, workplaces, or clinics, and through the mass media. A procedural model for systematically designing nutrition education is described later in this book. Such systematically planned nutrition education should be distinguished from incidental nutrition education that is carried out by other institutions in society such as families, businesses, newspapers, magazines, and radio and television stations. The latter type of education is labeled as *informal* nutrition education. TV food commercials, claims on food product packages, newspaper articles, and popular diet books are all examples of informal nutrition education.

Facilitate is used to emphasize the fact that educators can only *assist* people to make diet-related changes: people make changes when they see the need and want to do so. Motivations ultimately come from within individuals themselves, and actions with respect to food are voluntarily chosen in the light of individuals' values and larger life goals and situations. Education about foods and nutrition, then, is about increasing awareness, promoting active contemplation, and enhancing people's motivations through self-understanding and deliberation. It is also about facilitating the ability to take action through acquisition of knowledge and skills related to food and nutrition and through self-regulation and self-directed behavior or agency. Finally, it is also about engaging in coalitions with others to promote supportive food environments, systems, and policies where appropriate and possible.

Voluntary means recognizing and respecting that human beings have agency and free will and make choices in light of their own personal goals and values (Bandura, 1997; Rothschild, 1999; Deci & Ryan 2000; Bandura 2001; Buchanan, 2004). It means the program is conducted without coercion and with the full understanding of the participants about the purpose of the nutrition education activities. Individuals are both "the changers" and "the changed." Voluntary does not mean that the only appropriate approach is one limited to information dissemination only. Health psychologist Leventhal (1973) noted some years ago that "the decision to avoid coercion does not free one of the obligation to state facts, warn, and argue skillfully." By "arguing skillfully," he meant skillfully bringing to the people's attention the importance of specific issues or the potential consequences of their health actions. This means making the case for an issue or concern. An example is the message we described earlier making the case for eating more fruits and vegetables. The message was disseminated through various channels in the United States, such as television, grocery bags, or printed materials: "Eating 5 fruits and vegetables is one of the most important choices you can make to help maintain your health—National Cancer Institute." Another example is the message "Think globally, eat locally." The notion of voluntarism, human agency, or choice is not violated when nutrition educators increase awareness of an issue or make the case for using considerations of health or food system sustainability in making food choices.

Indeed, it can be argued that truly informed choice can be made by consumers *only* when they have the benefit of understanding arguments from all sides. Without the benefit of health communications from nutrition educators, consumers would receive only the arguments of all the other forces in society, such as food advertising and promotion activities, that are providing messages urging people to choose foods for reasons other than nutrition and health, such as taste or fun. Thus nutrition educators have an obligation to bring food and health concerns to the attention of individuals and to make a case for these concerns. Making the case is not limited to a discussion of benefits. It can also involve providing food tastings that demonstrate that healthful foods taste good, organizing a tour to show that shopping at a farmers' market can be convenient, or organizing a company "fun run" to show that exercise can be enjoyable. In other words, nutrition education strategies can be designed in such a way as to integrate the health-promoting role of nutrition educators with the notion of free will and agency on the part of individuals.

Behaviors are the food choices and other food- and nutrition-related actions that people undertake in order to achieve an intended effect and are the direct focus of nutrition education. For example, eating fruits and vegetables, a lower-fat diet, calcium-rich foods, or local foods or breastfeeding can be referred to as behaviors. The term *actions* is used synonymously with *behaviors*, although the former term can also refer to specific actions or sub-behaviors that constitute behaviors. For example, the behavior of eating more fruits and vegetables may involve the specific actions of shopping for fruits and vegetables, adding orange juice at breakfast, including a vegetable at lunch, and so forth. The word *practices* is also used interchangeably with *behaviors* and *actions*, although the term *practices* tends to refer to more general and continuing behaviors, such as food-related parenting practices, eating balanced meals, or buying foods at farmers' markets.

The terms *health* and *well-being* refer to both the nutritional health of individuals and an overall sense of well-being; both absence of disease and possession of positive attributes of being healthy, such as optimal functioning or high-level wellness. For some nutrition educators, the concept of health and well-being extends to include the health and sustainability of the food systems on which we all depend.

Multiple venues refers to the fact that systematically planned nutrition education can be delivered through multiple channels, such as group sessions and other in-person activities, newsletters, printed materials, visuals in formal settings such as schools and colleges or in nonformal settings such as community centers, food banks, workplaces, supermarkets, food stamp offices, WIC clinics, or outpatient clinics, and through mass media, billboards, and social marketing approaches.

Activities at the community and policy levels can promote environments supportive of healthful food choices and diet-related behaviors. *Environment* refers to the food, physical, social, informational, and policy environments external to a person that are relevant to the behavior or practices at issue. Taking action and maintaining a behavioral change is much more likely if the relevant environment is supportive. Promoting supportive environments usually requires nutrition educators to educate a different audience—providers of food

and services, key decision makers, and others with influence—and to work in coalition with them to achieve food and nutrition goals (and physical activity goals, where relevant). These individuals and organizations might include community leaders, food service personnel, school principals, workplace managers, and policy makers at local, state, and national levels, as well as the media, government agencies, and nongovernmental or private voluntary organizations. Promoting supportive environments may also mean engaging in activities to influence policy makers about nutrition, food, and health.

Summary

In sum, person and environment are closely interrelated. In some cases, people have the needed resources and the knowledge, skills, and confidence in their ability to effect change in themselves and in the environment, but they do not have a desire to do so. In other cases, people may be motivated to eat foods that will improve their own health or the health of their community, or promote a sustainable food system, but they do not have the environmental supports to act on their motivation.

Motivation is so important in diet-related behaviors that its role in nutrition education must be specifically recognized and addressed. Individuals are more likely to take action or change a practice if they understand the factors, environmental as well as personal, that have sustained or even encouraged their current way of living. They are also more likely to take action if they have had opportunity to examine and talk about food and health issues in relation to their own larger life goals (Campbell, 1988; Antonovsky, 1995; Deci & Ryan, 2000; Buchanan, 2004). Change grows out of a person's understanding of "the problems behind the problems." It also grows out of people's interest in their own well-being, health related or otherwise.

Nutrition education can help people understand that diet is related to their health and can provide information on what foods to eat for health, but it can go further: it can assist people to consider their food choices in relation to more fundamental issues in their *near environments*, such as personal relationships, home and work situations, economic and time pressures on decision making, and community structures and other conditions of living. It can also help them understand the influences on their diet-related practices of elements of the *far environment*, such as grocery store or food industry practices, government policy, food (and beverage) advertising, the general economic climate, and agricultural and trade practices. It can help people understand that the way food is grown, marketed, and consumed has an impact on the food system and has social consequences as well as nutritional ones. Finally, it can also assist people to take action on the environment through coalition building, empowerment, and collective action.

The view of nutrition education described here is in keeping with the vision of the foremost nutrition education professional organization, the Society of Nutrition Education (SNE), which defines its mission as being to "advance the food and nutrition education profession to impact healthful food choices and lifestyle behaviors at the individual, community and policy levels. SNE offers opportunities for members to share best practices, evidence-based knowledge and diverse perspectives" (SNE, 2006) (Box 1-1). It is also in keeping with the position statements of the American Dietetic Association (2003).

Is Nutrition Education Effective?

A number of reviews have been conducted to examine the question of whether nutrition education is effective, based on the above view of nutrition education. One such review used the statistical method of meta-analysis to examine 303 studies conducted over a 70-year period from 1910 to 1984 that included a total of 4,108 separate findings (Johnson & Johnson, 1985). The meta-analysis found that, overall, nutrition

> ### BOX 1-1 Society for Nutrition Education Mission and Identity Statements
>
> **Mission**
> The Society for Nutrition Education (SNE) advances the food and nutrition education profession to impact healthful food choices and lifestyle behaviors at the individual, community and policy levels. SNE offers opportunities for members to share best practices, evidence-based knowledge, and diverse perspectives.
>
> **Identity Statement**
> SNE is an international organization of nutrition education professionals who are dedicated to promoting healthful sustainable food choices and who share a vision of healthy people in healthy communities. Our members conduct research in education, behavior, and communication; develop and disseminate innovative nutrition education strategies; and communicate information on food, nutrition and health issues to students, professionals, policy makers, and the public. SNE members share ideas and resources through our journal, newsletter, annual conference, and the members-only listserve. Our Divisions offer networking opportunities for members with similar interests and expertise.
>
> *Source:* Society for Nutrition Education. 2006. http://www.sne.org.

education increased knowledge by 33 percentiles, attitudes by 14 percentiles, and behaviors by 19 percentiles.

A review by Contento and colleagues of 217 well-designed nutrition education intervention studies conducted between 1980 and 1995 found that nutrition education was a significant factor in improving dietary practices when behavioral change was set as the goal and when the educational strategies employed were designed with that as a purpose (Contento et al., 1995). In the studies reviewed, interventions did not always achieve across-the-board success on all criteria used to judge effectiveness, and often intervention effects were not large. In addition, where many components were involved, nutrition education often achieved positive results in some components and not in others. Nevertheless, overall, nutrition education did contribute significantly to change in a variety of food- and nutrition-related behaviors. Reviews of school-based studies also found positive effects of nutrition education (Lytle & Achterberg, 1995; McArthur, 1998).

The efficacy of interventions to modify dietary behaviors related to cancer risk was examined by reviewing well-designed and controlled studies conducted from about 1975 to 2000 (Ammerman et al., 2002). The review found positive effects of interventions to reduce fat intake and to increase intake of fruits and vegetables. There was a modest increase in both the average number of fruits and vegetables eaten each day and of the percentage of people who met the goal of eating five or more servings of fruits and vegetables a day. Media campaigns and randomized trials to increase fruit and vegetable consumption were evaluated in another study, providing estimates of the changes in intake that could be attributed to the interventions (Potter et al., 2000). A review of interventions conducted worldwide to increase fruit and vegetable consumption found that significant increases were achieved through a variety of venues: face-to-face education, counseling, telephone motivational interviewing, computer-tailored information, and community-based multicomponent programs (Pomerleau et al., 2005).

Cost-benefit analyses have also been conducted for nutrition education programs. This type of analysis compares the economic benefits of a nutrition education program for participants to the actual costs of delivering the program. It was found in one program that for every dollar in costs, the mean benefit to participants was about $10, ranging from about $3 to $17 (Rajopal et al., 2002). In another, for each dollar in costs, the mean benefit was about $3.60 (Schuster et al., 2003).

Thus, the evidence from these reviews and cost-benefit analyses of intervention studies demonstrates that nutrition education programs can make a significant contribution to improving dietary practices when they use appropriate strategies.

What Do Nutrition Educators Do? Settings, Audiences, and Scope for Nutrition Education

As we have seen, the rise in chronic disease and obesity has led to an increased interest in nutrition among consumers in recent decades. In addition, there has been an upsurge of interest in local and organic food and foods perceived to be high quality. Since nutrition can be seen as the link between agriculture and health, intentional education about food and nutrition covers a wide range of issues and takes place in a variety of settings, with different audiences.

Settings: Where Is Nutrition Education Provided?

Nutrition education is provided in many settings. Some of them are described in the following sections. More examples are given throughout this book and in Nutrition Education in Action 1-1.

Communities

Much nutrition education for the public at large occurs in communities through programs sponsored by the U.S. Department of Agriculture (USDA), such as Cooperative Extension programs. Each county in the United States is served by a Cooperative Extension office funded jointly by federal, state and county monies. The Cooperative Extension Service provides nutrition education activities to adults, families, and children to assist them to eat healthfully, through programs such as the Expanded Food and Nutrition Education Program (EFNEP). Special emphasis in recent years has been placed on assisting food stamp recipients to eat more healthfully through the Food Stamp Nutrition Education program. Most states have developed extensive nutrition education programs for food stamp participants. USDA's Women, Infants, and Children (WIC) program provides nutrition education to its participants in addition to providing food. The Head Start program provides both food and nutrition education to preschool children. The Administration on Aging provides meals to low-resources seniors in a group setting and serves most communities in the nation. Nutrition education is a required component of the program.

Many other agencies and private voluntary and nonprofit organizations, such as heart associations, cancer societies, and food banks, also provide nutrition education. Social marketing campaigns focusing on nutrition and physical activity have become more common within communities.

Food- and Food-System-Related Community and Advocacy Organizations

Community nutritionists work in emergency food organizations such as food pantries and soup kitchens, providing needed education to low-resources audiences. Community nutritionists also work in organizations that seek to enhance the availability and accessibility of affordable, nutritious food to individuals and communities by linking food producers to consumers through such programs as farmers' markets, community-supported agriculture, and farm-to-institution programs. Most of these programs include special outreach efforts to low-income communities. Nutrition educators provide educational sessions in these settings, take people on tours of farmers' markets and farms, and work with community policy makers.

Schools

Nutrition education is taught as a part of school health education in many states. In these instances, classroom teachers deliver the nutrition education. The role of the nutrition educator is to develop good curricular materials, provide professional development to teachers, and help teachers provide nutrition education, usually through specific funded projects. In addition, school food service personnel often provide informal nutrition education through posters and food-related activities in the lunchroom. Numerous school-based nutrition education research interventions have been conduced in schools in recent decades with funding from federal agencies such the National Institutes of Health and the USDA.

Workplaces

In recent decades, workplace health promotion has grown considerably, usually incorporating nutrition education, weight control, and physical activity along with other health education efforts to reduce the risk of chronic disease, such as cardiovascular disease and cancer. These efforts have been directed at both the general population of employees and high-risk individuals. Nutrition educators often assist in designing the programs and delivering them.

Health Care Settings

Although one-on-one nutrition counseling is the norm in health care settings, many medical centers provide outpatient nutrition education to at-risk individuals served by the center. Health maintenance organizations and health insurance plans often provide nutrition education to their membership. Nutrition educators also work in physician practices, weight control programs, and eating disorders clinics.

Audiences for Nutrition Education

Nutrition education is provided to a wide range of audiences who differ on many counts, including age, life stage, socioeconomic status, cultural background, and other characteristics.

Life Stage Groups

Nutrition education programs have been developed and delivered to people throughout the entire life span: preschool children and their caregivers; school-aged children through school curricula or after-school activities; college students through nutrition or health courses, cafeteria interventions,

NUTRITION EDUCATION IN ACTION 1-1

Nutrition Education Programs in Different Settings

Kids CATCH Heart-Healthy Habits at School and Home

A nutrition education program for third to fifth graders was developed to reduce the risk of heart disease through healthy eating and increased physical activity. CATCH (Child and Adolescent Trial for Cardiovascular Health) involves classroom curricula, physical education, food service changes, and family involvement. The third-grade program, Hearty Heart and Friends, features stories in the curricula and on videocassettes starring characters from planet Strong Heart. Their adventures emphasize the value of good health. Go for Health for grades 4 and 5 uses enjoyable activities such as preparing healthful snacks. Eat Smart helps cafeterias prepare more healthful meals, and

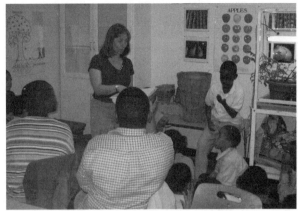

Learning about where food comes from: Examining soil.

the Home Team involves Family Fun Night activities and home activities that children and their parents can do together.

"5 A Day the Color Way" Campaign for Healthier Eating

The 5 A Day the Color Way program is a campaign to assist Americans to eat more fruits and vegetables with a simple and direct call to action: Eat Your Colors Every Day to Stay Healthy and Fit. It includes a website, booklets, TV and radio public service announcements, print ads, school cafeteria posters, and programs in stores to highlight fruits and vegetables. There is also a National 5 A Day month during which nutrition educators in many states provide food demonstrations and presentations at worksites, have the states' premier chefs demonstrate recipes for people to sample, or design floats at state or county fairs to promote fruits and vegetables.

Theater for Kids

Foodplay, a live theater performance for school assemblies or conferences and special events, was developed by a nutrition educator and has been presented all over the Northeast. These performances by nutrition educators on important current issues are complemented with school activity kits, supplementary material handouts, and newsletters that schools can use as follow-ups. Website: www.foodplay.com.

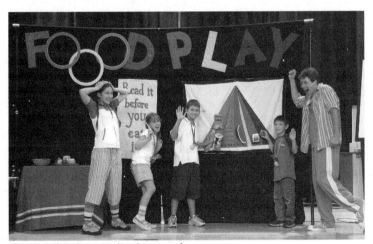

Nutrition education using live theater performances.

Community Gardens

Can community gardens thrive in a large city? The members of many low-income communities in large cities have decided that growing their own gardens is an important way to improve the quality of fresh foods available to them, fight hunger, and promote community-based entrepreneurship and economic opportunity. With names such as Garden of Happiness, Garden of Union, and New Perspectives Community Garden, these inner-city farms produce food not only for those who work in them but also to sell at farmers' markets and other fairs and to donate to soup kitchens and related organizations. Nutrition education is provided at many of these sites. The website for one such program can be found at www.justfood.org.

and student health center activities; adults through community or workplace programs; pregnant and lactating women through WIC and other programs; and older adults through a variety of specifically targeted programs.

Diverse Cultural Groups

Some nutrition education programs are developed specifically for different cultural groups, such as programs for African American churches, Latino/Latina groups, or recent immigrants speaking a variety of languages.

Socioeconomic Background

Socioeconomic status (SES) has been linked to health status, with those of low SES experiencing more health problems and greater premature death than those of higher SES. Many government programs are designed to reduce these health disparities through food assistance activities such as the food stamp and WIC programs or public health programs. Head Start seeks to reduce educational inequities by providing free schooling to eligible preschoolers. Nutrition education is an important component of all these programs, assisting low-resources participants to eat more healthfully.

Gatekeepers: Decision Makers and Policy Makers

Traditionally, the term *gatekeepers* referred to those in the family (usually the mother) who purchased and prepared the food, since such people controlled what the family ate. However, the term can be used more broadly. Today, individuals receive food from a variety of sources. Gatekeepers include individuals or organizations that provide food or services or have some policy-making role in the accessibility and availability of food- or nutrition-related services in organizations, communities, and local and national government. Gatekeepers may also be those who influence social and informational environments, such as the mass media. Given the important role of the environment in facilitating healthy eating, nutrition educators can educate not just individual consumers but policy makers, the mass media, the food industry, and those in the economic, agricultural, and political spheres who make decisions that affect dietary practices. Nutrition educators can educate these gatekeepers about current food and nutrition conditions (e.g., anemia, food insecurity, obesity) and make the case for the relevance of nutrition education and policy alternatives, so as to encourage policy makers to take actions that are more supportive of healthful eating and sustainable food systems.

Scope of Nutrition Education

The major function of nutrition education activities is to assist people to eat and enjoy healthful food by increasing awareness, enhancing people's motivations, facilitating the ability to take action, and improving environmental supports for action. But nutrition education can expand its scope not only in terms of appropriate audiences but also in terms of the content to be addressed and the nature of the strategies to be used.

Nutrition education can address an extremely wide range of content issues related to food and nutrition. The primary content issues are, of course, related to personal health, such as the relationship between diet and health, healthful eating as recommended by the *Dietary Guidelines* and MyPyramid, how to get the best nutrition within one's budget, food safety, breastfeeding, how to get ones' children to eat more healthfully, eating breakfast, balancing eating and physical activity, reducing diet-related chronic disease, and so forth. Indeed, any given nutrition education program can address any issue of concern or interest.

In recent years, there has been an increase in interest among consumers about food safety, spurred by concerns about the increasing incidence of foodborne illness, or about genetically engineered food, bovine growth hormone in milk, and so forth. Nutrition educators need to be prepared to assist consumers to evaluate these issues so they can make informed decisions. Other consumers—and nutrition professionals—have become interested in issues related to how and where food is produced, believing that eating fresh and local food is good for personal health, for farmers, and for the environment (Gussow, 2006). Farmers' markets have emerged in many communities. To increase the accessibility and affordability of local foods to low-resources individuals, the USDA has made it possible for such individuals to use food stamp coupons at farmers' markets. Various community organizations have also worked to link food banks and soup kitchens to local farmers. Nutrition professional organizations have also suggested that nutrition education in schools be linked with work in school gardens and other strategies to help children develop a deeper appreciation for the environment and food systems (American Dietetic Association, 2003).

Some consumers are interested in what are called social justice and sustainability issues related to food (Table 1-2). Indeed, the *Wall Street Journal* and the *New York Times* have noted that some surveys suggest that about one third of consumers are motivated in their purchases by concern for the environment as well as for their health, and mainstream food producers are beginning to cater to this segment (McLaughlin, 2004; Burros, 2006). Consequently, the scope of nutrition education can be expanded to address these content issues as well. Numerous other issues of interest and concern will no doubt emerge that can be addressed by nutrition educators.

Nutrition educators can embark on a wider variety of activities beyond mass media campaigns, lectures, group discussions, workshops, health fairs, or newsletters, videos, brochures and other print and audiovisual materials. They can use a critical consciousness-raising approach, originally proposed by Freire (1970), in which people participate in a process involving a careful analysis of the causes of the food or health issue facing the group and of the structure of power, and then plan ways to organize to take action. This approach has been used in nutrition education to assist low-resources groups identify the causes of their problems of access to food, and to take political and economic actions to reduce nutritional inequities (Travers, 1997).

Nutrition educators can also use a growth-centered educational approach, which seeks to foster self-reliance by building on the abilities and assets of the participants and providing opportunities for self-directed learning and activities and building social support (Arnold et al., 2001). Both of these approaches are related to an empowerment process through which individuals, communities, and organizations gain mastery over their lives (Israel, 1994; Kent, 1988; Rody, 1988; Minkler & Wallerstein, 2002). And indeed, an aim of nutrition education is for individuals in our programs to become less dependent on our activities over time and more able to take control of their own food choices and practices and to take collective action regarding their environments to make them more supportive—in short, to become more empowered.

Nutrition educators can also work in coalitions with other professionals, organizations, and governmental agencies to increase the accessibility and affordability of foods for low-resources audiences; promote environments at the institutional and community levels that foster attitudes and behaviors conducive to health; encourage the development of social networks and social support; build food and nutrition programs that involve genuine community participation and control; and promote policies at local, state, and national levels that are supportive of food- and nutrition-related health.

In sum, nutrition education can encompass a wide range of content, issues, and activities, ranging from group sessions about heart disease risk reduction to assisting low-resources audience to eat better, from helping schools and community groups to grow vegetable gardens to fostering school, worksite, and community food policy councils, and educating and building coalitions with decision makers and policy makers to increase opportunities for all people, but particularly low-resources audiences, to take action about food and nutrition issues (Figure 1-9).

Nutrition Education, Public Health Nutrition, and Health Promotion: The Roles and Context of Nutrition Education

Nutrition education that addresses both environmental and personal factors and includes expanded audiences and strategies begins to overlap public health nutrition and health promotion efforts. To make the situation even more complex, we should note that dietary interventions are often integrated with interventions directed at other health-related behaviors. Many cardiovascular disease risk reduction programs involve interventions directed not only at dietary changes but also at smoking cessation, blood pressure control, and increased physical activity. Within the context of today's emphasis on

TABLE 1-2 Are Your Groceries Sustainable and Fairly Traded?

Food product labels can now help consumers who wish to include considerations of social justice and sustainability in their grocery shopping practices. A variety of labels exist. Here are some of the commonly seen terms and what they mean.

Term	What It Is	What It Means
Sustainable	An unofficial, uncertified term	Food is produced in a way that is environmentally sound, beneficial to local communities, and profitable.
Certified sustainable	Certification licensed by various nonprofit organizations	Food production practices aim to protect the environment, treat workers well, and benefit local communities
Local	An unofficial, uncertified term	Food was grown nearby—no distance specified.
Fair trade certified	Products that comply with standards set by Transfair USA the Fair Trade Labeling Organization International	Farm inspections required. Growers are guaranteed above-commodity prices; men and women are paid equal wages; no child labor is used. Some environmental protections.
Rainforest Alliance Certified	A term licensed by Rainforest Alliance, a New York–based nonprofit organization dedicated to protecting biodiversity.	Farm inspections performed. Farming practices are environmentally sound and fair to workers.

Source: McLaughlin, K. 2004, February 17. Food world's new buzzword is "sustainable" products; fair trade certified mangos. *Wall Street Journal.* Used with permission.

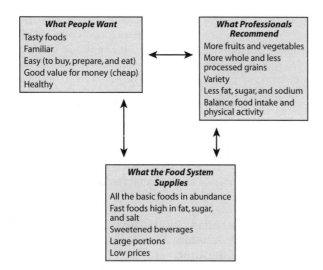

What People Want	What Professionals Recommend
Tasty foods Familiar Easy (to buy, prepare, and eat) Good value for money (cheap) Healthy	More fruits and vegetables More whole and less processed grains Variety Less fat, sugar, and sodium Balance food intake and physical activity

What the Food System Supplies

All the basic foods in abundance
Fast foods high in fat, sugar, and salt
Sweetened beverages
Large portions
Low prices

FIGURE 1-9 Why nutrition education is so exciting and challenging.

health promotion and disease prevention, the roles of nutrition education, public health nutrition, health education, and health promotion are indeed overlapping and intertwined.

At the same time, the scope of nutrition education is broader than educating about nutrition in relation to personal health. Nutrition has often been defined as the link between agriculture and health. Some nutrition educators are concerned about the agriculture-to-nutrition component of the link as well as the nutrition-to-health component. Thus, nutrition education can address such concerns as food safety and how to ensure the availability and accessibility of nutritious and wholesome food for all, poor and rich alike. As we have seen, for some nutrition educators and consumers, considerations about how food is produced are also important. Nutrition education can thus be visualized as including the overlapping portion of several intersecting circles, as shown in Figure 1-10.

Clearly, nutrition education by itself cannot accomplish everything needed for improved nutritional well-being for all people. It must be conducted in conjunction with many other related strategies, some not educational in nature. Facilitating individual behavior change and bringing about change in the environment are both important and interactive. Nutrition education is directed primarily at individual and group behaviors through activities that enhance motivations, knowledge and skills, and social support. However, it also includes nutrition education activities directed at decision makers and policy makers so as to promote specific environmental supports that make it easier for the public to engage in healthy behaviors. Public health nutrition efforts and food assistance programs, on the other hand, are directed primarily at environmental, systemic, and policy factors such as the availability and accessibility of food, access to nutritional services within the health care system, policy, and legislation and secondarily at personal, behavioral factors. In addition, those in nutrition education, public health nutrition, and health promotion share an interest in fostering collective efficacy and capacity building in communities so that communities will become empowered to act on their own food and nutrition issues for the long term.

Purpose of This Book

This book is intended to be a guide to designing and implementing effective nutrition education interventions and behavior change strategies. Effective interventions and strategies are those that effectively enhance people's motivation, ability, and opportunities to eat well. The book's focus is a system for designing, implementing, and evaluating nutrition education that focuses on behavior, is evidence based, and is grounded in the integration of theory, research, and practice.

We have seen that nutrition education can be delivered through multiple venues and that its scope is very broad. One book cannot cover all aspects of nutrition education. Consequently, this text focuses on designing and implementing the types of educational interventions and programs that the vast majority of nutrition educators offer on an ongoing basis in their places of work: *providing site-based, in-person educational activities with groups* in a variety of settings, such as communities, outpatient clinics, health maintenance organizations, fitness centers, schools, or workplaces, or private nonprofit organizations; *developing accompanying materials and activities,* such as printed materials, visual media, mass media and social marketing activities, or health fairs; and *engaging in activities and coalitions* to promote environments and policies that are supportive of the public's ability to eat healthfully.

Many factors in the larger society, such as public policy, systems, and structural changes, have important impacts on food- and nutrition-related behaviors and practices. Designing interventions to change these larger environmental forces operating at the community and national level is the subject of many available health promotion planning and social marketing books and is beyond the scope of this book. The focus of this book is on how to design and implement educational sessions that may be conducted within, or in collaboration with, these larger programs. At the other end of the spectrum, working with individuals one on one, as in nutrition counseling, is also the subject of available texts and will thus not be addressed in this book.

This is an exciting time in the field of nutrition education. The public is interested in food and nutrition. Research is very active, drawing investigators from a variety of fields. Such research has generated considerable evidence about effective approaches to nutrition education and has produced usable theories to guide practice. The remainder of this book is devoted to discussing theories, emerging nutrition educa-

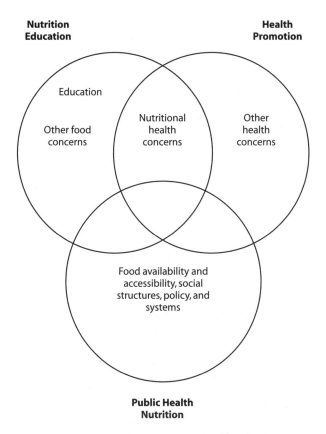

Nutrition
Education

Health
Promotion

Education

Other food
concerns

Nutritional
health
concerns

Other
health
concerns

Food availability and
accessibility, social
structures, policy, and
systems

**Public Health
Nutrition**

FIGURE 1-10 The overlapping roles of nutrition education, public health nutrition, and health promotion.

tion research evidence, and practical techniques for increasing awareness and enhancing motivation, facilitating the ability to take action, and promoting supportive environments so as to assist people to adopt and maintain food- and nutrition-related practices conducive to long-term health.

To design effective nutrition education, we need first to understand more fully the many influences on food choices and nutrition-related behaviors and the dietary change process. Part I of this book provides the background in behavioral nutrition and nutrition education research and theory for understanding the determinants of food choices and the process of dietary behavior change, as well as an overview of how research and theory can enhance nutrition education practice. Part II presents a six-step process for designing practical nutrition education strategies that are based on theory and research evidence, and Part III describes the nuts and bolts of implementing nutrition education and making theory and research practical.

Questions and Activities

1. State five reasons why nutrition education for the public is needed.
2. Describe three reasons why it is difficult for people to eat healthfully, despite the abundance of choices.
3. Social and behavioral factors are implicated in a broad range of diseases in the United States. What are the implications for nutrition education?
4. Three approaches to nutrition education are described in this chapter: information dissemination only; facilitating behavior change, and focusing on environmental change. Describe briefly the central tenets and criticisms of each approach.
5. Review what you wrote before you read the chapter.
   - What is your definition of nutrition education now? How does your definition relate to the three approaches described in the chapter?
   - In light what you have read, what do you now think the goals of nutrition education should be? What kinds of content do you think are appropriate for nutrition education?

REFERENCES

Agricultural Research Service, U.S. Department of Agriculture. 2000. *Continuing survey of food intakes by individuals 1994–1996 (CSFII 1994–1996)*. Washington, DC: Author.

Allegrante, J.P., and L.W. Green. 1981. Sounding board: When health policy becomes victim blaming. *New England Journal of Medicine* 305:1528–1529.

American Dietetic Association. 1990. Position of the American Dietetic Association: Nutrition education for the public. *Journal of the American Dietetic Association* 90(1):107–110.

American Dietetic Association. 2003. Nutrition services: An

essential component of comprehensive health programs. *Journal of the American Dietetic Association* 103:505–514.

Ammerman, A.S., C.H. Lindquist, K.N. Lohr, and J. Hersey. 2002. The efficacy of behavioral interventions to modify dietary fat and fruit and vegetable intake: A review of the evidence. *Preventive Medicine* 35(1):25–41.

Antonovsky, A. 1995. The moral and the healthy: Identical, overlapping or orthogonal? *Israel Journal of Psychiatry and Related Sciences* 32:5–13.

Arnold, C.G., P. Ladipo, C.H. Nguyen, P. Nkinda-Chaiban, and C.M. Olson. 2001. New concepts for nutrition education in an era of welfare reform. *Journal of Nutrition Education* 33:341–346.

Astrand, P. 1982. Diet, performance, and their interaction. In *The Psychobiology of Human Food Selection*, edited by L.M. Barker, 17–32. Westport, CT: Avi Publishing Company.

Balzer, H. 1997. *The NPD Group's 11th annual report on eating patterns in America: National Eating Trends tracking*. Port Washington, NY: The NPD Group.

Bandura, A. 1986. *Foundations of thought and action: A social cognitive theory*. Englewood Cliffs, NJ: Prentice-Hall.

———. 1997. *Self-efficacy: The exercise of control*. New York: WH Freeman.

———. 2001. Social cognitive theory: An agentic perspective. *Annual Review of Psychology* 52:1–26.

Bastiosis, P. P., A. Carlson, S.A. Gerrior, W.Y. Juan, and M. Lino. 2004. The Healthy Eating Index, 1999–2000: Charting dietary patterns of Americans. *Family Economics and Nutrition Review* 16(1):39–48.

Becker, W.C. 1986. *Applied psychology for teachers: A behavioral cognitive approach*. New York: Macmillan. (Originally published by Science Research Associates.)

Birch, L.L. 1999. Development of food preferences. *Annual Review of Nutrition* 19:41–62.

Blanchette, L., and J. Brug. 2005. Determination of fruit and vegetable consumption among 6- to 12-year-old children and effective interventions to increase consumption. *Journal of Human Nutrition and Dietetics* 18(6):431–443.

Brillat-Savarin, A.S. 1825. *The physiology of taste: Meditations on transcendental gastronomy*. Reprint. Translated by M. F. K. Fisher. New York: Heritage Press, 1949. Reprinted Washington, DC: Counterpoint Press 2000.

Buchanan, D. 2004. Two models for defining the relationship between theory and practice in nutrition education: Is the scientific method meeting our needs? *Journal of Nutrition Education and Behavior* 36:146–154.

Burros, M. 2006, January 11. Idealism for breakfast: Serving good intentions by the bowlful. *New York Times*, p. F1.

Campbell, C.C. 1988. Fostering a supportive environment for health. In *Professional Perspectives*. Ithaca, NY: Division of Nutritional Sciences, Cornell University.

Campbell, M.K., W. Demark-Wahnefried, M. Symons, et al. 1999. Fruit and vegetable consumption and prevention of cancer: The Black Churches United for Better Health project. *American Journal of Public Health* 89(9):1390–1396.

Center for Nutrition Policy and Promotion, U.S. Department of Agriculture. 2001, September. *Report card on the diet quality of children ages 2 to 9* (Nutrition Insights 25). Alexandria, VA: Author.

Center for Science in the Public Interest. 2003. *Pestering parents: How food companies market obesity to children*. Washington, DC: Author.

Clancy, K. 1999. Reclaiming the social and environmental roots of nutrition education. *Journal of Nutrition Education* 31(4):190–193.

Contento, I. 1980. Thinking about nutrition education: What to teach, how to teach it, and what to measure. *Teachers College Record* 81(4):422–424.

Contento, I., G.I. Balch, S.K. Y.L. Bronner, et al. 1995. The effectiveness of nutrition education and implications for nutrition education policy, programs, and research: A review of research. *Journal of Nutrition Education* 27(6):279–418.

Cook, A.J., and J.E. Friday. 2004. *Pyramid servings intakes in the United States 1999–2002, 1 day* (CNRG Table Set 3.0). Beltsville, MD: U.S. Department of Agriculture, Agricultural Research Service, Community Nutrition Research Group. http://www.ba.ars.usda.gov/cnrg.

Davis, C.M. 1928. Self selection of diet by newly weaned infants. *American Journal of Diseases of Children* 36:651–679.

Deci, E.L., and R.M. Ryan. 2000. The "what" and "why" of goal pursuits: Human needs and the self-determination of behavior. *Psychological Inquiry* 11(4):227–268.

Dietary Guidelines Alliance. 1996. It's all about you [Fact sheet]. Dietary Guidelines Alliance.

Drewnowski, A., N. Darmon, and A. Briend. 2004. Replacing fats and sweets with vegetables and fruits—a question of cost. *American Journal of Public Health* 94(9):1555–1559.

Elitzak, H. 2001. Food marketing costs at a glance. *Food Review* 24(3):47–48.

Flegal, K.M., M.D. Carroll, C.L. Ogden, and C.L. Johnson. 2002. Prevalence and trends in obesity among US adults, 1999–2000. *Journal of the American Medical Association* 288:1723–1727.

Food Marketing Institute. 2004. *Supermarket facts: Industry overview 2003*. Washington, DC: Author.

Food and Nutrition Board, National Research Council. 1989. *Diet and health: Implications for reducing chronic disease risk*. Washington, DC: National Academy Press.

Frazão, E. 1996. The American diet: A costly health problem. *Food Review* 19(1):1–6.

———. 1999. High costs of poor eating patterns in the United States. In *America's eating habits: Changes and consequences*, edited by E. Frazão. Washington, DC: U.S. Department of Agriculture.

Friere, P. 1970. *Pedagogy of the oppressed*. New York: Continuum.

Gallo, A.E. 1998. *The food marketing system in 1996*. Washington, DC: USDA Economic Research Service.

Gillespie, A.H. 1987. Communication theory as a basis for nutrition education. *Journal of the American Dietetic Association* 87(Suppl.):S44–52.

Green, L.W., and M.W. Kreuter. 1999. *Health promotion planning: An educational and ecological approach*. 3rd ed. Mountain View, CA: Mayfield.

Gussow, J.D. 1999. Dietary guidelines for sustainability: Twelve years later. *Journal of Nutrition Education* 31(4):194–200.

Gussow, J.D. 2006. Reflections on nutritional health and the environment: The journey to sustainability. *Journal of Hunger and Environmental Nutrition* 1(1):3-25.

Gussow J.D., and K. Clancy. 1986. Dietary guidelines for sustainability. *Journal of Nutrition Education* 18(1):1–4.

Gussow J.D., and I. Contento. 1984. Nutrition education in a changing world. *World Review of Nutrition and Diet* 44:1–56.

Hedley, A.A., C.L. Ogden, C.L. Johnson, M.D. Carroll, L.R. Curtin, and K.M. Flegal. 2004. Prevalence of overweight and obesity among US children, adolescents and adults, 1999–2002. *Journal of the American Medical Association* 291:2847–2850.

Hegsted, M. 1979, March 26. Interview quoted in *Nutrition and Health*. In *Chemical and Engineering News*, 27.

Hill, J.O., H.R. Wyatt, G.W. Reed, and J.C. Peters. 2003. Obesity and the environment: Where do we go from here? *Science* 299(7):853–855.

IFIC Foundation. 1999, September/October. Are you listening? What consumers tell us about dietary recommendations. *Food Insight: Current Topics in Food Safety and nutrition*.

Institute of Medicine. 2000. *Promoting health: Intervention strategies from social and behavioral research*, edited by B.D. Smedley and S.L. Syme. Washington, DC: Division of Health Promotion and Disease Prevention, Institute of Medicine.

Israel, B.A., B. Checkoway, A. Schulz, and M. Zimmerman. 1994. Health education and community empowerment: Conceptualizing and measuring perception of individual, organizational, and community control. *Health Education Quarterly* 21:149–170.

Johnson, D.W., and R.T. Johnson. 1985. Nutrition education: A model for effectiveness, a synthesis of research. *Journal of Nutrition Education* 17(Suppl.):S1–S44.

Kent, G. 1988. Nutrition education as an instrument of empowerment. *Journal of Nutrition Education* 20:193–195.

Leading advertisers. 2001, September 24. 100 leading advertisers. pp. 1–36.

Leiss, W. 1976. *The limits to satisfaction: An essay on the problem of needs and commodities*. Toronto: University of Toronto Press.

Leventhal, H. 1973. Changing attitudes and habits to reduce risk factors in chronic disease. *American Journal of Cardiology* 31:571–580.

Levy, L., R.E. Patterson, and A.R. Kristal. 2000. How well do consumers understand percentage daily value on food labels? *American Journal of Health Promotion* 14(3):157–160.

Lipton, K.L., W. Edmondson, and A. Manchester. 1998. *The food and fiber system: Contributing to the U.S. and world economies*. Washington, DC: Economic Research Service, U.S. Department of Agriculture.

Luepker, R.V., C.L. Perry, et al. 1996. Outcomes of a field trial to improve children's dietary patterns and physical activity. The Child and Adolescent Trial for Cardiovascular Health. CATCH Collaborative Group. *Journal of the American Medical Association* 275(10):768–776.

Lytle, L., and C. Achterberg. 1995. Changing the diet of America's children: What works and why. *Journal of Nutrition Education and Behavior* 27:250–260.

Mayer, J. 1986. Social responsibilities of nutritionists. *Journal of Nutrition Education* 116:714–717.

McArthur, D.B. 1998. Heart healthy eating behaviors of children following a school-based intervention: A meta-analysis. *Issues of Comprehensive Pediatric Nursing* 21(1):35–48.

McKenzie, T.L., P.R. Nader, P.K. Strikmiller, et al. 1996. School physical education: Effect of the child and adolescent trial for cardiovascular health. *Preventive Medicine* 25(4):423–431.

McKinley, J.B. 1974. A case for refocusing upstream—the political economy of illness. In *Applying behavioral science to cardiovascular risk*, edited by A.J. Enelow and J.B. Henderson. Seattle, WA: American Heart Association.

McLaughlin, K. 2004, February 17. Food world's new buzzword is "sustainable" products; fair trade certified mangos. *Wall Street Journal*.

McNeal, J.U. 1992. *Kids as customers: A handbook of marketing to children*. New York: Lexington Books.

Minkler, M., and N.B. Wallerstein. 2002. Improving health through community organization and community building. In *Health behavior and health education: Theory, research, and practice*, edited by K. Glanz, B.K. Rimer, and F.M. Lewis. San Francisco: Jossey-Bass.

Moliter, G.T.T. 1980. The food system in the 1980s. *Journal of Nutrition Education* 12(Suppl.):103–111.

Monteiro, C.A., W.L. Conde, and B.M. Popkin. 2004. The burden of disease from undernutrition and overnutrition in countries undergoing rapid nutrition transition: A view from Brazil. *American Journal of Public Health* 94(3):433–434.

National Center for Health Statistics. 2003. *Deaths: Final data for 2001* (National Vital Statistics Report). Hyattsville, MD: National Center for Health Statistics, Division of Vital Statistics.

Pomerleau J., K. Lock, C. Knai, and M. McKee. 2005. Interventions designed to increase adult fruit and vegetable intake can be effective: A systematic review of the literature. *Journal of Nutrition* Oct;135(10):2486–2495.

Potter, J.D., J.R. Finnegan, J.X. Guinard, et al. 2000. *5 A Day for Better Health program evaluation report*. Bethesda, MD: National Institutes of Health, National Cancer Institute.

Rajopal, R., R.H. Cox, M. Lambur, and E.C. Lewis. 2003. Cost-benefit analysis indicates the positive economic benefits of the Expanded Food and Nutrition Education Program related to chronic disease prevention. *Journal of Nutrition Education and Behavior* 34:26–37.

Reed, D.B., M.K. Bielamowicz, C.L. Frantz, and M.F. Rodriguez. 2002. Clueless in the mall: A Web site on calcium for teens. *Journal of the American Dietetic Association* 102(3 Suppl.):S73–S76.

Rody, N. 1988. Empowerment as organizational policy in nutrition intervention programs: A case study from the Pacific Islands. *Journal of Nutrition Education* 20:133–141.

Rolls, B. 2000. Sensory-specific satiety and variety in the meal. In *Dimensions of the meal: The science, culture, business, and art of eating*, edited by H.L. Meiselman. Gaithersburg, MD: Aspen Publishers.

Rothschild, M.L. 1999. Carrots, sticks, and promises: A conceptual framework for the management of public health and social issue behaviors. *Journal of Marketing* 63:24–37.

Rozin, P. 1982. Human food selection: The interaction of biology, culture, and individual experience. In *The psychobiology of human food selection*, edited by L.M. Barker. Westport, CT: Avi Publishing Company.

Schuster, E., Z.L. Zimmerman, M. Engle, J. Smiley, E. Syversen, and J. Murray. 2003. Investing in Oregon's Expanded Food and Nutrition Education Program (EFNEP): Documenting costs and benefits. *Journal of Nutrition Education and Behavior* 35:200–206.

Sims, L. 1987. Nutrition education research: Reaching towards the leading edge. *Journal of the American Dietetic Association* 87(Suppl.):S10–S18.

Society for Nutrition Education. 1995. Joint position of Society for Nutrition Education, the American Dietetic Association, and the American School Food Service Association: School-based nutrition programs and services. *Journal of Nutrition Education* 27(2):58–61.

———. 2006. Society for Nutrition Education mission and identity statement. Indianapolis, IN: Author. http://www.sne.org.

Stewart H., N. Blisard, and D. Jolliffe. 2006. Let's eat out: Americans weigh taste, convenience, and nutrition. Economic Information Bulletin No. EIB-19.

Travers, K.D. 1997. Reducing inequities through participatory research and community empowerment. *Health Education and Behavior* 24:344–356.

U.S. Department of Health and Human Services. 1979. *The surgeon general's report on health promotion and disease prevention*. Washington, DC: Author.

———. 1988. *The surgeon general's report on nutrition and health*. Washington, DC: Author.

———. 2000. *Healthy People 2010: Understanding and improving health*. 2nd ed. Washington, DC: Government Printing Office.

———. 2001. *The surgeon general's call to action to prevent and decrease overweight and obesity*. Washington, DC: Author.

Yudkin, J. 1978. *The diet of man: Needs and wants*. London: Elsevier Science.

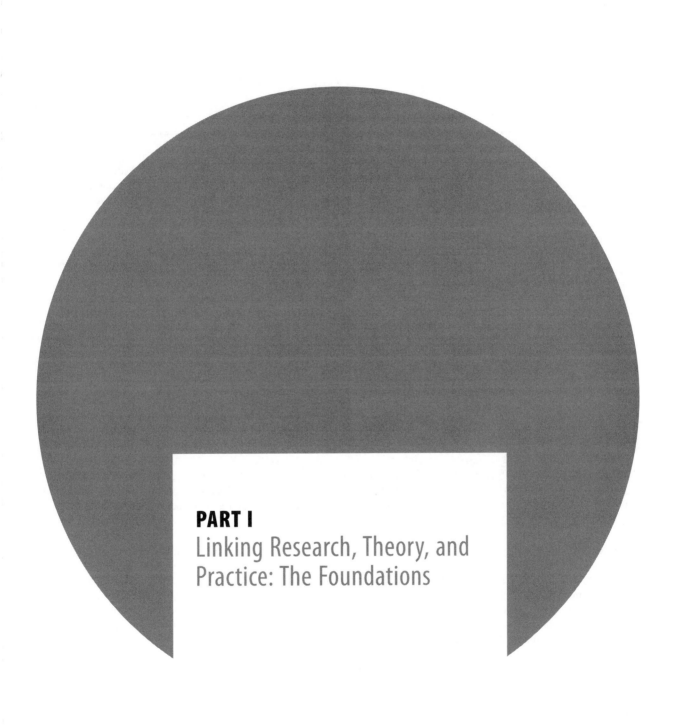

PART I
Linking Research, Theory, and
Practice: The Foundations

An Overview of Food Choice and Dietary Change:
Implications for Nutrition Education

OVERVIEW   This chapter provides readers with an overview of the numerous influences on food choice and dietary practices and their implications for nutrition education. It also provides a description of the desired competencies outlined by professional nutrition societies for nutrition education specialists.

OBJECTIVES   At the end of the chapter, you will be able to

- Describe three categories of influences on food choice and dietary behaviors: food, person, and environment
- Describe the research evidence for the influences of biological predispositions, experience with food, personal factors, and environmental factors on human food choice and dietary behaviors
- Understand the key role of intra- and interpersonal processes in food choice and dietary behaviors
- Appreciate the importance of these understandings for nutrition educators
- State the competencies needed to be an effective nutrition educator

SCENARIO

Think about all the food choices that you made yesterday. List on a sheet of paper 5 to 10 factors that influenced when you ate, what you ate, how much you ate, and with whom. Keep this list with you as you read this chapter. Compare your list with the factors discussed in this chapter as influences on our food choices.

Introduction

We've all known people like Alicia: she knows a lot about nutrition, and in particular she knows that she should eat more fruits and vegetables. She just can't seem to do it. Or Ray, who wants to lose weight and knows what he is supposed to do, but just can't seem to get to it. Or maybe it is ourselves—there is some eating habit we want to change but don't.

Nutrition education is often seen as the process of translating the findings of nutrition science to various audiences using methods from the fields of education and communication. If only the public knew all that we did, nutrition educa-

tors think, surely they would eat better. Thus we believe that our task is to provide the public with information to eat well. We plan sessions on MyPyramid and food label reading. We provide lists of high-fat or high-fiber foods, or food sources of nutrients such as calcium or vitamins. We discuss managing food budgets. However, studies show that simply providing this kind of knowledge is not enough. People often know to eat well but do not—just like Alicia or Ray.

A survey by a consumer research group has found that whereas about one quarter of the public consider nutrition to be very important and are very careful about what they eat, the rest fall almost equally into two groups that either don't want to be bothered or that know what they ought to do but will not or cannot do it (Balzer, 1997). A U.S. Department of Agriculture (USDA) analysis found that 40% of the people surveyed said their diet needed no improvement. Of the remaining 60%, 23% were interested in improving their diet, whereas 37% were not (USDA, 2000). Similarly, another survey found that 7 of 10 consumers said their diet needed some improvement. Guilt, worry, fear, helplessness, and anger were the primary emotions expressed about their diets. However, they said they knew enough about nutrition: "Don't tell us more" (IFIC Foundation, 1999). Clearly, then, although many Americans say their diets need improvement, they also indicate that they are knowledgeable about nutrition and are just unable to change or are uninterested in changing. Thus, many other factors besides knowledge must influence their food choices and diet-related behaviors.

This is not to say that knowledge is not important: knowledge in some form is a prerequisite for intentional healthful eating. However, food is more than nutrients, and eating is about more than health. Eating is a source of pleasure and is related to many of life's social functions. Eating behaviors are acquired over a lifetime, and changing them requires alterations in these behaviors for the long term—indeed, permanently. Unlike other health-related behaviors such as smoking, eating is not optional. We have to eat, and any changes we make are undertaken with a great deal of ambivalence. We want to eat to satisfy our physical hunger and psychological desires and yet we want to be healthy, which may require adopting eating patterns that conflict with these desires.

Nutrition education ultimately has to be about food and eating. Understanding people, their behavior, and the context of their behavior is one of the keys to effective nutrition education programs. Thus it is very important for nutrition educators to understand the various forces that influence an individual's or a community's decision to eat in a particular way. This chapter provides a brief overview of the factors influencing food choice and dietary behaviors for the purpose of helping us design more effective nutrition education programs.

Influences on Food Choice and Diet-Related Behavior: An Overview

We all make decisions about food several times a day: when to eat, what to eat, with whom, and how much. Whether the act of eating is a meal or a snack, the decisions are complex and the influences many. Biologically determined behavioral predispositions such as liking of specific tastes are, of course, important influences. However, these can be modified by experience with food as well as by various intrapersonal and interpersonal factors. In addition, the environment either facilitates or impedes the ability of people to act on their biological predispositions, preferences, or personal imperatives. The influences are so numerous as to be overwhelming to try

to understand! This chapter simplifies matters by examining these influences in three categories that are commonly used in studying food choice: factors related to food, to the individuals making the choices, and to the external physical and social environment—factors related to food, person, and environment (Shepherd, 1999). This scheme is shown in Figure 2-1.

Many factors within each of these categories influence our eating. Figure 2-2 shows the complexity of the influences on food choice and dietary behavior. These influences are explored in greater detail in the following sections.

Food-Related Factors: Biology and Learning

When asked, most people say their food choices are largely determined by "taste" (Food Marketing Institute [FMI], 2002; Glanz, 1998; Clark, 1998). By *taste,* they mean *flavor,* which includes smell and the oral perception of food texture as well (Small & Prescott, 2005). Sensory-affective responses to the taste, smell, sight, and texture of food are a major influence on food preferences and food choices. What are we born with and what is learned?

Biologically Determined Behavioral Predispositions

Humans appear to be born with unlearned predispositions toward liking the sweet taste and rejecting sour and bitter tastes, as can be seen from the facial expressions of newborn infants in response to such substances, work with preterm infants, and other evidence (Desor, Mahler, & Greene, 1977; Mennella & Beauchamp, 1996). The liking for salt seems to develop several months after birth, when infants have matured somewhat (Bernstein, 1990). It has been suggested that these predispositions may have had adaptive value: the liking for the sweet taste because it signaled a safe carbohydrate source of calories, and the rejection of bitterness because it may have signaled potential poisons.

Influences on Eating Behavior

FIGURE 2-1 Influences on eating behavior.

Influences on Eating Behavior

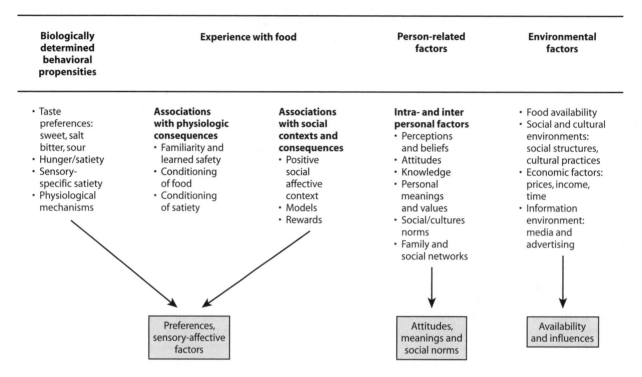

FIGURE 2-2 Complexity of factors that influence eating behavior.

The liking for the sweet taste remains throughout life and appears to be universal to all cultures. However, young children and adolescents are more likely to prefer intensely sweet sugar solutions (Desor, Mahler, & Greene, 1977; Pepino & Mennella, 2005), whereas adults prefer a range of intensities. We shall see later that such preferences can be modified through experience. Although we have a physiological need for salt, adolescents prefer higher levels of saltiness than adults. Preference for fat appears early in infancy or childhood. Fat is less a flavor than a contributor to texture. It imparts different textures to different foods: it makes dairy products such as ice cream seem creamy, meat juicy and tender, pastries flaky, and cakes moist. Many high-fat foods are those in which fat is paired with sugar (desserts) or salt (potato chips), enhancing their palatability. Foods containing fat are more varied, rich tasting, and higher in energy density than nonfat foods and hence are more appealing.

A fifth taste has been proposed: umami, a Japanese word for deliciousness, which is associated with the brothiness of soup or the meatiness in mushrooms. It seems to be related to glutamate, an amino acid, and captures what is described as the taste of protein in food (De Araujo et al., 2003). In addition, because some taste buds are surrounded by free nerve endings of the trigeminal nerve, people are able to experience the burn from hot peppers and the coolness of menthol (Mela & Mattes, 1988). However, the liking for specific tastes may be masked or altered when other flavors are added. For example, adding sugar to bitter-tasting foods (e.g., adding sugar to coffee) makes them more acceptable or even liked (Nasser et al., 2000), and salt can cut bitterness. This masking effect tends to occur for most mixed foods.

There are some genetic differences in sensitivity to tastes. Research shows that people differ in their responses to two bitter compounds called phenylthiocarbamide (PTC) and 6-n-propylthriouracil (PROP). When given PTC-impregnated paper, or PROP in liquid form, some people cannot taste it and are labeled nontasters, others are medium tasters, and still others are supertasters. These individuals differ in the number of fungiform taste buds they have, with supertasters having the most taste buds and nontasters the least (Tepper & Nurse, 1997). Such differences between individuals may be related to differences in being able to discriminate between the fat content of different food and differences in liking for certain foods, such as some bitter, fatty, or sugary foods (Duffy & Bartoshuk, 2000; Tepper & Nurse, 1997; Kaminski, Henderson, & Drewnowski, 2000). It has been suggested that such differences may be related to food patterns (Tepper 1998; Keller & Tepper, 2004).

There has been some discussion about whether certain foods contain chemicals that make them biologically "addictive," such as chocolate (most common for women) or meat (most common for men), which would then influence food choices. However, the evidence seems to suggest that liking, or craving, for such foods is most likely due to the oro-sensory experience of eating the food—its aroma, texture, and taste. Liking may also be linked to associations with past pleasant experiences and other psychological processes (Michener & Rozin, 1994; Rogers & Smit, 2000). Such associations, arising from associative conditioning, can be very strong, leading to difficulties in changing patterns of eating these foods.

There are, of course, many genetic and biological mechanisms that control hunger and satiety, mechanisms that ensure people will eat enough to meet their energy needs (DeCastro, 1999). Throughout most of human history, getting enough food was the primary challenge. The human body developed to function in an environment where food was scarce and high levels of physical activity were mandatory for survival. This situation resulted in the development of various physiological mechanisms that encourage the deposit of energy (i.e., fat) and defend against energy loss. These mechanisms behave as though we have some kind of "thrifty genotype," helping the body to hoard fat stores for times of famine (Neel, 1962; Eaton, Eaton, & Konner, 1997; Lowe, 2003; Chakravarthy & Booth, 2004). Today's environment, however, is one in which food is widely available, inexpensive, and most often high in energy density, while minimal physical activity is required for daily living. Researchers have proposed that the "modern environment has taken body weight control from an instinctual (unconscious) process to one that requires substantial cognitive effort. In the current environment, people who are not devoting substantial conscious effort to managing body weight are probably gaining weight" (Peters et al., 2002). This means that nutrition education has an important role.

Humans also appear to have a built-in biologically determined sensory-specific satiety mechanism whereby they get tired of one taste and move on to another one over a short time span, such as while eating a meal (Rolls, Engell, & Birch, 2000). Such a mechanism probably had adaptive value for humans because it ensured that people would eat a variety of different-tasting foods and thus obtain all the nutrients they needed from these foods. Studies also reveal that for adults, the variety of foods available influences meal size, with greater variety stimulating greater intake. Again, this mechanism might have been very useful in a situation of scarce food supply. However, in today's food environment, the variety possible in meals because of the wide array of foods available may contribute to overweight.

BOX 2-1 Meditation on Taste: A Nineteenth-Century Viewpoint

Taste, such as Nature has given to us, is yet one of our senses (among others such as hearing and sight) that, all things considered, procures to us the greatest of enjoyments:

1. Because the pleasure of eating is the only one that, taken in moderation, is never followed by fatigue;
2. Because it belongs to all times, all ages, and all conditions;
3. Because it occurs necessarily at least once a day, and may be repeated without inconvenience two or three times in this space of time;
4. Because it can be combined with all our other pleasures, and even console us for their absence;
5. Because the impressions it receives are at the same time more durable and more dependent on our will;
6. Finally, because in eating we receive a certain indefinable and special comfort, which arises from the intuitive consciousness that we repair our losses and prolong our existence by the food we eat.

Brillat-Savarin, A.S. 1825. *The physiology of taste: Meditations on transcendental gastronomy*. Reprint. Translated by M. F. K. Fisher. New York: Heritage Press, 1949. Reprinted Washington, DC: Counterpoint Press 2000.

These biologically determined predispositions contribute to some degree to preference and to food intake, particularly in children. However, as we shall see in the next section, most preferences are learned or conditioned—which is good news for nutrition educators, because that means they can be modified.

Experience with Food
Research in this area suggests that people's food preferences and food acceptance patterns are largely learned (Birch, 1999; Mennella, Griffen, & Beauchamp, 2004; Pepino & Mennella, 2005). Such learning begins early—in fact, prenatally. In studies, infants born to mothers fed carrots during pregnancy liked their cereal with carrot juice more than with

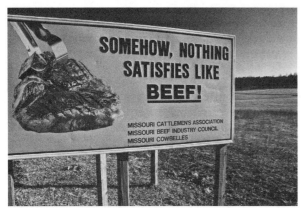

The number of influences on our diet choices is endless.

water at weaning (Mennella, Jagnow, & Beauchamp, 2001). At the second week of life, infants accepted a formula made of an unpleasant-tasting, sour and bitter protein hydrosylate as well as they accepted milk. However, when tested with the hydrosylate formula at 7 months, those fed the hydrosylate for 7 months drank it well, whereas those fed milk formula rejected it (Mennella, Griffen, & Beauchamp, 2004). Infants fed hydrosylate liked sour tastes into childhood (Liem & Mennella, 2002).

Thus, what humans seem to inherit primarily is the innate capacity to learn about the consequences of eating particular foods. By *learning* in this context, we do not mean cognitive learning, but rather physiological learning or conditioning arising from the positive or negative consequences that people experience from eating a food. Conditioning of food preferences continues throughout life, but early experience with food and eating is especially crucial in the development of eating patterns, in terms of both the kinds of food people come to prefer and the amount they eat. Experience with food influences the development of eating patterns of children and adults in several ways.

Exposure, familiarity, and learning to accept new foods. Humans, like other omnivores, experience the "omnivore's dilemma": they need to seek variety in their diets to meet nutritional requirements, but ingesting new substances can be potentially dangerous (Rozin, 1988). Although food neophobia, or negative reactions to new foods, is minimal in infants, it increases through early childhood so that 2- to 5-year-olds, like other young omnivores, demonstrate neophobia (Birch, 1999). This would have adaptive value because infants are fed by adults, but toddlers are beginning to explore their world and have not learned yet what is safe to eat and what is not. However, neophobia can be reduced by experience with food (Birch & Marlin, 1982; Birch, 1998), probably through a "learned safety mechanism." That is, when eating a food is not followed by negative consequences, increased food acceptance results. Studies with children show that

preference increases with repeated opportunities to sample new foods, sometimes requiring 12 to 15 exposures (Birch, 1999). Once the foods are familiar, the preferences tend to persist (Skinner et al., 2002). Similar results have been found for adults (Pliner, Pelchat, & Grabski, 1993; Pelchat & Pliner, 1995). In addition, tasting or actual ingestion was found to be necessary—not just looking at or smelling the food (Birch et al., 1987a).

In sum, with repeated consumption, preference for initially novel foods tends to increase. Thus, if children are exposed to many high-sugar, high-fat, and high-salt foods at home, at school, and in other settings, then these foods will become more familiar and will become preferred over those that remain relatively unfamiliar, such as vegetables or whole grains.

Likewise, biologically determined behavioral propensities can be modified through familiarity and learned preference mechanisms. For example, those who eat lower-salt diets come to like them more (Beauchamp, Bertine, & Engelman, 1983; Mattes, 1997). The dislike for bitterness can be overcome, as shown by the infant studies described earlier and by the fact that people come to like a variety of bitter tastes, such as coffee, dark chocolate, or bitter vegetables such as broccoli. Sour tastes, such as vinegar and grapefruit, can also become liked. Regarding the liking for fat, one study found that those who switched from a high-fat diet to one lower in fat for 12 weeks came to like the fat taste less if they ate naturally low-fat foods such as grains and vegetables (Mattes, 1993). This change in hedonic liking for the fat taste did not occur if the individuals ate lower-fat versions of the same foods made with fat substitutes such that the taste or mouthfeel remained the same. The former involved a change in behavior; the latter did not. Maintaining these changed preferences involves continuing to eat these new foods.

Learning from the physiological consequences of eating: preferences, aversions, and conditioned satiety. The physiological consequences of eating a food have a powerful impact on our food preferences. These consequences can be positive or negative. If eating is followed by negative effects, such as a feeling of nausea, a conditioned aversion follows. Conditioned aversions can be quite powerful. A one-time experience of illness following eating a food can turn individuals off that food for decades. On the other hand, preferences for foods usually develop more slowly through a process of *learned* or *conditioned preference*, whereby repeated eating of a food is followed by pleasant consequences such as a feeling of fullness or satiety. Such learning by association of a food flavor with its consequences is called *associative conditioning* (Birch, 1999; Sclafani, 2004, Sclafani & Ackroff, 2004).

People can learn to prefer new flavors by pairing them with an already preferred taste, such as the sweet taste, in what is called *flavor–flavor learning*. An example is a study in which people came to like a specifically flavored tea when it was served with sugar. Associating coffee with sugar and cream is a common practice. People also learn to like new flavors if they are associated with energy density (or calories), in what is called *flavor–nutrient learning*. For example, children have been shown to develop increased liking or preference for novel flavors (e.g., chocolate-orange) associated with high-calorie versions (whether through high starch or high fat) versus low-calorie versions of the same food, because the high-calorie versions were perceived as pleasantly filling, particularly when the children were hungry (Birch & Deysher, 1985; Johnson, McPhee, & Birch, 1991; Birch, 1992).

Research shows that in both young children and adults, satiety or the sense of fullness is influenced by associative learning and can be conditioned (Johnson, McPhee, & Birch, 1991; Birch & Fisher, 1995). Young children who learn that one flavor of pudding is high in calories and another is low will adjust the amount they eat of a meal served to them subsequent to eating the specific pudding. If they are given pudding of the same flavor as the one that was previously high in calories but which is now low in calories, they will eat amounts of the subsequent meal as though they had eaten the high-calorie pudding. This ability to learn about the satiety value of familiar foods may explain how meals can be terminated before people have yet experienced the physiological cues that signal satiety. Thus, as a result of repeatedly consuming familiar foods, people learn about the "filling" and the "fattening" quality of familiar foods and normally make adjustments in what they eat in anticipation of the end of the meal (Stunkard, 1975).

Humans also learn to prefer calorie-dense foods over calorie-dilute versions of the same foods. Such learned preferences for calorie-dense foods was first shown in rats (Sclafani, 1990) and then in young children (Birch et al., 1987b). When children have repeated opportunities to eat either a calorie-dense, high-fat food or a calorie-dilute, fat-free version of the same food, they learn to prefer the calorie-dense version of the food over the calorie-dilute version of the same food (Birch, 1992). The biological mechanism that assists people to like calorie-dense foods was very adaptive when food, and especially calorie-dense food, was scarce and probably explains the universal liking for calorie-dense foods in adults. The finding that tasty high-fat and high-sugar foods induce overeating and obesity in animals (Sclafani, 2004) suggests that this feature is less adaptive for humans in today's environment, where calorie-dense foods are widely available.

In sum, these studies show that food preferences and sense of fullness are learned through repeated exposure to the foods and from the physiological consequences of eating those foods.

Social-affective context, food preferences, and quantify of intake. The social environment also has a powerful impact on food preferences and on the regulation of how much to eat. Food is eaten many times a day, providing opportunities

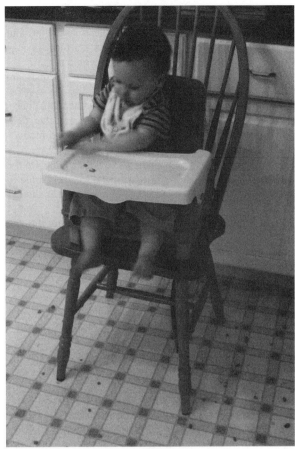

Neophobia increases through early childhood.

for people's emotional responses to the social context of eating to become associated with the specific foods being eaten. This is particularly true in children. Children's preferences are influenced by peer and adult models (Birch, 1999). Familiar adults have been found to be more effective than unfamiliar ones, and having the adults themselves eat the same foods is more effective than when adults offer the foods without eating the foods themselves (Harper & Sanders, 1975; Addessi et al., 2005). Food preferences also increase when adults offer the foods in a friendly way (Birch, 1999).

However, the use of rewards is more complex (Birch, 1999). If a food is given as a reward, there is a significant *increase* in preference: "You did a good job cleaning up the toys. Here, have some peanuts." The opposite is true if the child is asked to eat a food in order to obtain a reward: "If you eat your spinach, you can watch TV." In particular, requiring eating of a less-liked food in order to obtain a better-liked food ("You can have dessert if you eat your spinach") can *decrease* even further the liking for the initially less-liked food because children reason (as do adults) that the food must taste bad if they have to be bribed to eat it. In addition, because the foods used as rewards are typically those high in sugar, fat, and salt (e.g., desserts and salty snacks), such a practice may enhance even further the preference for these items.

Given that energy-dense, high-fat, high-sugar foods are widely available in our environment, tend to be used as rewards, are most often offered in positive social contexts such as celebrations and holidays, are liked by other family members, satisfy biological predispositions, and produce positive feelings of being full, it is not surprising that they become highly preferred by adults and children alike. On the other hand, fewer opportunities are provided for people to learn to like whole grains, fruits, and vegetables in similar social contexts.

Regarding quantity of intake, young children learn through associative conditioning about the fillingness of familiar foods, as we have seen, and can learn to self-regulate how much they eat. However, parenting practices and influences in the social environment can modify and interfere with that learned responsiveness. For example, children who are led to pay attention to their internal cues (feelings of hunger and being full) are more likely to be able to regulate appropriately the amount of food they eat than those who are asked to focus on externally oriented cues such as the time of day or the amount of food remaining on the plate (Birch et al., 1987b; Birch, 1999). Children at age 3 eat about the same amount regardless of the portion size of the food offered. However, by age 5, children eat more when they are offered more (Rolls, Engell, & Birch, 2000).

Children who have greater body fat stores have been found to be less able to regulate their calorie intake accurately, and when parents are more controlling, children have less ability to self-regulate energy intake (Johnson & Birch, 1994). Restricting foods can make the restricted foods more attractive. Thus, highly restrictive parental controls limit the opportunities for children to practice self-regulation and maintain a healthy weight (Birch, Fisher, & Davison, 2003; Faith et al., 2004). Overeating in the absence of hunger is also conditioned (Birch, Fisher, & Davison, 2003). On the other hand, parents' own practices in terms of eating more fruits and vegetables highly influence what their daughters eat (Fisher, 2002). However, in some populations, mothers' own flexible restraint can result in more healthful food choices for themselves and their children (Robinson et al., 2001; Contento, Zybert, & Williams, 2005), this control being interpreted as expressing parental responsibility and caring (Lin & Liang, 2005). It has been concluded that the best practice is for adults to offer an array of *healthful* foods and for children to choose which of them to eat (Satter, 2000). Thus, the practices of parents, child-care centers, and nutrition educators who work with young children can have important influences on the children's body weight and eating habits (Birch & Fisher, 2000). Many of these same findings apply to

adults as well and can inform the work of nutrition educators (Pliner, Pelchat, & Grabski, 1993).

Summary. Physiological mechanisms, genetically determined behavioral propensities, and conditioning through experience with food all influence our sensory experience of food and food preferences. These influences are summarized in Figure 2-2. Food preferences have a very direct impact on children's intakes because children tend to eat the foods they like and reject the foods they do not like in terms of taste, smell, or texture. The relationship between taste preferences and food choices is more indirect in older children and adults, because experience with food and beliefs about the impact of food on weight, appearance, health, or other valued outcomes can modify their propensity to act on their preferences for high-fat and high-sugar foods. These considerations may lead individuals to eat more healthful diets even if these are not the most appealing, as we discuss in the next section.

Person-Related Factors

Intrapersonal Factors
Perceptions, beliefs, and attitudes. Our biologies and our personal experiences with food are not the only influences on our food intake. We also develop perceptions and expectations about foods: how foods should taste and what impacts they will have on our sense of well-being. These perceptions can be called *sensory-affective responses* to food.

We may value some aspects of food over others. In the United States, the major values in choosing foods are taste, convenience, and cost (Glanz, Basil, Maibach et al., 1998). In Europe, the major values are quality/freshness, price, nutritional value, and family preferences, in that order (Lennernas, Fjellstrom, Becker, et al., 1997). We acquire beliefs about foods, some accurate, and some not. We also develop attitudes toward food- and diet-related issues, such as regarding eating meat or breastfeeding, and some of these may be deeply held. We may invest specific foods with personal meanings. For example, eating chocolate is very pleasurable for many people, addictive even, and is associated with intense emotions and personal meanings (rewarding oneself, memories, etc.). These perceptions, attitudes, beliefs, values, and personal meanings are all powerful influences on food choice and dietary behavior, as are individuals' interactions with others in their social environment.

Food rejections are also highly influenced by psychological processes, based on both previous experience and beliefs. Rozin and Fallon (1987) placed the motivations for rejecting foods into three main categories: (1) sensory-affective beliefs (e.g., the food will smell or taste bad) that lead to *distaste,* (2) anticipated consequences or beliefs about the possible harmful outcomes of eating certain foods (e.g., vomiting, disease, social disapproval), leading to *danger,* and (3) ideation or ideas about the origin or nature of foods, leading to *disgust.*

Knowledge regarding all these numerous person-related factors is crucial for nutrition educators so that we can better understand our audiences and assist them to eat more healthfully.

Because the process of procuring, preparing, and consuming food is a universal human behavior, the influences on food-related behavior have been studied by researchers in many disciplines in the behavioral sciences, ranging from anthropology to economics. Their findings can be helpful to nutrition educators. Because food is also related to health, research findings in the fields of health psychology, health education, and health promotion can also provide an understanding of health behavior that can be directly useful to the work of nutrition educators.

There are many schools of thought within the behavioral sciences about the determinants of human behavior. Several of the predominant ones relevant to nutrition education are sketched here in brief. One school that was especially dominant earlier viewed human behavior as motivated by internal forces such as needs, drives, and impulses that frequently operated below the level of consciousness. Later, Maslow (1968) proposed that once basic needs are met, people are motivated by needs for affection, self-esteem, and self actualization. This *humanistic* or *self-actualization school* views people as autonomous, thinking and choosing entities who are basically good and rational, acting in their own best interest as they perceive it. According to this school, given acceptance and freedom of choice, people will adopt those behaviors that are healthy and self-actualizing.

In contrast, many psychologists of the same period, led by Watson (1925) and Skinner (1953, 1971), came to favor the view that there is no such thing as an autonomous inner being. According to this school, we can only measure what is observable, hence statements about the causes of behavior can only come from what is observable and measurable. Feelings, attitudes, intentions, and ideas simply accompany or follow behavior; they do not cause behavior. Instead, human behavior is determined by environmental stimuli or by the consequences or reinforcement of behavior. That is, those behaviors that are reinforced or rewarded by the environment are more likely to be performed again. In simple terms, "behavior is determined by its consequences." Because both stimuli and reinforcement occur in the outer environment, it is the environment that shapes and changes behavior. This is the *behaviorist school*. From this point of view, the role of nutrition education is to structure (or change) the environment or social conditions in such a way so as to change or shape peoples' behavior by using the principles of behaviorism. Many early weight control programs run by nutritionists were based on behavior modification principles derived from this school. Clients or program participants were trained to use smaller plates, eat more slowly, make sure there were no tempting foods in the house, and so forth.

In anthropology, too, there have been two major schools of thought on the determinants of human behavior. The *ideational* or *mentalistic school* viewed culture as an overarching construct based on a system of ideas; differences in human behavior were a result of differences in idea systems. Changes in people's food-related behaviors would thus require changes in their culture and their ways of thinking. On the other hand, the *behaviorist-materialist school* viewed people's behavior as largely determined by material conditions such as access to resources, technological and energy factors, and biological features. Changes in behavior are thus considered more likely to result from changes in material conditions, such as initiation of a farmers' market program in the community, than from changes in ideas and beliefs, such as the importance of eating food from local farms (Pelto, 1981).

However, there is increasing recognition among psychologists that "human behavior is no more the exclusive function of some hypothetical entity called willpower or self-actualizing drive than it is the sole consequence of external stimuli in the physical environment. Instead, human behavior is partly determined by internal, covert processes . . . and physiological responses as well as by external events" (Thorsen & Mahoney, 1974). This has led to various cognitive behavioral and social cognitive approaches to understanding behavior that take into consideration both personal thoughts and environmental influences (e.g., Lewin, 1936; Bandura, 1986). Anthropologists, too, have come to a more holistic or systems view of human nature, in which ideas and beliefs as well as material, economic circumstances are important. Consequently, most behavioral scientists would now agree that behavior is the result of interactions between individuals and their environments and that these interactions can be quite complex.

This more comprehensive view of the determinants of human behavior can be applied to people's dietary behaviors. Our food choices and dietary practices are influenced by a variety of personal factors, such as our beliefs about what we will get from these choices. We want our foods to be tasty, convenient, affordable, filling, familiar, or comforting. Our food choices may be determined by the personal meanings we give to certain foods or practices, such as chicken soup when we are ill, or chocolate when we feel self-indulgent. We may also be motivated by how the food will contribute to how we look, such as whether it will be fattening or, in contrast, good for our complexion. Our food- and nutrition-related behaviors are also determined by our attitudes toward them—for example, our attitudes toward breastfeeding or certain food safety practices. Our identity in relation to food may also influence our behaviors. For example, some teenagers may see themselves as health conscious, but many others may see themselves as part of the junk-food-eating set. We may see that there are health benefits to eating more healthfully but consider the barriers, such as high cost or the effort required to prepare the foods in healthful ways, just too great to take action. Or perhaps we lack confidence in preparing foods in ways that are tasty and healthful. Or again, we may have specific culturally related health beliefs that influence what we eat. For example, although the concepts of balance and moderation are common among many cultures, individuals may come from cultures in which foods are believed to have hot and cold qualities and must be eaten in such a way as to balance cold and hot body conditions. These cultural beliefs can have a major influence on food choices.

These personal factors interact with environmental factors. For example, we may see a news story on the role of fruits and vegetables in reducing cancer risk, or a friend of ours develops colon cancer (external stimuli). We process such environmental stimuli or external events both cognitively and affectively. These stimuli are filtered through a host of internal personal reactions of the kind listed previously, such as our perceptions, beliefs, values, expectations, or emotions, and together these filters determine what actions we will take. For example, we may process the idea of eating more fruits and vegetables in terms of taste, convenience, expected benefits, perceived barriers, or what our friends and relatives do, in addition to our concerns about getting cancer. Consequently, our decisions about whether to eat more fruits and vegetables to reduce cancer risk are based on our beliefs and knowledge about *expected consequences* (of eating fruits and vegetables), our motivations and values about *desired consequences* (reduced risk of cancer), and our *personal meanings and values* (with respect to developing cancer).

In the food choice process, most times we will also need to make trade-offs among various criteria or reasons for food choice, such as among health considerations, taste, and cultural expectations. People may also trade off between items within a meal or between meals. For example, individuals may choose an item for its fillingness (e.g., a donut) but then balance it with something perceived as more healthful (e.g., orange juice). Or individuals may choose a "healthy" dinner to balance what they consider to have been a less than healthful lunch (Contento et al., 2006).

People's food-related knowledge and skills also influence what they eat. In particular, their misconceptions may play an important role. For example, a national survey found that about one third of individuals thought that the recommended number of servings of fruit and vegetables per day was one, and another third thought it was two; only 8% thought it was five (Krebs-Smith et al., 1995). Many consumers have major misconceptions about the amounts of fat and energy in many common foods and in their own diets (Mertz, 1991; Mela, 1993, Brug, Glanz, & Kok,1997). Lack of skills in preparing foods also influences what individuals eat.

Social and cultural norms. Humans are social creatures. We all live in a social and cultural context and experience social norms and cultural expectations, which can be extraor-

dinarily powerful. We feel compelled to subscribe to these norms and expectations to varying degrees. For example, teenagers may feel pressure to eat less-nutritious fast food items in a choice situation with peers (e.g., after school), or individuals may experience family members' expectations that they will eat in a certain way. Whether to breastfeed may be influenced very much by the desires of a woman's family. Our perceptions of our status and roles in our communities are also important. The food choices and eating patterns of celebrities create social expectations for us all. What others in our community think are appropriate foods to eat in various situations may also create social pressures. Thus, our choice of foods may be heavily influenced by our perceptions of the *social and cultural expectations* of those around us.

Interpersonal Factors
Within societies, we all participate in a network of social relationships, the extensiveness and density of which vary among individuals. These networks involve family, peers, coworkers, and those in various organizations to which we belong. For example, in one study, food choices were 94% similar between spouses, 76% to 87% similar between adolescents and their parents, and 19% similar between adolescents and their peers (Feunekes et al., 1998). Food choices and eating patterns are also influenced by the need to negotiate with others in the family about what to buy or eat (Connors et al., 2001; Contento et al., 2006). Relationships with peers and those with whom we work also have an impact on our day-to-day choices (Devine et al., 2003).

Indeed, eating contexts and the management of social relationships in these numerous contexts play a major role in what we eat. For example, if a woman becomes motivated to reduce her fat intake by using 1% or nonfat milk instead of whole milk, she may find that other family members like whole milk and do not want to switch. She will have to decide whether to go along with family wishes or to buy low-fat or nonfat milk separately for herself. She will also need to consider whether she has the space in the refrigerator to keep both types of milk, which then becomes a barrier to change.

The intra- and interpersonal factors that influence food choice and dietary behaviors are summarized in Figure 2-2.

Environmental Factors
Environmental factors are powerful influences on food choice and nutrition-related behaviors and must be considered by nutrition educators in planning programs.

Physical Environment: Food Availability and Accessibility
In developed countries and increasingly in less developed countries, food and processed food products are available in an ever-widening array of choices. More than 50,000 food items are available in U.S. supermarkets, and about 9,000 new brand-name processed food products are introduced

each year (Gallo, 1998; Lipton, Edmondson, & Manchester, 1998). The typical shopper averages 2.2 trips to the supermarket each week (FMI, 2005). Overall *availability* may be described as the array of food options that are present in the food system that are acceptable and affordable. *Accessibility* may be thought of as "immediate" availability, referring to the readiness and convenience of a food—whether the food requires little or no cooking, is packaged in a convenient way so that it can be eaten anywhere, or whether it can be stored for some time without spoilage. Studies have shown that the availability of more healthful options in neighborhood grocery stores, such as fruits and vegetables or low-fat milk, is correlated with these foods being more available in the homes, which in turn is related to a higher quality of food choices and intakes (Cheadle et al., 1991; Morland, Wing, & Diez Roux, 2002). Thus, what is available in the community influences what is purchased and eaten. The availability and accessibility of fruits and vegetables at home and school enable their consumption by children (Hearn et al., 1998).

Accessibility is also dependent on where sources of food are physically located. Supermarkets, where a wide range of foods is available, may require transportation to reach, limiting the accessibility of food for many people, such as older people who are no longer able to drive or lower-income people without cars. The types of foods that are readily available in the local grocery stores, small corner stores, and restaurants within a given community will depend on potential profits, consumer demand, and adequate storage and refrigeration facilities. The foods served or products stocked in them thus tend to be those that sell well, which are not always the most nutritious. Farmers' markets provide fresh, local foods but may require transportation to reach and are often only seasonal. Hence, some foods that are very important for health, such as fruits and vegetables, may not be readily accessible or are available only at a higher cost.

Foods available at or near workplaces also tend to be those that are convenient, low in cost, and will sell well. In most schools, food is available and accessible. The National School Lunch Program provides meals that conform to federal guidelines that specify nutritional standards to be met. Increasingly, however, à la carte offerings, vending machines, and school stores compete for student participation; the foods available from these sources are not subject to these guidelines. Participation in the School Lunch Program declines with age, so that by high school, two thirds of students are obtaining their lunch from other sources. The majority of competitive foods in these other venues have been found to be high-fat and high-sugar items, including snack chips, candy, and soft drinks. Within the home, accessibility means that a vegetable is not just available in the refrigerator but is already cut up and ready to eat, or fruit has been washed and is sitting on the counter ready to eat. The limited accessibility

of healthful, convenient foods in many settings may narrow good choices and make it difficult to eat healthfully.

Social Structures and Cultural Environment

Social environments and cultural contexts are no less important than the physical environment. Social influences and cultural practices all influence food choice and dietary behavior (Rozin, 1996).

Social influences. Society has been described as a group of people interacting in a common territory who have shared institutions, characteristic relationships, and a common culture. Most eating occurs in the presence of other people. The effect can be positive or negative in terms of healthful eating, in part because family and friends serve as models as well as sources of peer pressure. For example, there is evidence that eating with others can lead to eating more food compared with eating alone, especially when the others are familiar people (DeCastro, 1995, 2000). Spending more time at a meal eating with others also increases intake. Eating with others can result in pressure to eat higher-fat foods. On the other hand, eating with others can also result in pressure to try new foods that are healthy (MacIntosh, 1996). Parents' own eating patterns likely influence that of their children (Fisher et al., 2002 Contento, Zybert, & Williams, 2005), and it has been shown that children and adolescents who eat with their families most days each week have better-quality diets than those who eat with their families less frequently (Gilman, Rifas-Shiman, & Frazier, 2000).

Influence of cultural practices and family of origin. Culture has been described as the knowledge, traditions, beliefs, values, and behavioral patterns that are developed, learned, shared, and transmitted by members of a group. It is a worldview that a group shares, and hence it influences perceptions about food and health. Cultural practices and family of origin have an important impact on food choices and eating practices

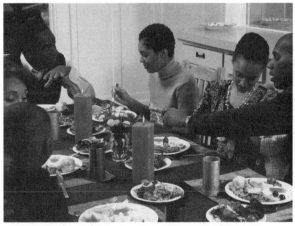

Families who eat together generally have better-quality diets.

even in modern, multiethnic societies where many different types of cuisine are available. Those from different regions of the country may have different practices. For example, for those from the South a home-style meal is chicken-fried steak, mashed potatoes, corn bread, and bacon- and onion-laden green beans, with pie for dessert, whereas those who live in Texas may expect to eat barbecue or Tex-Mex foods that are hot and spicy. Those who have immigrated from different countries from around the world maintain some of their cultural practices in varying degrees, and these traditions influence eating patterns.

Cultural rules often specify which foods are considered acceptable and preferable, and the amount and combination of various categories of foods that are appropriate for various occasions. The cultural practices of family and friends, especially at times of special celebrations and holidays, provide occasions to eat culturally or ethnically determined foods and reinforce the importance of these foods. If dietary recommendations based on health considerations conflict with family and cultural traditions, individuals wanting to make dietary changes may find themselves having to think about and integrate their cultural expectations with their concern about their personal health. All of these considerations influence individuals' willingness and ability to make changes in their diets. These beliefs and practices must be carefully understood so that nutrition educators can become culturally competent and can design culturally sensitive nutrition education programs.

Social structures: organizations and institutions. The organizations to which we belong can have a profound effect on our eating patterns. Some are voluntary organizations, such as religious, social, or community organizations; others include our places of work and professional associations to which we must belong. Their influence on us comes from the social norms of these institutions as well as their policies and practices.

Economic Environment
Many factors in the economic environment influence food choices and dietary practices, among them price of food,

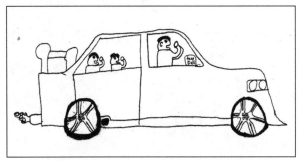

This child was asked to draw a picture of her family eating their favorite meal together. (Courtesy of Cooking with Kids)

income, time, and formal education. These factors need to be considered when nutrition education programs are designed.

Prices. Economic theory assumes that relative differences in prices can partially explain differences among individuals in terms of their food choices and dietary behaviors.

The price of food as purchased is usually per item, unit weight, or volume. However, price can also be thought of as the amount of food energy obtained per dollar. Processed foods with added fats and sugar are cheaper to manufacture, transport, and store than are perishable meats, dairy products, and fresh produce. This is partly because sugar and fat on their own are both very inexpensive, due in part to government agricultural policies. A diet made up of refined grains and processed foods with added sugar and fats can be quite inexpensive (a days' worth of calories for one to two dollars). Beans cost about the same, but animal protein sources may cost 5 to 10 times more per calorie, and fruits and vegetables (except potatoes and bananas) can cost some 50 to 100 times more per calorie than high-fat, high-sugar, mass-produced food products (Drewnowski & Barrratt-Fornell, 2004). When freely chosen diets were studied, it was found that adding fats and sweets was associated with a 5% to 40% decrease in food costs, whereas adding fruit and vegetables was associated with a 20% to 30% increase in food costs (Drewnowski, Darmon, & Briend, 2004). Not surprisingly, low-income individuals eat fewer fruits and vegetables. These disparities in cost may also contribute to the higher prevalence of obesity in those of lower socioeconomic status.

Income. People in the United States spend only about 10% of their disposable income on food prepared and consumed at home, compared with 15% in Europe and Japan, 35% in middle-income countries, and 53% in low-income countries (Seale, Regmi, & Bernstein, 2003). However, this is an average. The amount of money spent on food depends on income level. Upper-income individuals spend more money on food, but it is a smaller proportion of their income—about 8%. Lower-income households economize by buying more discounted items and generic brands and thus spend less on food; despite this, food accounts for 20% to 35% of their income (Putnam & Allshouse, 1999). Compared with other economic variables, income has the strongest marginal impact (i.e., additional effect) on diet behavior: those with higher incomes eat a higher-quality diet (Mancino, Lin, & Ballinger, 2004).

In this context, statistics show that about 11% to 12% of American households are *food insecure*, meaning that they do not have access, at all times, to enough food for an active, healthy life for all household members. The prevalence of food insecurity with hunger is about 3% to 4%, hunger being defined as the uneasy or painful sensation caused by lack of food (Food Research and Action Center, 2005).

Time use and household structure. Many people with whom nutrition educators work today say they are too busy to prepare healthful foods or to cook at all. Surveys and time use diaries show that the amount of time people spend on food-related activity in the home depends on many factors, including whether men or women are employed outside the home and whether they have children (Robinson & Godbey, 1997; National Pork Producers Council, 2002; Cutler & Glaeser, 2003). Between 1965 and 1985, the time spent preparing food and cleaning up after meals averaged about 40 minutes per day for single women and then declined to 30 minutes in 1995. During the same period, married women working outside the home decreased their time spent on these tasks from 1 hour to 40 minutes, and women *not* working outside the home decreased the time spent from 2 hours to 1 hour. Men on average spent from 10 to 18 minutes a day on these activities between 1965 and 1995. In both 1965 and 1995, men and women both reported spending about 7 to 8 hours a week eating. In the same time period, television viewing increased from about 9 hours to 15 hours a week for women and from about 12 to 17 hours a week for men. Time spent on household shopping has remained about the same, at 3 to 4 hours a week. People seem to be replacing time spent on food-related tasks with more time spent watching television. Thus, with the mass production of food, the time cost for obtaining food has declined (Cutler & Glaeser, 2003). According to economic theory, people should thus eat more, especially those who used to spend the time in food preparation and do not need to do so now, for example, women. This seems to be the case.

Time is scarce for all households, regardless of income. For some households, time constraints may limit personal investments in healthier behaviors. For example, it has been found that men and women who are married with children have a higher-quality diet than single parents, probably because they are better able to attend to their own health (Mancino, Lin, & Ballinger, 2004). These time constraints need to be considered in the development of nutrition education interventions.

Education. In general, more highly educated individuals eat a higher-quality diet and are less sedentary, due in large measure to watching less TV (Mancino, Lin, & Ballinger, 2004). People with more education may be better able to obtain, process, interpret, and apply information that will make them more able to eat healthfully. They may also be more forward looking and optimistic about their future and thus willing to seek health information and make greater investments in their health (Mancino, Lin, & Ballinger, 2004).

Grocery shopping trends. The influences described earlier impact how people shop for food. Surveys of grocery shoppers have found that about one third of shoppers are *economizers*, who are budget conscious and usually come from lower-income households. They plan weekly menus, check for sales, and use coupons. Another third are *carefree*

spenders, who are the least price conscious and least likely to compare prices and use coupons. The final third are *time-challenged* shoppers who are obsessed with convenience due to their hectic, multitask lifestyles. They have the largest households and are most likely to have preteen children (FMI, 2002).

Information Environment

Knowing one's audience is important in order to design messages and programs that are appropriate.

Media. We all live in a media-saturated environment that has undergone revolutionary changes in the past two decades, resulting in the availability to individuals and households of numerous television channels, radio stations, websites, and other emerging communication routes. Time spent on these various media is high: children aged 2 to 4 are exposed to about 4 hours a day of various media. This increases to 8 hours a day in middle school, when one considers that adolescents often use several media simultaneously. TV viewing is dominant and increases to 25 hours through childhood and

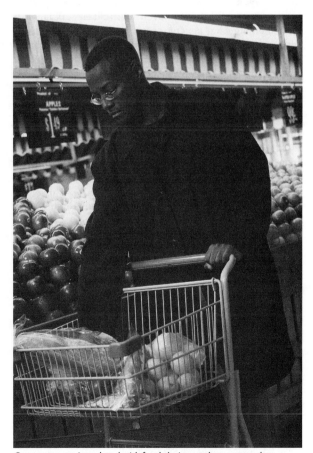

Consumers are inundated with food choices at the supermarket.

then declines somewhat in adolescence to 19 hours a week as music becomes more important. As noted earlier, adults spend about 15 to 17 hours a week on television viewing. The media are the main source of information about food and nutrition for many people, making them collectively a major source of informal nutrition education. Information about food and nutrition is now widely covered in newspaper articles, magazines, and television programs. Many magazines are devoted to health and nutrition, and entire channels on TV are devoted to food-related shows.

Advertising. The media have demonstrated a powerful capacity to persuade. Information on the impact of advertising on sales of food products is not easily available because it is considered proprietary information, but it is reasonable to suppose that advertisers would not spend $26 billion a year on something that had no effect. One study that was publicly reported showed that advertising was effective (Levy & Strokes, 1987). In addition, federally sponsored promotions of commodities such as milk, cheese, grapefruit juice, and orange juice resulted in greater sales (Gallo, 1996).

The U.S. food system is the economy's largest advertiser (Gallo, 1995). The food industry spends about $26 billion per year on marketing and advertising (Elitzak, 2001), with $15 billion aimed at children. Most of this is spent by companies that produce high-fat and/or high-sugar products that are highly processed and packaged; examples include $150 million for candy bars, $580 million for soft drinks, and more than $1.5 billion for fast foods (Center for Science in the Public Interest, 2003). These marketing activities clearly influence food choices (Institute of Medicine, 2006). Just for comparison, the National Cancer Institute's budget for its 5 A Day program is $4 million, and the National Heart, Lung, and Blood Institute spends $1.5 million on its National Cholesterol Education Program. The ubiquity of advertising, together with the amount of time people spend watching television and are exposed to marketing, makes these influences considerable.

The environmental influences on food choice and dietary behavior are summarized in Figure 2-2.

Summary

Figure 2-3 schematically represents the ways in which food, personal, and environmental factors influence food choice and diet-related practices as a series of concentric circles to show that they are not independent of each other but all related, each larger circle encompassing the influences in the smaller circles. These concentric circles reflect levels of influence or overlapping spheres of influence.

We have seen that genetically determined predispositions and experience with foods lead to taste preferences and the sense of satiety. There are also physiological mechanisms that regulate hunger, satiety, and body weight, promote variety in the diet, and maintain equilibrium. Although these mechanisms influence eating behaviors directly, they also exert their influence through psychological processes that can be perhaps even more powerful. People develop perceptions regarding foods—they expect the foods to taste a certain way and to have certain impacts on well-being. These preferences and sensory-affective responses to food influence food choices and eating behaviors, as shown earlier in Figure 2-2. At the same time, individuals develop attitudes toward foods, values, beliefs, and personal meanings, and these intra- and interpersonal factors also influence food choices and eating patterns.

We have also seen that the external environment influences food choices and dietary behaviors through such factors as the availability and accessibility of food, social networks, cultural practices, economic factors, and information. However, these environmental factors are also filtered by people's attitudes, beliefs, and values, which in turn influence food choices and dietary behavior. For example, availability may mean different things to different people. Recent immigrants may consider familiar food products "available" even if a long car or subway ride is needed to get to stores where they are stocked. For others, a food is not available if it cannot be cooked in the microwave and ready to eat in 5 minutes. Such differences in the interpretation of availability will influence individuals' food choices.

Likewise, the economic environment is based on the analyses, values, and interpretations of individuals, all of which have an impact on dietary choices. Economics is a behavioral science based on the fundamental notion that human wants are infinitely expansible, whereas the means to satisfy them are finite. Human wants always exceed the means to satisfy them, and there is therefore scarcity. (This has been simplified to the statement that human greed is infinite whereas the means to satisfy that greed is finite.) Economics is the study of people's reaction to the fact of scarcity—how people make choices when they must choose among alternatives to satisfy their wants. Economics is concerned with desired *scarce* goods, not free goods, such as air in natural settings, because free goods do not present a problem of choice. Cost can be seen as the sacrifice, or what needs to be exchanged, in order to obtain what is desired. In this context, the full price of a food or dietary practice is not just its monetary price but includes all the costs or sacrifices individuals make, such as travel costs, time, or child-care costs while shopping. For example, a person may be willing to exchange money for time by purchasing a food that is already prepared. Nutrition educators need to learn about the sacrifices individuals are willing to make in order to engage in a healthy behavior. How willing are they to sacrifice convenience for more healthful meals?

In the same way, although time for food-related tasks such as cooking or eating can be easily quantified in hours and minutes, the *perception* of time and its worth to individuals

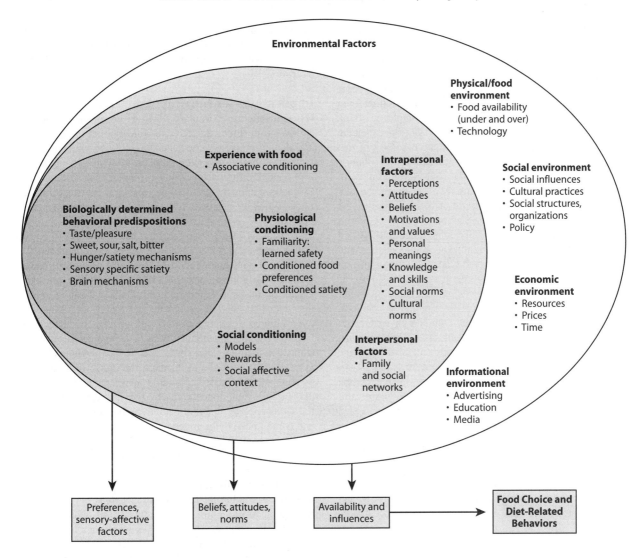

Environmental Factors

Physical/food environment
• Food availability (under and over)
• Technology

Experience with food
• Associative conditioning

Intrapersonal factors
• Perceptions
• Attitudes
• Beliefs
• Motivations and values
• Personal meanings
• Knowledge and skills
• Social norms
• Cultural norms

Social environment
• Social influences
• Cultural practices
• Social structures, organizations
• Policy

Biologically determined behavioral predispositions
• Taste/pleasure
• Sweet, sour, salt, bitter
• Hunger/satiety mechanisms
• Sensory specific satiety
• Brain mechanisms

Physiological conditioning
• Familiarity: learned safety
• Conditioned food preferences
• Conditioned satiety

Economic environment
• Resources
• Prices
• Time

Social conditioning
• Models
• Rewards
• Social affective context

Interpersonal factors
• Family and social networks

Informational environment
• Advertising
• Education
• Media

Preferences, sensory-affective factors

Beliefs, attitudes, norms

Availability and influences

Food Choice and Diet-Related Behaviors

FIGURE 2-3 Factors influencing food choices and dietary behaviors

for different tasks varies considerably. It is this perception that will affect food choices and dietary practices. Time is socially constructed. All living creatures, including humans, experience daily, seasonal, and annual cycles, and early conceptions of time were based on such natural cycles. However, in the West, as time and history became seen as linear rather than cyclical, with a beginning and an end, time became a finite commodity (Robinson & Godbey, 1997). The clock, which made industrial work possible, also made time scarce, and hence an economic issue. Time has no elastic boundaries. With enough money, people can expand boundaries for some commodities before scarcity arises. For example, people can have TVs in every room and multiple telephones or cars. We can also join numerous clubs or serve on numer-

ous committees. Time, however, cannot be extended. Efficiency—packing more productivity or activities into a unit of time—has thus become an important value. Time and motion studies in the 1890s made factory work more efficient. The notion of efficiency was soon extended even to homemaking, cooking, and kitchen design.

Even as efficiency increased, making more time available, the time required to make decisions about food also increased, because information became more complex. For example, there are about 50,000 items in the market to choose from, and about 9,000 new food items are introduced each year that people must learn about. No longer do people choose from three or four types of cold breakfast cereal, but from whole supermarket aisles of cereals. This takes time.

In addition, people have become more avid consumers, and consumption takes time: it takes time to use all the gadgets and objects that people have acquired. People believe they can have it all and are reluctant to pay the costs or sacrifices related to time. To overcome the scarcity of time, people do more than one thing at once, multitasking. Rather then either/or, people want both/and—for example, working full time and going to school full time, using their "leisure time" to do so. Add to that the economic necessity of two jobs for many and it is not surprising that the perception is that there is not just scarcity of time, but a time famine. In a survey, about 30% of people said they feel always rushed, and 55% felt sometimes rushed; only 17% almost never felt rushed (Robinson & Godbey, 1999). Thus, scarcity of time is both a reality and a perception. Feeling rushed and harried is an intrapersonal factor related to expectations, values, and meanings that must be considered when designing nutrition education activities.

Income also influences choices and decisions. As individuals' wages increase, they have more money to spend on everything, including higher-quality food and physical activity. Increased wages also make their time more valuable. This increase raises the cost of ill health, so individuals have more incentives to invest in their own health, such as eating more healthfully or being more physically active. On the other hand, as time spent on their jobs becomes more valuable, individuals may devote more time to work and spend less time being physically active; they may feel compelled to purchase foods that are more convenient and more highly prepared. If these foods are high in calories or less nutritious or both, then there may be negative impacts on health. Again, understanding the considerations and trade-offs that individuals make is important in designing nutrition education. Thus, environmental forces influence our food choices and dietary behaviors not only directly but also through our thinking, interpretations, and decisions.

This notion of multiple and overlapping influences can be applied to the example of trying to understand the low rate of breastfeeding in the United States. One study found that all levels of influence had an effect on breastfeeding among low-income women (Bentley, Dee, and Jenson 2003). This study is discussed in Nutrition Education in Action 2-1. The media images and messages, policy, and community-level influences were important. But interpersonal factors related to family, and intrapersonal factors such as personal beliefs, were dominant, often influenced by interpretations of the larger societal values, media messages, and policy.

The point that is important for nutrition educators is that although food-related factors and environmental context have important independent influences on diet, they also influence the development of beliefs, attitudes, interpretations, feelings, and meanings, which in turn influence behavior. It becomes clear, then, that perceptions, attitudes, beliefs, and meanings play a central role in food-related behaviors. This is good news for nutrition educators because these perceptions, attitudes, and beliefs are to some extent modifiable through education.

Implications for Nutrition Education

Nutrition education is more likely to be effective when it addresses all three categories of influence on food choices and dietary practices—food, person, and environment—and recognizes that food factors and environmental factors are also mediated through personal psychological processes. As Epictetus said many hundreds of years ago, "We are troubled not so much by events themselves but by the views we take of them."

Addressing food-related factors is very important in nutrition education. Food is a powerful primary reinforcer that produces instant gratification in taste and a sense of satisfaction and fullness. Because taste or preference are also shaped by repeated experience with foods and eating, nutrition educators working with any age group need to create opportunities to offer nutritious and healthy foods such as fruits and vegetables frequently in a positive social affective context so that individuals will come to like nutritious foods. Similarly, interventions to decrease the intake of food components such as fat or salt should help people adopt eating plans that include foods naturally low in these components for a long enough time that people can become used to them and come to like them. Indeed, in a long-term nutrition education intervention with women, those who were able to stay with a low-fat diet for 2 years or more were those who came to dislike the taste of fat (Bowen, 1994).

The use of foods in positive contexts as rewards or treats will enhance liking for those foods, whereas having people eat a food in order to obtain a reward will likely produce a decline in liking for that food. Because foods high in fat, sugar, and salt are widely available, particularly in positive social affective contexts such as celebrations, nutrition educators need to help people recognize the impact of such social environmental forces on their eating patterns and acquire the competencies to address them.

Nutrition education also needs to address environmental factors, by promoting the increased availability and accessibility of wholesome and healthful options and by taking into account the resources people have, their social networks and relationships, and the influence of media and advertising. We also need to be mindful of people's real and perceived time constraints and how they make choices in light of these constraints. Another important consideration is people's reaction to real and perceived economic scarcity. Nutrition educators need to learn about the exchanges or sacrifices that individuals are willing to make in order to engage in a healthy behavior. Some examples of nutrition education activities are discussed in Nutrition Education in Action 2-2.

NUTRITION EDUCATION IN ACTION 2-1

Multiple Influences on Breastfeeding: A Study of Low-Income Mothers

Media influences: TV shows and print media foster the perception that formula feeding is the norm whereas breastfeeding is not. Instead, women's breasts are used to advertise lingerie, perfume, or alcohol: these images influence personal beliefs.

Policy influences: There is legislation that supports breastfeeding in the work setting. Legislation also requires low-income mothers to work, thus making breastfeeding difficult.

Community and organizational factors: Workplaces can be supportive or not. Baby-friendly hospitals can encourage breastfeeding, whereas free infant formula packages on discharge do not. Returning to work predicts quitting breastfeeding after having initiated it in the hospital.

Interpersonal factors: The father of the baby can be a major influence, followed by the mother's mother. Cultural beliefs are also a factor, such as the belief that women may not have enough milk, particularly when babies are "greedy."

Personal factors: Beliefs, knowledge, and skills. The study found that cultural beliefs positive to breastfeeding were often outweighed by personal beliefs or anticipation that breastfeeding would be painful. There were also concerns about the appropriateness of feeding in public settings because of sexual images in the media, or the disapproval of the baby's father.

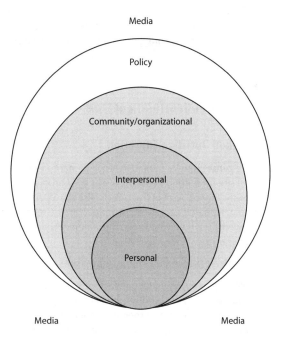

Source: Bentley, M.E., D.L. Dee, and J.L. Jensen. 2003. Breastfeeding among low-income, African-American women: Power, beliefs and decision-making. *Journal of Nutrition* 133:305S–309S. Used with permission of the American Society for Nutrition and the authors.

Person-related factors such as perceptions, beliefs, and attitudes play a central role in influencing eating patterns and food-related behaviors, as we have seen. Hence these perceptions and attitudes form the central focus of much of nutrition education. Thus, nutrition education can be seen as the process shown in Figure 2-4. How the influencing factors can be effectively addressed through nutrition education activities is described in the remaining chapters in this book.

Implications for Competencies and Skills for Nutrition Educators

Nutritionists and dietitians are well grounded in nutrition science and clinical nutrition and are anxious to transmit what they know to a variety of audiences in exciting ways. They are less well grounded in the social sciences, particularly the behavioral sciences and the field of communications. Yet as we have seen, food choices and dietary behaviors are influenced by a multitude of factors. Understanding behavior and

its context is crucial for effective nutrition education. One approach might be to deliver nutrition education through the use of teams, in which nutritionists would focus only on the nutrition science content, and behavioral specialists would actually design and deliver the educational sessions. However, that is neither practical nor desirable. What the field needs is nutritionists who are sufficiently conversant with the relevant fields of behavioral science and communications to be able to design effective nutrition education programs.

The Society for Nutrition Education's Competencies for Nutrition Education Specialists

The Society for Nutrition Education (SNE) has adopted a list of the competencies that nutrition education specialists should have (SNE, 1987). The society believes that nutrition education specialists should be competent in the following five areas:

1. *Food and nutrition content:* Understanding the fundamentals of nutrition science, food science, and clinical nutrition; having the ability to accurately assess nutritional status of individuals and groups; applying appropriate

dietary guidelines in making dietary recommendations
2. *Eating behavior:* Understanding the complexities of food supply systems and their effects on food selection; understanding the physiological, psychological, and environ-

NUTRITION EDUCATION IN ACTION 2-2

Barbershop Nutrition Education

Prostate cancer is twice as high in African American men as in white men. Eating fruits and vegetables may help to reduce risk. A novel site for nutrition education was the barbershop. A program was delivered to African American men while they were waiting for service. A set of five true or false statements was developed about the rate of prostate cancer in men and the role of fruits and vegetables in cancer risk reduction. The men were asked to answer them, and then the nutrition educator went over the answers. The men could keep the statements and the answer sheet. This simple intervention increased awareness of both prostate cancer and ways to reduce risk.

People at Work: 5 A Day Tailgate Sessions

Because many people working in factories and other similar locations do not have time to go to a different site for nutrition education sessions, the nutrition educator can go to them. At one sawmill, the workers ate their lunches from coolers in their cars. The nutrition educator therefore met them in the parking lot and provided monthly tailgate sessions over the course of a year (including through the midwestern winter), providing a food each time that involved interesting ways to use fruits and vegetables (such as baked apples, chili, or vegetable wraps). The focus was on how to incorporate fruits and vegetables into meals and snacks. The results showed that the workers' interest and motivation were enhanced, as were skills in incorporating more fruits and vegetables in their diets.

Operation Frontline

Share Our Strength's Operation Frontline is a nationwide nutrition education program developed to address the root causes of hunger in the United States. Operation Frontline enables chefs, nutritionists, and dieticians to share their strengths by teaching interactive six-week classes on nutrition and food budgeting to adults and children who are at risk of hunger. Operation Frontline classes make a concrete difference in the lives of program participants. The impact may be as basic as learning how to get a child to eat vegetables or how to cut up a chicken, or can be as profound as providing a starting point for a career in the culinary industry. One special feature is that after each class, each participant receives a bag of groceries containing all the ingredients needed to make that classes' meal at home. Class participants then report to the instructors during the next class session on their success with making a meal at home, and their families' reactions. Since its inception in 1993, more than 31,000 people have participated in Operation Frontline classes and an additional 89,000 have received nutrition information through nutrition fairs and events.

Community-Supported Agriculture

Community-supported agriculture (CSA) helps support family farms that are struggling to stay in business, while providing city people, particularly those in low-income neighborhoods, with access to high-quality, locally grown, affordable produce. During the winter and spring, the CSA farmer sells shares in his or her farm's upcoming harvest to individuals, families, or institutions. The shares go to the cost of producing the food. Each week, usually from June through November, the CSA farmer delivers the week's share to a central neighborhood distribution site. Organizations in cities are available to assist low-income individuals to purchase shares. These organizations usually provide food education during the harvest season on how to use the foods that individuals receive.

Sources: Magnus, M.H. 2004. Barbershop nutrition education. *Journal of Nutrition Education and Behavior* 36:45–46; Benepe, C. 2003. Presentation at the annual meeting of the Society for Nutrition Education, Philadelphia, PA; Share Our Strength. n.d. What we do. http://www.strength.org/what/operationfrontline.

mental (social, cultural, and economic) determinants of eating behavior

3. *Behavioral and educational theory:* Ability to apply learning theory, instructional theory, and behavior change theories in nutrition education; in particular, use of theories and techniques from the behavioral sciences for modifying food behavior

4. *Research methods and program evaluation:* Ability to analyze and evaluate both popular and scientific literature, and to use appropriate designs and methods to conduct research and program evaluations in nutrition education

5. *Design and delivery of nutrition education:* Designing nutrition education programs, curricula, and materials; delivering nutrition education programs, including the ability to communicate with individuals, small groups, organizations, and mass audiences, to write clearly, and to use supplemental materials appropriately; implementing and administering nutrition education programs

American Dietetic Association's Competencies

The American Dietetic Association's standards for the education of entry-level dietitians (ADA, 2002) include some competencies that are relevant for nutrition education as well:

1. Communications
   - Graduates will have *knowledge of* negotiation techniques, lay and technical writing, media presentations, interpersonal communication skills, counseling theory and methods, interviewing techniques, educational theory and techniques, concepts of human and group dynamics, public speaking, and educational materials development.
   - Graduates will have *demonstrated the ability to* use oral and written communications in presenting an educational session for a group, counsel individuals on nutrition, document appropriately a variety of activities, explain a public policy position regarding dietetics, use current information technologies, and work effectively as a team member.

2. Social sciences
   - Graduates will have *knowledge of* public policy development, psychology, and the health behaviors and educational needs of diverse populations.

3. Nutrition
   - Graduates will have *knowledge of* health promotion and disease prevention theories and guidelines.

Conclusion

This text seeks to provide you with sufficient background in behavioral and educational theories and in behavioral nutrition and nutrition education research so that you can apply this knowledge to the design, implementation, and evaluation of nutrition education sessions and programs that are

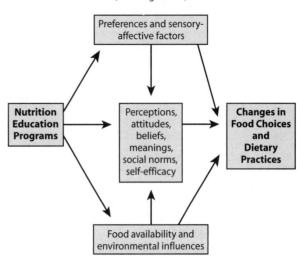

FIGURE 2-4 The process of nutrition education.

evidence based and more likely to be effective. Nutrition education research is active and ongoing. You can broaden your understanding and deepen your skills by reading current journal articles in nutrition education research and by learning about best practices at the same time that you are reading this book.

Questions and Activities

1. List at least five biological predispositions we are born with, and describe each in a sentence or so. Are they modifiable? If so, provide the evidence. How can the information be useful to nutrition educators?

2. One often hears parents say that their child will just not eat certain healthful foods, such as vegetables. They believe that such dislikes cannot be changed. Based on the evidence, what would you say to such a parent?

3. How can nutrition educators help young children learn to self-regulate the amount of food they eat?

4. "You can have dessert if you eat your spinach." Is this a strategy you would recommend to parents and child-care personnel to use to get children to like spinach? Why or why not?

5. Influences on dietary behavior arising from within the person have been stated to be central to our food choices and dietary practices. Why is this so? Describe three of these influences in a sentence or so each and indicate why they are so important. How might understandings of these personal factors help us make dietary changes?

6. Distinguish between food availability and food accessibility. How can they influence food choice? How might nutrition educators address these issues?

7. People live within social networks and may experience cultural expectations about how and what they eat. Since these can't be changed by nutrition education, why should we be interested in such information about our intended audience?

8. Describe four environmental factors that influence people's food choices and dietary practices. What can nutrition educators do with such information?

9. Review the list of potential influences on your eating and physical activity behavior that you wrote at the beginning of this chapter. Compare them to the categories of influences described in this chapter. Into which categories did the items on your list fall? Were there some surprises? How would you describe the motivations for your eating patterns?

10. In reviewing the competencies suggested by the Society for Nutrition Education for a nutrition educator, which competencies do you believe that you already possess? Which ones would you like to develop further? Keep these in mind as you read the remainder of this book.

REFERENCES

Addessi, E., A.T. Galloway, E. Visalberghi, and L.L. Birch. 2005. Specific social influences on the acceptance of novel foods in 2–5-year-old children. *Appetite* 45:264–271.

American Dietetic Association. 2002. *CADE accreditation handbook.* Chicago: American Dietetic Association, Commission on Accreditation for Dietetics Education (CADE).

Balzer, H. 1997. *The NPD Group's 11th annual report on eating patterns in America: National Eating Trends tracking.* Port Washington: The NPD Group.

Bandura, A. 1986. *Foundations of thought and action: A social cognitive theory.* Englewood Cliffs, NJ: Prentice-Hall.

Beauchamp, G.K., M. Bertino, and K. Engelman. 1983. Modification of salt taste. *Annals of Internal Medicine* 98(5 Pt 2):763–769.

Bentley, M.E., D.L. Dee, and J.L. Jensen. 2003. Breastfeeding among low-income, African-American women: Power, beliefs, and decision-making. *Journal of Nutrition* 133:305S–309S.

Bernstein, I. 1990. Salt preference and development. *Developmental Psychology* 2(4):552–554.

Birch, L.L. 1992. Children's preferences for high-fat foods. *Nutrition Reviews* 50:249–255.

———. 1998. Psychological influences on childhood diet. *Journal of Nutrition* 128:407S–410S.

———. 1999. Development of food preferences. *Annual Review of Nutrition* 19:41–62.

Birch, L.L., and M. Deysher. 1985. Conditioned and unconditioned caloric compensation: Evidence for self regulation of food intake by young children. *Learning and Motivation* 16:341–355.

Birch, L. L., and J.A. Fisher. 1995. Appetite and eating behavior in children. In *The pediatric clinics of North America: Pediatric nutrition*, edited by G.E. Gaull. Philadelphia: WB Saunders.

Birch, L.L., and J.O. Fisher. 2000. Mothers' child-feeding practices influence daughters' eating and weight. *American Journal of Clinical Nutrition* 71(5):1054–1061.

Birch, L.L., J.O. Fisher, and K.K. Davison. 2003. Learning to overeat: maternal use of restrictive feeding practices promotes girls' eating in the absence of hunger. *American Journal of Clinical Nutrition* 78(2):215–220.

Birch, L.L., and D.W. Marlin. 1982. I don't like it; I never tried it: Effects of exposure on two-year-old children's food preferences. *Appetite* 3:353–360.

Birch, L.L., L. McPhee, B.C. Shoba, E. Pirok, and L. Steinberg. 1987a. What kind of exposure reduces children's food neophobia? *Appetite* 9:171–178.

Birch, L.L., L. McPhee, B.C. Shoba, L. Steinberg, and R. Krehbiel. 1987b. Clean up your plate: Effects of child feeding practices on the conditioning of meal size. *Learning and Motivation* 18:301–317.

Bowen, D.J., M.M. Henderson, D. Iverson, E. Burrows, H. Henry, and J. Foreyt. 1994. Reducing dietary fat: Understanding the success of the Women's Health Trial. *Cancer Prevention International* 1:21–30.

Brug, J., K. Glanz, and G. Kok. 1997. The relationship between self-efficacy, attitudes, intake compared to others, consumption, and stages of change related to fruit and vegetables. *American Journal of Health Promotion* 12(1):25–30.

Center for Science in the Public Interest. 2003. *Pestering parents: How food companies market obesity to children.* Washington, DC: CSPI.

Chakravarthy, M.V., and F.W. Booth. 2004. Eating, exercise, and "thrifty" genotypes: Connecting dots toward an evolutionary understanding of modern chronic diseases. *Journal of Applied Physiology* 96:3–10.

Cheadle, A., B.M. Psaty, S. Curry, et al. 1991. Community-level comparisons between the grocery store environment and individual dietary practices. *Preventive Medicine* 20:250–261.

Clark, J.E. 1998. Taste and flavour: Their importance in food choice and acceptance. *Proceedings of the Nutrition Society* 57:639–643.

Connors, M., C.A. Bisogni, J. Sobal, and C.M. Devine. 2001. Managing values in personal food systems. *Appetite* 36:189–200.

Contento, I.R., S.S. Williams, J.L. Michela, and A. Franklin. 2006. Understanding the food choice process of adolescents in the context of family and friends. *Journal of Adolescent Health* 38:575–582.

Contento I.R., P.A. Zybert, and S.S. Williams. 2005. Relationship of cognitive restraint of eating and disinhibition to the quality of food choices of Latina women and their young children. *Preventive Medicine* 40:326–336.

Cutler, D.M., and E.L. Glaeser. 2003. *Why have Americans become more obese?* Cambridge, MA: Harvard Institute of Economic Research, Harvard University.

De Araujo, I.E., M.L. Kringelbach, E.T. Rolls, and P. Hobden. 2003. Representation of umami taste in the human brain. *Journal of Neurophysiology* 90:313–319.

De Castro, J.M. 1995. The relationship of cognitive restraint to the spontaneous food and fluid intake of free-living humans. *Physiology and Behavior* 57:287–295.

———. 1999. Behavioral genetics of food intake regulation in free-living humans. *Journal of Nutrition* 7/8:550–554.

———. 2000. Eating behavior: Lessons learned from the real world of humans. *Nutrition* 16:800–813.

Desor, J.A., O. Mahler, and L.S. Greene. 1977. Preference for sweet in humans: Infants, children and adults. In *Taste and development of the genesis of the sweet preference*, edited by J. Weiffenback. Bethesda: U.S. Department of Health, Education and Welfare.

Devine, C.M., M.M. Connors, J. Sobal, and C.A. Bisogni. 2003. Sandwiching it in: Spillover of work onto food choices and family roles in low- and moderate-income urban households. *Social Science and Medicine* 56(3):617–630.

Drewnowski, A., and A. Barrett-Fornell. 2004. Do healthier diets cost more? *Nutrition Today* 39:161–168.

Drewnowski, A., N. Darmon, and A. Briend. 2004. Replacing fats and sweets with vegetables and fruits—a question of cost. *American Journal of Public Health* 94:1555–1559.

Duffy, V.B., and L.M. Bartoshuk. 2000. Food acceptance and genetic variation in taste. *Journal of the American Dietetic Association* 100(6):647–655.

Eaton, S.B., S.B. Eaton III, and M.J. Konner. 1997. Paleolithic nutrition revisited: A twelve-year retrospective on its nature and implications. *European Journal of Clinical Nutrition* 51:207–216.

Elitzak, H. 2001. Food marketing costs at a glance. *FoodReview* 24(3).

Faith, M.S., K.S. Scanlon, L.L. Birch, L.A. Francis, and B. Sherry. 2004. Parent-child feeding strategies and their relationships to child eating and weight status. *Obesity Research* 12(11):1711–1722.

Feunekes, G.I.J., C. De Graff, S. Meyboom, and W.A. Van Staveren. 1998. Food choice and fat intake of adolescents and adults: Association of intakes within social networks. *Preventive Medicine* 26:645–656.

Fisher, J.O., D.C. Mitchell, H. Smiciklas-Wright, and L.L. Birch. 2002. Parental influences on young girls' fruit and vegetable, micronutrient, and fat intakes. *Journal of the American Dietetic Association* 102(1):58–64.

Food Marketing Institute. 2002. *Shopping for health 2002.* Washington, DC: Author.

———. 2005. *Supermarket facts: Industry overview 2004.* Washington, DC: Author.

Food Research and Marketing Center. 2005, December. Hunger in the U.S. http://www.frac.org/html/hunger_in_the_us/hunger_index.html.

Gallo, A.E. 1995. *The food marketing system in 1994* (Agricultural Information Bulletin No. 717). Washington, DC: U.S. Department of Agriculture.

———. 1996. *The food marketing system in 1995* (Agricultural Information Bulletin No. AIB731). Washington. DC: U.S. Department of Agriculture.

———. 1998. *The food marketing system in 1996* (Agricultural Information Bulletin No. AIB743). Washington, DC: U.S. Department of Agriculture Economic Research Service.

Gillman, M.W., S.L. Rifas-Shiman, and A.L. Frazier. 2000. Family dinner and diet quality among older children and adolescents. *Archives of Family Medicine* 9:235–240.

Glanz, K., M. Basil, E. Maibach, J. Goldberg, and D. Snyder. 1998. Why Americans eat what they do: Taste, nutrition, cost, convenience, and weight control concerns as influences on food consumption. *Journal of the American Dietetic Association* 98(10):1118–1126.

Harper, L.V., and K.M. Sanders. 1975. The effect of adults' eating on young children's acceptance of unfamiliar foods. *Journal of Experimental Child Psychology* 20:206–214.

Hearn, M.D., T. Baranowski, J. Baranowski, et al. 1998. Environmental influences on dietary behavior among children: Availability and accessibility of fruits and vegetables enable consumption. *Journal of Health Education* 19:26–32.

IFIC Foundation. 1999, September/October. Are you listening? What consumers tell us about dietary recommendations. *Food Insight: Current Topics in Food Safety and Nutrition.*

Institute of Medicine. 2006. *Food marketing to children and youth: Threat or opportunity?* Washington, DC: Institute of Medicine, National Academy Press.

Johnson, S., and J. Birch. 1994. Parents' and children's adiposity and eating style. *Pediatrics* 94(5):653–661.

Johnson, S.L., L. McPhee, and L.L. Birch. 1991. Conditioned preferences: Young children prefer flavors associated with high dietary fat. *Physiology and Behavior* 50:1245–1251.

Kaminski, L.C., S.A. Henderson, and A. Drewnowski. 2000. Young women's food preferences and taste responsiveness to 6-n-propylthiouracil (PROP). *Physiology and Behavior* 68:691–697.

Keller, K.L., and B.J. Tepper. 2004. Inherited taste sensitivity to 6-n-propylthiouracil in diet and body weight in children. *Obesity Research* 12:904–912.

Krebs-Smith, S.M., J. Heimendinger, B.H. Patterson, A.F. Subar, R. Kessler, and E. Pivonka. 1995. Psychosocial factors associated with fruit and vegetable consumption. *American Journal of Health Promotion* 10:98–104.

Lennernas, M., C. Fjellstrom, W. Becker, I. Giachetti, A. Schmidt, A. Remaut de Winter, and M. Kearney (AU: Is Giachetti a separate reference?). 1997. Influences on food choice perceived to be important by nationally-representative samples of adults in the European Union. *European Journal of Clinical Nutrition* 51(Suppl. 2):S8–S15. Levy, A., and R. Strokes. 1987. Effects of a health promotion advertising campaign on sales of ready-to-eat cereals. *Public Health Reports* 102:398–403.

Lewin, K. 1936. *Principles of topological psychology.* New York: McGraw-Hill.

Liem, D.G., and J.A. Mennella. 2002. Sweet and sour preferences during childhood: Role of early experiences. *Developmental Psychobiology* 41:388–395.

Lin, W., and I.S. Liang. 2005. Family dining environment, parenting practices, and preschoolers' food acceptance. *Journal of Nutrition Education and Behavior* 37(supplement 1):P47.

Lipton, K.L., W. Edmondson, and A. Manchester. 1998. *The food and fiber system: Contributing to the U.S. and world economies.* Washington, DC: Economic Research Service, U.S. Department of Agriculture.

Lowe, M.R. 2003. Self-regulation of energy intake in the prevention and treatment of obesity: Is it feasible? *Obesity Research* 11(Suppl.):44S–59S.

MacIntosh, W.A. 1996. *Sociologies of food and nutrition.* New York: Plenum Press.

Mancino, L., B.H. Lin, and N. Ballenger. 2004. *The role of economics in eating choices and weight outcomes* (Agriculture Information Bulletin No. 791). Washington DC: U.S. Department of Agriculture, Economic Research Service.

Maslow, A.H. 1968. *Towards a psychology of being.* Princeton: Van Nostrand Reinhold.

Mattes, R.D. 1993. Fat preference and adherence to a reduced-fat diet. *American Journal of Clinical Nutrition* 57(3):373–381.

———. 1997. The taste for salt in humans. *American Journal of Clinical Nutrition* 65(2 Suppl.):692S–697S.

Mela, D. 1993. Consumer estimates of the percentage energy from fat in common foods. *European Journal of Clinical Nutrition* 47:735–740.

Mela, D.J., and R.D. Mattes. 1988. The chemical senses and nutrition: Part 1. *Nutrition Today* 23(March/April):4–9.

Mennella, J.A., and G.K. Beauchamp. 1996. The early development of human flavor preferences. In *Why we eat what we eat,* edited by E.D. Capaldi. Washington, DC: American Psychological Association.

Mennella, J.A., C.E. Griffen, and G.K. Beauchamp. 2004. Flavor programming during feeding. *Pediatrics* 113:840–845.

Mennella, J.A., C.P. Jagnow, and G.K. Beauchamp. 2001. Prenatal and postnatal flavor learning by human infants. *Pediatrics* 107:e88.

Mertz, W., J.C. Tsui, J.T. Judd, et al. 1991. What are people really eating? The relationship between energy intake derived from estimated diet records and intake determined to maintain body weight. *American Journal of Clinical Nutrition* 54(2):291–295.

Michener, W., and P. Rozin. 1994. Pharmacological versus sensory factors in the satiation of chocolate craving. *Physiology and Behavior* 56:419–422.

Morland, K., S. Wing, A. Diez Roux. 2002. The contextual effect of the local food environment on residents' diets: The atherosclerosis risk in communities study. *American Journal of Public Health* 92:1761–1767.

Nasser, J.A., H.R. Kissileff, C.N. Boozer, C.J. Chou, and X. Pi-Sunyer. 2000. PROP status and oral fatty acid perception. *Eating Behaviors* 2:237–245.

National Pork Producers Council. 2002. The kitchen survey. In *The kitchen report.* Urbandale, IA: Author.

Neel, J.V. 1962. Diabetes mellitus a "thrifty" genotype rendered detrimental by "progress"? *American Journal of Human Genetics* 14:352–353.

Pelchat, M., and P. Pliner. 1995. Try it. You'll like it. Effects of information on willingness to try novel foods. *Appetite* 24:153–166.

Pelto, G.H. 1981. Anthropological contributions to nutrition education research. *Journal of Nutrition Education* 13(Suppl.):S2–S8.

Pepino, M.Y., and J.A. Mennella. 2005. Factors contributing to individual differences in sucrose preference. *Chemical Senses* 30(Suppl. 1):i319–i320.

Peters, J.C., H.R. Wyatt, W.T. Donahoo, and J.O. Hill. 2002. From instinct to intellect: The challenge of maintaining healthy weight in the modern world. *Obesity Reviews* 3:69–74.

Pliner, P., M. Pelchat, and M. Grabski. 1993. Reduction of neophobia in humans by exposure to novel foods. *Appetite* 7:333–342.

Putnam, J.J., and J.E. Allhouse. 1999. *Food consumption, prices, and expenditures, 1970–97* (Statistical Bulletin No. 965). Washington, DC: U.S. Department of Agriculture, Food and Rural Economics Division, Economic Research Service.

Robinson, J.P., and G. Godbey. 1997. *Time for life: The surprising ways Americans use their time*. University Park, PA: Pennsylvania State University Press.

———. 1999. *Time for life: The surprising ways Americans use their time*. 2nd ed. University Park: Pennsylvania State University Press.

Robinson, T.N., M. Kiernan, D.M. Matheson, and K.F. Haydel. 2001. Is parental control over children's eating associated with childhood obesity? Results from a population-based sample of third graders. *Obesity Research* 9:306-312.

Rogers, P.J., and H.J. Smit. 2000. Food craving and food addiction: A critical review of the evidence from a biopsychosocial perspective. *Pharmacology, Biochemistry and Behavior* 66:3-14.

Rolls, B.J., D. Engell, and L.L. Birch. 2000. Serving size influences 5-year-old but not 3-year-old children's food intakes. *Journal of the American Dietetic Association* 100:232-234.

Rozin, P. 1988. Social learning about food by humans. In *Social learning: Psychological and biological perspectives*, edited by T.R. Zengall and G. G. Bennett. Hillsdale, NJ: Lawrence Erlbaum Associates.

———. 1996. Sociocultural influences on human food selection. In *Why we eat what we eat: The psychology of eating*, edited by E.D. Capaldi. Washington, DC: American Psychological Association.

Rozin, P., and A.E. Fallon. 1981. The acquisition of likes and dislikes for foods. In *Criteria of food acceptance: How man chooses what he eats*, edited by J. Solms and R.L. Hall. Zurich: Forster Verlag.

———. 1987. A perspective on disgust. *Psychology Review* 94(1):23-41.

Satter, E. 2000. *Child of mine: Feeding with love and good sense*. 3rd ed. Boulder, CO: Bull Publishing Co.

Sclafani, A. 1990. Nutritionally based learned flavor preferences in rats. In *Taste, experience, and feeding*, edited by E.C.T. Powley. Washington, DC: American Psychological Association.

———. 2004. Oral and post-oral determinants of food reward. *Physiology and Behavior* 81:773-779.

Sclafani, A., and K. Ackroff. 2004. The relationship between food reward and satiation revisited. *Physiology and Behavior* 82(1):89-95.

Seale, J. Jr., A. Regmi, and J. Bernstein. 2003. *International evidence on food consumption patterns* (Technical Bulletin No. 1904). Washington, DC: U.S. Department of Agriculture, Economic Research Service.

Shepherd, R. 1999. Social determinants of food choice. *Proceedings of the Nutrition Society* 58:807-812.

Skinner, B.F. 1953. *Science and human behavior*. New York: Macmillan.

———. 1971. *Beyond freedom and dignity*. New York: Knopf.

Skinner, J.D., B.R. Carruth, W. Bounds, and P.J. Ziegler. 2002. Children's food preferences: A longitudinal analysis. *Journal of the American Dietetic Association* 102:1638-1647.

Small, D.M., and J. Prescott. 2005. Odor/taste integration and the perception of flavor. *Experimental Brain Research* 166:345.

Society for Nutrition Education. 1987. Recommendations of the Society for Nutrition Education on the academic preparation of nutrition education specialists. *Journal of Nutrition Education* 19(5):209-210.

Stunkard, A. 1975. Satiety is a conditioned reflex. *Psychosomatic Medicine* 37:383-389.

Tepper, B.J. 1998. 6-n-Propylthiouracil: A genetic marker for taste, with implications for food preference and dietary habits. *American Journal of Human Genetics* 63:1271-1276.

Tepper, B.J., and R.F. Nurse. 1997. Fat perception is related to PROP taster status. *Physiology and Behavior* 61:949-954.

Thorsen, C., and M. Mahoney. 1974. *Behavioral self-control*. New York: Holt, Rinehart, & Winston.

U.S. Department of Agriculture. 2000. *Beliefs and attitudes of American towards their diet* (Nutrition Insight No. 19). Washington, DC: Center for Nutrition Policy and Promotion, U.S. Department of Agriculture.

Watson, J.B. 1925. *Behaviorism*. New York: Norton.

An Overview of Nutrition Education:
Facilitating Why and How to Take Action

OVERVIEW   This chapter introduces readers to behavior-focused nutrition education and provides on overview of how behavioral science theory and nutrition education research can help increase nutrition education effectiveness.

OBJECTIVES   At the end of the chapter, you will be able to

- Explain what is meant by a behavior- or action-focused approach to nutrition education
- Appreciate the primary role of nutrition education in addressing the influences on behavior
- State how nutrition behavior theory and nutrition education research can provide a map for how to design effective nutrition education
- Critique the importance of theory in research and practice
- Describe the three components of nutrition education and the educational goal for each
- Describe a conceptual framework for theory-based nutrition education

SCENARIO

Remember Alicia and Ray from the last chapter? Alicia is a 19-year-old high school graduate who is working in a busy doctor's office as an administrative assistant. She knows she should eat lots of fruits and vegetables, but at lunch time she likes to eat food that is filling and can be picked up fast and eaten quickly. She would also much rather eat a slice of apple pie than an apple. Besides, she is not overweight and feels fine and doesn't see much need to change.

Ray is in his mid-forties. His weight just crept up on him, a pound or two each year, and now he is about 40 pounds overweight and is at risk for diabetes. His doctor tells him

he should lose weight to help reduce the risk. He really wants to, but it seems so hard. After a day at his job as a salesman in a store, where he is mostly on the phone or stands around and is not very active, he wants to just sit and watch TV when he comes home. His wife is interested in eating more healthfully, but he likes a hearty meal with lots of meat and always a dessert.

If nutrition education is a combination of strategies to facilitate behaviors conducive to health, what can we as nutrition educators do to assist Alicia or for Ray to eat more healthfully?

Introduction

When health professionals first became interested in promoting health and facilitating change in health-related behavior, the emphasis was on providing information to patients and to the public. The assumption was that when individuals such as Alicia and Ray became well informed, they would take the necessary actions to avoid disease and improve their health,

such as getting vaccinations, eating healthfully, attending health screenings, or stopping smoking. However, analyses of the results of health campaigns revealed that information alone was not sufficient to lead to the desired behavior. For most people, health is not an end in itself but a means to an end: the ability to do what they want to do in life to achieve the goals they have. Thus, taking actions related to health in the absence of symptoms is not a high priority for most. In the area of food, too, eating healthfully is not an end in itself for most people. Eating is about providing essential nourishment for life's many other activities and is a source of pleasure and enjoyment. So the question is, how can nutrition education programs best assist people to eat more healthfully? How can healthful eating become a source of pleasure and enjoyment? What factors contribute to making health behavior change programs more effective?

These are questions that the nutrition profession has grappled with for decades. Nutrition education in the United States and many other Western nations began as a formal activity in the early 1900s with the identification of food components such as vitamins and the recognition of their importance for health. In 1965, McKenzie and Mumford reviewed the published literature about nutrition education around the world and were able to find only 22 research studies in which objective evaluations were included. They found that success or failure depended "on the methods used, the personalities involved and the circumstances prevailing in the area. . . . However, we are not as yet in a position to isolate these factors more clearly . . . partly because so few evaluated studies have been done . . . and partly because the purely technical devices for use in evaluation have not been fully developed" (McKenzie & Mumford, 1965). In a more comprehensive review of nutrition education around the world between 1900 and 1970, Whitehead (1973) came to some very broad conclusions: nutrition education was a factor in improving dietary practices when changing behavior was clearly specified as a goal, when appropriate educational methods were used, when individuals themselves were actively involved in problem solving, and when an integrated community approach was used. However, she too noted that there was a need for better-designed studies to provide specific information on effective methods and techniques for nutrition education.

Increased interest in health promotion and chronic disease prevention led to the publication by the U.S. government of the first *Dietary Guidelines for Americans* in 1980, the Food Guide Pyramid in 1993 (now MyPyramid), and the first Healthy People policy document in 1990, all focusing on assisting the public to eat more healthfully to improve health and prevent chronic disease. Whereas prevention of nutrient deficiencies involved *adding* specific foods to the diet, health promotion and chronic disease prevention require *changes* in what is eaten and how much—a much more difficult task. A burst of activities on the part of nutrition education professionals also took place in the 1980s and 1990s—workshops and conferences made up of behavioral nutrition experts, nutrition education researchers, behavioral scientists, and nutrition practitioners, and reviews of the literature—as nutrition educators began to seek to understand not just what works, but *why* and *how* (e.g., Contento, 1980; Olson

& Gillespie, 1981; Zeitlin & Formation, 1981; Gussow & Contento, 1984; Johnson & Johnson, 1985; Contento, Manning, & Shannon,1992). These conferences and reviews all called for more research in nutrition education and for more systematic application of theories and results from food choice studies, health education, and behavioral science research to bring about more effective nutrition education.

Researchers have been very active in the past two decades, encouraged largely by government research funding and programs because the government has become concerned about chronic disease prevention as well as overweight prevention. Such research has generated findings that are very useful for nutrition education practice (Achterberg & Lytle, 1995; Contento et al., 1995; Potter et al., 2000; Ammerman et al., 2002; Bowen & Beresford, 2002; Baranowski et al., 2003; Pomerleau et al., 2005; Doaket al., 2006). These studies extend the earlier findings of Whitehead in a number of ways. They all agree that nutrition education is more likely to be effective when it does the following:

- Focuses on specific behaviors or practices rather than merely disseminating general information.
- Makes its central mission to identify and address influences on these behaviors that have personal relevance to a particular group. These influencing factors are those that motivate, reinforce, and enable behavior and are called determinants of behavior or potential mediators of diet-related behavior change or action.
- Designs educational strategies to address these potential mediators of behavior change, based on theory and research in nutrition education, behavioral nutrition, and related areas.
- Attends to the multiple levels of influences on food choice and eating behavior and uses multiple channels to convey messages over a sufficient period of time.

These elements of effectiveness are explored in the following sections. They also form the foundation of this book.

Nutrition Education: A Focus on Behaviors and Their Influences

A Focus on Behaviors or Actions

Nutrition education is more likely to be effective when it is behavior focused. What do we mean by that? A *behavior-focused approach* to nutrition education means that the central focus of the program or activities is on addressing the specific individual food choice behaviors, nutrition-related actions, or community dietary practices that influence health and well-being rather than on simply disseminating food or nutrition information in a general manner. A behavior-focused approach to nutrition education is one that uses a set of educational strategies, accompanied by relevant environmental supports, to facilitate dietary behavior changes or actions that are conducive to health. Nutrition-related behaviors can include the following:

- Food choices or observable behaviors related to health, such as eating sufficient fruits and vegetables a day, a lower-fat diet (specified as to what that means), smaller portions of food, or even eating breakfast
- Behaviors and practices related to food safety, food preparation or cooking, managing food-related resources, foods from farmers' markets, and other food-related concerns
- Behaviors related to other nutrition-related concerns, such as breastfeeding
- Specific physical activities, such as running, bicycling, or playing softball, because maintaining a healthy weight involves considerations of energy balance

Thus, if an intervention seeks to reduce cardiovascular and cancer risk, it might focus on the behaviors of eating more fruits, vegetables, and whole grains and fewer foods high in saturated fats. If the intervention seeks to reduce gain in weight, it can focus on the behaviors just mentioned along with the behaviors of controlling portions of high-energy density foods and increasing physical activity. A behavior-focused approach means that the outcomes expected are changes in behaviors or practices. The desired long-term outcomes are improvements in health or in quality of life, or both.

The behaviors to be addressed are identified from the needs, perceptions, and desires of the intended audience, as well as from national nutrition and health goals and nutrition science–based research findings. Behaviors must of course be addressed and framed within their social context, because behaviors both influence and are influenced by their social and environmental context.

Focusing on specific individual behaviors and community practices is especially important now that promoting health and reducing chronic disease and obesity have become major aims of nutrition education. As one research scientist said at the time the first *Dietary Guidelines* came out: "In the past, the message was, in essence, to eat more of everything. Now we are faced with the difficult problem of teaching the public to be more discriminating. Increasingly, the message will be to eat less" (Hegsted, 1979). Being more discriminating and eating less may mean improving the quality and reducing the quantity of food eaten to make them more healthful. Given our biological predispositions and early conditioning to prefer sweet and energy-dense foods, and given an environment in which such foods are widely available and highly promoted, making such changes is not easy. Researchers have noted that human physiology developed to function within an environment where food was scarce and physical activity was high, but the opposite now pertains (Peters et al., 2002). Thus the modern environment has taken body weight control from an instinctual (unconscious) process to

one that requires substantial cognitive effort. People who are not devoting substantial conscious effort to managing body weight are probably gaining weight. The same applies to eating a high-quality diet. As we saw in the last chapter, there is no biological mechanism automatically ensuring that people will select nutritious diets from today's food supply. It requires conscious effort.

Information about good eating in general, the food groups, and nutrients and their effects on the body is too diffuse by itself to really help people make changes in their behavior. For nutrition education to have an impact, it must focus on specifically defined behaviors or community practices. To illustrate, we can take the example of the Children and Adolescent Trial for Cardiovascular Health (CATCH) study for third- to fifth-graders (Luepker, Perry, & McKinlay, 1996). The nutrition education intervention encouraged eating a healthy diet and increasing physical activity. It focused on choosing foods low in fat and high in fiber. Results showed that the program had a positive impact on the behaviors of focus. When the data were then analyzed to see whether the program had also had an impact on consumption of fruits and vegetables (which were included in the category of high-fiber foods but were not a focus of the intervention), the results were negative (Perry, Lytle, & Feldman, 1998). Later, a separate program directed specifically at fruits and vegetables and using similar approaches did result in increased fruit and vegetable intake (Perry & Bishop, 1998), illustrating the importance of being specific.

A behavior-focused approach does *not* mean that food and nutrition information is not important. Indeed, for many complex food and nutrition behaviors, a good deal of information may be needed, along with critical thinking skills. However, it does mean that the information provided by the intervention should be relevant to the behaviors and practices being targeted and should be designed to assist individuals to become willing and able to take action. Nor does it mean that nutrition education should be directed at manipulating people's behaviors to make them more healthful in the old behaviorist sense. Individuals change their behaviors only when they themselves see a need to do so and want to make a change. Nutrition education must both honor and foster such autonomy and self-responsibility through dialogue and debate (Buchanan, 2004). Popular author John C. Maxwell (2000) put it this way: people change when they hurt enough that they have to, learn enough that they want to, and receive enough that they are able to.

Addressing the Influences on Behavior and Behavior Change

Research tells us that nutrition education is more likely to be effective when it addresses the many influences on behaviors, rather than merely disseminates general information about healthy eating. A behavior-focused approach thus means that the focus of nutrition education is on understanding the influences on behavior and facilitating behavior change. As has been noted, "it is a major paradigm shift to change the target of nutrition education from the goal of increasing knowledge to that of modifying factors that influence dietary behaviors" (Baranowski et al., 2003). Indeed, the central mission of nutrition education is to design activities that address the many influences on behavior that have personal relevance for a particular group.

Consequently, we must first understand people's food-related behaviors and how they change if we are to design nutrition education programs that are effective. Behavioral science research has been most helpful here. Such research helps us understand why knowledge-based nutrition education does not generally lead to change in dietary behaviors. In Chapter 2 we saw that there are numerous influences on food choice and nutrition-related behaviors in addition to knowledge. Consequently nutrition education must address these many influences if it is to be effective. These influences go by many names. Influences on why we eat what we do are usually called *determinants of behavior*. In the context of nutrition education, this means *modifiable* determinants such as perceptions, attitudes, or feelings as opposed to non-modifiable ones such as socioeconomic status or educational level. We seek to understand not only the determinants of people's current eating patterns but also determinants of why and how people make changes in their eating patterns. When these determinants of change are addressed in a nutrition education program, they are often called *potential mediators of behavior change*. The most effective way to assist people to make changes in their dietary practices is to identify the determinants of their current diets as well as the determinants that can mediate behavior change.

In nutrition education the word *behavior* refers to the actions people take to improve their health. Such actions can be referred to as a behavior or behavior change depending on how the action is stated. For example, if our intervention seeks to encourage people to eat recommended servings of fruits and vegetables, we can talk about the behavior as *taking action* and the influences as *determinants or mediators* of action. Or we can ask people to eat *more* fruits and vegetables, in which case we can talk about the behavior as *behavior change* and the influences as *mediators of behavior change*. Both these terms will be used where appropriate.

The last chapter demonstrated that there are many overlapping spheres of influence on behaviors. Thus nutrition education must address these multiple influences, as shown in Figure 3-1. More specifically, we saw in the last chapter that evidence from research tells us that food, physiological factors, and environmental factors exert their influence on food choice and dietary practices not only directly but also through our interpretations of the world. These powerful psychological processes (perceptions, beliefs, values, and attitudes) are key influences on what we do. Nutrition education is thus directed primarily at these powerful influences on behavior, along with supportive activities in the environment.

The primary task of nutrition education is to design activities that bring to individuals' awareness the many factors influencing their dietary behavior, and to activate contemplation, build skills, and provide supports so that individuals have the motivation, ability, and opportunity to change these behaviors if they choose (see Figure 2-4).

A more detailed look is shown in Figure 3-2. Starting from the right, we can see that nutritional well-being is dependent on nutritional status and chronic disease risk factors, which in turn are very much influenced by food- and nutrition-related behaviors. These in turn are influenced by numerous factors. In Chapter 2 we saw that these influences on behaviors can be placed into three categories: food, person, and environment. Food- and person-related factors are often placed together because our predispositions and experience with food lead to sensory-affective responses that are individual and intrapersonal. Figure 3-2 acknowledges that biological factors such as age, gender, and genetics, and some external physical factors such as physical activity, concurrent infections, or other issues also have impacts on health and on behaviors that are not modifiable by nutrition education. At the same time, our behaviors will have effects on the kinds of food system we have, through consumer demand. For example, if we make our food choices based primarily on taste, low cost, and convenience, then that is what our food system will provide for us. If we make choices based on quality or concern for the viability of local farms, then our food system will reflect those choices. Our food-related behaviors and practices also have impacts on society, such as on farmers, farm workers, and how food-related social structures and communities will be organized. Figure 3-2 shows that behaviors are the focus of nutrition education and that addressing the influences on these behaviors or mediators of behavior change is the central mission of nutrition education.

To design and conduct nutrition education, therefore, the influences on dietary behaviors and potential mediators of behavior change must be identified for a given group and prioritized so that strategies can be developed to address them.

Using Theory and Evidence to Guide Nutrition Education

So how shall we go about designing these educational strategies and environmental support activities? What principles will guide us? Just knowing a list of the determinants of behavior or of potential mediators of behavior change does not necessarily help us design more effective nutrition education strategies. Some factors are more important than others in truly mediating behavior change for a given group or for a specific behavior. Given limited time and resources, we must

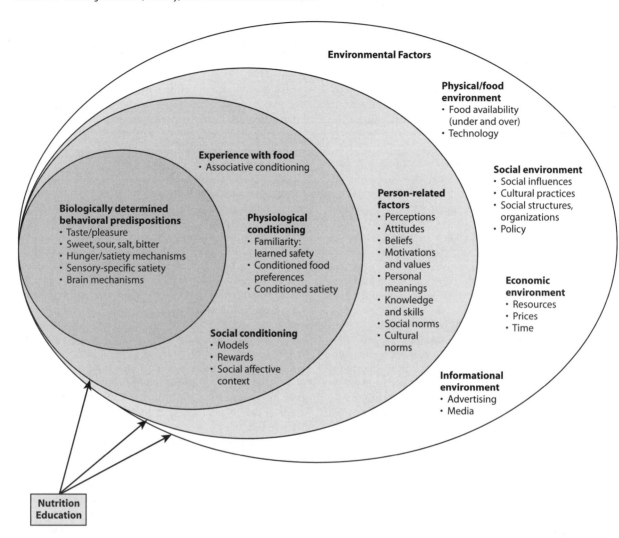

FIGURE 3-1 Factors influencing food choice and dietary behaviors and the role of nutrition education.

choose the factors that are most relevant in mediating dietary change and target them using appropriate educational strategies. How do we know which of the potential mediators are more important than others? Are these mediators related to each other? And if so, how do we know their relationships to each other?

This is where theory comes in to act as a guide. The purpose of theory is to tell us the nature and strength of the relationships of these potential mediators to the behavior change or action. Theory is based on evidence from research in the field of nutrition education, yet nutrition practitioners often express the opinion that research and theory are too abstract and impractical for day-to-day nutrition education—that they are not "real." They think of the word *theory* as referring to the realm of abstract speculation or ideal circumstances,

as when members of the general public say, "In theory, it should take only a week, but in reality it will take two to three weeks." Not surprisingly, nutrition education practitioners say they get impatient with discussions of theory.

However, as nutrition educators, we all use theory and research or evidence to guide our work, whether we are aware of it or not. For example, there are hundreds of possible nutrition issues to discuss with consumers, students, or clients, and there are dozens of methods of doing so; the moment we choose a topic or a method, we are demonstrating that we have used a set of assumptions, or theory, to guide our choices and have drawn upon accumulated experience, or evidence. Indeed, it is impossible *not* to employ some kind of theory when making choices of what to cover and how. Such theory may be derived from professional experiences

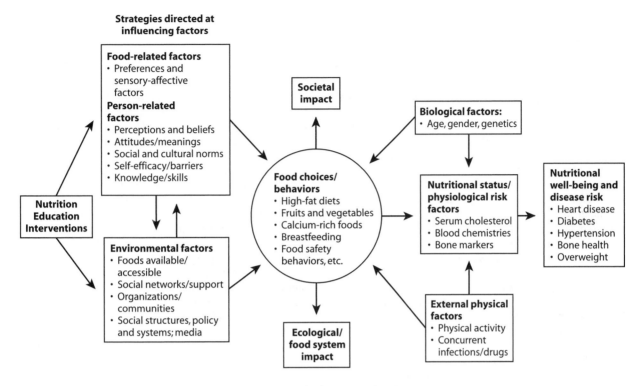

FIGURE 3-2 Factors influencing nutritional well-being and the role of nutrition education.

and can be described as *practice theory* (Gillespie & Gillespie, 1991). Theories used in the service of everyday living can be referred to as *everyday theory*, as when we use certain strategies to get our children to eat their vegetables. These generalizations or rules of thumb (or "theories") derived from experience (or "research") are often unconsciously applied and are not thought of as theories, yet they are essential for our very existence. We do not have time to observe, analyze, and then make judgments about every person or every situation separately; we have to develop generalizations about how the world seems to work or what human beings seem to be about. The type of theory that people usually think of as theory refers to *scientific theory*. Scientific theories differ from everyday and practice theories only in that they have been more systematically defined, tested, and refined.

What Is Theory?

Just as a physical map is an abstract representation of some geographical space, so theory, in its simplest terms, is a *mental map* derived from evidence that helps us understand how some part of the physical, biological, psychological, social, or political world works. Just as in a physical map, squares and other shapes connected by double lines represent buildings connected by roads, so theory consists of concepts linked to each other in some manner. In our case, theory

provides a mental map linking concepts, referred to as "constructs," together to explain our food choices and nutrition-related behaviors and how they change. Social psychologists describe theory as an abstract, symbolic representation of what is conceived to be reality; that is, a set of abstract statements or concepts designed to fit some portion of the real world (Zimbardo et al., 1977). A more comprehensive, and widely used, definition in the social sciences is that theory is a set of interrelated constructs (or concepts) that presents a systematic view of phenomena (e.g., eating fruits and vegetables) by specifying relations among the constructs, with the purpose of explaining and predicting these phenomena (Kerlinger, 1986). Theory in the area of behavioral nutrition and physical activity has also been described more simply as "a generalized and carefully interpreted, systematic summary of empirical evidence" (Brug, Onema, & Ferreira, 2005).

As we can see, all the definitions focus on theory as a *mental map*, *conceptual model*, or *picture* of some part of the world that (1) is derived from empirical evidence, (2) provides an abstract representation of some aspect of reality, and (3) specifies how concepts (constructs) within this representation relate to each other. In its simplest terms, theory in nutrition education is a mental map, where "constructs" are the abstract representations of real world "potential mediators of behavior or behavior change." Theory, derived from evidence, thus helps us understand how potential mediators (constructs) are related to food- and nutrition-related behavior change.

Thus, theory tells us how the many determinants of our food choices or mediators of food- and nutrition-related behavior change, such as the beliefs, attitudes, and cultural norms shown in Figure 3-1, are related to each other and to behavior. As just noted, these potential mediators of action or behavior change in the real world are called *constructs* in theories. Behavioral nutrition and nutrition education research evidence then tells us which of these mediators or constructs are more important than others for which behaviors and with which people. For example, theory might say that both our beliefs about the benefits of taking a given action and our perceived peer pressure are very important in our taking health-related actions. Evidence might then tell us that for behaviors such as eating fruits and vegetables, beliefs about benefits are more important than peer pressure. However, for breastfeeding, peer pressure is more important than beliefs about the benefits of breastfeeding. This kind of information is very important so that we can supply nutrition education that is appropriate.

Do We Really Need Theory?

A founder of the field of social psychology, Kurt Lewin, said, "There is nothing so practical as a good theory" (Lewin, 1935). However, there are some who think that theory is more limiting than useful. Indeed, there has been some discussion and debate about the predictiveness, usefulness, and appropriateness of theory for understanding nutrition-related behavior.

Yet clearly theory is useful, for at least two main reasons. The first is that use of theory can help us design nutrition education that is more effective. The second is that we all use theory anyway, whether we are aware of it or not, and our interventions are likely to be more effective if we understand our own theories! We will explore these reasons in greater detail.

Conducting nutrition education requires considerable resources in terms of time, money, and personnel, which are all usually in short supply. Thus, we want to conduct nutrition education activities that make the most effective use of these resources. We can do that only if our nutrition education programs are based on evidence. If theory is the interpreted summary of evidence, presented in the form of a conceptual map, then we need theory to guide our work. Evidence can come from quantitative studies or from interpretative studies (described later in this chapter). If we do not use evidence-based theories, we must rely on our everyday and practice theories. These might be very effective, but they might not be—we usually do not have the evidence to know. In some cases, evidence accumulates from practice and can be generalized as "best practices" that can be useful to others.

Most behavioral science theories use experimental designs to test cause-and-effect relationships between potential mediators and behavior. In studies of nutrition education interventions, the randomized control trial is often considered the gold standard because it can control for confounding factors. In this type of study, people are randomly selected from a larger population and randomly assigned to groups, one of which receives the nutrition education intervention; the other group does not and serves as the control group. Pretests and post-tests are administered to both groups and compared. Changes in the intervention group that are statistically significantly greater than changes in the control group provide an indication of the effectiveness of the intervention.

Researchers in the area of education have argued, however, that other empirical designs may be more suitable for studies of educational interventions in field settings (Chatterji, 2004). In particular, sound field experiments require that researchers formally study and take into consideration contextual and site-specific factors in the organizational or community settings in which the education takes place and use multiple research methods.

Still others have argued that because humans have agency, or free will, and are able to make choices based on moral reasoning or values, their decisions and actions defy prediction. Thus their likely behaviors cannot be captured in theories or models of health behavior based on the scientific method but are more likely to be captured by a humanistic approach. Buchanan (2004) argues that people choose foods and behaviors on the basis of what they think is right and what they ought to do. They choose what they want to do, including whether to act on these wants or desires. In this formulation, theories are not developed for their predictive power but because they can be used to help people come to a clearer understanding of their own life situations or to see themselves and their world in a new light, which might move them to act differently. For this purpose, grounded theory or interpretative approaches are considered more appropriate. Here, instead of reducing the information acquired from research into a small set of constructs and examining the quantitative relationships among them, in-depth interviews and other qualitative methods are used to generate a rich description of the ways people engage with food, incorporating their own meanings and understandings (Strauss & Corbin, 1990). Themes that emerge are recorded, analyzed, and interpreted. Various procedures are used to ensure that findings are trustworthy.

Interpretative studies can indeed provide rich descriptions of food-related motivations and behaviors. For example, such studies have provided a model of the food choice process and how people use the process in making food choices (Furst et al., 1996; Blake & Bisogni, 2003). In one study, interviewers found that many people were moved to eat everything on their plates to avoid wasting food. To leave food on the plate, they felt, would be violating an important larger value for them—that they should not waste resources (Pelican et al., 2005). Because both the experimental and interpretative approaches are attempting to understand more clearly our motivations and actions with respect to food and nutrition and are empirical in nature, both approaches are important to use, and they often converge. For example, the finding about not wasting food is similar to the construct of *moral and ethical responsibility* used in some theories. Even human agency is a major thrust of social cognitive theory (described in the next chapters), which also provides strategies for how human agency can be fostered in individuals and communities (Bandura, 2001).

Thus, experimental and interpretive studies can both generate theories or abstract representations—conceptual models or mental maps—of some aspect of reality that can help nutrition educators better understand the world of the people with whom they work and better assist these people in attaining their own health and life goals. Such mental maps are useful rather than limiting. Indeed, reviews of nutrition education conclude that programs are more likely to be successful when they use appropriate theory and evidence to guide their choice of activities (Achterberg and Lytle, 1995; Contento et al., 1995; Baranowski, 2001; Baranowski et al., 2003). This chapter and the ones to follow describe several theories that have been generated from both qualitative and quantitative research and are helpful in guiding nutrition education planning.

None of the research and the theories derived from them provides a complete explanation of food choice and dietary behavior change. Researchers can only infer the true reasons why people do what they do from what people say and what they do. Members of the public are not necessarily being untruthful about why they eat what they do; rather, people often do not know why they do what they do or how to go about making healthful changes. For example, individuals, particularly adolescents, insist that they are not influenced by others in their environment. Yet we know that we all are. Knowing ourselves is not easy! In addition, our reasons for what we do may change from time to time and differ by specific behavior.

Most theories provide 30% to 50% of the explanation for the food and nutrition behaviors under study, depending on the theory and the behavior (Staffleu et al., 1991–1992; Baranowski, Cullen, & Baranowski,1999). When the theories are more complete (i.e., incorporate more of the influencing factors) or when the behavior is more specific (such as soda drinking), their explanatory power tends to be greater. Although this leaves some part of eating behavior still unexplained, human behavior is complex and dynamic and behavior change is not easily explained, especially in the short time period usually used in studies. This degree of explanation for food-related behaviors is similar to that found

for other behaviors and provides a good foundation for helping us design nutrition education.

A second reason that use of theory is important in nutrition education is that, as noted earlier, all researchers and practitioners use theory to guide their work, whether they make it explicit or not. It is helpful for nutrition educators to make explicit the theory guiding their work, because they then have the opportunity to build in specific components based on the theory and to observe which components are useful and which are not. For example, will adding a module dealing with peer pressure, which theory suggests is important, enhance breastfeeding outcome compared with teaching only the basic module about the nutritional benefits of breast feeding? Making a theory explicit also helps practitioners develop appropriate teaching activities (e.g., role playing of peer pressure situations and group suggestions of how to respond) and evaluation instruments (e.g., measurements of peer pressure as well as nutrition knowledge). The result is that conclusions can be drawn that will be helpful the next time around.

The importance of making underlying assumptions or theories explicit is illustrated by a comprehensive review and meta-analysis of 303 nutrition education studies and programs by Johnson and Johnson (1985). They noted that although nutrition education was found to be effective to some extent overall, the studies and programs conducted up to the time of their review generally did not clearly lay out a theoretical framework or research-based rationale that guided the selection of factors to target in the educational intervention. The result was that even when the programs were successful, the researchers had not measured factors that could have explained *how* or *why* the educational efforts were successful. Thus the results of the studies were not as helpful as they could have been in providing guidance on how to make nutrition education more effective in the future.

Why Are There So Many Theories and Models?

The question often comes up, why are there so many different theories of dietary behavior? Why not just one? Most of the theories used in nutrition education originated in the behavioral sciences, food choice research, health education, or related fields. They were developed to explain specific kinds of behavior that were of interest for different reasons. For example, a few theories were developed by psychologists interested in public health specifically to explain why people did or did not take some action that might prevent a negative health condition, such as participation in immunizations to prevent polio or screenings for HIV infection. These theories emphasized health beliefs. At the same time, others were interested in food choice. These researchers were not necessarily interested in health. They wanted to find out what people wanted in their foods—taste, cost, convenience, texture, and so forth. Health might or might not have been an important concern. These researchers produced theories of food choice (Conner & Armitage, 2002). Still other theories were originally developed to explain social behaviors, such as purchasing various goods, voting, participating in organizations, and so forth. These theories sought to identify and understand both intrapersonal and interpersonal influences on social behavior.

As nutrition educators, we recognize that eating behavior is complex, involving many settings and situations and influenced by many internal and external factors that often conflict with each other. We are interested in people's health beliefs with respect to food, nutrition, and physical activity. But we are also interested in why and how people make food choices in general. Because food is most often eaten in social contexts and may involve negotiations with others, we are keenly interested in theories of social interactions as well. Thus we have to draw on all these theories to provide a more complete picture of why people eat what they do and how they change.

In addition, the factors that influence behavior changes that involve *adding* foods to the diet, such as fruits and vegetables or calcium-rich foods, may be different from those involving *modifying* our habits, such as reducing foods high in saturated fat. No single behavioral theory, as an abstract representation of reality, may be able to capture all these factors. Different theories may be useful for different behaviors and different settings. We shall see, however, that there is some overlap among the various theories. Consequently, there has been a call for the use of multiple theories (Achterberg & Miller, 2004) and more comprehensive theories (Triandis, 1979; Kok et al., 1996; Fishbein, 2000; Institute of Medicine, 2002).

Recall that each of these influences is a determinant of behavior or a potential mediator of behavior change and hence can be represented as a construct in a theory. Some theories are more complex than others, and some have been more thoroughly conceptualized and intensively studied than others. Each theory uses unique terms to describe the factors influencing behavior or specific concepts that are important for the theory based on its origins. Often these terms are similar across theories; we will make a note of this where appropriate. Some of the themes generated from interpretive studies are also similar to constructs in standard health behavior change theories. Some clarifications are provided here.

Constructs and variables. The influences on behavior that we have described so far as determinants of behavior or potential mediators of behavior change, such as beliefs, benefits, emotions, or attitudes, are the building blocks of theories. When they are systematically used in a particular theory they are called *constructs*, or mentally constructed ideas about unobservable, intangible attributes (beliefs, attitudes) that are part of the theory. They exist in the mind as abstractions about some aspect of human experience. No one

has observed "beliefs" about salt in the diet, or "attitudes" toward breastfeeding. Yet we can talk about them and measure them. For example, if a person believes that there are benefits to taking a specific health action, such as reducing salt intake will reduce risk of hypertension, this belief will influence whether she or he will add salt to food. This belief about benefits becomes the "perceived benefits" construct in the health belief model.

The term *variable* is often used synonymously with *construct*, but variables are really the operational definitions of constructs, specifying how a construct is to be measured for a specific situation. They are "variables" because they can vary in value. Thus, the perceived benefits of taking a specific action (e.g., the benefit of eating fruits and vegetables to reduce cancer risk) can be measured on a 1 to 5 scale. Individuals may judge the same specific benefit differently: some individuals may judge eating fruits and vegetables to reduce cancer risk as highly beneficial, giving it a score of 5, whereas others as only moderately so, giving it a score of 2 or 3. Constructs or variables are thus names, such as "perceived benefit," given by a particular theory, in this case the health belief model, for given determinants of behavior. These constructs are content-free, in that the theory does not specify what the benefits are. Information about each construct must be obtained from any given audience or group through means such as in-depth interviews or quantitative surveys. For example, the benefits of eating fruits and vegetables for adults may be their role in prevention of chronic disease, but for adolescents the benefits may be clear skin and help in controlling weight.

Theory, conceptual model, and theoretical framework. The terms *theory, model, conceptual model,* and *theoretical framework* are often used to describe similar ideas. *Model* or *conceptual model* usually describes relationships between two or more constructs, focusing on *how* they relate. *Theory* is often used to describe a clearly stated set of relationships among core constructs, such as beliefs or emotions, to *explain* behavior or behavior change. *Theoretical framework* refers to a description of a set of concepts in relation to each other. It tends to be less formal than a theory. However, these terms are similar to each other and overlapping, and definitions are not standardized. In this book, we use the terms as given by the researchers who developed and tested them. That is, if they refer to their mental map as a theory (e.g., the "theory of planned behavior"), we use the word *theory;* if they use the term *model* (e.g., the "health belief model"), we use the word *model.* The term *theory,* when used in a general sense in this book, refers to all these specific theories and models.

Several of the mental maps that are described in later chapters illustrate these definitions. The health belief model, for example, provides a description or mental map of how various determinants of a health action or behavior are related to each other and to behavior. The theory of planned behavior attempts to explain behavior and provides mathematical relationships, based on research evidence, between the mediators of behavior and behavior itself.

Moderators. Sometimes mediating variables such as beliefs may be important for one group of people but not another. For example, in one study "overall health concern" was found to be an important determinant of food choice for husbands but not wives, whereas the opposite was true for the determinant "beliefs about convenience." In this case, gender was a moderator of the influence of the mediators "health concern" and "convenience" on the outcome, food choice. Thus, *moderators* are factors that modify the influence of a determinant or potential mediator on the behavior. Examples of other possible moderators are ethnicity or educational level. That is, a nutrition education intervention may work in one ethnic group but not in another, or with those at some educational levels but not others.

Relationships Among Research, Theory, and Practice

Research has been defined as "careful or diligent search; investigation or experimentation aimed at the discovery and interpretation of facts; revision of accepted theories or practical application of such new or revised theories" (Merriam-Webster, 2003). Research and theory are thus closely interrelated. Theory is a dynamic entity. Research generates theory; at the same time, theory is guided by, and tested through, research and practice. Stated more simply, theory is not divorced from practical experience but is in fact experience that has been systematically explored and reflected upon.

Quantitative research based on epidemiological data, survey methods such as questionnaires or interviews, experimental studies, or randomized control trials, in which numerical data are analyzed quantitatively, can be used to test theory and explore its generalizability to various populations. Interpretative research using detailed interviews, case studies, focus groups, or direct observation can provide rich descriptions of the way people think, feel, and act. Themes generated from such descriptions can lead to what is called *grounded theory,* which is also useful for nutrition education practice. Research and theory thus interact to generate results that can be used to enhance the practice of nutrition education. At the same time, theory can be tested, refined, and modified as it is applied in interventions in practice settings and its effectiveness is evaluated (Rothman, 2004). Thus theory, research, and practice all need each other.

Using Theory in Nutrition Education

Theories are not meant to be applied mechanically in the design of nutrition education but to be used as the basis for a range of activities that help individuals gain clarity and insight into the reasons and values underlying their behaviors. Theory-based activities can increase an awareness of the roles and functions of food and the food system in today's

> ### BOX 3-1 Why Theory Is Important to Nutrition Educators: A Summary
>
> Theory is a conceptual model or a mental map representing how potential mediators influence behavior or behavior change. Mediators in real life are represented as constructs or variables in a theory. Theory is important to nutrition educators for the following reasons:
>
> - Theory provides a mental map of *why* a behavior or behavior change occurs. It is not just a list of influences on behavior or behavior change. Such a map helps nutrition educators identify the specific set of mediators of behavior change that should be addressed in a nutrition education intervention.
> - Theory specifies the *kinds of information* that need to be gathered before designing an intervention. It helps us separate relevant from irrelevant mediators for a given group and behavior.
> - Theory also provides us guidance on exactly *how to design* the various intervention components and educational strategies in order to reach people more effectively.
> - Theory provides guidance on exactly what to *evaluate* to measure the impact of the intervention, and how to design accurate measuring instruments.
> - Theory is generated from research in nutrition education and related fields, using both qualitative and quantitative approaches.

society, promote active contemplation, activate decision making, and facilitate the ability to engage in voluntarily chosen change. One nutrition education researcher has pointed out that "nutrition educators should not consider theories as a definitive 'recipe' that, if followed closely and precisely, will result in a highly predictable outcome, but rather as the conceptual grounding or structural blue-print for designing strong, practical programs that can be adapted to help individuals and populations be healthier" (Lytle, 2005).

An Overview of Theory for Understanding Dietary Behavior and Behavior Change

What can the theories generated from research tell us about health and nutrition behaviors and behavior change that are useful for nutrition education? This section provides a general overview of relevant theory. Specific theories and their use in nutrition education are explored in greater detail in the following chapters.

Theories of Behavior and Behavior Change

The Knowledge-Attitude-Behavior Model

An approach commonly used in nutrition education, whether it is made explicit on not, is the knowledge-attitude-behavior (KAB) model. This model proposes that as people acquire knowledge in the nutrition and health areas, their attitudes change. Changes in attitude then lead to changes in behavior. Thus, the role of nutrition education is to provide a target audience with new information about nutrition or health, with the assumption that this information will lead to changes in attitudes, which in turn will result in improved dietary behavior or practices. The primary motivator is assumed to be accumulation of knowledge. This would seem to be logical, since knowledge at some level is essential for making healthful choices. The importance of information seems to be corroborated when millions can switch from eating "low-fat" diets to eating "low-carb" diets or the other way around in a matter of weeks, based on news reports that one is supposed to be better than the other for weight control. However, this phenomenon is really more about people's interest in the quick fix than about changed behaviors resulting from new scientific evidence or information. Witness the difficulty of getting people to eat more fruits and vegetables, despite health campaigns.

Because we are thinking beings, all of our actions are related in some way to knowledge and understanding, often accompanied by feelings and emotions (Bandura, 1986). However, there are many ways to conceptualize knowledge. In most nutrition education programs, *knowledge* refers to understanding basic facts about food and nutrition, such as food groups or balanced diets, knowing the key features of MyPyramid, being able to read food labels, identifying food sources of nutrients, knowing how to store and prepare foods, shopping wisely, managing food budgets, and so forth. This kind of knowledge can be described as *instrumental* or *"how-to" knowledge*. It is essential for those already motivated to eat healthfully or who perceive some personal health risk. It may also be motivating for people who are highly disciplined or those who will eat according to accumulating scientific knowledge, who may be called cognitive or conscientious eaters. In this context, it should be noted that misinformation and misconceptions about food and nutrition can cause problems for those wishing to eat healthfully.

For most people, however, this kind of knowledge is not motivational. Such how-to knowledge is unlikely to lead to improved attitudes or behaviors in those who are not interested or motivated (Backett, 1992; Moorman & Matulich, 1993). Indeed, the scientific evidence for the link between the knowledge component of the KAB model and behavior is weak (Baranowski et al., 2003). In nutrition education intervention studies in which the "dissemination of information" or "teaching of skills" models were effective, the audiences were self-selected and already motivated (Contento et al., 1995).

On the other hand, knowledge can be motivating and may lead to changes in attitudes and behaviors when it is about the consequences of the actions of individuals and communities. Thus, knowledge can be motivating when it is nutrition science–based information that eating certain foods, nutrients, or according to certain patterns is related to specific health outcomes. For example, information from studies showing a relationship between antioxidants in food and reduced risk of cancer, or between calcium intake and bone health, can be very motivating, depending on the audience. The outcomes can be positive, such as the improved heart health and body functioning and assistance with weight control that result from eating fruits and vegetables. The outcomes can also be negative, such as the increased heart disease risk from diets high in saturated fat, the dental problems in children resulting from high intakes of sweetened drinks, or the poor bone health related to low intakes of calcium. For some audiences, information on how eating locally can help sustain local farms can also be motivating.

Science-based information that has motivational power may be described as *"why-to" knowledge* because it provides reasons that we can give to individuals about *why to* make a particular food choice or dietary change, such as why to eat more fruits and vegetables, why to eat more calcium-rich foods, or why to buy from local farmers. Such reasons are also called *outcome beliefs* because they are beliefs about the outcomes of a specific nutrition action such as eating fruits and vegetables. These beliefs constitute a key construct in many theories about motivations for health behaviors and behavior change. But as we noted earlier, beliefs about social outcomes, and personal and self-evaluative outcomes are also important. Thus, behavior change is more complex than a straightforward factual knowledge-to-attitudes-to-behavior framework would suggest.

Why-to knowledge is an important basis of motivation for individuals. Consequently, we need detailed information about what motivates people so that we can help them see why to take action. We need theories that incorporate but expand on these basic notions about knowledge, attitudes, behavior, and their interrelationships, providing much more detailed explanations and complex descriptions of dietary and health behavior. These more complex and precise descriptions are essential for nutrition education design and are described below.

Social Psychological Theories of Health Behavior and Behavioral Change

Much of the work in the health behavior area that provides a rich description and explanation of health behavior is based on the pioneering thinking of Kurt Lewin, a leading social psychologist who emphasized that the function of social psychology is to understand the relationships between an individual and the social environment (Lewin et al., 1944).

He took a phenomenological approach, which emphasized that it is the world as it is perceived by the individual perceiver that most powerfully influences what the individual will do. He was thus interested in developing a psychological approach that explained both inner experiences and observable behavior from the person's own point of view. The environment or situation was also important. He held that "every psychological event depends upon the state of the person and at the same time on the environment, although their relative importance is different in different cases" (Lewin, 1936).

The social psychological approach emphasizes the following:

- *The power of the situation*. We are creatures of our cultures and social contexts.
- *The power of the person*. At the same time, we construct our social world and have an impact on it. Facing the same situation, different people may react differently.
- *The power of cognition*. Our beliefs or cognitions about the world powerfully influence how we react to it. Social reality is something we subjectively construct. Our beliefs about ourselves also matter.

In other words, "people's social behavior is best understood by examining their beliefs about their behavior in a social context, and their social perceptions and representations" (Rutter & Quine, 2002). When it come to food, the social psychological approach (sometimes referred to as the social cognition approach) is concerned with understanding how thoughts, feelings, and values affect food choices and dietary behaviors and with how the interactions with others and with the social environment can influence what and how much individuals eat (Conner & Armitage, 2002). The purpose of understanding social psychological processes is not to manipulate individuals to make changes in their diets but rather to facilitate individuals' voluntary adoption of healthful behaviors by helping to increase awareness and reduce barriers to action, both personal and environmental.

Many theories in this area are *expectancy-value theories*, or theories of decision-making under conditions of uncertainty. The basic premise is that we all have internally determined goals. Prediction of behavior depends on the value we place on the goal (the "pull" or desirability of the goal) and our expectations, or beliefs and estimates, that the given behavior will lead to this desired goal (Lewin et al., 1944). For example, some of us may want to look attractive (the goal or value). If we expect or anticipate that exercising (the action or behavior) will lead to the desired goal of looking attractive, then we will embark on the action. In making our estimates of the effectiveness of the given behavior (exercising), we weigh the costs and benefits of the behavior (e.g., the inconvenience and exertion involved in exercising versus the improved muscle tone and decreased weight). The outcome of such cost-benefit analyses determines whether we will take action. In general, we are motivated to maximize the chances of desirable outcomes occurring and minimize the chances of undesirable outcomes occurring. That is, we ask the question "What's in it for *me* (or for my family or my community)?" Only when people are convinced that there is something in it for them personally will they be motivated to act. Goals can be short term and immediate or may be more long term and global, involving values and ethics.

The theories that we discuss in this book all have as a premise that people will engage in a behavior if they believe it will bring about outcomes that they desire, called *outcome expectations,* and that the benefits of taking action will outweigh barriers (see Box 3-2). Some important outcomes are as follows:

- *Health outcomes*. Researchers who have studied health behaviors found that an additional construct was important: individuals had to first feel a certain degree of threat of disease in order for them to consider whether the benefits of taking action would outweigh the barriers to reducing the threat of disease (e.g., health belief model).
- *Social outcomes*. Researchers who have studied a variety of social behaviors, such as voting in elections or participating in a worksite health program, have found that in addition to outcome expectations, social norms are important. These are what others will think of their performing the behavior (e.g., theory of planned behavior).
- *Self-evaluative outcomes*. Self-evaluative outcomes, such as self-esteem or self-image, are also important for certain behaviors or situations.

Researchers who have studied a variety of social behaviors have found that in addition to outcome expectations, individuals' estimate of whether they will be *able* to perform the behaviors are extremely important. This construct is called *self-efficacy* and is central to many theories (e.g., social cognitive theory).

These theories acknowledge that many factors influencing health behaviors, such as genetics, age, and gender, are not modifiable. Some of these factors may be moderators of the influences on behavior, as we saw earlier. For example, men and women may perceive certain events differently, or certain health beliefs may differ by ethnicity or cultural context. These differences moderate the influence of beliefs on behavior.

Other factors that are not directly changeable by a nutrition education program, such as past experiences, life stage and life trajectories, personality, socioeconomic factors, place of residence, and social and cultural context, are not specifically part of these theories. However, expectancy-value theories propose that although early childhood experiences with food, past life experiences, life stage, place of residence, or cultural context cannot be changed, they do—if they are

> ▶ **BOX 3-2 Expectancy-Value Theories of Motivation: The Foundation of Social Psychological Theories**
>
> Expectancy-value theories posit that we will engage in a behavior if we believe it will bring about outcomes that we desire.
>
> Motivation = Beliefs about *expected* outcomes of behavior × the *values* we place on those outcomes.
>
> That is,
>
> $$\text{Motivation} = \text{Expectancy} \times \text{Values}$$
>
> We want to maximize positive outcomes and minimize negative outcomes:
>
> - *Health outcomes:* Scientific data about the relationships between food choice or diet and health or disease (perceived risk)
> - *Social outcomes:* Social pressure
> - *Self–evaluative outcomes:* Self image; self-esteem, self-efficacy.
>
> These desired outcomes may serve larger goals and values that we possess.

currently salient to the individual—influence behavior by influencing *current* preferences, beliefs, attitudes, values, expectations, motivations, sense of efficacy, or habits. These current beliefs, attitudes, and values can be captured by theory and research.

In general, social psychological theory proposes that although behavior certainly leads to objective consequences, it is the *interpretation* of these consequences by the individual that influences the person's intention to perform the behavior in the future (i.e., will reinforce the behavior). Peer and family opinions are also important: these constitute the construct of *social norms*. Other social environmental and cultural forces also exist. However, social psychologist Triandis (1979) suggests that for any given individual, even such "external" factors as culture and social situations influence behavior because they are internalized by each individual. Thus, culture and social situations exist not only "out there" but also "in here," as subjective culture and subjective social situations that serve as mental maps that guide our behavior by influencing our values, norms, roles, and so forth. All in all, then, a person's perception of the world appears to be a powerful influence on behavior. Indeed, often what people will or will not do is influenced more by their *perception* of reality than by reality itself (Lewin et al., 1944; Bandura, 1986).

In its simplest terms, then, research and theory suggest that for a particular dietary behavior to occur, we need to possess the following convictions about the particular behavior, such as eating more fruits and vegetables, referred to here as *X*. The first belief is

 I want to do X because it leads to the consequences I value.

That is, we need to care about taking a particular action and feel that it is in our interest to do so. This statement is an expression of a *determinant* of behavior or a mediator of behavior change; it is the building block of several theories and is given the name *outcome expectation* or *behavioral belief.*

The next belief is

 I can do X.

Once we are convinced that taking action has desired consequences for us, once we *care*, once we are motivationally ready, we need to feel confident that we can carry out the action to obtain these benefits. This too is a construct that is common to most contemporary health behavior theories and is referred to as *self-efficacy*.

If both these convictions are strong, the likelihood is increased that we will decide or intend to eat more fruits and vegetables. This is called a *behavioral intention* or *goal intention:*

 I will do X.

The role of other people is also important:

 Other people who are important to me think I should do X, and I value their opinion.

However, translating such intentions to action requires yet another step, the development of *implementation intentions* or an *action plan:*

 I will do X three times this coming week.

Translating intentions into action also requires that we have the needed food and nutrition knowledge and skills to carry out the action. For example, we need to know how many servings of fruits and vegetables to eat, the need for eating a variety of colors, how to store fruits and vegetables so that they will last longer, or how to prepare them in a way that tastes good to us.

Maintaining the behavior over the long term requires a further step: the development of self-regulatory skills. Here we set small achievable goals to achieve the outcomes we desire (such as "I will eat one extra serving of vegetable at lunch time each day this week") and monitor our actions to evaluate how well we are fulfilling our action plans or goals. We then take corrective actions as necessary.

Behavior Change as a Process: Phases of Change

When we look closely at how nutrition education is often conducted, we see that it seems to be based frequently on the assumption that diet-related change is a quick, one-step process. One day individuals are eating unhealthful diets, and the next day, after "nutrition education," they are model eaters. This assumption leads professionals into expecting that people change quickly and thus into expecting that the typical four- to six-session program can change lifelong dietary habits. This is an unrealistic view of how people make changes in their lives, and it places unrealistic expectations on health promotion and nutrition education programs—and on ourselves.

When we carefully examine research in the health behavior and behavioral nutrition domains, it becomes evident that behavior change is a process. It may be a short one for some individuals or for some behaviors, and a long one for others. Although the process is continuous, with many factors interacting with each other, it can be described as occurring in two main phases: a motivational, pre-action or *thinking* phase and an action or volitional or *doing* phase (Conner & Norman, 1995; Norman, Abraham, & Conner, 2000; Schwarzer & Fuchs, 1995).

The Motivational, Pre-action Phase

In the motivational, pre-action phase (or thinking phase), beliefs and attitudes or feelings are most important: beliefs such as whether individuals feel a sense of risk or threat regarding an issue; expectations about the outcomes of taking action, including perceived benefits and barriers; expectations of family and friends; and self-efficacy. These beliefs and attitudes can result in motivational readiness to take change, expressed in the form of a *behavioral intention*, or choice of a specific behavioral goal. This phase is described in greater detail in Chapter 4.

The Action Phase

In the action phase (or doing phase), individuals make *action plans* so that intentions can be translated into action. An action plan might be "I will add to my diet a fruit for a snack three days this coming week." In the early action phase, individuals may need to learn new food and nutrition information and new skills, such as learning about what constitutes a serving of fruits and vegetables, how to store and prepare them, how to read food labels, and how to handle family conflicts over food. However, behaviors need to be maintained for the long term, indeed for the rest of the individual's life, if individuals and communities are to see the benefits of

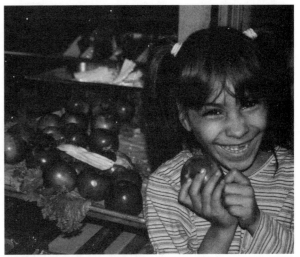
Parents and other family members can play a role in encouraging kids' behavior and goal intentions.

these changes. For actions that are complex, as they are for dietary change, *maintenance* of the behaviors over the long term requires an additional set of skills involving a variety of self-management and self-regulation processes. This phase is described in greater detail in Chapter 5.

Other Phases

Other research has suggested that the process can be divided into more specific phases or stages. Horn (1976) proposed a model of personal choice regarding health behavior in which the process of behavior change was seen as involving four stages: contemplation of change, the decision to change, short-term change, and long-term change. More recently, Prochaska and DiClemente (1982) proposed that change takes place through the stages of precontemplation, contemplation of change, the decision or preparation to change, action, and maintenance.

Other psychologists and sociologists have also proposed various stages of change. For example, the diffusion of innovations framework (Rogers, 1983) proposes that the process of change is initiated when individuals first become aware of the new idea or practice and gain some understanding of it. At the persuasion stage, individuals form a favorable or unfavorable attitude toward the practice. In the decision stage, individuals engage in activities, such as evaluating alternatives that lead to a choice to adopt or reject the new idea or practice. The individual may then go through a stage of trial adoption or implementation during which the innovation is tried out on a small scale before moving on to the final stage of full adoption or confirmation.

Understanding that dietary change occurs in phases or stages permits us to better understand individuals' specific level of motivational readiness to take action, and to tailor nutrition education to their stage in the change process. The theory also proposes that individuals at different stages use different experiential and behavioral processes to make changes. The theory is described in more detail in a later chapter.

Application to Different Population Groups

As described earlier, theories are abstract, symbolic representations of what is conceived to be reality based on evidence from research. As such, these theories can be used in nutrition education for a variety of different population and cultural groups. For different population groups, the beliefs about desired outcomes may be different, based on cultural expectations, past life experiences, life stage (e.g., mothers of young children, postmenopausal women), or role in life (e.g., mothers, husbands, businesspeople). These beliefs must be carefully explored in formative research using these theories in order to understand the behavior from the perspective of the intended audience.

Researchers believe that when properly understood and applied, these theories can be used with many different cultural groups. Fishbein (2000) notes that each of the variables of the theory of planned behavior, for example, can be found in any culture, and that an integrative theory based on this theory has been used in HIV programs in over 50 countries in both the developing and developed world. In the area of diet, the relative importance of the variables may differ for different groups (e.g., Liou & Contento, 2001). For some groups, cultural beliefs regarding food may be more important than convenience. For others, taste preferences are more important for motivating behavior change than health considerations, self-efficacy, or skills. For others, the influence of family may override all other considerations.

The nature of the specific behavior is also important. Some behaviors may be more complex. For example, reducing saturated fat intake requires reducing intake of certain high-fat foods, avoiding fat as a condiment, substituting high-fat foods with specifically manufactured alternatives (low-fat salad dressings, low-fat milk), substituting high-fat foods with fruits and vegetables, and so forth. Such changes may require more skills than motivation. Other behaviors may be easier, such as eating fruits and vegetables, and may require more motivation than skills.

Addressing Multiple and Overlapping Influences on Behavior

An important conclusion from recent research, which also supports the early conclusions of Whitehead (1973), is that nutrition education is more likely to be effective when it addresses the many levels of influences on behavior, ranging from food preferences and the sensory-affective responses to food to personal factors such as beliefs and attitudes and to the environmental context.

For intentions or decisions to be translated into action and for the actions to be maintained for the long term, a supportive social and physical environment is required. At first individuals may adopt the behavior only on a trial basis. Long-term maintenance of the behavior depends on whether they can fit it into their daily lives, whether there is social support for the behavior, and whether material conditions or social structures are in place or can be modified in some way to make it possible to carry out this new practice. Nutrition education programs thus seek to provide environmental support to individuals to enable them to act on their motivations and apply their skills.

As we saw in Figure 3-1, the role of nutrition education is to address the multiple and overlapping spheres of influence on food choices and dietary behaviors that we identified in Chapter 2. To do this, nutrition education needs to develop programs at the several levels of intervention (Figure 3-3):

- *Individual or intrapersonal level:* Focusing on the psychobiological core of experience with food, food preferences and enjoyment of food, beliefs, attitudes, values, knowledge, social and cultural norms, or life experience
- *Interpersonal level:* Focusing on family, friends, peers, interactions with health professionals, social roles, and social networks
- *Institutional/organizational level:* Focusing on rules, policies, and informal structures in workplaces, schools, or religious and social organizations to which individuals belong
- *Community level:* Focusing on social networks, norms, and community expectations, grocery stores, or restaurants
- *Social structure, policy, and systems level:* Focusing on policies and structure that regulate health actions

This approach is called the *social-ecological model* (McLeroy et al., 1988). The idea of directing interventions at various spheres of influence is now widely used in health promotion (Green & Kreuter, 1999; Booth et al., 2001; Gregson et al., 2001; Wetter et al., 2001).

Thus, nutrition education is more likely to be effective when it

- Focuses on specific individual behaviors and community practices that are of importance to the individuals themselves, to communities, or to larger society. These behaviors may also serve larger goals of value to the individual or community.
- Clearly identifies the factors influencing the behaviors of the intended audience, and makes modifying these influencing factors (or potential mediators of the desired behavior change) the direct target of nutrition education interventions rather than merely providing general information.

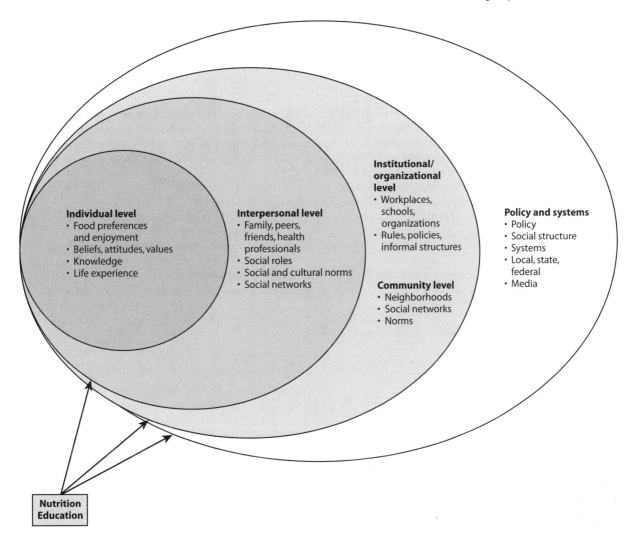

FIGURE 3-3 Social-ecological model: Levels of intervention for nutrition education.

• Develops strategies to address the identified determinants of behavior or potential mediators of change and the environmental contexts of behavior and behavior change at various levels of influence.

An example of a program that focuses on behaviors and their contexts is the U.S. Department of Agriculture's Team Nutrition program for schools (see Nutrition Education in Action 3-1). Clearly such an approach requires teamwork on the part of many besides the nutrition educator, such as teachers, school administrators, parent and community organizations, and various agencies.

Nutrition Education as Facilitating Why to and How to Take Action

The goal of nutrition education is to facilitate the adoption and maintenance of behaviors conducive to health and well-being, as we have noted. To do so effectively, we must shift the focus of nutrition education from simply increasing knowledge to addressing additional factors, both personal and environmental, that influence dietary behavior. As we have seen, these factors are determinants that can serve as potential mediators of behavior change. These determinants must be identified and prioritized so that educational strategies for addressing them can be designed. Theories from behavioral nutrition and nutrition education research help us

NUTRITION EDUCATION IN ACTION **3-1**

Team Nutrition: A Comprehensive Program

The U.S. Department of Agriculture (USDA)'s Team Nutrition is an integrated, comprehensive plan for promoting nutritional health in the nation's schools. This plan involves schools, parents, and the community in efforts to continuously improve school meals, and to promote the health and education of 50 million school children in more than 96,000 schools nationwide. The goal of Team Nutrition is to improve children's lifelong eating and physical activity habits through nutrition education based on the principles of the Dietary Guidelines for Americans and MyPyramid.

Team nutrition uses three strategies to change behavior:

1. Training and technical assistance for Healthy School Meals
   - Planning and preparing healthful meals that appeal to ethnic and culture taste preferences in all Child Nutrition Programs;
   - Linking meal programs to educational activities, such as learning in the classroom and developmental progress in child care;
   - Providing nutrition expertise and awareness to the school or child care community; and
   - Using sound business practices to assure the continued availability of healthy meals and the financial viability and accountability of school meal programs
2. Nutrition Education
   Through fun, interactive nutrition education children are encouraged to:
   - Eat a variety of foods.
   - Eat more fruits, vegetables, and whole grains.
   - Eat lower-fat foods more often.
   - Get your calcium-rich foods
   - Be physically active
3. School and Community Support
   School and community support for healthy eating and physical activity focuses on three behavior outcomes for school and community leaders:
   - Adopting and implementing school policies that promote healthful eating and physical activity.
   - Providing school resources adequate to achieve success.
   - Fostering school and community environments that support healthful eating and physical activity.

Broad support is needed to provide nutritious meals, nutrition education, and healthy school and community environments. Adults can provide this support and positive messages in a variety of ways, through their actions and decisions.

Communication Channels

The nutrition education messages delivered through Team Nutrition's six reinforcing communication channels not only reach children where they live, learn, and play, but also the adults who care for them and can influence their behavior. These channels are:

- Food Service Initiatives
  The dining room offers a positive atmosphere that reinforces nutrition education messages and provides opportunities for students to practice skills learned in the classroom.
- Classroom Activities
  Interactive classroom activities that incorporate nutrition education across the curriculum not only teach students about nutrition, but also provide opportunities to develop skills necessary to form lifelong healthy eating habits.
- School-Wide Events
  Nutrition education activities that all students, school personnel, parents, and the community can enjoy (a school garden project, nutrition fair, or school play) are fun learning opportunities for everyone and reinforce the value of healthy eating and physical activity.
- Home Activities
  Home activities for children and their parents strengthen the messages that children learn at school and in the community. Through their positive example, parents help children learn to make good choices for healthy eating and

(continued)

NUTRITION EDUCATION IN ACTION **3-1** *(continued)*

physical activity. Home activities also provide opportunities for students to influence parental shopping and food preparation decisions.

- Community Programs and Events
  Individuals and organizations develop community-wide education initiatives that emphasize nutrition and physical activity. Joint efforts by schools and communities expand the reach of Team Nutrition messages.
- Media Events and Coverage
  Media coverage of school and community events helps ensure that Team Nutrition messages are repeated and are received by wide audiences. Press releases, PSAs, and other news features are appropriate tools for disseminating nutrition messages and enhancing community support for Team Nutrition goals (http://www.fns.usda.gov/tn).

Evaluation of the program finds that fostering teamwork and collaboration is quite labor intensive and time-consuming and requires a combination of skills to coordinate. But such collaboration can bring about changes that no one individual group can. And all involved believe the effort is worthwhile in fostering awareness and interest in healthful eating and physical activity.

Sources: Levine, E., C. Olander, C. Lefebvre, et al. 2002. The Team Nutrition pilot study: Lessons learned from implementing a comprehensive school-based intervention. *Journal of Nutrition Education and Behavior* 34:109–116; and United States Department of Agriculture. 2006, October. Food and nutrition services. http://www.fns.usda.gov/tn.

---

identify and prioritize these determinants because the determinants are constructs within these theories, and these theories are our mental maps.

As we have seen, there is an emerging consensus that health behavior change by individuals can be seen as a process, involving a pre-action, thinking, or motivational phase and a postdecision, action, or doing phase. Prochaska's stage of change model subdivides these phases further into precontemplation, contemplation, preparation, action, and maintenance, as noted earlier. Beliefs, attitudes, and feelings predominate as determinants of behavior in the pre-action, motivational phase, and food- and nutrition-related knowledge and skills and self-regulation processes predominate as mediators of behavior in the action phase.

Food and nutrition information that has a motivational role can be considered to be why-to knowledge—the reasons *why to* take action or make changes, such as information on a health risk or about the anticipated benefits of taking action. Information that increases the ability to act can be considered as how-to knowledge, such as what constitutes a serving of fruit or vegetables, understanding the food label information on fat content, or eating according to MyPyramid. Why-to knowledge is more important in the pre-action, motivational phase of dietary change, whereas how-to information is more important in the action phase of change.

Why-to and How-to Knowledge

Why-to knowledge is often based on information from nutrition science studies about the health outcomes of taking action based on the relationship of nutrients or foods to health, such as the latest information on calcium and bone health or on antioxidants and reduced cancer risk. The stronger the evidence for health benefits, the more convincing will be the case you can make to your audience for taking action. Using the term why-to knowledge is a useful way to communicate to the lay public the kind of information that is motivational in nature and can serve as potential mediators of change. Why-to information also includes non health-related information on other types of motivators of behavior that are of personal importance, such as perceptions of convenience, taste, or cost; beliefs, attitudes, and feelings; values and personal meanings; social and cultural norms; and individual and ethnic identities.

Why-to information may be particularly important for issues new to your audiences, such as safe food handling practices or the importance of foods containing omega-3 fatty acids for health. Sometimes why-to nutrition science knowledge seems not to have motivational value. This may be because this kind of information, such as on perceived benefits or expected health outcomes, is so commonly known and accepted (e.g., eating fruits and vegetables is good for your health) that it seems to have lost its motivational power. Nevertheless, that does not undermine the importance of the "why-to knowledge" category for enhancing motivation. It just means that ways of freshening why-to nutrition messages must be found from time to time. For example, the 5 A Day program changed its message from "Five a day for better health" to "Eat your colors," which focuses on the importance of variety. Issues of taste can also be addressed by providing taste tests of healthful foods so that individuals can enjoy the new foods and develop the additional reason of taste preference for making changes.

How-to knowledge includes information on basic facts about food and nutrition, such as knowing the key features of MyPyramid, knowing what is meant by balanced diets, being able to read food labels, identifying food sources of nutrients, shopping wisely, being able to practice safe food preparation methods and so forth. Such knowledge is vital to those who want and are ready to make changes but is not as useful to those who are not motivated or not yet ready to make a change.

Theories of the Problem and Theories of the Solution

Some theories help us understand why people do or do not eat healthfully; these are often referred to as *theories of the problem.* They are useful to nutrition educators for the why-to phase of nutrition education because they can provide a mental map to help us understand why individuals do or do not take action, such as breastfeeding, eating sufficient calcium-rich foods, or practicing proper food safety behaviors. Thus, they can be used to help us identify determinants of behavior, such as individuals' perceptions, beliefs, attitudes, or values, that contribute to the problem. These theories can also be used to provide us with a framework for developing strategies to modify these determinants so that they can become mediators of behavior change. The theories described in Chapter 4 are useful theories of the problem.

Some theories are useful for the action phase of nutrition education as well as for the motivational phase; these are often referred to as *theories of the solution.* These theories provide a framework for developing strategies that will facilitate the ability to take action in individuals who are motivationally ready to do so. They are thus especially important in the how-to phase of nutrition education. In this phase we provide needed how-to knowledge and skills in the food and nutrition areas, and these theories provide guidance to us

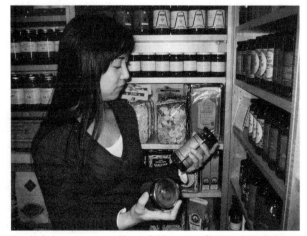

Food labels serve as a readily available source of how-to knowledge.

on how to assist people to develop skills for self-regulating their own behaviors. These types of theories are described in Chapter 5.

Although phases of change have been proposed and have been supported by evidence, the factors predicting behavior are all closely related to each other. Hence the motivational and action phases—thinking and doing—can also be thought of as *components* of the change process rather than phases. Either way, separating these two aspects of dietary change is conceptually useful and has heuristic value when designing nutrition education. It reminds us that to be effective, nutrition education must have a *motivational role* as well as a *facilitating action/providing skills role.* In addition, nutrition education must promote *environmental opportunities* to take the chosen action. The framework also reminds us that individuals may be at different stages in the change process at any given time. Nutrition education can thus be conceptualized as consisting of three components with differing but complementary roles, all serving the educational or intervention goals of the program (Figure 3-4).

The Motivational, Pre-action Phase or Component: A Focus on Why to Take Action

During the motivational, pre-action phase, the behavior change process going on within the individual focuses on becoming motivated to consider action and deciding whether to take action. Many factors influencing motivational readiness to take action are important at this time and are listed in Figure 3-4. Theory and evidence from research suggest that the influencing factors, or potential mediators of behavior change, include awareness of risk or threat, beliefs about taking action, feelings about taking action, beliefs about self-efficacy, and beliefs about social environments. Decision making is influenced by an analysis of the positive and negative outcomes or of benefits versus the costs of taking action and by clarification of one's values. When a decision is made, an intention is formed to take action. The educational goal during this phase is to increase awareness, promote contemplation, enhance the motivation to act, and facilitate the intention to take action. The focus of nutrition education strategies is on why to take action. The specific theories and research that are useful to guide this phase or component of nutrition education are described in Chapter 4.

The Action Phase or Component: A Focus on How-to Take Action

During the action phase, the behavior change process going on within the individual focuses on initiating action and maintaining it for the long term. Theory and evidence from research suggest that developing implementation and action plans is crucial for translating intentions into action. Food- and nutrition-related knowledge and cognitive, affective, and behavioral skills are also important, as are self-regulation

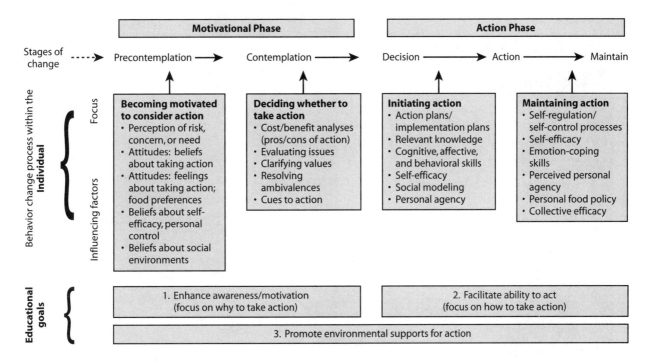

FIGURE 3-4 Conceptual framework for nutrition education.

skills. These result in self-efficacy and a sense of personal agency that can lead to development of personal food policies and to acting with others to make changes in the community. The educational goal during this phase is to increase the individual's ability to act. The focus of nutrition education strategies is on how to take action. The specific theories and research that are useful to guide this phase or component of nutrition education are described in Chapter 5.

The Environmental Support Phase or Component
A supportive environment is important throughout the dietary change process. The nutrition education intervention goal is to educate decision makers, policy makers, and others who have power and authority to make changes in the environment about the importance of nutrition and health concerns and, where possible and appropriate, to work in collaboration with them to promote more supportive environments. The specific research that is useful to guide this phase or component of nutrition education is described in Chapter 6.

Putting It All Together
The conceptual framework just described can be used to develop activities for individual nutrition education sessions or entire programs. It should be noted that for any given program or set of sessions or media materials, nutrition educators need to identify which of the educational goals should

predominate, based on the intended audience's stage of readiness to change. For an audience primarily in a pre-action phase, activities to increase awareness and enhance motivation should predominate. The health belief model, the theory of planned behavior, and other social cognition theories are particularly useful here and are described in Chapter 4. For those who are already motivated, behavior change and self-regulation strategies should predominate. Social cognitive and other self-regulation theories are especially useful here and are described in Chapter 5. In most audiences or groups, people will be at different phases in the change process. Thus, nutrition education should generally begin with awareness and motivational activities. This should be followed by strategies to provide skills and information to assist individuals to take action. For all audiences, but particularly those ready to take action, environmental supports are important.

An example of how why-to information and how-to information can be presented is provided by the Sisters Together campaign sponsored by the Weight-control Information Network (WIN) of the National Institute of Diabetes and Digestive and Kidney Diseases. Information from its website (also a flyer) is reproduced in Nutrition Education in Action 3-2. You can see that the flyer begins with motivational, pre-action-phase nutrition education strategies focusing on why-to information such as the positive outcomes or benefits to be expected from taking action. The website then focuses on per-

NUTRITION EDUCATION IN ACTION 3-2

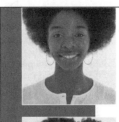
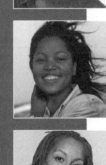
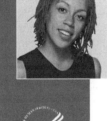
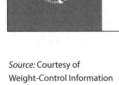

Sisters Together: Move More, Eat Better

Celebrate the Beauty of Youth!

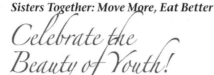

Want to feel better, look better, and have more energy? Moving more and eating better is the best place to start.

Why Move More and Eat Better?

Being physically active and making smart food choices is good for your health. But that is not the only reason to move more and eat better. You can:

- have more energy
- look good in hip, trendy clothes
- tone your body (without losing your curves!)
- reduce stress, boredom, or the blues
- feel good about yourself.

Celebrate the Beauty of Youth's WIN program encourages women to work together to improve their health and nutrition.

Tips on Moving

Physical activity can be fun. Try:

- dancing
- rollerblading
- fast walking

If you can, be physically active with friends. You can cheer each other on, have company, and spend time outdoors. Find a local park where you can take a stroll in a local park.

Think you do not have time? You can fit in a little more by making small changes.

- Get off the bus or subway stop on the way (be safe though!).
- Park your car a little farther away.
- Walk to the store.

Look Good

If you avoid wearing clothes that you like because you do not want others to see your body, try:

- a n...
- a s...
- a...

Tips on Eating Better

Eating right can be hard when you do not feel like cooking or there is a fast-food place on every corner. Here are some simple things you can do to eat better:

- Start every day with breakfast. Try a low-fat whole-grain breakfast bar, nonfat or low-fat yogurt, or whole-grain toast or bagel spread with a little peanut butter, jam, or low-fat cream cheese.
- Eat more fruits and vegetables, and choose whole grains like 100 percent whole wheat bread, oatmeal, or brown rice instead of refined grains like white bread and white rice.
- Choose low-fat or nonfat milk instead of whole milk or a milkshake.
- Order a plain hamburger (without sauce or mayonnaise) or a grilled (without sauce or sandwich. Skip the fries and try a salad with fat free or low-fat dressing instead.
- Do not let sugary soda or other sweets crowd out healthy foods and beverages.

TIP: Many food labels say "low-fat," "reduced fat," or "light." That does not always mean the food is low in calories. Sometimes fat free or low-fat muffins or desserts have even more sugar than the full fat versions. Remember, fat free and calorie free and calories do count!

Many people think that bigger is better. We are so used to value-sized servings that it is easy to eat more than our bodies need. Eating smaller portions will help you cut down on calories and fat (and might save you money too!).

Even take-out and high-fat foods can be part of a balanced diet — if you do not eat them every day

and do not eat too much of them. Here are sensible serving sizes for some favorite foods:

- French fries: 1 small serving (equal to a child's order)
- Shrimp fried rice (as a main dish): 1 cup
- Cheese pizza: 2 small slices or 1 large slice.

TIP: Do you eat in front of the TV out of habit? Do you eat when you are bored, nervous, or sad? Be aware of when, where, and why you eat, and try to eat balanced meals throughout the day. Instead of reaching for that cookie, do something else like call a friend or take a walk.

Out 'n About

You can hang out with your friends and still make healthy food choices. Try these tips when you are out 'n about:

- Order vegetable toppings on pizza instead of salty, high-fat meats like pepperoni or sausage.
- Share popcorn (and skip the added butter) at the movies instead of getting your own bag, or order the smallest size—you will save money too!
- Choose bottled water instead of sweetened soda.
- Munch on pretzels or vegetables at parties instead of fried chips or fatty dips.
- If you drink wine, beer, or other alcohol, limit yourself to one drink—alcohol has lots of calories and little nutritional value.

You Can Do It!

Set doable goals. Move at your own pace. Celebrate your successes. Allow for setbacks. Let your family and friends help you. And keep trying—you can do it!

NIDDK
National Institute of Diabetes and Digestive and Kidney Diseases
NIH Publication No. 04-4903
Reprinted June 2004

Source: Courtesy of Weight-Control Information Network.

ceived barriers to taking action and how to overcome them. It continues with action-phase nutrition education strategies, focusing on how-to information such as relevant food- and nutrition-related knowledge and skills, and concludes with the action-phase nutrition education strategy of goal setting.

Chaos Theory

Some researchers note that behavior change in individuals does not always follow paths as linear as the theories and models suggest. Through our nutrition education efforts, individuals may become aware of their own motivations or their behaviors, but they do not immediately take action; when they do, they may not make the decision in the orderly sequence laid out previously and as described in various models. Researchers have suggested that chaos theory from physics can help us understand these phenomena (Resnicow and Vaughan, 2006). It is known, for example, that smokers on average make eight attempts to quit before they successfully do so. They cannot usually explain why they were successful this particular time. The theory constructs are still important and, on average, may work well. But for any given individual, the new information given about outcome expectations, the new feelings engendered, or the new skills provided may need to percolate in what may appear to be a chaotic fashion. From numerous occasions of nutrition education or individual counseling, after much rumination about the influences on their dietary or physical activity patterns and about what the individual wants out of life, may come action. Because we do not know when or why any given individual may choose to take action, we must, as nutrition educators, use theory-based interventions to keep providing opportunities for individuals to contemplate and decide (Brug, 2006).

The Case of Alicia and Ray

Let us now examine the case of Alicia and Ray. Alicia is not very concerned about her diet. She appears to be in a pre-action mode. Yet the nutrition science literature suggests that this is the time when she should be getting plenty of calcium-rich foods and that eating fruits and vegetables could make a big difference in her health in the future. So pre-action, motivational-phase nutrition education would likely be most appropriate for her, with an emphasis on why-to information and activities. These may stimulate her to actively contemplate her situation, and should emphasize benefits that are important for her and what is in it for her if she takes action.

Ray, on the other hand, has thought about his situation, and his physician has provided a strong cue to action. His problem seems to be related to how to translate interest and intention into action. For Ray, action-phase nutrition education may be more appropriate, with an emphasis on translating intention into action through setting realistic goals and following them up.

The next few chapters describe theory and evidence from nutrition education and health behavior research that will help us determine the kinds of strategies that might work for Alicia and Ray.

A Framework for Planning Nutrition Education: A Logic Model Approach

Where and how, then, to begin? The task of nutrition education seems daunting, so we will need some systematic way to help us plan it effectively. Many planning models are used in different health-related programs, from the PRECEDE-PROCEED model (Green & Kreuter, 1999) to various health communications models (e.g., NCI Health Communications, CDCenergy) to social marketing models (Andreasen, 1995). None of these is quite right for what we want to do in this book—provide a way to assist nutrition educators to develop, deliver, and evaluate the kinds of educational interventions and programs that the vast majority of us conduct on an ongoing basis in our places of work.

A tool that is being used in many fields and has been applied to nutrition education programs is helpful to us here: the *logic model,* which is a simplified but very logical model of how to plan a nutrition education program (Medeiros, Butkus, & Chipman, 2005). It shows that in our planning we need to think about the following:

- The resources that will go into a program (the *inputs*)
- The activities the program will undertake (the *outputs*)
- The changes or benefits that result (the *outcomes*)

In its simplest form, it thus consists of the components shown in Figure 3-5.

Based on our discussions so far, we can use the logic model as follows. We first identify the specific behaviors or practices that we want to address. Then, having considered what our resources are, we design a set of activities that will directly address the potential mediators of change for the specific behaviors or practices that we have identified.

The logic model and other planning models, however, do not—and are not designed to—tell us *exactly how* to design the outputs component. That is, the model does not tell us exactly how we should develop the educational activities and materials for which specific behaviors, directed at which multiple levels of influence, and on what basis. This book is designed to fill this important gap. We will thus incorporate this component into a logic model, as shown in Figure 3-6.

We first determine the behaviors or practices that will be the focus of the program, based on concerns or needs arising from nutrition science evidence, health policy, assessment of the intended audience, and other considerations. With the behavioral focus clearly delineated, we now consider the inputs, outputs, and outcomes.

FIGURE 3-5 Components of the logic model.

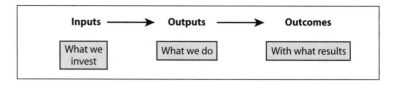

- *The inputs are what we invest.* These consist of the staff and volunteers of the program, time, materials, money, space, and partners and collaborators.
- *The outputs are what we do.* These consist of the activities that we are familiar with: we conduct classes, facilitate groups, and develop material, products, and other resources; we work with families, community partners, and public policy makers; and we work with media. But what we are less familiar with is the fact that these activities must be directed at the identified potential mediators of change that are suggested by theory. This means that these activities must be theory based, not just whatever is informative, fun, engaging, or familiar to us. How to design theory-based nutrition education intervention strategies, or outputs, is the major focus of this book. Developing motivation-phase, action-phase, and environmental support strategies is part of the outputs component of the logic model planning tool. The next three chapters explore each of these components of the nutrition education framework in more detail.
- *The outcomes are the results we obtain from the theory-based strategies that we designed and implemented.*

These outcomes become the basis of our evaluation. Although the ultimate desired outcomes are improved health, decreased disease risk, or other long-term benefits, such as community actions or revised policies to support the program's targeted core behaviors, most nutrition education programs are not intense enough or long enough to achieve such improvements. Therefore they aim for changes in behaviors, which are often considered to be medium-term outcomes. They may even have to be satisfied with improvements in the mediating variables themselves, such as increased knowledge or more positive attitudes. These are considered short-term outcomes.

The Cooking with Kids Logic Model

How the logic model is used to plan nutrition education directed at several levels of influence is illustrated by the Cooking with Kids program, shown in Figure 3-7. The program consists of individual–level activities directed at students in the classroom; family-level activities; and institutional–levels activities designed to improve foods offered at school. The program is described in Nutrition Education in Action 3-3.

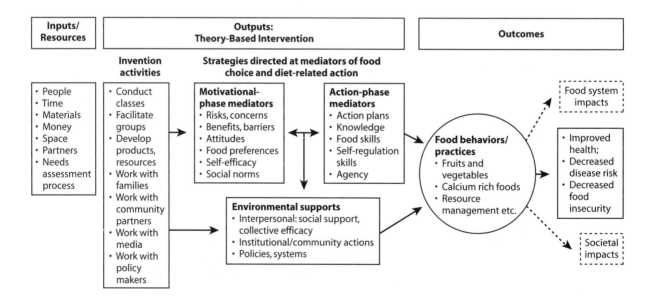

FIGURE 3-6 A logic model framework for theory-based nutrition education.

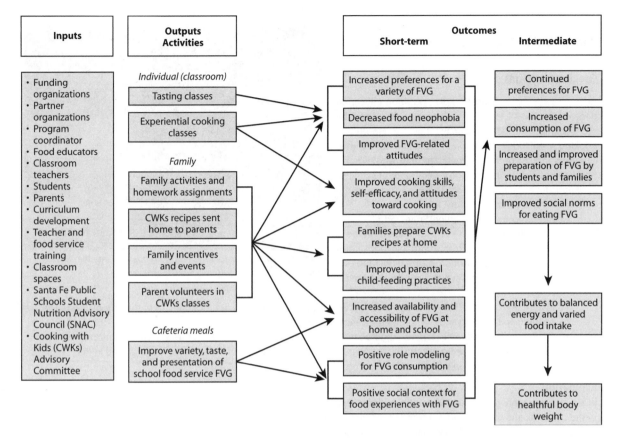

FIGURE 3-7 Logic Model for Cooking With Kids. *Source:* Logic model developed by L. Cunningham-Sabo and N. Hood. Presented by Walters, L., J. Stacey, and L. Cunningham-Sabo. 2005. Learning Comes Alive Through Classroom Cooking: *Cooking with Kids.* Presented at the annual meeting of the Society for Nutrition Education. Orlando, FL. Used with the permission of L. Cunningham-Sabo.

Focus of This Book

The focus of this book is on providing you with the motivation, knowledge, and skills to

- *Use theory and research evidence to identify and design strategies* to address the determinants of behavior that can serve as potential mediators of behavior change so as to achieve the behavioral goals of a given program.
- *Attend to the multiple and overlapping levels of influences* on food choice and eating behavior and use multiple channels to convey messages. In particular, to
  - ▶ *Design, deliver, and evaluate direct education through site-based, in-person educational activities with groups in a variety of settings,* such as communities, outpatient clinics, health maintenance organizations, fitness centers, schools, workplaces, or private nonprofit organizations.

  - ▶ *Develop and use indirect methods through multiple venues,* such as printed materials, curricula, newsletters, visual media, health fairs, and population-based activities, including mass media communications or social marketing activities.
  - ▶ *Engage in activities and coalitions with organizational, community, and other partners* to promote policies and environments that are supportive of the public's ability to eat healthfully.

The next three chapters provide the background in terms of theory and evidence for designing nutrition education activities and materials. This may be considered information on *why to* conduct behavior-focused, theory- and evidence-based nutrition education. Part II of this book then describes a six-step process for translating theory and evidence into specific practical educational strategies for the outputs and impacts components of the logic model. This may be considered how-to information.

NUTRITION EDUCATION IN ACTION 3-3

Cooking with Kids

How the logic model is used to plan nutrition education directed at several levels of influence is illustrated by the Cooking with Kids™ program, shown in Figure 3-7. Cooking with Kids is a program designed to improve children's intakes of fruits, vegetables, and whole grains (the targeted behaviors) through several kinds of activities at various levels of intervention. These are shown in the logic model and described below:

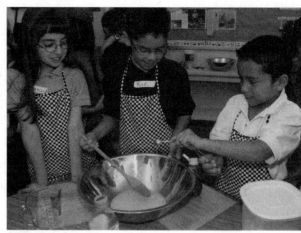
Cooking with Kids incorporates nutrition education into the classroom curriculum.

- *Individual-level intervention:* Fruit- and vegetable-tasting activities for students in the classroom; cooking fresh, affordable foods from diverse cultures; nutrition information; foods in history; food journal activities; and take-home recipes.
- *Family-level activities:* Volunteer participation; activities such as families getting together at the school during the evening and cooking and eating together; events; and incentives.
- *Institutional or environmental level:* Improvements in the meals offered at school through collaboration with others, such as farm-to-table organizations; locally grown produce included in school meals; foods cooked in the classroom adapted and served in school meals.

Evaluation

In a pilot evaluation, more than 80% of the students reported liking the foods cooked in the classroom, 75% chose the foods in the cafeteria, and 60% ate half or more of the lunch. About 50% of the parents reported that they used Cooking with Kids recipes at home, and 65% said their children now ate more fruits and vegetables at home.

Source: Walters, L., J. Stacey, and L. Cunningham-Sabo. 2005. Learning comes alive through classroom cooking: *Cooking with Kids.* Presented at the annual meeting of the Society for Nutrition Education. Orlando, FL; Walters, L., and J. Stacey. Cooking with Kids. www.cookingwithkids.net.

Questions and Activities

1. Describe what is meant by "behavior-focused" nutrition education. Is it the same thing as a behaviorist approach? How or how not?

2. Describe four key elements that contribute to the effectiveness of nutrition education, based on research.

3. Define *theory*. Give three reasons why theory is considered important in nutrition education.

4. What do we mean by the term *theory construct*? How is it related to the term *variable*?

5. Think back to a specific instance in which you gave a nutrition education session or discussed nutrition informally with others. Do you think you used theory? If so, describe the key features of your theory. If you did not use theory, explain what guided your session.

6. To what extent are you personally convinced that the use of theory and evidence will help you design more effective nutrition education? Why or why not?

7. The knowledge–attitude–behavior (KAB) model of behavior change is quite commonly used. How effective has it been in nutrition education? Why?

8. Describe what is meant by expectancy-value theories. How might they differ from the KAB model?

9. Distinguish between why-to knowledge and how-to knowledge in the area of nutrition education.

10. We have described nutrition education as consisting of two phases or components, accompanied by environmental supports. What are they and what is the primary focus of each phase?

11. Describe the key features of the logic model. If you have provided nutrition education before, no matter how small (e.g., one session) or large in scale, map it out according to the logic model. What are some of your reflections on the experience?

REFERENCES

Achterberg, A., and C. Miller. 2004. Is one theory better than another in nutrition education? A viewpoint: More is better. *Journal of Nutrition Education and Behavior* 36:40–42.

Achterberg, C., and L. Lytle. 1995. Changing the diet of America's children: What works and why? *Journal of Nutrition Education* 27(5):250–260.

Ammerman, A.S., C.H. Lindquist, K.N. Lohr, and J. Hersey. 2002. The efficacy of behavioral interventions to modify dietary fat and fruit and vegetable intake: A review of the evidence. *Preventive Medicine* 35(1):25–41.

Andreasen, A.R. 1995. *Marketing social change: Changing behavior to promote health, social development, and the environment.* Washington, DC: Jossey-Bass.

Backett, K. 1992. The construction of health knowledge in middle class families. *Health Education Research* 7:497–507.

Bandura, A. 1986. *Foundations of thought and action: A social cognitive theory.* Englewood Cliffs, NJ: Prentice-Hall.

———. 2001. Social cognitive theory: An agentic perspective. *Annual Review of Psychology* 52:1–26.

Baranowski, T., K.W. Cullen, and J. Baranowski. 1999. Psychosocial correlates of dietary intake: Advancing intervention. *Annual Review of Public Health* 19:17–40.

Baranowski, T., K.W. Cullen, T. Nicklas, D. Thompson, and J. Baranowski. 2003. Are current health behavioral change models helpful in guiding prevention of weight gain efforts? *Obesity Research* 11(Suppl.):23S–43S.

Blake, C., and C.A. Bisogni. 2003. Personal and family food choice schemas of rural women in upstate New York. *Journal of Nutrition Education and Behavior* 35:282-293.

Booth, S.L., J.F. Sallis, C. Ritenbaugh, et al. 2001. Environmental and societal factors affect food choice and physical activity: Rationale, influences, and leverage points. *Nutrition Reviews* 59(Suppl):S21–S39.

Bowen, D.J., and S.A. Beresford. 2002. Dietary interventions to prevent disease. *Annual Review of Public Health* 23:255–286.

Brug, J. 2006. Order is needed to promote linear or quantum changes in nutrition and physical activity behaviors. *International Journal of Behavioral Nutrition and Physical Activity* 3:29.

Brug, J., A. Oenema, and I. Ferreira. 2005. Theory, evidence and intervention mapping to improve behavioral nutrition and physical activity interventions. *International Journal of Behavioral Nutrition and Physical Activity* 2(2).

Buchanan, D. 2004. Two models for defining the relationship between theory and practice in nutrition education: Is the scientific method meeting our needs? *Journal of Nutrition Education and Behavior* 36(3):146–154.

Chatterji, M. 2004. Evidence on "what works": An argument for extended-term mixed-method (ETMM) evaluation

designs. *Educational Researcher* 33(9):3–13.

Conner, M., and C.J. Armitage. 2002. *The social psychology of food.* Buckingham, UK: Open University Press.

Conner, M., and P. Norman. 1995. *Predicting health behavior.* Buckingham, UK: Open University Press.

Contento, I. 1980. Thinking about nutrition education: What to teach, how to teach it, and what to measure. *Teachers College Record* 81(4):422–424.

Contento, I.R., G.I. Balch, Y.L. Bronner, et al. 1995. The effectiveness of nutrition education and implications for nutrition education policy, programs, and research: A review of research. *Journal of Nutrition Education* 27(6):277–422.

Contento, I.R., A.D. Manning, and B. Shannon. 1992. Research perspective on school-based nutrition education. *Journal of Nutrition Education* 24:247–260.

Doak C.M., T.L.S. Visscher, C.M. Renders, et al. 2006. The prevention of overweight and obesity in children and adolescents: A review of interventions and programs. *Obesity Reviews* 7;111-136.

Fishbein, M. 2000. The role of theory in HIV prevention. *AIDS Care* 12(3):273–278.

Furst, T., M. Connors, C.A Bisogni, J. Sobal, and L.W. Falk. 1996. Food choice: A conceptual model of the process. *Appetite* 26: 247-266.

Gillespie, G.W., and A.H. Gillespie. 1991. Using theories in nutrition education: is it practical? Paper presented at the annual meeting of the Society for Nutrition Education.

Green, L.W., and M.W. Kreuter. 1999. *Health promotion planning: An educational and ecological approach.* 3rd ed. Mountain View, CA: Mayfield.

Gregson, J., S.B. Foerster, R. Orr, et al. 2001. System, environmental, and policy changes: Using the social-ecological model as a framework for evaluating nutrition education and social marketing programs with low-income audiences. *Journal of Nutrition Education* 33:S4-S15.

Gussow, J.D., and I. Contento. 1984. Nutrition education in a changing world. *World Review of Nutrition and Diet* 44:1–56.

Hegsted, M. 1979, March 26. Interview quoted in *Nutrition and Health. Chemical and Engineering News*, edited by Anders, H.J., 27.

Institute of Medicine. 2002. *Speaking of health: Assessing health communication strategies for diverse populations.* Washington, DC: National Academy Press.

Horn, D.S. 1976. Model for the study of personal choice health behavior. *International Journal of Health Education* 19:89–98.

Johnson, D.W., and R.T. Johnson. 1985. Nutrition education: A model for effectiveness, a synthesis of research. *Journal of Nutrition Education* 17(Suppl):S1–S44.

Kerlinger, F.N. 1986. *Foundation of behavioral research.* 3rd ed. New York: Holt, Rhinehart and Winston.

Kok, G., H. Schaalma, H. De Vries, G. Parcel, and T. Paulussen. 1996. Social psychology and health. *European Review of Social Psychology* 7:241–282.

Lewin, K.T. 1935. *A dynamic theory of personality*. New York: McGraw-Hill.

———. 1936. *Principles of topological psychology*. New York and London: McGraw-Hill.

Lewin, K., T. Dembo, L. Festinger, and P.S. Sears. 1944. Level of aspiration. In *Personality and the behavior disorders*, edited by J.M. Hundt. New York: Roland Press.

Liou, D., and I.R. Contento 2001. Usefulness of psychosocial theory variables in explaining fat-related dietary behavior in Chinese Americans: Association with degree of acculturation. *Journal of Nutrition Education* 33:322-331.

Luepker, RV., C.L. Perry, and S.M. McKinlay. 1996. Outcomes of a field trial to improve children's dietary patterns and physical activity: The Child and Adolescent Trial for Cardiovascular Health (CATCH) collaborative group. *Journal of the American Medical Association* 275:768–776.

Lytle, L.A. 2005. Nutrition education, behavioral theories and the scientific method: Another viewpoint. *Journal of Nutrition Education and Behavior* 37:90–93.

Maxwell, J.C. 2000. *Failing forward: Turning mistakes into stepping stones for success*. Nashville: Thomas Nelson Publishers.

McKenzie, J.C., and P. Mumford. 1965. The evaluation of nutrition education programmes: A review of the present situation. *World Review of Nutrition and Dietetics* 5:21–31.

McLeroy, K.R., D. Bibeau, A. Steckler, and K. Glanz. 1988. An ecological perspective on health promotion programs. *Health Education Quarterly* 15:351–377.

Medeiros, L.C., S.N. Butkus, H. Chipman, et al. 2005. A logic framework for community nutrition education. *Journal of Nutrition Education and Behavior* 37:197-202.

Merriam-Webster. 2003. *Merriam-Webster's collegiate dictionary*. 11th ed. Springfield, MA: Merriam-Webster

Moorman, C., and E. Matulich. 1993. A model of consumers' preventive health behaviors: The role of health motivation and health ability. *Journal of Consumer Research* 20:208–228.

Norman, P., C. Abraham, and M. Conner. 2000. *Understanding and changing health behavior: From health beliefs to self-regulation*. Amsterdam: Harwood Academic Publishers.

Olson, C.M., and A.H. Gillespie. 1981. Workshop on nutrition education research: Applying principles from the behavioral sciences. Proceedings of a workshop. *Journal of Nutrition Education* 13(1, Suppl. 1):S1–S118.

Pelican S., F. Vanden Heede, B. Holmes, et al. 2005. The power of others to shape our identity: Body image, physical abilities, and body weight. *Family and Consumer Sciences Research Journal* 34(1):57-80.

Perry, C.L., and D.B. Bishop. 1998. Changing fruit and vegetable consumption among children: The 5-a-Day Power Plus program in St. Paul, Minnesota. *American Journal of Public Health* 88(4):603–609.

Perry, C.L., L.A. Lytle, and H. Feldman. 1998. Effects of the Child and Adolescent Trial for Cardiovascular Health (CATCH) on fruit and vegetable intake. *Journal of Nutrition Education* 30:354–360.

Peters, J.C., H.R. Wyatt, W.T. Donahoo, and J.O. Hill. 2002. From instinct to intellect: The challenge of maintaining healthy weight in the modern world. *Obesity Reviews* 3:69–74.

Pomerleau, J., K. Lock, C. Knai, and M. McKee. 2005. Interventions designed to increase adult fruit and vegetable intake can be effective: A systematic review of the literature. *Journal of Nutrition* 135:2486–2495.

Potter, J.D., J.R. Finnegan, J.X. Guinard, E. Huerta, S.H. Kelder, and A.R. Kristal. 2000. *5 A Day for Better Health program evaluation report*. Bethesda, MD: National Institutes of Health, National Cancer Institute.

Prochaska, J.O., and C.C. DiClemente. 1982. Transtheoretical therapy: Toward a more integrative model of change. *Psychotherapy: Theory, Research, Practice* 19:276–288.

Resnicow, K., and R. Vaughan. 2006. A chaotic view of behavior change: a quantum leap for health promotion. *International Journal of Behavioral Nutrition and Physical Activity 3:25*.

Rogers, E.M. 1983. *Diffusion of innovations*. New York: Free Press.

Rothman, A.J. 2004. "Is there nothing more practical than a good theory?" Why innovations and advances in health behavior change will arise if interventions are used to test and refine theory. *International Journal of Behavioral Nutrition and Physical Activity* 1(11).

Rutter, D.R., and L. Quine. 2002. *Changing health behaviour: Intervention and research with social cognition models*. Buckingham, UK: Open University Press.

Schwarzer, R., and R. Fuchs. 1995. Self-efficacy and health behaviors. In *Predicting health behavior*, edited by M. Conner and P. Norman. Buckingham, UK: Open University Press.

Staffleu, A., C. de Graaf, W.A. Van Staveren, and J.J. Schroots. 1991–1992. A review of selected studies assessing social psychological determinants of fat and cholesterol intake. *Food Quality and Preferences* 3:183–200.

Strauss, A.L., and J. Corbin. 1990. *Basics of qualitative research: Grounded theory procedures and research*. Newbury Park, CA: Sage Publications.

Triandis, H.C. 1979. Values, attitudes, and interpersonal behavior. In *Nebraska symposium on motivation*, edited by H.E. How Jr., Vol. 27, 195–259. Lincoln: University of Nebraska Press.

Walters, L., J. Stacey, and L. Cunningham-Sabo. 2005. Learning comes alive through classroom cooking: *Cooking with Kids.* Presented at the annual meeting of the Society for Nutrition Education. Orlando, FL.

Wetter, A.C., J.P. Goldberg, A.C. King, et al. 2001. How and why do individuals make food and physical activity choices? *Nutrition Reviews* 59(Suppl):S11–S20.

Whitehead, F. 1973. Nutrition education research. *World Review of Nutrition and Dietetics* 17:91–149.

Zeitlin, M., and C.S. Formation. 1981. *Nutrition intervention in developing countries. Study II. Nutrition education.* Cambridge, MA: Oelgeschlager, Gunn & Hain.

Zimbardo, P.G., E.B. Ebbeson, and C. Maslach. 1977. *Influencing attitudes and changing behavior.* Reading, MA: Addison-Wesley.

Foundation in Theory and Research:
Increasing Awareness and Enhancing Motivation

OVERVIEW   This chapter describes key theories and research that help readers understand the important role of motivation in food choice and nutrition-related behaviors and examines their implications for effective nutrition communication and education. It focuses on motivation to act and the key role of beliefs, feelings, and attitudes in providing *why-to* nutrition education.

OBJECTIVES   At the end of the chapter, you will be able to

- Describe key theories that help us understand motivation for health and nutrition behaviors, in particular the health belief model and the theory of planned behavior
- State key concepts in these theories and their practice applications
- Describe how these theories have been used in research to investigate determinants of food choice and nutrition-related behaviors
- Discuss how theories and research have been used in nutrition education programs to enhance motivation in food choice and nutrition-related behaviors
- Demonstrate understanding that the major task of nutrition education is to use theory to identify determinants that potentially mediate behavior change and design strategies to address these potential mediators of change
- Identify implications for nutrition education design and effective communication to increase interest, enhance motivation, promote active contemplation, and facilitate formation of intentions to take action

SCENARIO

If you were asked to design some sessions for a group of young people rather like Alicia from the last chapter, you would first need to know what kinds of reasons, insights, or feelings would motivate them to think seriously about *why to* take action now about eating more fruits and vegetables. Write a list of the reasons you think would ring true for them. Remember they are in their late teens; they feel fine and are not overweight. Although they are not entirely satisfied with how they are eating, they see no need to change. What do you think would be the barriers this group would experience? Write these down as well. As you read the chapter, try to match up these reasons or motivations with the constructs of the theories described here. From your list, think of what kind of nutrition education might be effective with people like Alicia.

Introduction: Increasing Awareness and Enhancing Motivation: Why to Take Action

Our food choices and eating patterns have developed over a lifetime and are embedded in many aspects of our lives. Many of us, like Alicia, may not be entirely satisfied with how we are eating, but our patterns generally work for us, given our life circumstances and the trade-offs we need to make. Given the many competing desires and priorities in our lives, health is not always uppermost. The first crucial step in making specific changes is to become aware of a need to change and to see what's in it for us to do so. When aware, interested, and motivated, we are more ready for information and skills that will assist us to take action.

We saw in the last chapter that the accumulated evidence from health behavior research suggests that the adoption and maintenance of health behaviors is a process involving two main phases: a decision-making or deliberative phase and an action or implementation phase (Schwarzer, 1992; Abraham & Sheeran, 2000). This suggests that nutrition education programs should consist of both a motivational pre-action component and a postdecision action and maintenance component. It is recognized, of course, that we are thinking, feeling, and acting wholes, so that motivation or willingness to take action and the ability to act are closely related, each enhancing the other. It may be that for many individuals, problems with getting started and maintaining action rather than motivation or forming intentions prevent them from engaging in recommended healthful behaviors. Nevertheless, thinking about the behavior change process as two phases or components helps with the conceptualization and design of nutrition education programs.

This chapter focuses on the first phase or component. It examines what nutrition behavior research and theory can tell us about how individuals become aware, interested, and motivated so that nutrition education programs can be designed to assist individuals move from not even considering taking action to deliberating about it and taking action if they see the need and choose to do so.

We saw in the last chapter that cognitive-motivational factors or social cognitions—our beliefs, values, feelings, attitudes, and perceptions of social and cultural norms—influence our health behaviors. These cognitive-motivational factors come from cultural, social, family, or personal sources. Most theories also note the importance of prior life experiences, life stage, personality, family structure, and sociodemographic and historic factors that may influence behavior. These, of course, are not modifiable by educational means. However, these factors affect *current* beliefs, attitudes, or self-identities that influence behavior, and these *can* be addressed by nutrition education.

Cultural Context

Consideration of cultural context is important in planning nutrition education. All humans are cultural creatures. We experience culture from the moment we are born: for example, in some cultures girl babies get pink clothes and boy babies, blue. As noted in Chapter 2, culture is concerned with shared knowledge and shared meanings, where "meanings" implies some complexity of belief or knowledge and a connection of values or feelings with beliefs (D'Andrade, 1984). Cultural knowledge and values develop over time for the group or society in ways that help to promote its survival (LeVine, 1984). Food, which is essential to survival, is not surprisingly very much part of culture. Our culture defines what we should or should not eat and prescribes how to prepare food; where, when, and with whom it should be eaten; who does the shopping and cooking; and whose opinions are most important in the choice of family meals (Rozin, 1982; Sanjur, 1982; Kittler & Sucher, 2001).

Differences in cultural values about health in general can also influence dietary practices. For example, some cultures, such as mainstream American culture, emphasize personal responsibility or self-help in promoting individual health or preventing illness, whereas others may believe that chance or fate is more important. Although mainstream culture may emphasize personal choice in matters of food and eating, others emphasize the role of family in decisions related to food and health. Some of these differing cultural norms are shown in Table 4-1.

Children acquire their cultures' beliefs and values both directly and indirectly (Spiro, 1984). Direct influence occurs when the child is told explicitly about "facts," norms, values, and so forth about the culture (e.g., "We don't eat pork"). Indirect acquisition occurs through observing what other people do (norms), whether in interpersonal settings or through media such as television, and making inferences from norms and cultural artifacts about the values of the culture. For example, if families within a culture spend a lot of time to prepare healthful food (norms), or if their kitchens are equipped for making healthful foods (artifacts), children growing up in that culture are likely also to value healthful food. Anthropologists suggest that this outcome is likely in part because there is a tendency for the descriptive understanding of one's culture—how things are—to become fused with a normative understanding—how things should be. LeVine (1984) comments, "The fusion of what is and ought to be in a single vision . . . gives distinctive cultural ideologies their singular psychological power, their intimate linkages with individual emotion and motivation" (p. 78).

Given these definitions and observations, culture can be seen as connected intimately with the intra- and interpersonal cognitive-motivational factors in food choice that are discussed later in this chapter. That is, the beliefs, attitudes, and values to be discussed there are the same ones under discussion here; culture may be considered their primary source. The relation of culture to the food and physiological factors discussed in earlier chapters has been explored by

Rozin (1982), who describes how mild social pressure may maintain the consumption of initially unpalatable foods until preference becomes internalized by liking for the taste, as with chili, or by other factors, such as addiction to coffee.

Social pressure of this kind tends to be consistent with the beliefs, values, and practices of the culture or subculture (e.g., adolescents or ethnic groups). However, cultural and social influences are distinguishable to some degree through the concept of internalization. Culture involves beliefs and values that are internalized or believed in widely among members of the group; as children acquire these beliefs and values, we say they become acculturated. Two kinds of social influence have been distinguished by Deutsch and Gerard (1955). With *normative* social influence, people conform to others' wishes in order to gain social acceptance. Conformity to the family's wishes is of some importance earlier in life; later, the key reference group consists of our peers. With *informational* social influence, people learn about reality from what others say and do. This learning then also influences people's values, attitudes, and actions

Researchers point out that culture "out there" is interpreted by the family and passed down to their children as family cultural traditions (Birch, 1999). Children in turn filter these family cultural traditions through their own personal experience with food to develop their own interpretations of their culture (Rozin, 1982). Likewise, traditional cultures of immigrants and subcultures are interpreted by communities and families to varying degrees. Individuals filter these family and community interpretations of traditional culture through their own experiences with food and mainstream culture to come up with their own personal or family interpretations of their traditions and cultures.

For example, some cultures believe that foods have "hot" and "cold" (or yin and yang) qualities and must be eaten to balance hot and cold body conditions in order to maintain health. However, individuals within a culture differ in the strengths of their beliefs about this interpretation of health and consequently on the extent to which these beliefs influence their health behaviors. Knowledge about the strength of these beliefs for a given audience can be useful in planning nutrition education (Liou & Contento, 2004). Likewise, fate in some cultures is an important determinant of health behaviors. Again, members of the culture may differ considerably in the strength of this belief. For other subcultures, where religiosity, racial pride, sense of time, or sense of community are important, individual differences exist and individual cognitive-motivational factors remain very important (Kreuter et al., 2003). In the case of breastfeeding, although cultural and family expectations are very important, individuals *still* differ in their opinions about these expectations (Bentley, Dee, & Jensen, 2003).

All these considerations help us recognize that individuals *internalize* the beliefs, norms, and values of their culture, and it is these personal interpretations that are powerful in people's lives (Triandis, 1977). Some of these internalized cultural beliefs, norms, and values can be considered to be determinants of behavior and can be included as constructs in the theories and models described in this chapter, which can then be addressed in nutrition education activities directed at individual change. Other cultural values may need to be more specifically addressed in nutrition education.

TABLE 4-1 Comparison of Some Common Cultural Values Relevant to Dietary Behavior

Mainstream American Culture	Some Other Cultural Groups
Health and illness are located in the person.	Health and illness are long-term, fluid, and continuous expressions of relationships between the individual and others.
Illness is caused by natural etiological agents such as genes, viruses, bacteria, or stress.	Illness is caused by quasi-natural agents such as weather or various states of one's blood (e.g., thin, weak, or bad), or by violations of religious or moral expectations, emotions such as envy or jealousy, or punishment for misconduct.
Personal responsibility for health; importance of sense of control.	Chance, fate, God influence health, illness, and healing.
Nutritional health is due to deficiencies and imbalances in food components and nutrients in food.	Health is due to the balance of forces in body, such as hot-cold; imbalances cause illness, and health can be restored by balancing of hot and cold foods.
Self-help	Societal or community obligation to assist
Emphasis on individualism/privacy	Welfare of the group; interpersonal harmony important
Time highly important	Personal interactions highly important
Future orientation	Past or present orientation; tradition is important
Interactions emphasize directness and openness	Interactions emphasize indirectness, importance of "face"
Informality and egalitarianism	Status, formal relationships important

Understanding Motivations for Health Behavior Change

Centuries ago, the Greeks described both *logos* (reason) and *pathos* (emotion) as important in the human experience and key bases for action. Social psychological theories address both aspects of human motivation. The next several chapters describe several theories that are especially useful for nutrition educators. Why are there several theories? Why not one? As we saw in the last chapter, some theories were developed because researchers were studying health-related behaviors specifically, whereas others were investigating other social behaviors (such as consumer behaviors, including food choice) not necessarily related to health.

For example, the health belief model was developed specifically to understand and predict health behaviors. Its main constructs—perceived threat, perceived benefits, and perceived barriers (to be described in greater detail later in this chapter)—have proved to be very important and are widely used in interventions. However, the theory was developed to predict simple health behaviors such as whether people would go for immunizations, and therefore does not explain more complex behaviors such as how to bring about dietary change. The model also does not help us understand food choices and dietary behaviors that are undertaken for a variety of reasons other than health. For such understanding, we need to turn to attitude-change theories and other related social psychological theories.

Researchers in the early 1900s became interested in the construct of attitude as a predictor or determinant of behavior (Zimbardo, Ebbesen, & Maslach, 1977; Ajzen, 2001). Marketers were particularly interested because they found that by using communication strategies designed to change attitudes toward products or actions, they could change behaviors. The attitude-change theories they developed are not specially designed for health-related behaviors and hence are also incomplete. Still, these attitude-change theories are very useful for designing nutrition education activities to increase interest and assist people to acquire the motivation to move from nonaction to the intention to take action on food- and nutrition-related issues. They are useful not only for group settings, but also for mass media health communication campaigns. Key among these theories is the theory of planned behavior, which is described later in this chapter.

We recognize that although these theories are very useful in helping us understand motivation and to design activities and media messages on why to take action, they, too, are incomplete. They generally do not provide sufficient information on how to help individuals translate intention into action for complicated behaviors such as dietary behaviors and to maintain the behaviors for the long term. For this, we turn to still other theories, such as self-efficacy and self-regulation theories. The next chapter describes those theories, research, and strategies that are particularly useful in facili-

tating the adoption and maintenance of diet-related behaviors for the long term.

We know from research that those who develop strong and stable intentions will be more likely to take action on

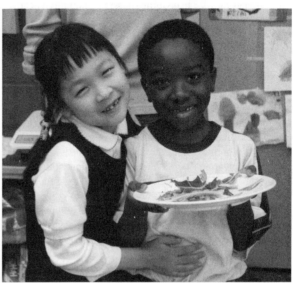

Attitude-change theories can help develop nutrition education activities to motivate students in group settings.

▶ BOX 4-1 The Role of Theory

Theory in nutrition education provides a conceptual map, derived from evidence, to help us understand how the various influences on food and nutrition-related behavior change are related to each other and to behavior itself. These influences or potential mediators of change in the real world are thus "constructs" in the conceptual maps or theories.

Mediators of behavior change = Constructs in theories

Some theories were developed to explain behaviors undertaken for health reasons (e.g., health belief model). Other theories are needed to understand food choices and dietary behaviors undertaken for a variety of reasons in addition to health (e.g., attitude-change theories, theory of planned behavior). Still other theories are needed to understand how individuals can translate attitudes and intention into long-term dietary change (e.g., self-regulation models, social cognitive theory).

their intentions. Most of us have intentions for many health-related behaviors, but the intentions are not always very strong—as seems to be the case for Alicia and Ray. We want to eat more healthfully, be more active, or get more sleep. Yet food choice and nutrition-related behaviors are complex, each competing with many other possible alternative actions, such as eating fruit *or* cake for dessert, going for a run *or* watching television. For any given action there are also many competing beliefs and emotions (cake is tasty but fattening; walking is healthy but takes time and effort). Thus it is not always easy to develop strong and stable intentions.

Acting on these weak health intentions is made even more difficult in the face of strong environmental forces to act otherwise, from television advertising or the conveniently located less-than-healthful foods at work to the family members with whom we eat who have other needs and tastes. Thus a motivational component in nutrition education is important for all: (1) those who are not aware of the importance of specific food-related actions that they could take to protect their health, (2) those who are aware but are uncommitted to taking action, and (3) those with weak intentions, whom we can stimulate to reexamine their intentions and assist to develop stronger intentions. The theories described in this chapter help us understand how to help our audiences develop strong intentions for given behaviors.

The Health Belief Model

The health belief model is a framework for understanding individuals' psychological readiness or intention to take a given health action. It was one of the earliest conceptual models to address health behavior specifically and is the most well-known theory in the field of public health. The model was developed in the 1950s by social psychologists working in the Lewin tradition, who were interested in using social science to solve practical public health problems (Becker, 1974; Rosenstock, 1974). They were committed to building theories for long-term use and not merely to solving practical health problems one at a time. The model has been widely accepted and used by health professionals to design interventions in many parts of the world. It is intuitively appealing, easy for nonpsychologists to understand and apply, and inexpensive to implement. Its commonsense constructs (beliefs) are clearly stated, manageable in number, and easily measured in a variety of ways, from interviews to surveys. The model focuses health professionals' attention on modifiable factors influencing behavior.

Like the other theories, this model proposes that considerations of the perceived benefits versus perceived barriers of taking action are important motivators of behavior. But, as a model focused on health, it proposes that we need to perceive a threat regarding a health condition before we consider the benefits and barriers of taking action to reduce the risk of the health condition.

Constructs of the Model

More specifically, the model proposes that our likelihood of taking a specific health-related action is primarily motivated by the following perceptions or considerations:

- *Perceived threat or risk of a condition.* Examples are cancer, osteoporosis, and the lack of safety of our food. Risk in turn is determined by our perceptions about the severity or seriousness of the personal impact of the condition, and our own personal susceptibility or risk for contracting the condition. These concerns result in our readiness to act.
- *Perceived benefits and barriers.* Perceived benefits are our perceptions that a preventive action is available, such as eating fruits and vegetables, that is likely to be beneficial or effective to reduce the threat. Perceived barriers are our perceptions of the difficulties of performing the behavior, both psychological, such as our perceptions of the cost and inconvenience of eating fruits and vegetables, and the actual, if some fruits and vegetables may not agree with us physiologically. Changing these beliefs through nutrition education, such as by increasing the perceived benefits and decreasing perceived barriers, should change the likelihood of our taking a given health action.
- *Self-efficacy.* The health belief model was originally developed to explain simple health behaviors such as vaccinations or screenings, and hence did not include the influence of other people in the environment or the role of perceived skill or ability to perform the behavior (called self-efficacy). The role of self-efficacy has now been added to the model to explain long-term behaviors such as dietary behaviors. Self-efficacy is the

---

▶ BOX 4-2   The Health Belief Model in Practice

The health belief model proposes that readiness to take action is based on the following beliefs or convictions:

- I am susceptible to this health risk or problem.
- The threat to my health is serious.
- I perceive that the benefits of the recommended action outweigh the barriers or costs.
- I am confident that I can carry out the action successfully.
- Cues to action are present to remind me to take action.

confidence we have that we can perform the behavior (such as selecting, storing, and preparing fruits and vegetables in a tasty way). Lack of self-efficacy is thus a barrier to taking action.

- *Cues to action.* External events, such as the illness of a friend or family member or news stories on a scientific study about the issue, or internal events, such as personal symptoms and pains, are cues that remind us to act. These cues may influence our perceived threat for the condition and increase the likelihood that we will take action.

The model also postulates that demographic variables such as age, sex, and ethnicity indirectly influence behavior through their impact on perceived threat or perceived benefits and barriers. Likewise, sociopsychological variables such as personality, socioeconomic status, and peer and reference group pressure also influence behavior indirectly through their impact on perceived threat or perceived benefits and barriers.

A summary of the model is shown in Figure 4-1, and practice applications of the main constructs of the theory are listed in Table 4-2. An example of how this theory was used in developing educational materials for those with HIV/AIDS (Hoffman et al., 2005) is described in Nutrition Education in Action 4-1.

Evidence from Research and Intervention Studies

Because the health belief model is concerned with beliefs and concerns that can be changed through the means of communications or education, the model has been used as a

framework to guide a variety of health behavior and nutrition education investigations.

Research Studies Using the Model

In a comprehensive review of 29 prospective and retrospective health belief model–related investigations undertaken during the decade following the publication of the health belief model in 1974, Janz and Becker (1984) found that the determinants most powerful in predicting health behavior across all studies were as follows: perceived barriers to taking action (significant in 91% of studies), perceived benefits of taking action (81%), perceived susceptibility to the condition (71%), and perceived severity of the condition (59%). A study examining the differences between those who had voluntarily made dietary changes suggested by the *Dietary Guidelines for Americans* and those who had not discovered that the main differences were the perceived benefits of taking action, followed by perceived susceptibility, and then by overall health concern (a mediating determinant sometimes included in the health belief model) (Contento & Murphy, 1990). Another study found that the health belief model was a moderately good predictor of fat intake, accounting for about 30% of the variance in behavior between groups (Shafer, Keith, & Schafer, 1995). This model included the construct of self-efficacy, with items stated in terms of difficulty: "Even though I know that my way of eating is not good for me, I just can't seem to change my habits."

In a study of individuals' likelihood or intention to reduce their fat intake in order to reduce heart disease risk, perceived barriers also emerged as most important, followed by self-efficacy (Liou & Contento, 2001). A study to understand

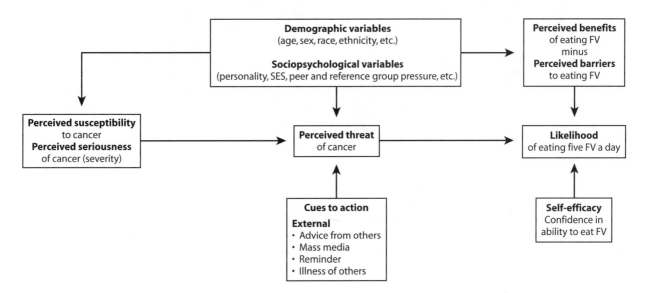

FIGURE 4-1 Health belief model (FV = fruits and vegetables).

TABLE 4-2 Health Belief Model: Major Concepts and Implications for Nutrition Education Interventions

Construct of Theory/Mediator of Behavior Change	Practice Applications
Perceived threat or sense of risk	Messages about risk for conditions such as diabetes or heart disease, based on scientific research evidence on diet–disease relationships.
Perceived severity	Messages about the serious personal impacts (medical and social) of conditions such as heart disease or diabetes.
Perceived susceptibility	Messages or activities to personalize risk for individuals based on family history or behavior through self-assessment tools.
Perceived benefits of behavior in reducing the risk	Messages about benefits of engaging in a behavior to reduce risk based on scientific evidence on the efficacy of the behavior to reduce risk; other benefits, such as taste or convenience.
Perceived barriers to engaging in the behavior	Identify and reduce perception of barriers. For example, fruits and vegetables can be inexpensive if eaten in season and can be filling. Provide messages about how to store them. Correct misconceptions, such as need for only one or two servings of fruit and vegetables a day.
Self-efficacy	Messages that provide guidance on how to make behavior easy to do.
Cues to action	Provide reminders about the behavior: posters, community billboards, and media campaigns.
Future orientation	Past or present orientation
Interactions emphasize directness and openness	Interactions emphasize indirectness, importance of "face"
Informality	Status, formality

factors that would influence pregnant women to permanently follow a high-folate diet found that all the health belief model factors were important, but the perceived benefits construct was the most predictive (Kloeblen & Batish, 1999). In a study with older adults, the perceived threat of foodborne illness was important, but safe food handling behaviors were most strongly influenced by the cues to action from news stories or labels on food packages (Hanson & Benedict, 2002). Perceived seriousness and perceived susceptibility, knowledge of risk factors, and general health motivation predicted heart disease prevention behaviors in a sample of women (Ali, 2002). These studies show that although most health belief model constructs are important mediators of dietary behavior, their relative importance differed by study, most likely reflecting the specific behavior in question and the nature of the particular groups of people in the different studies. This is suggested by a study that found that for wives the costs of a healthy diet in terms of expense, time, unpleasantness, and confusion about recommendations had a significant effect on fat intake, whereas for their husbands, perceived threat of disease and self-efficacy had a significant effect (Shafer, Keith, & Schafer, 1995).

Taken together, these studies suggest that both a sense of threat or perceived risk of disease (e.g., heart disease) *and* perceived benefits of taking action are important. Benefits in

this context are effective responses or actions individuals can take to reduce the threat or avoid the danger—actions such as eating a healthier, low-fat diet or eating organic foods. Hence the term *response efficacy* is also used. An understanding of barriers to action and a feeling of self-efficacy in overcoming barriers are also paramount. The perceived seriousness of various diet-related chronic conditions, such as heart disease, did not always appear significant in these studies, but that is because these conditions are considered severe by most people and hence beliefs were not different between people who had made dietary changes and those who had not. Those who made changes were those who believed these conditions were serious but *also* that they themselves were personally at risk. Cues to action can come from many sources but can also be effective motivators.

Intervention Studies Using the Model
Numerous intervention programs based on the health belief model have been developed and implemented in the public health arena, including dietary change. Indeed, the constructs of *benefits* and *barriers* are widely used in interventions. We shall see later that they are similar to constructs in other theories, such as the pros and cons of change in the transtheoretical model, and beliefs about outcomes (or *outcome expectations*) in the theory of planned behavior and

NUTRITION EDUCATION IN ACTION 4-1

Use of the Health Belief Model in the Development of Food Safety Materials for People with HIV/AIDS

Theory Construct/Determinant or Mediator of Behavior	Application to Food Safety Materials
Perceived susceptibility	Provided statistics and stated that people living with HIV/AIDS are more at risk for foodborne illness
Perceived severity	Stated that a foodborne illness can result in long-term health problems and even death
Perceived benefits	Provided positive, action-oriented effects of properly preparing and eating food safely; gave information on how to act, what to do
Perceived barriers	Gave enough information on food preparation and pathogens to correct misinformation; gave information to assist in properly preparing; gave reassurance
Cues to action	Gave explanations for issues brought up in discussion groups, for example, why some foods are risky, how to reduce risk for some foods by reheating, and substitutes for risky foods
Self-efficacy	Provided positive, action-oriented food selection and handling tips designed to reduce anxiety, and guidance in performing food safety actions to prevent foodborne illness

Source: Modified from Hoffman, E.W., V. Bergmann, J. Armstrong Schultz, P. Kendall, L.C. Medeiros, and V.N. Hillers. 2005. Application of a five-step message development model for food safety education materials targeting people with HIV/AIDS. *Journal of the American Dietetic Association* 105:1597–1604. Used with permission of the American Dietetic Association.

social cognitive theory. What the health belief model adds is the construct of perceived risk, which is regarded as the motivational factor that initiates the psychological readiness to take action.

A study with older Americans focused on increasing consumption of whole-grain foods by older adults (Ellis et al., 2005). The program was delivered in congregate meal sites and consisted of five sessions based on the health belief model:

- *Perceived susceptibility and severity:* Emphasizing the health conditions that occur frequently in older people that are associated with low intake of whole grains
- *Perceived benefits:* Describing the potential benefits in terms of decreasing the risk of certain health conditions
- *Perceived barriers:* Providing information on how to overcome barriers; taste testing many different whole-grain foods to overcome the barrier of taste
- *Self-efficacy:* Demonstrating and reinforcing during the sessions various ways to include whole-grain foods, teaching label reading skills, and correcting misinformation about the labeling of whole grains
- *Cues to action:* Recipes, tip sheets, and other handouts to provide continuing cues to action at home

The program resulted in increases of the frequency of eating whole-grain foods based on the mean intakes of the three-whole-grain food with the largest increases. The participants' knowledge improved (although it was high to begin with), and they believed more strongly than before that whole-grain foods would reduce risk of disease.

Likewise, an eight-session program with university employees that focused on perceived risk for cardiovascular disease and cancer, perceived benefits to taking action, and perceived barriers resulted in significant behavioral change in terms of reduced intakes of calories, fat as a percentage of calories, saturated fat, and cholesterol (Abood, Black, & Feral, 2003). Intakes of fruits and vegetables also increased but did not reach significance. An intervention involving a television program series resulted in significant improvements in people's belief that there were more benefits and fewer barriers to healthful eating, which along with cues to action (including viewing the TV series) boosted viewers' self-efficacy and behavior change (Chew et al., 2002).

A national social marketing campaign was designed to promote low-fat eating: Project LEAN (Low-fat Eating for Americans Now) (Samuels, 1993). The program consisted of several components, including media strategies to heighten public awareness about the risk of diets high in dietary fat, especially saturated fat; participation of chefs and food journalists to demonstrate to health professionals how to help the public appreciate the taste of low-fat foods; and community programs and private voluntary organization activities to reinforce the message. Dietary fat was chosen because of its health risks and because surveys showed it was a concern of the public. A series of 10 focus group interviews revealed that knowledge of sources of fat was high. However, convenience, habit, and taste were major obstacles. It was decided that the media component would consist of a national public service advertising campaign based on the health belief model and sponsored by the Advertising Council. Given that lack of motivation was considered the major obstacle to eating lower-fat foods, the campaign consisted of two components: motivational messages to enhance the sense of perceived risk (why to change) and a toll-free hotline (1-800-EATLEAN) that people could call to receive a booklet that provided information on effective actions individuals could take to reduce the risk, including recipes (how to change). The 15- and 30-second television spots used a Hitchcock-like, humorous approach to emphasize the impact of fat in the diet. The print ads are shown in Nutrition Education in Action 4-2. The messages were broadcast through various channels, including television, radio, newspapers, and media events. It was estimated that the public service advertising component reached 50% of the viewing audience, and the print publicity more than 35 million readers. The hotline received more than 300,000 calls, and numerous local campaigns were implemented.

Another social marketing campaign based on the health belief model focused on the positive message of how to reduce barriers. It was called Pick a Better Snack and was conducted in Iowa. See Nutrition Education in Action 4-3 for a description.

In sum, most of the individual concepts in the model have received empirical support even though the relationships among the concepts have not been clearly specified. As noted earlier, the model was originally developed for simple health behaviors and hence did not include concepts that address maintenance of behavior change. For that, it has had to incorporate the self-efficacy concept from social cognitive theory (Bandura, 1997), which is described in the next chapter. The model also did not provide guidance on how to adopt and maintain health behavior. The model is thus most useful in the design of the motivational component of nutrition education.

NUTRITION EDUCATION IN ACTION 4-2

Public Service Advertisements for Project LEAN

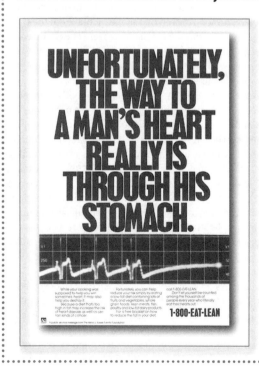

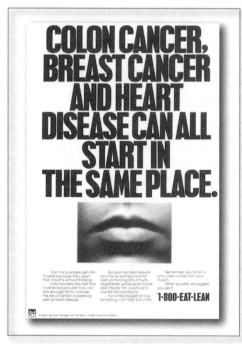

Source: Levine Huntley Schmidt and Beaver for the Advertising Council. Reprinted with the permission of the Ad Council.

NUTRITION EDUCATION IN ACTION 4-3

The Pick a Better Snack Campaign

The Pick a **better** snack campaign was developed by the partners in the Iowa Nutrition Network to increase fruit and vegetable consumption among children in Iowa by promoting a switch from high-fat, low-nutrient snacks to nutrient-dense, low- or no-fat fruits and vegetables. Intended audiences were low-income parents, providers of early childhood education, and schools, as well as children themselves. The campaign included monthly classroom lessons that featured the fruits and vegetables most available or seasonal that month, as well as simple graphics with colorful fruits and vegetables that were used on recipe cards, posters, grocery-store signage, bookmarks, brochures, and billboards.

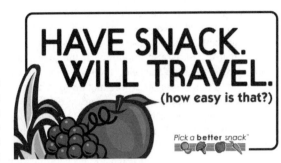

Theoretical framework

In terms of theory application, the Pick a **better** snack campaign originated from formative research, with the health belief model as the foundation. Social marketing research and materials from other states were reviewed, and campaign themes were selected for testing. Focus groups were then held. They included groups of low-income mothers, fathers, and child-care providers to determine their perceptions about motivations, benefits, barriers, and information channels. Pick a **better** snack was selected as a key message because it emphasized a simple action that can lead to increased consumption of fruit and vegetables.

- *Perceived benefits.* The focus was on the benefit that fruits and vegetables "taste good." The audience already knew the fact that fruits and vegetables are also good for your health. In the school component, students tasted different fruits and vegetables in monthly classes to increase familiarity with and enjoyment of the sensory-affective aspects of these foods.
- *Perceived barriers.* Messages through the mass media focused on making eating fruits and vegetables easy to do. Recipes were provided where appropriate.

Examples of messages are as follows:

Bananas: Peel. Eat. (how easy is that?)
Tomatoes: Slice. Eat. (how easy is that?)
Apples: Wash. Bite. (how easy is that?)

Evaluation

Two communities were selected for implementation of intense media efforts in early 2003 to determine which strategies would best reach the targeted low-income audience. Media buys were secured for billboards, bus signs, radio, and local shopper newspapers. Surveys were conducted in Food Stamp offices (n=600) and with customers in the front of grocery stores in low-income neighborhoods (n=500). Surveys indicated that the most effective implementation channels were billboards, schools, television, grocery stores, and WIC offices. Among survey respondents, 51% recalled hearing or seeing the campaign messages, 25% reported they were starting to eat more fruits and vegetables, and 36% were thinking about eating more fruits and vegetables because of Pick a **better** snack. Surveys of elementary age students (n=1455) receiving the classroom component showed a statistically significant improvement in attitudes toward fruit and vegetable snacks among these children.

More detailed information about the program, its partners, and its funding sources (Food Stamp Nutrition Education and other sources) can be found on the Pick a **better** snack website: http://www.idph.state.ia.us/pickabettersnack/default.asp.

Source: Logo and graphics used with permission of Iowa Department of Public Health and Iowa Department of Education, Bureau of Nutrition Programs and Transportation.

Perceived Personal Risk: Overcoming Optimistic Bias

The primary motivation to change in the health belief model is the level of perceived threat or risk of a specific condition, or sense of concern about an issue, as we have just seen. Perceived threat or risk is also important in the precaution adoption process model (Weinstein, 1988). In this model, the response to a risk is seen as proceeding through a series of stages, starting with persons being unaware of a risk or hazard (e.g., osteoporosis or heart disease), and then being aware but unengaged and believing that the risk may apply to other people but not to themselves. Here they have an *optimistic bias*. Individuals who reach the decision-making stage are engaged with the issue and are considering their response, such as whether to take calcium supplements or whether to reduce their saturated fat intake as a precaution. They can choose to take action or not to act. If they decide to act, they then initiate the behavior.

Based on these models, then, making people aware of threat or risk is an important task of nutrition education. Indeed, studies have found that many people are falsely optimistic about their diets (Shim, Variyam, & Blaylock, 2000). Many think that their diets are appropriately low in fat when in fact their diets are high in fat (Glanz & van Assema, 1997). Personal risk information through risk appraisals and self-assessments can be used. Such personalized feedback works probably because it counters people's tendency to be optimistically biased and encourages them to make changes in their dietary behaviors based on their true risk. Personal feedback about risk works best if the information is accompanied by information about how to deal with the threat. A review of studies found that knowing personal risk may indeed spur lifestyle changes. Giving people fitness tests plus a health hazard appraisal that estimated their risk of dying from preventable causes in the next 10 years spurred many to get more exercise. Such risk appraisals combined with information about available services showed even greater effects on people's behaviors (McClure, 2002).

Theory of Planned Behavior

The theory of planned behavior (Ajzen, 1991), derived from the earlier theory of reasoned action (Fishbein & Ajzen, 1975), was not originally developed to explain health behavior per se but has been found to be very useful for understanding food choice and health and dietary behaviors. The name of this theory would lead one to expect that it is a model for rational behavior. However, what the name really means is that this model, like other social psychological theories based on expectancy-value considerations, assumes that we make decisions in a reasonable manner; that is, that we are rational actors. The theory does not imply that our behaviors will necessarily be rational or appropriate from an objective point of view—only that they make sense to us. For example, eating a large piece of chocolate cake to make us feel good is rational

from our own point of view, whatever the nutritional merits of the act. The theory of planned behavior permits us to discern these underlying reasons by providing a framework for identifying and combining beliefs that are relevant to a given group. This allows us to understand the group's own reasons that motivate the behavior. The theory does not specify what these beliefs are, only the constructs to explore. It is thus a content-free model that can be used with a variety of health behaviors and groups. The actual beliefs must be obtained from the groups themselves, using open-ended elicitation interviews.

Nor does the theory imply that we consciously and systematically go through all the processes described here every time we act. Obviously many health-related behaviors have become automatic or habitual, such as smoking or eating cereal at breakfast. However, the theory does suggest that the attitudes and beliefs underlying these behaviors can be brought to awareness and hence changed. It is thus important for nutrition educators to understand the nature of attitudes and beliefs, how they are formed, and how they might be changed.

A summary of the model is shown in Figure 4-2, and practice applications of the main constructs of the theory are listed in Table 4-3.

Behavior

The theory of planned behavior calls for the behaviors to be stated specifically: the more specifically the behavior is stated, the more predictive the theory is of the behavior. Questions regarding very specific behavior are "How many times do you eat fruit as part of your noon day meal each month?" (Conner & Sparks, 1995) and "How often do you eat fruits and vegetables each week?" However, many studies state behaviors more generally, reflecting practical considerations, such as "eating a low-fat diet" or "eating a healthy diet" (and providing a definition of a healthy diet). In these examples, some sort of scale is used, such as a behavior frequency scale. In the area of diet, food frequency questionnaires or behavioral checklists are often used to measure behaviors. (Often, questionnaires such as these ask about behaviors in the past month or past week to make responses more accurate.) In cross-sectional studies, behaviors and the determinants of the behaviors (described later in this chapter) are measured at the same time, whereas in prospective studies, determinants are measured first, followed by the behavior some time later, such as the next day, or two or four weeks later, as specified.

Behavioral Intention

The theory of planned behavior proposes that we are more likely to engage in a behavior, such as eating low-fat foods, if we intend to do so. This most immediate mediator of behavior change is called *behavioral intention* (BI). That is, when we make plans to do something, we are more likely to do it than if we had not. This state of mind may be stated simply as *intentions*, such as "I intend to eat a low-fat diet over the next month" or "I intend to eat more fruits and vegetables and fewer high-fat snacks in the next month" (on a scale from "definitely do not" to "definitely do"). Sometimes stating intention in terms of *expected action* may be more appropriate for some behaviors, such as "How likely are you to eat foods produced by gene technology methods in the future?" or "How likely are you to support the use of gene technology in food production in the future?" (Sparks, Shepherd, & Frewer, 1995). It has been suggested that *desires* ("I would like to eat fruit as part of my midday meals") may be a precursor to behavioral intention or another way to state behavioral intention.

Research evidence based on the theories has found that reported intentions are reliably and moderately correlated ($r \cong 0.50$) with a range of health actions (Armitage & Conner, 2001). Although this means that other determinants, or mediators, of behavior need to be considered, nonetheless behavioral intention is a key mediator of behavior: it is a key indicator of level of commitment or motivation. We are certainly not likely to engage in a behavior if we do *not* intend to do so.

Attitudes

Behavioral intention is in turn determined by attitudes. Attitudes are our favorable or unfavorable judgments about a given behavior, such as "Eating fruits and vegetables would be good/bad; enjoyable/unenjoyable," rated on a 5- or 7-point scale.

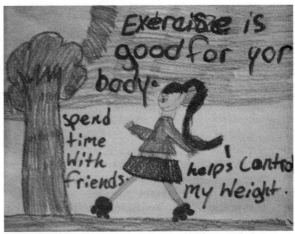

The theory of planned behavior allows us to understand what motivates us to exercise.

Attitudes have both a *cognitive/evaluative component*, such as how good or bad for health it would be to lose weight, and an *affective component*, such as how good or bad I would feel about myself losing weight. Both components influence intentions (Trafimow & Sheeran, 1998; Ajzen, 2001).

Cognitive/Evaluative Component

Attitudes are strongly influenced by our beliefs about the consequences of our actions or evaluations of the scientific evidence linking our actions to health and disease and how important these consequences are to us.

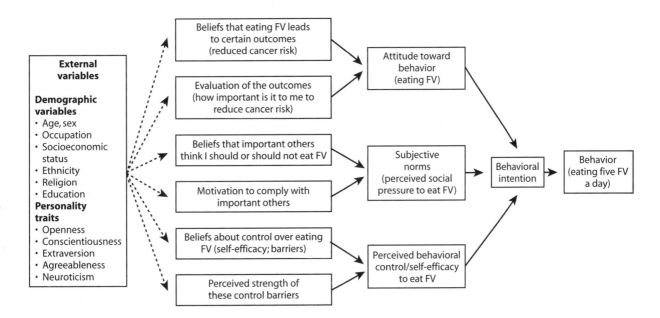

FIGURE 4-2 Theory of planned behavior: Example of behavior of eating fruits and vegetables (FV).

TABLE 4-3 Theory of Planned Behavior and Extensions: Major Concepts and Implications for Nutrition Education Interventions

Construct of Theory/ Potential Mediator of Behavior Change	Practice Applications
Attitudes	Messages and images showing healthful behavior in positive light to elicit positive feeling about it, such as a colorful, attractive group of F&V, and people expressing pleasure in eating them.
Outcome expectations (basis of attitudes)	Enhance positive expectations: Messages or strategies in groups to enhance people's expectations about taste, health benefits, and convenience of eating F&V, including through tasting, preparing, or cooking them. Decrease negative expectations: F&V can be inexpensive if eaten in season and can be filling; correct misconceptions.
Affect/sensory response to foods (physical outcome expectations)	Provide opportunities to experience and enjoy healthful food through food tastings, or food preparation and cooking experiences accompanied by eating the food prepared with others.
Subjective norms	For adolescents, show that eating F&V is cool; use peer or valued models to encourage eating F&V.
Descriptive norms	In groups, collect or give data showing that many teens do eat F&V and/or value health; correct misconceptions.
Perceived behavioral control (self-efficacy)	Messages that eating F&V can be easy and convenient (e.g., bananas: "Peel; eat; how easy is that!"). How to prepare F&V to carry to school or work.
Behavioral intention	Lead group through decision-making activities (pros and cons) to assess personal positive and negative expectations of change and commitment to try new fruits, vegetables, or recipes.
Personal norms (including perceived moral or ethical obligation)	Activities to assist group to clarify personal values and moral and ethical obligations relative to the behavior or issue.
Self-identity	Activity to bring to awareness individuals' self-identities: explore how they are related to health, community, or food system concerns.
Actual self versus ideal self	Messages or activities to bring to awareness individuals' ideals, where they come from, and how realistic or helpful they are.
Actual self versus ought-to-be self	Messages or activities to bring to awareness sources of "oughts" (e.g., being a good mom) and how to handle them.

F&V = fruits and vegetables.

Beliefs about outcomes of our behavior. Everything we do is a means to an end, and the end is the fulfillment of a value that has meaning for us. These values can be quite immediate or more enduring, more personal or more all-pervasive and global. The more immediate, or instrumental values, are our beliefs and expectations that a behavior (such as eating fruits and vegetables) will lead to certain outcomes, and are usually called *outcome beliefs* or *outcome expectations* (OEs). For example, "Eating fruits and vegetables will increase how much energy I have and reduce my risk of cancer." These beliefs about outcomes are really reasons why to engage in the behavior. Outcome beliefs are similar to the perceived benefits component of the health belief model and to the outcome expectancies component of social cognitive

theory. The more global, underlying values are described in the section "Values or Hot Buttons" later in this chapter.

Expected outcomes or reasons for a given action or behavior are of two major kinds: health outcomes based on scientific evidence and personally meaningful outcomes, including social and self-evaluative outcomes. Health outcomes are based on the scientific evidence on diet and health or diet and disease relationships, such as between eating calcium-rich foods and bone health, breastfeeding and the health of the infant, antioxidants in food and cancer, and so forth.

Personally meaningful outcomes might be taste, convenience, preparation/cooking needs, cost, good value for money, contribution to our looking better and having more energy, and so forth. Expected outcomes can be positive (e.g., good taste) or negative (e.g., high cost), as well as cognitive (e.g., "Eating fruits and vegetables will decrease my risk of cancer") and affective (e.g., "Eating fruits and vegetables will make me feel good about myself"). For example, those who believed that there was a connection between diet and cancer risk decreased their intake of fat over a three-year period (Kristal et al., 2000). These outcomes of behavior may also serve larger goals, such as empowerment of communities, support of local farmers, or social justice for those who work in the food system.

Evaluations of outcomes. Evaluations are our judgments about how desirable the outcomes of the behavior are for us. They are measured as the degree of importance of these outcomes to us, or the extent to which we desire or value them. An example is "How much energy I have is important to me," measured on some kind of scale, such as a rating from 1 to 5, with 1 meaning "not at all" and 5 meaning "extremely important."

Motivation to initiate a behavior depends on our beliefs about both the *likelihood* and the *value* to us personally of future outcomes from the behavior. Future events cannot serve as determinants of behavior in the present. However, their representations in our minds in the present can have powerful causal impacts on present action. That is, we want to maximize positive outcomes such as health, taste, or not wasting food and to minimize negative outcomes of engaging in food or nutrition behavior, such as cost or inconvenience.

Attitudes and Their Underlying Beliefs

Attitudes can be measured directly on some scale, such as the 1- to 5-point scale described earlier, or indirectly by multiplying beliefs about outcomes of our behavior and evaluations of those outcomes; that is, by combining the strength of our expectations about future outcomes of the behavior (expectancy) with the strength of the desirability of these outcomes (value). Attitudes are thus based on a theory of expectancy × value. A few aspects of attitudes and their underlying behavioral beliefs are important to keep in mind.

Attitudes toward a behavior can be considered our summaries of our decision-making processes about the behavior. We come to judge whether we are positively or negatively inclined toward a given behavior, such as eating lower-fat diets or breastfeeding, based on our underlying beliefs about the outcomes of the behavior. It has been found that attitudes and their underlying beliefs are often quite interchangeable in studies: they often yield the same predictive power (Schwarzer, 1992). Thus, beliefs about expected outcomes of behavior are major mediators of behavioral intention (through attitude formation) and hence are motivators of behavior.

In designing nutrition education interventions, we can assess and then design activities to address directly people's specific expectations about the outcome of the behavior, such as taste, cost, convenience, or wasting food. The cognitive/

evaluative component of attitudes is thus likely to be derived from communications or information about the likelihood of certain outcomes for the behavior.

Affective Component: Emotions and Enjoyment of Food

Although the cognitive component of attitudes based on beliefs about outcomes of a behavior is a major motivator of behavioral intention, the affective component of attitudes, reflecting our feelings or emotions, is also a powerful—some would say more powerful—motivator of dietary behaviors (Salovey & Birnbaum, 1989). Our emotions and feelings reflect our more enduring values, our hot buttons. Affective beliefs or feelings are more likely to be derived from direct experience, such as physiological reactions to food (e.g., taste, smell, sight, or fillingness of food) and familiarity. *Emotions* have been described as a state of arousal involving both conscious thought and physiological or visceral changes. The result of this internal process of emotion is a feeling toward a food, behavior, object, or situation.

Food preferences and enjoyment. We saw in Chapter 2 that familiarity or experience with food is a major determinant of food preferences and liking and that such sensory-affective responses to food powerfully influence food choice and dietary behavior. From their research, Rozin and Fallon (1981) found that people's sensory-affective responses to food formed a category separate from other anticipated consequences of eating. The importance of sensory-affective or emotional responses to food is quite clear to most consumers, who consistently rate taste preferences and liking as a leading motivator of their dietary choices. It was also demonstrated in a study using the theory of reasoned action to study the choice of low-salt breads (Tuorila-Ollokainen, Lahteenmaki, & Salovaara 1986). The theory predicted 38% of buying intentions and 21% of actual selections. However, the individuals were also given a taste test and asked to rate breads in terms of "liking." When this rating of liking was included in the theory, the values were improved to 52% and 32%, respectively. In fact, liking was by itself the best predictor of the behavior.

Feelings, emotions, and anticipated feelings. Another aspect of the affective component of attitudes is our feelings and emotions about a food, behavior, object, or situation and our involvement. For example, our attitude toward losing weight may be motivated not only by our belief that it will make us healthier or look better (the cognitive aspect of attitudes) but also that it will make us feel good about ourselves by being able to take control of our lives or some other personally meaningful feeling. Helping our children enjoy eating more vegetables may make us feel good about ourselves as parents.

Anticipated affect or feelings. Anticipated regret or worry about the consequences of acting or failing to act has also been shown to be a mediator of preventive health behavior. A study showed that anticipated affective reactions or feelings influenced the intention to eat junk foods (Richard, van der Pligt, & de Vries, 1996). Another example in the behavioral nutrition area might be our anticipated regret or worry that regularly eating foods high in saturated fat may increase our risk of getting heart disease later.

Relationship Between Cognitive and Affective Components

The cognitive and affective components are inextricably linked to each other. Development of preferences or feelings arises from both direct experience of food and at least some evaluation or thinking, just as expectation (thinking) about how a food will taste is based on some prior sensory-affective response to the food (Bandura, 1986). Studies have found that when beliefs and feelings are consistent with each other, both are equally good at predicting attitudes and behavior. However, where they are not consistent, feelings are primary (Ajzen, 2001).

Individuals may differ in their tendency to base their attitudes on beliefs or feelings. In studies on social issues, the attitudes of those identified as "thinkers" were better predicted by their beliefs than by their feelings, whereas the reverse was true for individuals identified as "feelers" (Ajzen 2001). In a parallel fashion, attitudes toward some foods or issues (e.g., specific foods such as chocolate) may be based largely on feelings, whereas attitudes toward others (e.g., eating foods produced through gene biotechnology) may be based largely on reasoning and the evaluation of scientific information.

Attitude Strength and Stability

Studies have shown that strong attitudes toward foods are more predictive of behavioral intentions than weak attitudes (Sparks, Hedderley, & Shepherd, 1992). Information of high personal relevance leads to the formation of stronger attitudes. Stronger attitudes are less susceptible to change. Stable attitudes are also more predictive of dietary behaviors. For example, stable attitudes were predictive of eating a low-fat diet three months later (Conner, Sheeran, & Norman, 2000) and of eating a healthier diet six years later (Conner, Norman, & Bell, 2002). More stable attitudes are also more resistant to persuasion. The downside of these findings is that strong and stable attitudes toward less nutritious foods or diets are less likely to be changed by nutrition education. The upside is that once people form strong and stable attitudes toward more healthful food practices—through nutrition education, for example—these are likely to last and to be predictive of behavior.

Attitudinal Ambivalence–Conflicting Attitudes

Beliefs about the outcomes of a behavior are numerous and may often be conflicting (Armitage & Connor, 2000a; Ajzen, 2001). Ambivalence may reflect the coexistence within individuals of both positive and negative beliefs about outcomes. This is especially true for food choices and dietary behaviors. For example, eating fruits and vegetables may be desirable because doing so reduces the risk of cancer, but fruits and vegetables may also be expensive and inconvenient to carry around or eat; animal products may taste good, but there may also be concern about animal welfare issues. Ambivalence may also result from a conflict between the cognitive component (chocolate cakes are fattening) and the affective component of attitudes (I love how I feel when I eat chocolate). The relative strengths of these thoughts and feelings will influence whether individuals will take action. For example, greater ambivalence about eating meat, vegetarian, or vegan diets resulted in weaker associations between attitudes and intentions (Povey, Wellens, & Conner, 2001). The same was found for ambivalence about eating chocolate or meat (Sparks et al., 2001). Ambivalent attitudes are weak and are more susceptible to persuasive communication.

Subjective Norms (Perceived Social Pressure)

Subjective norms, or perceived social pressure, are our beliefs that most people who are important to us either approve or disapprove of our performing a behavior (e.g., "People who care about me think that I should/should not eat fruits and vegetables"). Subjective norms are similar to social outcome expectations in social cognitive theory. Subjective norms are in turn determined by the following:

- *Normative beliefs:* The strength of an individual's beliefs that specific important people approve or disapprove of the behavior ("My close friends/parents think that I should/should not eat fruits and vegetables").
- *Motivation to comply:* The strength of the desire of an individual to comply with these people's opinions ("How much do you want to do what your friends think you should do?"). This strength may range from "not at all" to "very much." Because individuals' motivations may be related to the approval of a range of specific others, the variety of people (e.g., peers, family) whose approval is important for the particular behavior (e.g. eating fruits and vegetables or soda drinking) and the particular population (e.g., teenagers) must be assessed in order to design effective nutrition education.

Descriptive Norms

It has been shown that *descriptive norms* can be as important as injunctive ones in motivating health behaviors (Sheeren, Norman, & Orbell, 1999). Descriptive norms include beliefs about other people's *attitudes* toward the behavior in question (group attitude), such as attitudes toward drinking soda, and perceptions of other people's *behavior* (group behavior), such as how many in an individual's social circle drink soda.

Relationship Between Attitudes and Subjective Norms

Individuals differ on the relative weight they place on attitudes and on the opinions of others. These relative weights also differ across behaviors. For example, subjective norms may be more important in cultures that are more collectivist in nature, whereas attitudes may be more important in individualistic cultures (Ajzen, 2001). Some food behaviors (such as eating low-fat foods) may be more influenced by attitudes, whereas others (such as breastfeeding) are more influenced by social norms.

Perceived Behavioral Control

We also act in accordance with our perceptions of our control over the behavior, or *perceived behavioral control* (PBC). This mediator of behavior was added to the original theory of reasoned action to account for many behaviors over which we may not have full control, such as dietary behaviors. For example, healthier foods may not be easily available in our local grocery store, or we may not know how to cook. Perceived behavioral control influences both intention and behavior, probably because *perception* of control is likely to increase our effort to successfully carry out an intention and because perception of control may reflect *actual* control. (see Figure 4-2). Perceived behavioral control is individuals' perceptions about the degree to which they have some control over the behavior, can overcome barriers, or can perform the behavior.

Relationship of Perceived Behavioral Control to Self-Efficacy and Perceived Barriers

Perceived behavioral control is similar to the self-efficacy construct of social cognitive theory and as used in the health belief model (Armitage & Conner, 1999, 2001). Many researchers consider the terms to be interchangeable (Ajzen, 1991, 1998; Bandura, 2000; Fishbein, 2000), with some using the term *self-efficacy* (Fishbein, 2000) in models and others *barriers* (Lien, Lytle, & Komro, 2002; Kassem et al., 2003). Therefore, for most practical purposes in designing nutrition education interventions, using the term *self-efficacy* in this context is appropriate. However, you will see when you read the literature that there are some differences between constructs.

Whereas self-efficacy is generally defined in terms of personal competence or confidence in being able to carry out a given behavior ("I am confident that I could successfully eat five fruits and vegetables a day if I wanted to"), perceived behavioral control includes the notion of perceived difficulties, including personal resources and external barriers, tapped by such questions as "How much control do you feel you have over eating fruit and vegetables each day?" These two concepts can also be combined to have participants respond to such statements as "I am confident that I can eat fruit at work even if it is not readily available" or "I can avoid eating attractive, high-fat foods, even at a party."

> ### ▶ BOX 4-3 Theory of Planned Behavior in Practice
>
> The theory of planned behavior proposes that individuals are likely to take a specific action if they *intend* to take that action. Intention to take action is based on the following beliefs and feelings:
>
> - I believe that taking this action will lead to outcomes I desire.
> - I perceive that the positive outcomes of taking this action outweigh the negative outcomes.
> - I have positive feelings about taking this action, and taking action will make me feel good about myself.
> - People important to me think that I should take this action and their opinions are important to me.
> - I am confident that I can carry out the action, despite difficulties.

Extensions of the Theory of Planned Behavior: Personal Norms and Self-Representation

Research has led to investigations of possible extensions of the theory of planned behavior by incorporating mediators of behavior that reflect on the self, such as moral norms and self-identity. In the area of food and nutrition, these mediators have been found to make some additional independent contribution to the prediction of behavior. Figure 4-3 summarizes the many constructs of the extended theory of planned behavior and how they are related to and predict behavioral intentions and behavior. Table 4-3 shows how the constructs of the theory can be applied to nutrition education practice.

Personal Normative Beliefs: Perceived Moral or Ethical Obligation

A number of researchers have found that personal normative beliefs are important (Armitage & Conner, 2000b). This concept is similar to Bandura's notion of personal standards against which one judges oneself. An example might be "I feel I should breastfeed my baby." Studies have shown that moral and ethical considerations make some contribution to prediction of behavior, such as parents giving milk to their children ("I feel it is my moral obligation to feed my child milk/healthful foods") (Raats, Shepherd, & Sparks, 1995) or people's expectations about foods produced by biotechnology processes ("I feel that I have an ethical obligation to avoid eating food produced by gene technology" and "I feel that I have an ethical obligation to support the use of gene technology in food production") (Sparks, Shepherd, & Frewer, 1995). A review has found that moral norms are important in bridg-

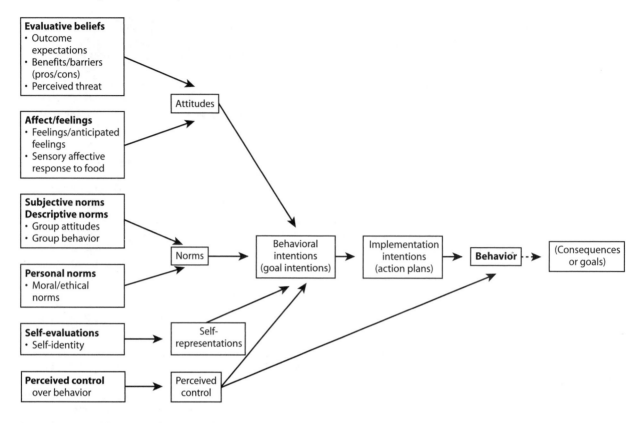

FIGURE 4-3 Extended theory of planned behavior

Source: Based on Abraham, C., and P. Sheeran. 2000. Understanding and changing health behaviour: From health beliefs to self-regulation. In *Understanding and changing health behaviour from health beliefs to self-regulation,* edited by P. Norman, C. Abraham, and M. Conner. Amsterdam: Hardwood Academic Publishers.

ing the intention–behavior gap (Godin, Conner, & Sheeran, 2005). A related concept is perceived personal responsibility, such as "I feel that I have a responsibility to buy organic foods to improve the health of the natural environment" (Bissonette & Contento, 2001).

Self-Identity

Related to the focus on personal norms are other thoughts we have about ourselves, including our self-concept or self-identity, referring to the relatively enduring characteristics people ascribe to themselves (Sparks, 2000). These *self-refer-ent factors* have been shown to contribute some additional predication of behavior: "I think of myself as someone who is concerned about environmental issues" (Sparks, Shepherd, & Frewer, 1995; Bissonette & Contento, 2001; Robinson & Smith, 2002); "I think of myself as someone who is very concerned with 'green' issues" (Sparks, Hedderley, & Shepherd, 1992), or "I think of myself as a health-conscious consumer."

Qualitative studies have found that individuals had identities in food choice related to personal traits, their reference

group, and social categories. These identities were both stable and dynamic over time and were shaped by life experiences (Bisogni et al., 2002). *Ideal-self versus actual-self discrepancies,* resulting in disappointment, sadness, or depression, and *ought-to-be self versus actual-self discrepancies,* resulting in fear and anxiety, have been studied in other domains (Abraham & Sheeran, 2000). In nutrition, surveys of consumers often reveal these kinds of considerations when individuals think about their diets. For example, one survey found that people's predominant emotions about their diets were guilt, worry, helplessness, anger, and fear: "I feel like a bad mom. I know that my kids should have better things to eat" (IFIC Foundation, 1999). These considerations are especially strong relative to weight issues.

Personality

The theory of planned behavior, like the health belief model, proposes that personality may have an indirect effect on health behaviors, being mediated through the more imme-diate cognitive-motivational variables such as beliefs and attitudes. Studies investigating personality effects in health behaviors show that of the personality traits commonly examined in studies (openness, conscientiousness, extraversion, agreeableness, and neuroticism) (McCrae & Costa, 1987), conscientiousness is the trait most likely to have an impact on health behavior; although it has a direct impact on exercise behavior, its effect on dietary behavior tends to be indirect, mediated by intention or attitude (Conner & Abraham, 2001; Chang, Contento, and Cheng 2003).

Implementation Intentions (Action Plans)
Personal experience suggests, and research confirms, that behavioral intentions are not sufficient to initiate difficult behaviors such as dietary change. Intentions are more likely to be carried out if they are first translated into *implementation intentions,* specifying exactly when, where, and how the particular behavior will be undertaken. In other theories these are called *action plans.* The general behavioral intention may be to eat five fruits and vegetables a day. However, to make that a reality, we will need to make more specific plans, such as "I will have a midmorning snack of fruit and add one vegetable to my lunch each day this week."

It is hoped that after the implementation intentions for a new healthy behavior have been carried out for some time, the behavior will become more automatic or habitual. It has be noted, however, that setting an implementation intention for a healthy behavior (e.g., eating more fruit for a snack) by itself does not necessarily drive out a habit that might be counter to this intention (e.g., eating fatty snacks and sweets) (Verplanken & Faes, 1999).

Evidence for the Theory from Research and Intervention Studies

Research on Food Choice and Dietary Behaviors
The theory of planned behavior (and the theory of reasoned action before it) has been studied extensively and rigorously in the social psychology field and used widely to understand health issues. It has also been used in numerous studies to investigate influences on food choice and dietary behavior. A review of studies using meta-analysis showed that the variables or constructs of the theory of planned behavior explained or predicted 41% of intentions and 34% of behaviors across a variety of health behaviors (Godin et al., 1996). This is considered very good for such studies. In food-related studies with adults, the theory of planned behavior explained (predicted) 57% of the intention to eat five servings of fruits and vegetables, and 32% of actual fruit and vegetable consumption (Povey, Wellens, & Connor, 2001). Among adolescents, the theory of planned behavior explained 34% of the variance in soft drink intake (Kassem et al., 2003) but only 17% of eating a healthful diet (defined in terms of calories,

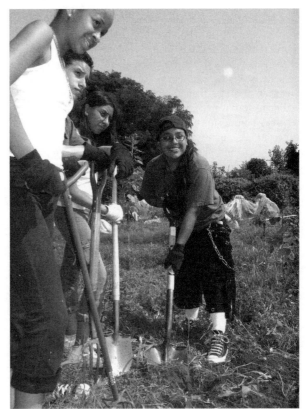

These students' self-referent factors encourage them to volunteer on weekends.

fat, and fruits and vegetables) (Backman et al., 2002). Soft drink intake is a very specific behavior, whereas a "healthful diet" is much more general, representing several behaviors. We have noted before that theories or models are better at explaining health behavior when the behavior is specifically focused or defined. The effectiveness of the model may thus depend on how specifically the behavior is defined as well as on the nature of the group.

A few specific studies are described here to indicate the range of behaviors and groups with whom the theories have been used. Each of these studies was preceded by extensive open-ended interviews or focus groups, or both, to gain insight into the factors important to the group with respect to food. As noted earlier, the theories are content-free: they do not specify what the specific beliefs are, only the constructs to explore, since the actual beliefs differ by group and by behavior.

The theory of reasoned action was used to investigate the dietary behaviors of college students. One study of fast food consumption found that the students' own beliefs were more important than the opinions of others, in particular, beliefs about whether the food at such establishments would be tasty, nutritious, of low quality, or limited in variety (Axelson, Brinberg, & Durand, 1983). In contrast, another study found that students' intention to reduce the fat and sugar in their diets was influenced by both subjective norms and personal attitudes, with norms, however, being more important than attitudes (Saunders & Rahilly, 1990). Interestingly, health majors were more influenced by beliefs and values, whereas non-health majors were more influenced by social expectations. Significant beliefs about the effectiveness of reducing fat and sugar in the diet included the following: would increase energy level, would feel good about self, and would avoid mood swings.

Studies with adolescents have examined a variety of behaviors. Eating chocolate and sweets, chips (french fries), and fruit at lunchtime was investigated in one study (Dennison & Shepherd, 1995). Attitudes and perceptions of control were most important in predicting intentions. Although social norms (which are injunctive—"My family/friends think I should eat chips at lunchtime") were not predictive, descriptive norms ("My friends eat chips at lunchtime") were. Self-identify as a health-conscious person was a determinant or mediator of behavior intention for girls, but not boys. Dietary restraint was not a significant influence. In another study, subjective norms and perceived behavioral control, measured as perceived barriers, were most predictive of intention to eat more fruits and vegetables and fewer high-fat foods, with the prediction of barriers being significant for both indirect effects through intentions and direct effects on behavior (Lien, Lytle, & Komro, 2002). A further study with adolescents, this time of "eating a healthful diet" (defined in terms of calories, fat, and fruit and vegetable consumption), found that the constructs of the theory of planned behavior together predicted 42% of intention and 17% of behavior (Backman et al., 2002). All three constructs of the theory of planned behavior were good predictors; the underlying outcome beliefs that were most important were as follows: like the taste of healthful foods, feel good about self, tolerate giving up liked foods, and lose or maintain a healthy weight.

For soft drink consumption, which is a very specifically defined behavior, the predictions (R^2) by the constructs of the theory of planned behavior were high: 64% for intention and 34% for behavior (i.e., soda consumption) (Kassem et al., 2003). The strongest predictors of soda consumption were attitude and the subjects' underlying outcome beliefs (feel healthy, become hyper, gain weight, quench thirst), followed by perceived behavioral control (availability at home and school, money) and subjective norms. One study examined the role of an expanded theory of planned behavior on buying or eating local and organic foods by adolescents (Bissonnette & Contento, 2001). It found that behavior was best predicted by behavioral intention, beliefs about outcomes, and perceived social influences. Also significant were perceived responsibility for buying and eating organic foods,

and self-identity for buying and eating local food. A study with adults had similar findings (Robinson & Smith, 2002).

Numerous studies with adults have been conducted using the theory of reasoned action and the theory of planned behavior in the area of food choice and dietary change. Beliefs about outcomes of behavior have been consistently demonstrated to be one of the most powerful motivators of behavior change. For example, those who believed that there is a connection between diet and cancer risk decreased their intake of fat over a three-year period (Patterson, Kristal, & White, 1996). The importance of eating vegetables, their health benefits, convenience, and the taste of vegetables were highly associated with eating vegetables in a variety of situations in another study (Satia et al., 2002). Intrinsic motivations or beliefs about outcomes, such as staying healthy, feeling better, preventing illness, and controlling weight, have been found to be more important than extrinsic motivations such as social norms and rewards (Trudeau et al., 1998).

Many other studies have shown that the constructs of these theories explain eating a low-fat diet (Conner, Norman, & Bell, 2002) and following meat, vegetarian, or vegan diets (Povey, Wellens, & Connor, 2001). These theories have also been used to explain behaviors related to the food system, namely, eating organic foods and being a green consumer (Sparks, Hedderley & Shepherd, 1992) and eating or supporting foods produced with gene biotechnology (Sparks, Shepherd, & Frewer, 1995). Constructs of the theory of planned behavior explained 40% of behavioral intention and 18% of actual fruit and vegetable consumption in older adults (Sjoberg, Kim, & Reicks, 2004).

The constructs of the theory of planned behavior (i.e., the determinants that mediate the behavior) explained 49% of milk consumption in a sample of pregnant women enrolled in or eligible for the Women, Infants and Children program (Park & Ureda, 1999). The most important reasons for—or outcome beliefs about—drinking milk were taste, quenching thirst, and perceived health consequences. Also important were the behavioral control beliefs of confidence in being able to keep milk fresh and having access to milk. Milk intake is, of course, important for pregnant women. Thus, understanding these beliefs or motivations can be used as the basis for designing nutrition education programs that are relevant to such women. This study is discussed in Nutrition Education in Action 4-4.

Intervention Studies

Using the theory of planned behavior to develop interventions involves two stages. In the first stage, the theory is used to identify which of the constructs or mediators of behavior are relevant for the target group and thus should be addressed. In the second stage, the message content is designed based on these relevant beliefs. If the model is used in a strict way, with all the variables, then both of these stages can be

NUTRITION EDUCATION IN ACTION 4-4

Using the Theory of Planned Behavior to Understand Milk Consumption Among Pregnant Women Enrolled in the Women, Infants and Children (WIC) Program

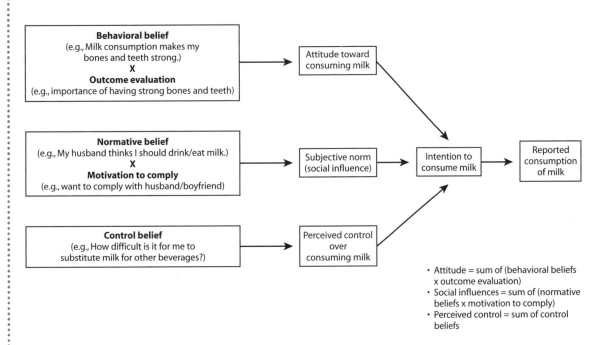

- Attitude = sum of (behavioral beliefs x outcome evaluation)
- Social influences = sum of (normative beliefs x motivation to comply)
- Perceived control = sum of control beliefs

Target Audience and Behavior
- *Audience:* Pregnant women enrolled in, or eligible for, the WIC program
- *Behavior:* Consumption of milk and of milk used in cooking or added to cereal, quantified as the number of cups per day

Theory Constructs/Mediators
- *Behavioral intention:* "How likely is it that you will drink at least 2 cups of milk a day (including milk from milk-containing foods) for the next month?" and "How often do you plan to drink/eat milk for the next month?"
- *Outcome expectations:* Fifteen belief items, such as taste, provides my baby with necessary nutrients, makes me fat, quenches my thirst, makes me feel great, good for my skin and hair.
- *Normative beliefs:* Six items, such as my best friend, mother/parents, sister/brother, or nurse/WIC staff/nutritionist think I should drink milk.
- *Beliefs about control:* Twelve items such as able to buy/get whenever I want, difficult to drink milk.

Results
The following beliefs were among the most predictive of milk consumption.
- *Behavioral beliefs:* Taste, provides my baby with necessary nutrients, quenches my thirst, makes me feel sick/upsets my stomach, makes my bones and teeth strong, causes constipation
- *Social influence:* None significant
- *Control beliefs:* Able to buy/get whenever I want, able to drink 2 cups per day, able to keep milk fresh, kept at home for me

Source: Park, K., and J.R. Ureda. 1999. Specific motivations of milk consumption among pregnant women enrolled in or eligible for WIC. *Journal of Nutrition Education* 31(2):76–86. Diagram used with permission of the Society for Nutrition Education.

quite labor intensive and time-consuming. However, numerous interventions have used the key elements of the theories with some success, focusing on outcome beliefs, social norms, and self-efficacy. Mass media campaigns have most often drawn on attitude-change theory to develop messages that are motivating. Messages are in essence "arguments" for the behavior, providing outcome expectation information, including perceived benefits.

Several national media-based interventions have used the theory of reasoned action or the theory of planned behavior. The Take Five program in the United Kingdom to increase fruit and vegetable consumption had a significant impact on several outcome beliefs, notably about the link between diet and cancer and the role of vegetables (Anderson et al., 1998). The 5 A Day fruits and vegetables national program in the United States also used outcome beliefs (or reasons for taking action) for its main message: eating five servings of fruits and vegetables daily can improve your health (Potter, 2000). The theory of reasoned action was used as the basis for a media campaign called "1% or Less" that encouraged people to switch from higher-fat milk to milk with 1% or less fat (Booth-Butterfield & Reger, 2004). The campaign targeted behavioral beliefs and found significant effects on intention, attitudes, and behavioral beliefs; these were related to changes in self-reported milk use. A brief telephone-delivered message followed up by three mailings compared beliefs regarding individuals' personal and social responsibility to eat five fruits and vegetables (Williams-Piehota et al., 2004). Both types of messages increased intake substantially, with the social message slightly more effective over a longer term.

5 A Day–Power Play, a social marketing program in California to encourage fourth and fifth graders to eat five servings of fruits and vegetables a day used constructs from several theories, including constructs listed earlier in this chapter and constructs from social cognitive theory and resiliency theory (Foerster et al., 1998). The program focused on school activities conducted over eight weeks. However, children in some schools received messages from other channels as well, including supermarkets, farmers' markets, community youth organizations, and media. Parents were involved in family fun nights. The program resulted in a significant increase in fruit and vegetable intake by students. The program is summarized in Nutrition Education in Action 4-5.

A worksite program measured beliefs, attitudes, and behavioral intention (motivation) and found a significant impact on these variables, accompanied by more healthful eating (Kristal et al., 2000). In addition, many studies have used an approach to intervention that involves tailoring the nutrition education to individuals by using theory of planned behavior constructs and stages of change and have found it an effective approach. Here individuals are given a questionnaire (by mail or on the Web); based on how the individuals

score on each of the variables, they receive messages that are personally tailored to the influences that are particularly relevant to them (Brug, Campbell, & van Assema, 1999).

Summary of Theory of Planned Behavior

The primary potential mediators of behavior change in the theory of planned behavior are as follows:

- Our desire to maximize positive outcomes (e.g., health, reduction of chronic disease risk, weight control) and to minimize negative outcomes (e.g., cost, inconvenience) of engaging in food- or nutrition-related behavior (e.g., eating more calcium-rich foods)
- Our desire to comply with the expectations of people who are important to us
- The feeling that we have control over the behavior and are self-efficacious

At some point in our thinking process, positive outcomes will sufficiently outweigh negative outcomes such that we will be willing to try to take action or will state an intention to do so, such as adding more calcium-rich foods to our diets or, for those concerned about food sustainability issues, buying local or certified sustainable foods. As noted in the previous chapter, chaos theory suggests that we may not know exactly when this point in thinking leading to intention and action occurs; however, if we have numerous opportunities to contemplate and weigh options and feelings, we are more likely to reach this point. The behavioral intention is translated into action through the development of specific implementation plans. The primary resource needed to engage in the behavior is our estimation of our perceived control over the behavior. The model implies a process approach to dietary change (outcome beliefs and attitudes, social norms, and beliefs about control lead to behavioral intention, which then leads to behavior) but does not provide any specific suggestions for processes that people can use to make changes.

Other Potential Mediators of Food Choice and Dietary Behavior Change

Values or Hot Buttons

Values are an important basis for action. The theories we use in the dietary change area are based on expectancy-value theory, which, as we have seen, posits that individuals are motivated to take action if the action will lead to outcomes or goals they value (Lewin et al., 1944). These valued goals may be quite immediate and instrumental, that is, important to achieve certain ends, such as taste, seeming cool, losing weight, or being liked by one's friends. We have called these goals *outcome expectations* in our discussion so far. Others are more global and are called *terminal* or *end-state values*. These are often set by our culture or subculture and are relatively enduring. A widely used set of end-state values is

NUTRITION EDUCATION IN ACTION 4-5

Five A Day–Power Play: A Program to Increase Fruit and Vegetable Consumption

This social marketing program was originally evaluated with fourth and fifth graders. It used constructs from several theories, including resiliency theory. It used five communications channels: schools, supermarkets, farmers' markets, community youth organizations, and media. Schools were assigned to a school-only condition, a school-plus-community condition, or a control condition.

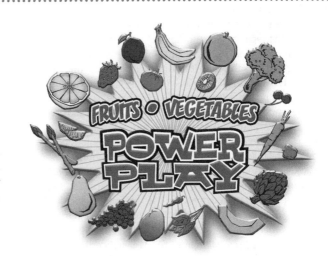

Behavior: Intakes of fruits and vegetables assessed through 24-hour food diaries

Classroom component: Classroom strategies to address theory constructs

- *Affect/motivation:* Taste testing, making fruit kabobs, singing or dancing to 5 A Day rap song.
- *Knowledge/outcome expectation:* Five A Day message through classroom activities (such as word scrambles), on all materials, and Supermarket Sleuth grocery store tours.
- *Skills:* Children learned to identify new foods and designed a meal for school cafeteria.
- *Social norms:* Students observed their peers eating and enjoying vegetables and fruits.
- *Bonding and belonging:* Children surveyed family about vegetable and fruit consumption and participated with family in family fun events.
- *Self-assessment:* Power Passport (2-week diary).
- *Reward and recognition:* Contests and recognition.

Other channels

- *In supermarkets:* Power Play! tours, posters, signs, grocery bags, and special games and contests for children.
- *Families:* Special family fun events for children and parents in school gymnasium; families made fruits and vegetables available at home.
- *Local television stations:* Aired Power Play! public service announcements.

Results: The mean intake of fruits and vegetables at the end of the program was as follows:

School-plus-community condition	3.3 servings a day
School condition	2.9 servings a day
Control condition	2.3 servings a day

Expansion to the California Children's 5 a Day-Power Play! Campaign

Since this study was conducted, the program has expanded to become state-wide, with the purpose of motivating and empowering California's 9- to 11-year-old children to eat three to five cups of fruits and vegetables and get at least 60 minutes of physical activity every day. The program also promotes environmental changes that make practicing these behaviors both easy and socially acceptable.

The campaign helps communities throughout the state to bring these messages to children through school classrooms and cafeterias; community youth organizations, including after-school and summer programs; farmers' markets; supermarkets; restaurants; and the media. The campaign has many partners and funding sources: It involves 400 schools, 3,000 teachers, and 500 community youth organizations, as well as media and public relations activities.

Source: Foerster, S.B., J. Gregson, D.L. Beall, et al. 1998. The California children's 5 a Day–Power Play! Campaign: Evaluation of a large-scale social marketing initiative. *Family Community Health* 21:46–64; and excerpts from http://www.dhs.ca.gov/ps/cdic/cpns/powerplay/download/PowerPlay_FactSheet.pdf Accessed 10/16/06. Logo used with permission.

that of Rokeach (1973): an exciting life, a world of beauty, inner harmony, a sense of accomplishment, social recognition, national security, a comfortable life, pleasure, a world at peace, equality, family security, freedom, happiness, mature love or sexuality, salvation, self-respect, true friendship, and wisdom. He did not include health as a value because he believed that health was important for everyone and thus did not differ among people. However, health was incorporated in the list of values in a food choice study for adolescents and was found to exert some influence on food choices (Williams, Michela, & Contento, Personal communication).

Marketers often use Kahle's list of values (Kahle, 1984; Andreason 1995): self-respect, sense of accomplishment, self-fulfillment, fun and enjoyment in life, security, being well respected, a warm relationship with others, and excitement. Other lists include additional values such as novelty, independence, or sense of belonging. You will notice that these values are based on our emotions or deepest feelings about our selves or the world around us. Consequently, they are often referred to as people's *hot buttons*. The relative importance of these values may differ at different times. Other values may also be important. For example, a study with adults found that individuals did not want to waste food because it was linked to a larger value of not wasting resources (Pelican, et al., 2005). Likewise, exercising just to exercise, such as taking a walk, seemed to counter the larger value that all physical activity should serve useful purposes.

Personal and Functional Meanings Given to Food

Out of these values may emerge very personal meanings we attach to the foods we eat, based on specific past experiences, the functions they serve in our lives, and feelings and values we have. Foods may be eaten because they are comfort foods for us or remind us of positive childhood experiences, or because we want to use them to manage feelings. Some of these meanings can also be seen as *outcome expectations* (e.g., if I eat this food, I will feel comforted or it will relieve my depression) or as *self-evaluations* (e.g., I deserve to eat this; I am worth it).

Although personal meanings given to food and eating are similar to expected outcomes of behavior, they are generally more intrinsic in character in that the meaning with which a behavior is imbued may be dissociated from the knowledge of outcomes that we have. For example, a study with teenagers found that although they knew that eating sweets might be unhealthy, bad for their teeth, or fattening, it was also a way to deal with frustration, stress, or anger (Spruijt-Metz, 1995). Eating junk food or skipping lunch was a way to assert their independence and personal will and to challenge (parental) authority and test boundaries. Studies with adults found that personal meanings included food as an enemy, being a picky eater or not liking to be told what to eat, and meanings related to their role in the family: the peacekeeper

whose needs were subordinated to those of others, or one who did not like to cook and would rather others do the cooking (Blake & Bisogni, 2003). These personal meanings of food must be explored and considered as we plan nutrition education programs.

Past Behavior, Habit, Routines, Automatic Behaviors

Many behaviors appear to occur without much thought. We do not seem to consciously and systemically go through a decision-making process based on beliefs and peer pressure every time we make a choice—for example, every time we approach a familiar cafeteria line, restaurant menu, or grocery store. We have routines or habits that seem to be automatic responses to situations and are often the driving force in behavior. Indeed, for many behaviors, past behavior has been shown to be a good predictor of future behavior (Triandis, 1977; Ajzen & Madden, 1986; Conner et al., 2000; Ajzen, 2001). This is especially true of frequently performed behaviors, in which the processes that initiate and control the performance of the behavior seem to become automatic, such as occurs in the area of food: one would expect past behavior to be a strong determinant of future behavior because of the habitual nature of much of eating behavior (Kumanyika et al., 2000).

Research suggests that this comes about because when we repeatedly perform a behavior in a particular context, both the overall motivation, such as our liking for cereal in the morning, and the instructions for its implementation—preparing the cereal—may become integrated in our thinking about the situation. Both the motivation and instructions for implementation are automatically triggered in memory when we are faced with the same situation. These automatic cue–response links facilitate action without deliberation and conscious decision making (e.g., eating cereal in the morning). This process may be the basis for the effects of familiarity and past behaviors. In addition, strongly held attitudes, or attitudes based on prior experience, can also result in "automatic" actions (Fazio, 1990). For example, when we pass an ice cream store, positive feelings based on prior experience may come to mind spontaneously, causing the ice cream to appear delicious and thus leading us to obtain and eat it. The various costs and benefits of eating the ice cream may not be considered at all or may be weighed only after it is eaten.

It has been suggested that reasoned processes are used under certain circumstances, and habitual or automatic processes in others (Fazio, 1990). For example, behavioral decisions may be more likely to be guided by deliberate processes of reflection when they are perceived to have serious personal consequences, such as the choice whether to breast-feed a baby. However, when consequences are perceived not to be very serious, as is the case of many everyday food choices, automatic processes will occur. The time available to make a decision may also be a factor. When there is very little time to make a decision, such as may occur in supermarket purchases, spontaneous processes may be more important than reasoning processes.

The downside of this aspect of behavior is that unhealthful eating practices may have become habitual. A key role for nutrition education in this case is to bring such habits and routines to individuals' awareness so that they can choose to change them if they wish. On the upside, it means that healthful eating patterns can also become automatic or habitual. Study findings indicate that although past health protection and exercise behaviors have some direct effect on future behavior, their effects are mostly mediated through variables of the theory of planned behavior and anticipated effects on feelings (Conner & Abraham, 2001). Another study showed that past behavior was predictive of eating a low-fat diet but that stable intentions were just as powerful, if not more so, in mediating future behavior than was past behavior (Conner et al., 2000). Taken together, these studies show that targeting both intentions and perceived control over the behavior is likely to influence behavior *despite* past behavior. Thus, nutrition education can assist individuals to make specific plans or make personal policy decisions about their habitual patterns in order to make them more healthful, such as to eat whole-grain cereals for breakfast rather than high-sugar cereals each morning. There is evidence that current habit strength can significantly predict healthful eating, such as of fruit (Brug et al., 2006).

Summary: An Integrative Model of Behavior Change

In summary, theories and the research based on them suggest that beliefs and affect are major motivational forces in food- and nutrition-related behaviors. The health belief model, theory of planned behavior, and related attitude-change models arose for different reasons, but they all seek to understand human motivation and hence are useful in this phase of nutrition education, where they can serve the needs of different interventions.

An intervention can be based on one specific theory or can integrate them. There is some debate about which is the best course of action. Many would argue that dietary behavior is too complex to be captured by any one theory and hence a combination of theories should be used (Achterberg & Miller, 2004). In addition, there are many overlapping constructs among the social psychological models used in nutrition education (Bandura, 1997, 2000; Brug, 2005). The major principle here is that if constructs are combined from several theories, they must be consistent with each other so that the constructs together provide a coherent explanatory model of dietary behavior and are based on research evidence showing their effectiveness in dietary interventions.

Indeed, because there are so many constructs in common, developers of the leading theories have proposed that, for most practical health communication and promotion purposes, the theories can be combined into a *general integrative model of behavior change* (Kok et al., 1996; Abraham & Sheeran, 2000; Fishbein, 2000; Institute of Medicine, 2002). This integrative model is shown in Figure 4-4. As you can see, the general integrated model proposes that changes in health behaviors ultimately depend on changes in behavioral outcome beliefs, normative beliefs, and beliefs about self-efficacy or control. The relative importance of each of the constructs will depend on the behavior and the population group. The translation of these beliefs into action is also influenced by skills and abilities and environmental constraints. This chapter has focused on the cognitive-motivational factors—beliefs influencing *why to* take action. The next chapter examines research and theory on facilitating the ability *how to* take action, and Chapter 6 examines how to make the environment more supportive of the desired behavior.

The constructs that are found in common among various theories and are part of the integrative model are briefly summarized in the following list.

- *Perceived risk or sense of concern.* Risk perceptions or concerns serve predominantly to set the stage for a thinking process or to initiate a state of readiness to take action. An increased sense of concern or risk (societal or personal) is important because believing that we are *not* vulnerable to a threat or that there are no negative consequences to individual or collective dietary behaviors is *not* likely to lead to any desire to change. However, mere acknowledgement of risk or concern is not sufficient to prepare one for action. The other beliefs listed here are also needed.
- *Outcome expectations, perceived benefits and barriers, or pros and cons.* These are beliefs about anticipated future outcomes stemming from the behavior and our evaluations about how desirable these outcomes are to us. Although future events cannot serve as determinants of behavior in the present, their representations in our thinking in the present *can* have important causal effects on present action. We desire to achieve *positive outcomes* that are important to us, such as eating fruits and vegetables to be good to our bodies and help control weight. We desire to avoid *negative outcomes*, such as cost, bad taste, inconvenience, or increase in weight. These outcomes may be more immediate, such as the food will taste good, or may serve larger goals, such as self-respect or social justice. Outcome expectations have been demonstrated in numerous studies to be one of the most powerful motivators of behavior change.
- *Affect or feelings about outcomes from the behavior.* The affective component of attitudes is also important. In the field of food and nutrition, a primary motivation for food choice is related to the sensory-affective

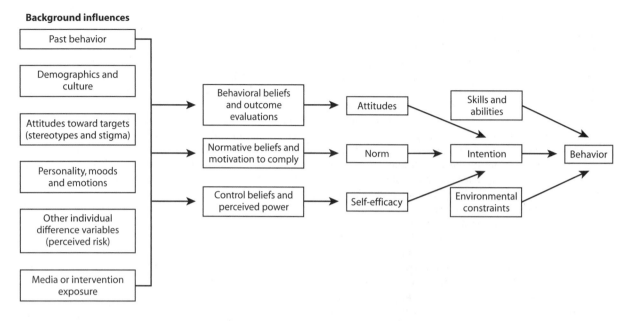

FIGURE 4-4 A general integrative model of the determinants of behavior change.

Source: Institute of Medicine. 2002. Speaking of health: Assessing health communication strategies for diverse populations. In *Improving the Health of Diverse Populations*. Washington, DC: Institute of Medicine, National Academy Press. Used with permission.

aspects of food—its taste, smell, flavor, and the physiological impact of the food on the body, such as sense of fullness. When the foods are eaten repeatedly and their effects are positive, they will become preferred or liked. This variable is included as a belief about expected outcomes of behavior in most theories. However, our reactions to food involve both beliefs (e.g., we may believe that spinach will taste bad, or that chocolate will taste good) and an affective response to food, from which we develop feelings about food. Tasting and eating food may influence our choices directly. Our sensory-affective response to food is an important motivator with a physiological basis, so it should be considered separately and planned for in nutrition education interventions. Likewise, we have many other feelings related to our dietary practices: eating a food may be a way to comfort ourselves, to show we are caring parents, or even to show defiance of authority.

- *Perceived behavioral control or self-efficacy.* This is individuals' confidence that they can carry out the behaviors, such as breastfeeding, despite obstacles or difficulties. This construct is considered so important that it has now been incorporated into most theories of behavior and behavior change. The concept carries with it the sense of personal control over one's thoughts, feelings, behaviors, and agency in the environment.

- *Social norms.* The theory of planned behavior suggests that social norms or social expectations are also important. Social influences are included in the cues to action construct of the health belief model.

Thus we can safely say that regardless of the specific theory chosen for the nutrition education intervention, the motivational phase of the intervention must at least include activities that will specifically target *outcome expectations*, *social norms*, and *self-efficacy*.

Other constructs are as follows:

- *Personal norms and beliefs about the self.* Personal norms or perceived responsibility, both personal and social, along with perceived moral obligation, may be important in some cases. For example, eating local or organic foods may be considered socially responsible, and not wasting food may be considered an important value or a moral obligation. Self-identity or social identity may influence motivation for some issues, such as self-identity as a vegetarian, a "green consumer," a health-conscious person, or a person committed to social justice issues, or identity as a member of a social/cultural or ethnic group.

- *Behavioral intention.* The motivational phase in dietary change can be considered to be concluded when individuals make a decision to take action. This decision point involves making a commitment to take action by stating a *behavioral intention.* (Other names for this construct are *goal intention* or *proximal goal.*)

Other factors may also be important for some groups and some food-related issues, such as habits, routines, or automatic processes. Behaviors sometimes seem to take place "spontaneously" as the result of strong attitudes and repeatedly performing the same behavior in the same context. Habit or routines are also important motivators of behavior. Some are more health-promoting than others.

The Case of Alicia

To determine the reasons, insights, or feelings that would motivate Alicia and individuals like her to think seriously about why to take action now about eating more fruits and vegetables, we would have to conduct some interviews. From these, the reasons or outcome expectations, attitudes or feelings, and hot buttons in the following list might emerge. Review the list of potential motivators of behavior that you wrote before you read this chapter. Modify and add to the following list those that you think would be powerful for Alicia and her friends.

- *Attitudes.* Their attitude toward eating fruits and vegetables is positive, but weakly so.
- *Outcome expectations.* There are competing beliefs or outcome expectations about eating fruits and vegetables: they are known to be healthful, but they don't taste as good as other foods, they are not convenient to eat during the day, and they are expensive.
- *Social norms.* Alicia and youth like her are busy, vibrant young people who do things together—eating fruits and vegetables is not one of them! It is just not part of their mind-set.
- *Values or hot buttons.* They feel they are now adults, able to make their own choices. Eating fruits and vegetables seems like what "good children" do. They are no longer children.
- *Self-identity.* They do not see themselves as "health-conscious eaters." They know people like that and don't want to be like them.

Nutrition education for this group thus needs to address all these determinants that are potential mediators of behavior change, helping Alicia and her friends to see "what's in it for me" to eat fruits and vegetables. The theory-based strategies described in the next section can help.

Implications for Motivational-Phase Nutrition Education: Emphasis on Why to Take Action

We have examined some of the key theories or models for understanding the motivation to act. What are the implications for nutrition education practice? How can we use this information to design nutrition education that emphasizes why to take action?

The major implication is that nutrition education programs need to address those determinants of behavior change that are related to motivation as delineated in the theories or models. A change in these determinants will in turn lead to changes in behavior, serving as mediators of behavior change, as follows:

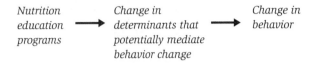

In order to address potential mediators that have motivational power, we must first identify them; only then can we select educational methods to address them. Theories are content-free and can thus help us to do two things:

1. *Identify potential mediators of change.* Theory assists us to carefully identify the key potentially relevant beliefs, attitudes, values, and other motivators of behavior change for the particular group, audience, or population with whom we plan to work. This process is called a *needs analysis* and can be done through surveys, focus groups, interviews, or other means of collecting information.
2. *Design nutrition education strategies to address potential mediators of change.* In particular, theory is used to do the following:
   - Carefully select from theory those theory constructs—or the mediators of change—that are most likely to influence behavior change for the given audience and the given intervention.
   - Match learning objectives and educational strategies to these mediators as appropriate for the audience.

How to design such theory-based nutrition educational strategies is described in great detail in Part II of this book.

A Conceptual Framework for Nutrition Education

Chapter 3 introduced the conceptual framework for nutrition education. This framework is based on the general integrative model of behavior change shown in Figure 4-4, but adds a time dimension. We noted earlier that research evidence suggests nutrition education can be conceptualized as consisting of two phases. Changes in beliefs, affect, and attitudes are essential and usually come first. Skills and abilities are also essential but usually come later. This chapter has explored the first phase—the motivational phase. Figure 4-5 presents a more detailed version of this phase, based on the theory and evidence that we have reviewed in this chapter.

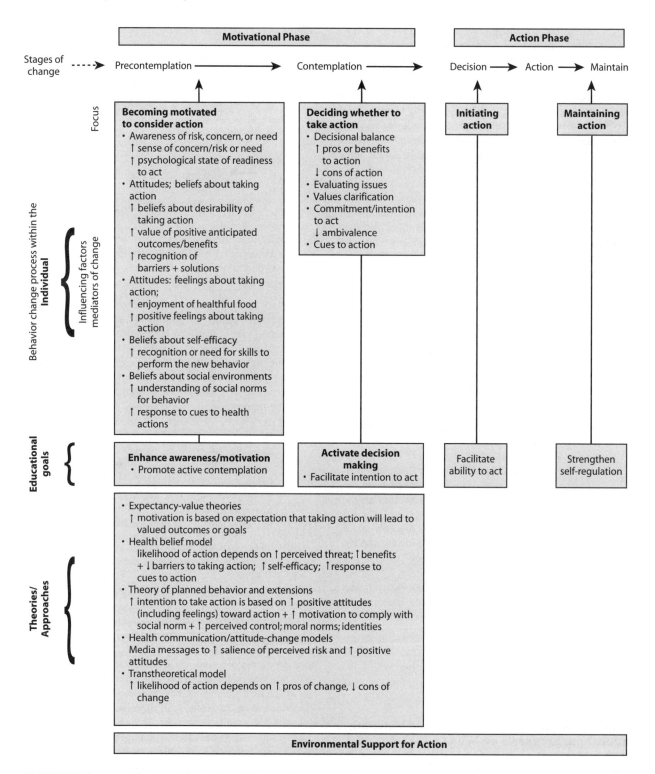

FIGURE 4-5 Conceptual framework for nutrition education: Considering action.

Influencing Factors or Mediators of Behavior Change
The dietary change process begins when individuals become motivated to consider taking action. As shown in Figure 4-5, some sense of concern about an issue or sense of personal risk may be important in order for individuals to be in a state of readiness to act. The evidence suggests that although necessary, perceived risk or concern may not be the most immediate or direct mediator of behavior change. It is a first step. In addition, individuals must also have positive attitudes toward taking action by believing that taking action will lead to outcomes they desire in terms of reducing the threat, addressing their concern, or enhancing health. Individuals also must feel that the behavior will help them achieve their values or goals. Individuals must also have self-efficacy, or confidence in their ability to carry out the necessary action. These mediators may lead individuals to a decision point about whether to take action.

Educational Goal
The educational goal of nutrition education during the motivational phase or component is to enhance awareness and motivation. We can do this by bringing to awareness the salience and personal importance of particular issues, behaviors, or practices for individuals, promoting active contemplation, and enhancing the motivation to act. By targeting potential mediators of behavior change, nutrition education interventions can assist individuals who are unaware or uninterested in an issue or behavior to become interested, think about the issue, understand the value of potential outcomes of the behavior to them personally, and increase their confidence in their own ability to obtain these outcomes. We can activate decision making by assisting individuals to clarify their values and understand and resolve their ambivalences. Finally, we can facilitate the formation of behavioral intentions and implementation plans among those who make a choice to take action.

Useful Theories
Figure 4-5 shows that several theories are particularly helpful for this phase or component of nutrition education, in particular the health belief model, the theory of planned behavior, health communication attitude-change models based on them, and the integrative model presented in Figure 4-4. These theories focus on motivational aspects of behavior change and do not provide extensive guidance on strategies for making changes. The motivational component can stand alone, as sometimes occurs in media campaigns, or as part of interventions that also provide opportunities for more extensive education, such as group nutrition education. Note that environmental supports are also important.

Translation of Behavioral Theory into Educational Strategies for Why to Take Action
Appropriate translation of information about potential mediators of behavior change into practical strategies to address them in an intervention, whatever the channel used, is a crucial process for the effectiveness of the nutrition education intervention. In this section we list the mediators of behavior change derived from theory along with potential practical, theory-based educational strategies that might be used to address them. You would only select those strategies that operationalize the theory-based potential mediators of change that you choose to use in designing your nutrition education program. The process of linking mediators of behavior change with educational practice is the central focus of this book and is described more fully in the nutrition education design process set forth in Part II.

Awareness of Risk, Concern, or Need
Interventions can be designed to make issues of concern more salient or to increase perceived risk related to personal health, community practices, or the sustainability of food system practices. People need enough knowledge of potential danger to warrant action but not so much as to paralyze them from action. It is often useful to start with, or include, educational strategies or messages to provide more accurate perceptions and understandings of risk or concern. Effective strategies might involve the following:

- *Increasing the salience of issues and problems.* Trigger films, striking national or local statistics, pictures and charts, personal stories, and other strategies can be used to make salient issues of concern, such as the increase in obesity rates, the rate of loss of farm land, how much of school lunches are thrown away, the portion sizes of food products, or the prevalence of bone loss and metabolic syndrome in adolescents.
- *Providing personal risk appraisal or self-assessment compared to recommendations.* Individuals could complete checklists, food frequency questionnaires, or 24-hour food intake recalls and compare intakes to a standard, such as number of fruits and vegetables, to give themselves an accurate picture of their intake. They could complete checklists to see how "green" their food shopping practices are (e.g., where the food comes from, or degree of packaging). Such personalized feedback helps counteract the tendency to be optimistically biased and encourage individuals to consider changes in their dietary behaviors based on their true risk. The personal feedback about risk works best if the information is accompanied by information about how to deal with the threat.

- *Making a community assessment of practices.* Information about community food practices could provide a true picture of the extent of risk or severity of an issue. Existing data or surveys, formal and informal, can be used.

Use of fear-based communications. The use of fear-based communications in health promotion activities to increase perceived risk has been the subject of some debate and discussion. Fear and threat are conceptually distinct: *fear* is defined as a negative emotion accompanied by a high level of arousal, whereas *threat* is a cognition. They are, however, intricately related, such that the higher the threat, the greater the fear experienced. Reviews of studies have found that overall, fear appeals have a moderate effect on changing attitudes, intentions, and behavior (Leventhal, 1973; Witte & Allen, 2000). Strong fear appeals produce high levels of perceived seriousness and susceptibility and are more persuasive than low or weak fear appeals—the stronger the fear aroused by a fear appeal, the more persuasive it is. However, fear appeals result in two competing responses that interfere with each other: an adaptive response to deal with the risk or danger, or a maladaptive response of denial or defensiveness. As a consequence, fear appeals are effective only if people also feel that they can do something to protect themselves. Thus, fear appeal messages are effective in bringing about behavior change when they (1) depict a significant and relevant threat, but only when the messages also (2) clearly specify that there are effective strategies in which people can engage to reduce the fear, and that (3) these strategies appear easy to accomplish. Specific instructions need to be provided on exactly when, where, and how to take action.

For example, a campaign providing cancer risk information should be accompanied by information on actions such people can take to reduce the risk, such as eating more fruits and vegetables, increasing physical activity, and getting regular checkups with physicians. The social contexts of individuals are also important to consider and should be explored with the intended audience in formative research (Salovey, Schneider, & Apanovitch 1999). How messages are framed in terms of gains and losses may be important. For example, there is some evidence that health communications about the need for people to get checkups (e.g., mammograms) are more persuasive if they are framed in terms of guarding against health losses (breast cancer), but that to get people to adopt preventive actions, communications are more effective if they are framed in terms of health benefits or gains.

Attitudes and Beliefs About Taking Action: Outcome Expectations and Perceived Benefits

A major task in enhancing motivation is to design activities that focus on beliefs about the potential desirable outcomes of behaviors, such as the benefits of eating healthful foods or food-related behaviors that contribute to the sustainability of food systems. Such beliefs are powerful motivators of behavior through their impact on attitudes, intentions, and formation of goals. As we have seen, attitudes and their underlying evaluative beliefs are often interchangeable in their impact as immediate or proximal mediators of behavior change. Thus, mass media messages or educational activities to enhance motivations or attitudes toward a given behavior (e.g., eating five fruits and vegetables) focus on *beliefs* about expected outcomes for the behavior, stated in the form of reasons or arguments for the action. Such beliefs constitute, of course, information or knowledge (that fruits and vegetables reduce chronic disease risk). However, note that it is information of the why-to category. Excluded here is knowledge of the how-to category, such as information on the nutrients in fruits and vegetables, or serving sizes in MyPyramid. Such how-to information will be needed to carry out the behavior but is not in itself motivational. Dissemination of such information is described in the next chapter.

The first step is to identify which *beliefs* and *attitudes or feelings* are relevant to the intention or goal to undertake the recommended nutrition- or food-related behavior in the given group through a thorough needs assessment. These beliefs and feelings can be identified by surveys, focus groups, interviews, or other methods. This is a crucial step and is similar to market research in the social marketing process.

A series of key beliefs underpinning intentions can then be selected as intervention targets. The relative importance of different beliefs, or reasons for action, will differ depending on the behavior and the group or audience. For example, in the case of eating fruits and vegetables, being cool may be important for teenagers, improving the health of the baby may be important for pregnant women, reducing cancer risk may be important in men, and ease of preparation may be important for women. In focus groups before the 5 A Day campaign was launched, the benefits of feeling better, health, and weight control were determined to be most salient to consumers. Despite scientific evidence, the stated benefit that eating fruits and vegetables would "cut my risk of getting cancer in half" was not considered credible or relevant to their eating choices (pollution and genetics were more important). Similarly, the benefit of "feeling less stress and a little more in control of my life" from eating fruits and vegetables was met with skepticism (Loughrey, Balch, Lefebvre, et al., 1997), affirming the importance of identifying motivating beliefs and attitudes from the audience before an educational program is designed.

These beliefs about valued outcomes, or perceived benefits, to be achieved from the recommended behavior (such as breastfeeding or eating fruits and vegetables) are then converted to messages for the mass media or into educational activities for groups. The elaboration likelihood model (ELM) proposes that individuals process messages through either a central route or a peripheral route (Petty & Cacioppo, 1986). The effectiveness or persuasiveness of our messages about the perceived benefits or desirability of the outcomes of the recommended behavior (breastfeeding, parents feeding their children healthy foods), whether delivered through group educational activities, mass media messages, or brochures and newsletters, depends on many factors, chief among them being whether the messages are constructed in such a way as to induce individuals to *think* about the messages or *elaborate* on them. In this "central processing" of the message, individuals understand and evaluate the benefits or other outcomes of behavior presented in the message or activities in light of their own established beliefs and attitudes. Beliefs and attitudes changed by this route are well thought out and become integrated into individuals' belief or attitude structure, such as "It is desirable for me to eat more locally grown foods because it will support local farmers."

Individuals are more likely to think about a given message if they judge it to be personally relevant and there are few barriers to in-depth processing of the message; that is, when the message is easy to understand, there is time to think about it, and there are not many distractions. When the message is difficult to process or does not seem relevant, individuals tend to judge the message by more superficial aspects, such as the attractiveness or credibility of the source or the associations of the food with other desirable attributes, such as a picture of a slender, attractive woman. This is the "peripheral," or "mindless," route to changes in beliefs and attitudes.

Attitudes and Feelings

As we have seen, affective attitudes and sensory-affective responses to food are powerful motivators or determinants of food choices. One important way to increase motivation to eat healthful food is to provide opportunities for individuals to experience and enjoy healthful food, for example through food tastings, or food preparation and cooking experiences in groups accompanied by eating the prepared food together. These food experiences need to be long term to have full impact. Repeated experiences and familiarity are more likely to lead to positive sensory-affective responses to new foods. Indeed, an intervention study found that after 16 weeks eating lower-fat foods, individuals' reported desires to eat low-fat foods increased and their desires to eat high-fat foods decreased (Grieve & Vander Weg, 2003). Where appropriate, groups can explore their feelings about food, understand them, and seek ways to enjoy substituting less healthful with more healthful foods. In addition, since our feelings and emotions are closely related to our deeply held values, emotion-based messaging has been proposed as a way to build on people's values and hot buttons, such as about being a good parent (McCarthy & Tuttelman, 2005).

Misconceptions

Misconceptions should also be identified through formal or informal assessment and addressed at this time. Very often behaviors are not initiated because of erroneous beliefs about expected outcomes, such as that whole grains and beans are difficult to digest. The 5 A Day campaign found that many of those surveyed believed people needed only one to two fruit and vegetable servings a day. Consequently, the need for five a day became a central message.

Social Norms and Social Expectations

Groups can be made aware of the influence of social norms on their behaviors through group activities identifying what important others think that target group members should be doing (e.g., perceptions of the spouse's or partner's approval or disapproval of breastfeeding). In addition, materials, films, and statistics can be used to indicate how individuals similar to the target group are engaging in the healthful behaviors, such as other WIC women breastfeeding, other teenagers drinking water, and so forth (descriptive norms).

Personal Norms or Internal Standards

Personal norms or internal standards and sense of responsibility can be explored through various values clarification activities. Individuals can reflect on and evaluate the importance of health in their lives and make choices about the values they wish to place on health.

Beliefs About Self-Efficacy or Perceived Behavioral Control: Barriers and Difficulties

Beliefs about self-efficacy or control over the behavior, as well as perceived barriers and difficulties in enacting the behavior, are important in the motivational phase of decision making about diet as well as in the postdecisional phase when individuals are attempting to carry out the behavior. In the motivational phase, self-efficacy can be seen as the mirror image of perceived barriers or difficulty in taking action. In group settings, perceptions of the barriers to taking action can be elicited from group members themselves, and then ways to reduce those barriers. Appropriate food- and nutrition-related knowledge and skills can also be useful here. In mass media approaches and materials, difficulties can be addressed in the messages. For example, a statewide program placed a series of messages on billboards about eating fruits and vegetables. These included pictures of bananas with the message "Peel, eat; how easy is that!" and tomatoes with the message "Slice, eat; how easy is that!" (www.idph.state.ia.us/pickabettersnack/default.asp).

Beliefs About the Self

As we have seen, many other related beliefs are also potential mediators of behavior change, such as perceived responsibility or moral obligation and personal meanings given to food and eating. These needs should be identified and addressed in the nutrition education activities where they are relevant and salient for a given audience. Such beliefs can be identified for a given group in a personal setting or through surveys, or information may be found in the published literature. The educational strategies used will also depend on the channel and on the behavior. Active methods of self-exploration and understanding are likely to be most effective. Films, discussions, or debates of the pros and cons of the behavior may be useful here. Self-presentations such as self-identity or social identity can be explored. Ideal-self versus actual-self discrepancies and ought-to-be self versus actual-self discrepancies can be explored through activities that bring to awareness these discrepancies, and strategies can be provided for handling them.

Addressing Habits or Routines

Many behaviors appear to occur without much thought. As we have seen, this results from the frequent pairing of foods and the situations in which they are consumed. Nutrition education can be directed at bringing such attitude–situation cues to awareness so that individuals can choose to change behaviors if they wish. Habit or routines are also important

motivators of behavior. Nutrition education activities can be designed to bring the less positive routines (e.g., being a couch potato) to consciousness so that they can be considered and replaced by more positive routines or habits. Since these may require more effort (e.g., exercising regularly), tip sheets, checklists, or activities can be designed to assist individuals to develop these new routines.

Overall

Taken together, it is clear that a major task in enhancing motivation is to design activities that focus on the benefits of healthful food choices and diet-related behaviors, help participants identify potential barriers to carrying out the behaviors, and explore ways to overcome barriers. Media communications is a useful strategy to deliver messages in this phase of nutrition education. Affect or feelings are particularly important in the case of food and eating. Thus, individuals should be provided with opportunity to taste and experience healthful foods, and their emotions with respect to food should be explored and understood. By addressing all these mediators of behavior change, nutrition education interventions can enhance motivation to act, activate decision making, and assist people to form intentions to act.

Questions and Activities

1. What do we mean by *theory constructs*? Describe in a few sentences.
2. Describe briefly what you think are the essential features of each of the following theories in terms of how they explain health motivations:
   a. The health belief model
   b. The theory of planned behavior
3. Describe in your own words the following theory constructs. How are the terms related to motivation?
   a. Outcome expectations
   b. Perceived threat
   c. Perceived susceptibility
   d. Perceived benefits
   e. Perceived barriers
   f. Attitudes
   g. Behavioral intentions
   h. Subjective norms
   i. Self-efficacy
   j. Self-identity
   k. Perceived behavioral control
4. Several of the constructs listed in Question 3 are similar in concept but have different names because of the different origins of the theories. Which are they?
5. Now that you have read the chapter:
   a. Can you match up *each* of the reasons and difficulties that you listed at the beginning of the chapter for a food-related change that you would like to make with at least *one construct* of one of the theories described?

Reasons and Difficulties You Stated	Name of Theoretical Construct	Justification for Assignment

   b. In what ways do the theories help you understand your food choices and eating behaviors better?
6. If you were asked to design media messages for a group of young people like Alicia, what do you think would be one key message you would want to get across?
7. If you were asked to design a session for the women enrolled in the WIC program described in this chapter, what would you focus on?
8. What do you think is the key take-away message in this chapter in terms of implications for nutrition education?

REFERENCES

Abood, D.A., D.R. Black, and D. Feral. 2003. Nutrition education worksite intervention for university staff: Application of the health belief model. *Journal of Nutrition Education and Behavior* 35:260–267.

Abraham, C., and P. Sheeran. 2000. Understanding and changing health behaviour: From health beliefs to self-regulation. In *Understanding and changing health behaviour from health beliefs to self-regulation*, edited by P. Norman, C. Abraham, and M. Conner. Amsterdam: Hardwood Academic Publishers.

Achterberg, A., and C. Miller. 2004. Is one theory better than another in nutrition education? A viewpoint: More is better. *Journal of Nutrition Education and Behavior* 36:40–42.

Ajzen, I. 1991. The theory of planned behavior. *Organizational Behavior and Human Decision Processes* 50:179–211.

———. 1998. Models of human social behaviour and their application to health psychology. *Psychology and Health* 13:735–739.

———. 2001. Nature and operation of attitudes. *Annual Review Psychology* 52:27–58.

Ajzen, I., and T.J. Madden. 1986. Prediction of goal-directed behavior: Attitudes, intentions and perceived behavioral control. *Journal of Experimental Social Psychology* 22:453–474.

Ali, N.S. 2002. Prediction of coronary heart disease prevention behaviors in women: A test of the health belief model. *Women Health* 35:83–96.

Anderson, A.S., D.N. Cox, S. McKellar, et al. 1998. Take Five, a nutrition education intervention to increase fruit and vegetable intakes: Impact on attitudes towards dietary change. *British Journal of Nutrition* 80:133–140.

Andreason, A.R. 1995. *Marketing social change: Changing behavior to promote health, social development and the environment.* Washington, DC: Jossey-Bass.

Armitage, C.J., and M. Conner. 1999. Predictive validity of the theory of planned behaviour: The role of questionnaire format and social desirability. *Journal of Community and Applied Social Psychology* 9:261–272.

———. 2000a. Attitudinal ambivalence: A test of three key hypotheses. *Personality and Social Psychology Bulletin* 26(11)1421–1432.

———. 2000b. Social cognition models and health behavior: A structured review. *Psychology and Health* 15:173-189.

———. 2001. Efficacy of the theory of planned behaviour: A meta-analytic review. *British Journal of Social Psychology* 40:471–499.

Axelson, M.L., D. Brinberg, and J.H. Durand. 1983. Eating at a fast-food restaurant: A social-psychological analysis. *Journal of Nutrition Education* 15(3):94–98.

Backman, D.R., E. H. Haddad, J.W. Lee, et al. 2002. Psychosocial predictors of healthful dietary behavior in adolescents. *Journal of Nutrition Education and Behavior* 34:184–192.

Bandura, A. 1986. *Foundations of thought and action: A social cognitive theory.* Englewood Cliffs, NJ: Prentice-Hall.

———. 1997. *Self-efficacy: The exercise of control.* New York: WH Freeman.

———. 2000. Health promotion from the perspective of social cognitive theory. In *Understanding and changing health behavior: From health beliefs to self-regulation*, edited by P. Norman, C. Abraham, and M. Conner. Amsterdam: Harwood Academic Publishers.

Becker, M.H. 1974. The health belief model and personal health behavior. *Health Education Monographs* 2(4):324–473.

Bentley, M.E., D.L. Dee, and J.L. Jensen. 2003. Breastfeeding among low-income, African-American women: Power, beliefs, and decision-making. *Journal of Nutrition* 133:305S–309S.

Birch, L.L. 1999. Development of food preferences. *Annual Review of Nutrition* 19:41–62.

Bisogni, C.A., M. Connors, C.M. Devine, and J. Sobal. 2002. Who we are and how we eat: A qualitative study of identities in food choice. *Journal of Nutrition Education and Behavior* 34:128–139.

Bissonnette, M.M., and I.R. Contento. 2001. Adolescents' perspectives and food choice behaviors in relation to the environmental impacts of food production practices. *Journal of Nutrition Education* 33:72–82.

Blake, C., and C.A. Bisogni. 2003. Personal and family food choice schemas of rural women in upstate New York. *Journal of Nutrition Education and Behavior* 35:282-293.

Booth-Butterfield, S., and B. Reger. 2004. The message changes belief and the rest is theory: The "1% or less" milk campaign and reasoned action. *Preventive Medicine* 39 (3):581–588.

Brug, J., M. Campbell, and P. van Assema. 1999. The application and impact of computer-generated personalized nutrition education: A review of the literature. *Patient Education and Counseling* 36(2):145–156.

Brug, J., E. de Vet, J. de Nooijer, and B. Verplanken. 2006. Predicting fruit consumption: Cognitions, intention, and habits. *Journal of Nutrition Education and Behavior* 38:73–81.

Brug, J., A. Oenema, and I. Ferreira. 2005. Theory, evidence and intervention mapping to improve behavioral nutrition and physical activity interventions. *International Journal of Behavioral Nutrition and Physical Activity* 2(2).

Chang, Y.P., I.R. Contento, and Y.Y. Cheng. 2003, July 29. The role of personality in dietary fat reduction. Presentation at the Annual Meeting of the Society for Nutrition Education. Philadephia, PA.

Chew, F., S. Palmer, Z. Slonska, and K. Subbiah. 2002. Enhancing health knowledge, health beliefs, and health behavior in Poland through a health promoting television program series. *Journal of Health Communications* 7:179–196.

Conner, M., and C. Abraham. 2001. Conscientiousness and the theory of planned behavior: Towards a more complete model of the antecedents of intentions and behavior. *Personality and Social Psychology Bulletin* 27:1547–1561.

Conner, M., P. Norman, and R. Bell. 2002. The theory of planned behavior and healthy eating. *Health Psychology* 21:194–201.

Conner, M., P. Sheeran, P. Norman, and C.J. Armitage. 2000. Temporal stability as a moderator of relationships in the theory of planned behaviour. *British Journal of Social Psychology* 39:469–493.

Conner, M., and P. Sparks. 1995. The theory of planned behaviour and health behaviours. In *Predicting Health Behaviour*, edited by M. Conner and P. Norman. Buckingham, UK: Open University Press.

Contento, I.R., and B.M. Murphy. 1990. Psychosocial factors differentiating people who reported making desirable changes in their diets from those who did not. *Journal of Nutrition Education* 22:6–14.

D'Andrade, R.G. 1984. Cultural meaning systems. In *Culture theory: Essays on mind, self, and emotion*, edited by R.A. Shweder and R.A. LeVine. Cambridge, UK: Cambridge University Press.

Dennison, C.M, and R. Shepherd. 1995. Adolescent food choice: An application of the theory of planned behaviour. *Journal of Human Nutrition and Dietetics* 8:9–23.

Deutsch, M., and H.G. Gerard. 1955. A study of normative and informational social influence upon individual judgement. *Journal of Abnormal and Social Psychology* 51:629–636.

Ellis, J., M.A. Johnson, J.G. Fischer, and J.L. Hargrove. 2005. Nutrition and health education intervention for whole grain foods in the Georgia Older Americans Nutrition Program. *Journal of Nutrition for the Elderly* 24:67–83.

Fazio, R.H. 1990. Multiple processes by which attitudes guide behavior: The MODE model as an integrative framework. In *Advances in Experimental Social Psychology*, edited by M.P. Zana. San Diego: Academic Press.

Fishbein, M. 2000. The role of theory in HIV prevention. *AIDS Care* 12(3):273–278.

Fishbein, M., and I. Ajzen. 1975. *Belief, attitude, intention and behavior: An introduction to theory and research.* Reading, MA: Addison-Wesley.

Foerster, S.B., J. Gregson, D.L. Beall, et al. 1998. The California children's 5 a Day–Power Play! campaign: Evaluation of a large scale social marketing initiative. *Family Community Health* 21:46–64.

Glanz, K., and P. van Assema. 1997. Are awareness of dietary fat intake and actual fat consumption associated? A Dutch-American comparison. *European Journal of Clinical Nutrition* 51:542–547.

Godin, G., M. Conner, and P. Sheeran. 2005. Bridging the intention-behavior "gap": The role of moral norm. *British Journal of Social Psychology* 44(Pt 4):497–512.

Godin, G., and G. Kok. 1996. The theory of planned behavior: a review of its applications to health related behaviors. *American Journal of Health Promotion* 11:87-98.

Grieve, F.G., and M.W. Vander Weg. 2003. Desire to eat high- and low-fat foods following a low-fat dietary intervention. *Journal of Nutrition Education and Behavior* 35:98–104. Hanson, J.A., and J.A. Benedict. 2002. Use of the health belief model to examine older adults' food-handling behaviors. *Journal of Nutrition Education and Behavior* 34:S25–S30.

Hoffman, E.W., V. Bergmann, J. Armstrong Schultz, P. Kendall, L.C. Medeiros, and V.N. Hillers. 2005. Application of a five-step message development model for food safety education materials targeting people with HIV/AIDS. *Journal of the American Dietetic Association* 105:1597–1604.

IFIC Foundation. 1999, September/October. Are you listening? What consumers tell us about dietary recommendations. *Food insight: Current topics in food safety and nutrition.*

Institute of Medicine. 2002. Speaking of health: Assessing health communication strategies for diverse populations. In *Improving the Health of Diverse Populations.* Washington, DC: Institute of Medicine, National Academy Press.

Janz, N.K., and M.H. Becker. 1984. The health belief model: A decade later. *Health Education Quarterly* 11:1–47.

Kahle, L.R. 1984. The values of Americans: Implications for consumer adaptation. In *Personal values and consumer psychology,* edited by R.E. Pitts Jr. and A.G. Woodside. Lexington, MA: Lexington Books.

Kassem, N.O., J.W. Lee, N.N. Modeste, and P.K. Johnston. 2003. Understanding soft drink consumption among female adolescents using the theory of planned behavior. *Health Education Research* 18(3):278–291.

Kittler, P.G., and K.P. Sucher. 2001. *Food and culture.* 3rd ed. Belmont, CA: Wadsworth/Thomson Learning.

Kloeblen, A.S., and S.S. Batish. 1999. Understanding the intention to permanently follow a high folate diet among a sample of low-income women according to the health belief model. *Health Education Research* 14:327–338.

Kok, G., H. Schaalma, H. De Vries, G. Parcel, and T. Paulussen. 1996. Social psychology and health. *European Review of Social Psychology* 7:241–282.

Kreuter, M.W., S.N. Kukwago, D.C. Bucholtz, E.M. Clark, and V. Sanders-Thompson. 2003. Achieving cultural appropriateness in health promotion programs: Targeted and tailored approaches. *Health Education and Behavior* 30:133–146.

Kristal, A.R., K. Glanz, B.C. Tilley, and S. Li. 2000. Mediating factors in dietary change: Understanding the impact of a nutrition intervention. *Health Education and Behavior* 27:112–125.

Kumanyika, S.K., L. van Horn, D. Bowen, et al. 2000. Maintenance of dietary behavior change. *Health Psychology* 19(Suppl.):42–56.

Leventhal, H. 1973. Changing attitudes and habits to reduce risk factors in chronic disease. *American Journal of Cardiology* 31:571–580.

LeVine, R.A. 1984. Properties of culture: An ethnographic view. In *Culture theory: Essays on mind, self and emotion,* edited by R.A. Shweder and R.A. LeVine. Cambridge, UK: Cambridge University Press.

Lewin, K., T. Dembo, L. Festinger, and P.S. Sears. 1944. Level of aspiration. In *Personality and the behavior disorders,* edited by J.M. Hundt. New York: Roland Press.

Lien, N., L.A. Lytle, and K.A. Komro. 2002. Applying theory of planned behavior to fruit and vegetable consumption of young adolescents. *American Journal of Health Promotion* 16(4):189–197.

Liou, D., and I.R. Contento. 2001. Usefulness of psychosocial theory variables in explaining fat-related dietary behavior in Chinese Americans: Association with degree of acculturation. *Journal of Nutrition Education* 33:322–331.

———. 2004. Health beliefs related to heart disease prevention among Chinese Americans. *Journal of Family and Consumer Sciences* 96:21–22.

Loughrey, K.A., G.I. Balch, C. Lefebvre, et al. 1997. Bringing 5 a day consumers into focus: Qualitative use of consumer research to guide strategic decision making. *Journal of Nutrition Education* 29:172-177.

McCarthy, P., and J. Tuttelman. 2005. Touching hearts to impact lives: Harnessing the power of emotion to change behaviors. *Journal of Nutrition Education and Behavior* 37(Suppl. 1):S19.

McClure, J.B. 2002. Are biomarkers useful treatment aids for promoting health behavior change? An empirical review. *American Journal of Preventive Medicine* 22(3):200–207.

McCrae, R.R., and P.T. Costa. 1987. Validation of the five-factor model of personality across instruments and observers. *Journal of Personality and Social Psychology* 54:81-90.

Park, K., and J.R. Ureda. 1999. Specific motivations of milk consumption among pregnant women enrolled in or eligible for WIC. *Journal of Nutrition Education* 31(2):76–86.

Patterson, R.E., A.R. Kristal, and E. White. 1996. Do beliefs, knowledge, and perceived norms about diet and cancer predict dietary change? *American Journal of Public Health* 86(10):1394–1400.

Pelican, S., F. Vanden Heede, B. Holmes et al. 2005. The power of others to shape our identity: Body image, physical abilities, and body weight. *Family and Consumer Sciences Research Journal* 34(1):57-80

Petty, R.E., and J.T. Cacioppo. 1986. *Communication and persuasion: Central and peripheral routes to attitude change.* New York:Springer-Verlag.

Potter, J.D., J.R. Finnegan, J.X. Guinard., et al. 2000. *5 A Day for Better Health program evaluation report.* Bethesda, MD: National Institutes of Health, National Cancer Institute.

Povey, R., B. Wellens, and M. Conner. 2001. Attitudes towards following meat, vegetarian and vegan diets: An examination of the role of ambivalence. *Appetite* 37:15–26.

Raats, M.M., R. Shepherd, and P. Sparks. 1995. Including moral dimensions of choice within the structure of the theory of planned behavior. *Journal of Applied Social Psychology* 25:484–494.

Richard, R., J. van der Pligt, and N. de Vries. 1996. Anticipated affect and behavioral choice. *Basic and Applied Social Psychology* 18:111–129.

Robinson, R., and C. Smith. 2002. Psychological and demographic variables associated with consumer intention to purchase sustainably produced foods as a defined by the Midwest Food Alliance. *Journal of Nutrition Education and Behavior* 34;316-325.

Rokeach, M. 1973. *The nature of human values.* New York: Free Press.

Rosenstock, I.M. 1974. Historical origins of the health belief model. *Health Education Monographs* 2:1–8.

Rozin, P. 1982. Human food selection: The interaction of biology, culture, and individual experience. In *The psychobiology of human food selection*, edited by L.M. Barker. Westport, CT: AVI Publishing.

Rozin, P., and A.E. Fallon. 1981. The acquisition of likes and dislikes for foods. In *Criteria of food acceptance: How man chooses what he eats*, edited by J. Sohms and R.L. Hall. Zurich: Forster Verlag.

Salovey, P., and D. Birnbaum 1989. Influence of mood on health-relevant cognitions. *Journal of Personality and Social Psychology* 57(3): 539-551.

Salovey, P., T.R. Schneider, and A.M. Apanovitch. 1999. Persuasion for the purpose of cancer risk reduction: a discussion. *Journal of the National Cancer Institute Monographs* 25:119-122.

Samuels, S.E. 1993. Project LEAN—lessons learned from a national social marketing campaign. *Public Health Reports* 108:45–53.

Sanjur, D. 1982. *Social and cultural perspectives in nutrition.* Englewood-Cliffs, NJ: Prentice-Hall.

Satia, J.A., A.R. Kristal, R.E. Patterson, M.L. Neuhouser, and E. Trudeau. 2002. Psychosocial factors and dietary habits associated with vegetable consumption. *Nutrition* 18:247–254.

Saunders, R.P., and S.A. Rahilly. 1990. Influences on intention to reduce dietary intake of fat and sugar. *Journal of Nutrition Education* 22:169–176.

Schwarzer, R. 1992. Self-efficacy in the adoption of maintenance of health behaviors: Theoretical approaches and a new model. In *Self-efficacy: Thought control of action*, edited by R. Schwarzer. Washington: Hemisphere.

Shafer, R.B., P.M. Keith, and E. Schafer. 1995. Predicting fat in diets of marital partners using the health belief model. *Journal of Behavioral Medicine* 18:419–433.

Sheeran, P., P. Norman, and S. Orbell. 1999. Evidence that intentions based on attitudes better predict behaviour than intentions based on subjective norms. *European Journal of Social Psychology* 29:403–406.

Shim, Y., J.N. Variyam, and J. Blaylock. 2000. Many Americans falsely optimistic about their diets. *Food Review* 23(1):44–50.

Sjoberg, S., K. Kim, and M. Reicks. 2004. Applying the theory of planned behavior to fruit and vegetable consumption by older adults. *Journal of Nutrition for the Elderly* 23(4):35–46.

Sparks, P. 2000. Subjective expected utility-based attitude-behavior models: The utility of self-identity. In *Attitudes, behavior and social context: The role of norms and group membership*, edited by D.J. Terry and M.A. Hogg. London: Lawrence Erlbaum.

Sparks, P., M. Conner, R. James, R. Shepherd, and R. Povey. 2001. Ambivalence about health-related behaviors: An exploration in the domain of food choice. *British Journal of Health Psychology* 6:53-68.

Sparks, P., P. Hedderley, and R. Shepherd. 1992. An investigation into the relationship between perceived control, attitude variability, and the consumption of two common foods. *European Journal of Social Psychology* 22:55–71.

Sparks, P., R. Shepherd, and L.J. Frewer. 1995. Assessing and structuring attitudes toward the use of gene technology in food production: The role of perceived ethical obligation. *Basic and Applied Social Psychology* 163:267–285.

Spiro, M.E. 1984. Some reflections on cultural determinism and relativism with special reference to emotion and reason. In *Culture theory: Essays on mind, self and emotion*, edited by R.A. Shweder and R.A. LeVine. Cambridge, UK: Cambridge University Press.

Spruijt-Metz, D. 1995. Personal incentives as determinants of adolescent health behavior: the meaning of behavior. *Health Education Research* 10:355-364

Trafimow, D., and P. Sheeran. 1998. Some tests of the distinction between cognitive and affective beliefs. *Journal of Experimental Social Psychology* 34:378–397.

Triandis, H.C. 1977. *Interpersonal behavior*. Monterey, CA: Brooks/Cole.

Trudeau, E., A.R. Kristal, S. Li, and R.E. Patterson. 1998. Demographic and psychosocial predictors of fruit and vegetable intakes differ: Implications for dietary interventions. *Journal of the American Dietetic Association* 98(12):1412–1418.

Tuorila-Ollikainen, H., L. Lahteenmaki , and H. Salovaara. 1986. Attitudes, norms, intentions, and hedonic responses in the selection of low salt bread in a longitudinal choice experiment. *Appetite* 7 (2):127-3.

Verplanken, B., and S. Faes. 1999. Good intentions, bad habits, and effects of forming implementation intentions on healthy eating. *European Journal of Social Psychology* 29:591–604.

Weinstein, N.D. 1988. The precaution adoption process. *Health Psychology* 7:355–386.

Williams, S.S., J.L. Michela, and I.R. Contento. Personal communication. Health value influences healthfulness of food choices among adolescents.

Williams-Piehota P.A. Cox, S.N. Silvera, et al. 2004. Casting health messages in terms of responsibility for dietary change: increasing fruit and vegetable consumption. *Journal of Nutrition Education and Behavior* 36(3):114-20.

Witte, K., and M. Allen. 2000. A meta-analysis of fear appeals: Implications for effective public health campaigns. *Health Education and Behavior* 27:591–615.

Zimbardo, P.G., E.B. Ebbeson, and C. Maslach. 1977. *Influencing attitudes and changing behavior*. Reading, MA: Addison-Wesley.

Foundation in Theory and Research:
Facilitating the Ability to Take Action

OVERVIEW This chapter describes key theories and research that help readers understand the behavior change process within individuals and the implications for nutrition education. The focus of this chapter is on the ability to act and the key role of self-regulation processes in providing *how-to* nutrition education.

OBJECTIVES At the end of the chapter, you will be able to

- Describe key theories of health behavior change, including social cognitive theory, self-regulation models such as the health action process model, and the transtheoretical model
- State key concepts in these theories and their implications for practice
- Compare theories in terms of their constructs
- Describe how theories and research have been used in interventions to assist people to make changes in their food choice and other nutrition-related behaviors
- Discuss how theory and research can be used to design nutrition education interventions to facilitate individuals' ability to take action

SCENARIO

Before you begin, interview two people who have attempted to take action on a food-related behavior in the past year: one who was successful at taking action and another who was not.

For the person who was successful, ask her or him, How did you go about taking action? Did you follow any particular plan? Did you use any special procedures or strategies to make the change? What was helpful and what was not? For the person who was not successful, ask him or her, What made it so difficult? What were the barriers? What would have been helpful? As you read the chapter, try to match up the successful strategies the person reported or barriers he or she experienced with the constructs of the theories described here.

Introduction: Facilitating the Ability to Take Action

Numerous factors influence our food choices and eating patterns on a daily basis, as we have seen. We have also developed many habits and routines that guide our behavior. It has been said that each of us probably eats only about twelve different meals or recipes. To take action or change our behaviors, we have to be convinced of the desirability, effectiveness, and feasibility of the change. Once convinced, we

may state an intention to carry out the behavior, but stating an intention to take action does not by itself lead to action. We still need a way to translate intentions into action.

Ray from our previous chapters illustrates this difficulty. Remember that Ray is in his mid-forties. His weight just crept up on him, a pound or two each year, and now he is about 40 pounds overweight and is at risk for diabetes. His doctor tells him he should lose weight to help reduce the risk. He really wants to, but it seems so hard. He is a salesman in a large appliance store, where he is mostly on the phone or standing around and is not very active. He keeps snacks at his desk, such as potato chips or cookies, which he eats when he is bored during down time or when he has to talk with clients during lunchtime. When he comes home, he wants to just sit and watch TV. His wife is interested in eating more healthfully, but he likes a hearty meal with lots of meat and always a dessert.

There are many people like Ray, including us at times, for whom problems with getting started and maintaining action rather than motivation prevent them from engaging in behaviors that they themselves have concluded are important to them (Gollwitzer, 1999; Gollwitzer & Oettingen, 2000). How can we help individuals such as Ray bridge the intention–behavior gap? How do we help them move from motivation to action, from intention to reality?

The major way to bridge the intention–behavior gap is to make the desired action easier to understand and do. We can do that in two major ways: we can build individuals' abilities and skills to act on their motivations, and we can make the environment more supportive of the behavior. Facilitating the ability to take action is the topic of this chapter. Making the environment more supportive is the subject of the next.

This chapter begins by describing the theories and research that are especially helpful in understanding how individuals translate motivations into action, and how they achieve and maintain personal change. This lays the foundation for designing strategies in nutrition education to facilitate the ability to take action. This is the how-to phase of nutrition education.

Theories and Research to Understand the Mediators of Action or Behavior Change

What can research and theory tell us that would be useful in assisting individuals and groups to translate these intentions or goals into action?

Research and theory suggests that just as the potential mediators of behavior change such as beliefs and affect or feelings predominate in the pre-action phase, so food- and nutrition-specific knowledge and skills and self-regulatory processes predominate in the action and maintenance phase of the behavior change process. Research also suggests that the tasks are somewhat different for initiating action and maintaining behavior change. The most useful theories or models for this phase of nutrition education are social cognitive theory, self-regulation models such as the health action process approach (Schwarzer & Fuchs, 1995; Sniehotta, Scholz, & Schwarzer, 2005) and others (Bagozzi, 1992; Gollwitzer, 1999), and the transtheoretical model or stages of change model (Prochaska & DiClemente, 1984). These models are similar to the ones discussed in the last chapter in that they identify factors that explain motivation for health behaviors. However, these theories in addition provide guidance on ways to facilitate our ability to take action and make changes in our behavior.

Again, the question might be: why are there several theories instead of just one? And again the reason is that they were developed under different circumstances to understand different behaviors. There is remarkable agreement among them, however, about the importance of the self-regulation process for taking and maintaining action. A few key theories that have been found useful to nutrition education are described here.

Social Cognitive Theory

Social cognitive theory, as proposed and developed by Bandura (1977, 1986) to analyze and understand human thought, motivation, and action in general, has become the most widely used theory for designing nutrition education and health promotion programs because it not only provides a unified conceptual framework for understanding the determinants of *behaviors*, but also describes potential mediators and mechanisms of *behavioral change* that can be used to design strategies to assist people to take action.

Social cognitive theory is a comprehensive theory describing a multifaceted causal structure for behavior involving numerous concepts, explained in detail over the course of several books (Bandura, 1977, 1986, 1997). Only the key concepts relevant to nutrition education are described here. Social cognitive theory proposes as a major organizing principle for understanding behavior the concept of reciprocal determinism, in which personal, behavioral, and environmental factors work in a dynamic and reciprocal fashion to influence health behavior. *Personal factors* involve our internal thoughts and feelings; *behavioral factors* include our food-, nutrition-, and health-related knowledge and skills, together called *behavioral capability;* and *environmental factors* include those factors external to us, such as the physical and social environment.

Social cognitive theory does not take a stage approach but instead focuses on the complexity of behavior and behavior change processes at all times. However, it acknowledges that in practice, some determinants that mediate behavior change may occur before others in the behavior change process (Bandura, 1986). Indeed, Bandura himself has noted the special importance of outcome and self-efficacy beliefs for motivating individuals to form goal intentions to initiate behavior and the importance of self-regulation processes for maintaining behavior, referring to these as "phases" of behavioral change (Bandura, 2000). Thus, social cognitive theory can help nutrition educators design activities that enhance the motivation to act as well as activities that facilitate the ability to take action.

Constructs of the Theory

The constructs of the model and their relationships to each other and to behavior are shown in Figure 5-1. Table 5-1 provides a summary of the constructs of the theory and how they can be applied in nutrition education.

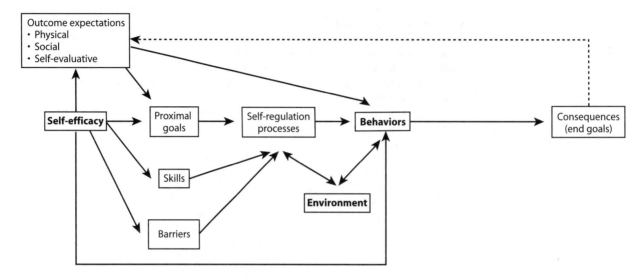

FIGURE 5-1 Social cognitive theory.

Source: Based on Bandura, A. 2000. Health promotion from the perspective of social cognitive theory. In *Understanding and changing health behavior: From health beliefs to self-regulation,* edited by P. Norman, C. Abraham, and M. Conner. Amsterdam: Harwood Academic Publishers.

Individual or Personal Factors

Social cognitive theory points out that our behavior is influenced by a host of self-referent thoughts or beliefs. We have the capacity to symbolize and thus translate our experiences into internal models that can guide future action. We demonstrate forethought and are thus capable of intentional or purposive action, which is related to our symbolic capability. Future events cannot serve as determinants of current behavior, but their cognitive representations in the present through our symbolic capability can have a strong motivating impact on current behavior. We are self-reflective and able to evaluate our actions, and we can exercise influence over our own behavior. We can recognize the importance of others in influencing our behaviors. Among the many person-related factors, two major constructs that are important in motivating behavior are outcome expectations and self-efficacy.

Outcome expectations. Social cognitive theory posits that much of our behavior is regulated by forethought or outcome expectations. These are our beliefs about anticipated outcomes from engaging in a behavior or health-related lifestyle (that is, reasons that make the behavior or lifestyle desirable). As such, they are similar to beliefs about outcomes of behavior in the theory of planned behavior and to perceived benefits of behavior in the health belief model. *Outcome expectancies* are the values we place on these outcomes and are also called *incentives* by Bandura (1986). Expectancies have a quantitative value that can be measured on a scale, and can be positive or negative. Similar to other social cognition theories, such as the theory of planned behavior, social

cognitive theory states that we will choose to perform an action, such as eating fruits and vegetables, that maximizes the positive outcomes (good for body functioning, helps me maintain my weight, reduces risk of cancer) and minimizes the negative outcomes (not tasty or filling). Outcome expectations can take three forms. With each form, anticipated positive outcomes serve as incentives, and negative outcomes serve as disincentives (Bandura, 2000). Although outcome expectancies have direct influences on behavior, they are also influenced by how we interpret information about the impact of our behavior in the environment, as shown in Figure 5-1.

- *Physical outcomes:* The physical and health effects that accompany the behavior. Positive outcomes include pleasant sensory experiences, such as from the pleasant taste of fruits and vegetables, and the recognition of chronic disease risk reduction; negative outcomes include aversive sensory experiences (e.g., vegetables may be considered bitter and unpleasant) and physical discomfort (e.g., from eating beans) According to Bandura (2000), negative physical outcomes also include risk of disease from not engaging in healthy behaviors, similar to the perceived seriousness and perceived susceptibility constructs of the health belief model, and positive outcomes are similar to the perceived benefits construct.
- *Social outcomes:* The social consequences of the behavior. These are similar to the social norm construct of the theory of planned behavior. Behaviors that fulfill social norms bring positive reactions, such as soda

TABLE 5-1 Social Cognitive Theory: Major Concepts and Applications to Nutrition Education Interventions

Theory Construct/ Potential Mediator of Behavior Change	Practice Applications
Outcome expectations	
Physical or material outcomes	Activities to enhance the importance of positive outcomes (perceived benefits) of taking action (e.g., eating fruits and vegetables [F&V]), such as messages about cancer risk reduction, and overcoming negative outcomes (perceived barriers), such as inconvenience or cost.
Social outcomes	Messages about social norms and activities on how to handle them (e.g., make eating F&V cool for teens).
Self-evaluative outcomes	Emphasize self-satisfaction and self-worth from behavior (e.g., "By eating F&V I am being good to myself").
Outcome expectancies	Assess the values individuals place on the expected outcomes (degree of motivation) and design activities to increase the value to them of healthful outcomes (e.g., teens can eat F&V for health and still be cool with peers).
Behavioral capability	Provide needed food and nutrition knowledge and cognitive skills needed for taking action through presentations, handouts, demonstrations, videos, and other channels, as well as discussions and debates to develop critical thinking skills. Also provide behavioral skills such as food purchasing and storage, cooking skills, safe food handling and preparation behaviors, and growing vegetables.
Observational learning/modeling	Conduct food demonstrations relating to the behavior being enacted, such as making a low-fat recipe. Provide opportunities for the group to practice the recipe, with guidance, to enhance mastery.
Self-efficacy	Assist individuals to achieve success by making change in small steps. Create modeling and mastery experiences about food and nutrition as above (e.g., cooking, gardening, advocacy). Provide feedback and encouragement. Assist individuals to correctly interpret physiological responses to the new food or behavior.
Reinforcements	Provide external reinforcement in the form of rewards or incentives, such as tee-shirts, key-chains, and raffle tickets, for goal attainment. Provide opportunities to develop internal or self-reinforcement by recognizing and appreciating individuals' own accomplishments.
Self-regulation/self-control	Provide instruction and practice opportunities for individuals to develop skills in self-control of behavior: assessing their values, self-monitoring, goal setting, self-rewards, and problem solving. Emotion-coping and stress-management skills are also included.

drinking among teenagers, whereas those that violate social norms bring social censure, such as breastfeeding in public in cultures where this is not the norm.

- *Self-evaluative outcomes:* The positive and negative self-evaluative reactions we have to our own behaviors. We engage in behaviors that bring satisfaction and a sense of self-worth; for example, "By eating fruits and vegetables I am being good to myself." We avoid behaviors that lead to dissatisfaction, such as "I avoid eating junk foods because if I eat them, I am not doing the right thing for myself." Bandura (2000) believes

that self-satisfaction for personal accomplishments, such as success in breastfeeding or growing one's own vegetables, is one of the more powerful regulators of behavior, often more important than tangible rewards.

Self-efficacy. Self-efficacy, or beliefs about personal efficacy is considered to be the major motivator of action and mediator of behavior change Bandura (2000) points out that knowledge about health outcomes or risks is usually high among the general public. Although such beliefs about the outcomes of behavior are a precondition for change, additional self-influences are needed to overcome impediments or barriers to adopting and maintaining healthy lifestyles. Chief among the self-influences is perceived self-efficacy, which is the confidence we have that we can carry out the intended behavior successfully or deal effectively with different situations, including confidence in overcoming barriers to engaging in the behavior. Examples might be our confidence that we can select and prepare vegetables, run three miles a day, change our eating patterns or shopping practices to be more supportive of sustainable food systems, or organize our work situation to be able to breastfeed even when it is difficult to do so.

Self-efficacy is considered to be domain or situation specific. For example, feeling self-efficacious in the food domain does not mean that we will feel the same way about exercise or other behaviors. Our judgments of our own self-efficacy have far-reaching influences on our thought patterns, emotional reactions, and behavior. Unless we believe that we can produce desired outcomes through our own actions, we have little incentive to take action. Extensive research indicates that the higher the level of perceived efficacy, the more effort individuals will expend and the longer they will persist in a new learned behavior, especially in the face of difficulties. According to Bandura (2000), such a sense of personal efficacy is not just confidence in our knowledge and skills to carry out a given action but is also the ability to regulate our own motivations, thought processes, feelings, and behavioral patterns or to change environmental conditions depending on what is needed in the context of this domain of action. In short, self-efficacy involves the exercise of personal control, requiring both skills and the confidence that we can effectively and consistently use them, even under difficult circumstances. Social cognitive theory thus views individuals as agents who are able to take charge of their lives. Behavior change involves the ability to exercise self-influence or self-control over our own behavior.

Beliefs in personal efficacy can be strengthened through four main sources of influence.

1. *Personal mastery experiences:* Learning to master the behavior by the setting and achieving of action goals despite obstacles. Practice is thus the most effective way of creating a strong sense of personal efficacy.
2. *Social modeling:* Observing others similar to ourselves succeed by sustained effort.
3. *Social persuasion:* Persuasion by others that we can succeed. Encouragement by others can overcome our self-doubts. Included here are also efforts to structure the situation so that we can succeed and to help us measure success against our own improvement.
4. *Modification of emotional or physical responses to the behavior:* We rely partly on information from our physiological states to judge our own abilities. Self-efficacy

can thus be strengthened by assisting us in modifying our emotional or physical responses to the behavior where these are stressful (e.g., physiological arousal and anxiety) or due to misinterpretations of the experience. For example, individuals who first start eating a lot of whole grains and beans may have physiological reactions that lead them to believe that they cannot eat these foods. Or individuals first attempting to become more physically active might read their fatigue, windedness, or aches and pains as signs that they are not able to do these activities. These (mis)perceptions can be corrected.

Self-efficacy has been shown through research to be especially important in the initiation, modification, and maintenance of complex behaviors such as healthful eating and physical activity. Thus the concept of self-efficacy has been incorporated into the more recent versions of other theories such as the health belief model, theory of planned behavior, and the transtheoretical model as they are applied to the area of diet and health.

Measurement of the construct of self-efficacy can consider the following three dimensions: *level of difficulty*, which is the ability to perform successively more difficult tasks ("I can eat three fruits and vegetables a day"; or five; or nine); *strength*, or level of confidence that we can perform the task at a given level (from not at all confident to very confident); and *generality*, or the perception of efficacy across several domains, such as negative feeling states (when feeling nervous or upset), positive social states (at a party), or availability ("I can stick to low-fat foods on a regular basis even when lots of rich desserts are available") (Bandura, 1997; Ounpuu, Woolcott, & Rossi, 1999; Chang et al., 2003).

Reinforcements. Reinforcements are the responses to a person's behavior that increase or decrease the likelihood of occurrence of that behavior. We tend to use this term in describing positive reinforcements or rewards, which can be external or internal. External reinforcement is providing an action or item that is known to have reinforcement value for the individual or group, such as gold stars for children completing a task in school, or tee-shirts or other rewards for completing a health program or a task such as goal setting. Internal reinforcement is individuals' own perceptions that the behavior had some value for them.

Impediments. Impediments are barriers to taking action (see Figure 5-1). In social cognitive theory, the construct of barriers is multifaceted. Some barriers are personal, including our assessment of our self-efficacy—or lack thereof—to surmount obstacles (such as lack of confidence to cook healthful foods) and negative expected outcomes associated with eating more healthfully (such as taking more time and effort). The anticipated negative outcomes are somewhat like the perceived barriers in the health belief model. According to Bandura (2000), assessing barriers is part of self-efficacy assessments, since they allow us to judge whether we will be able to carry out a behavior even under difficult circumstances, such as cooking a low-fat meal even when we are busy or tired from a day at work. Some impediments are external or reside in the environment, such as lack of availability or accessibility of healthful foods or lack of health resources.

Goals and goal intentions. The concept of goals in the health promotion and nutrition education literature can refer to different levels of intention. Goals can refer to more distal intentions that express valued end states that serve an orienting function for the long term, such as being healthy, enjoying a high quality of life, living an ethical life, and so forth. They are extremely important because they represent internal standards or values we develop from a variety of sources, against which we can judge our current behaviors; sometimes they may be too broad to guide specific actions.

Goals can also refer to goal intentions or proximal goals that will contribute to the overall goal. Such goals are similar to the behavioral intention construct of the theory of planned behavior and constitute the immediate or proximal mediator of behavior. For example, "My goal is to eat five fruits and vegetables a day" is the same as "I intend to eat five fruits and vegetables." In the context of a behavior change process, this represents a commitment to take action. When our outcome expectations are positive (perceived benefits) and self-efficacy is high, we will be motivated to form proximal goals. Achieving larger goals requires the setting of these proximal goals, or *subgoals* as Bandura calls them, and developing action plans to carry them out. This process is part of the self-regulation process described later in this chapter.

Relapse prevention. Relapse prevention focuses on strategies to maintain the new behaviors. These strategies include cognitive restructuring, which involves substituting alternative thoughts and behaviors for less healthful eating behaviors (often referred to as changing "self-talk"); controlling the environment by removing or avoiding cues to less healthful eating (such as avoiding going into the ice cream store) and adding cues for more healthful eating (such as leaving washed fruit out on the counter at home); and setting new goals.

Behavioral Factors

According to social cognitive theory, behavioral factors are equally important. Behavioral capabilities are the food-related knowledge and skills needed to engage in the behavior, such as eating low-fat foods, when desired. In addition, initiation and maintenance of the behavior for the long term requires self-regulation skills, including the ability to exercise influence and control over our own behavior.

Behavioral capabilities (knowledge and skills). These are the food- and nutrition-related knowledge and skills that individuals need to carry out the behavior or practice the

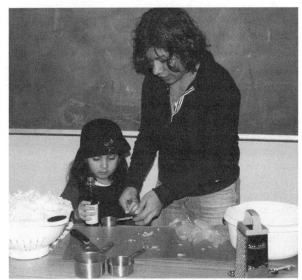

One mom helps her daughter cook at a WIC center.

behavioral goals they have selected. Here knowledge is of the instrumental or how-to kind, consisting of factual knowledge, procedural knowledge, and specific cognitive and behavioral skills.

Included in the *factual knowledge* category might be food and nutrition information and how to use it, such as information about carbohydrates, fats, proteins, vitamins and minerals, MyPyramid and the *Dietary Guidelines*, the differences between different weight loss diet plans, and so forth. The information must be specific to the behavior that has been chosen if it is to be helpful to the individuals attempting to carry out the behavior. This is the kind of information that nutritionists know a great deal about!

Procedural knowledge is the knowledge about *how* to do something, or decision rules for solving given cognitive tasks. Procedural knowledge or cognitive skills might encompass relatively simple skills, such as how to read food labels for the fat content of foods, and more complex skills, such as might be involved in critical thinking about issues such as evaluating the advantages and disadvantage of breastfeeding or of eating foods produced through gene biotechnology. It would also include information on how exactly to breastfeed or where to buy organic foods. Through the acquisition of such knowledge, we develop *knowledge structures*, or schemas—personal conceptual frameworks, if you will—for given areas of information. Factual and procedural knowledge together are well suited for cognitive problem solving. However, such knowledge and cognitive skills, although necessary, are insufficient for action in the area of food-related behavior, as in many other areas.

Additional mechanisms are needed to get from knowledge structures to skilled action. Enactive learning or physical enactment is the translating vehicle, according to Bandura (1986). In simpler language, this means we need to develop *behavioral skills* through performing the behaviors and practicing them ("learning by doing"), such as preparing healthful snacks, cooking low-fat recipes, practicing safe food handling behaviors, breastfeeding, or growing vegetables. Nutrition educators can facilitate the acquisition of such skills by first demonstrating the skills and then providing the opportunity for individuals to practice them. This is sometimes referred to as *modeling and guided practice*. With continued practice these skills can become easy to do and routinized and hence can be performed without much additional thought.

Self-regulation or self-control processes. According to social cognitive theory, we can change our behaviors by exercising self-influence, self-directedness, and self-control through self-regulatory processes. Motivation alone is not sufficient to initiate health-promoting personal change. Self-regulation, or the ability to direct and control our behavior, is also required. This is not achieved through willpower but through the development of self-regulation skills: we need to be taught skills for self-influence. Self-regulation or self-control of behavior involves the following components: we must first observe the behavior we seek to change (e.g., we observe that we eat only two servings of fruits and vegetables each day). This helps us identify the determinants of our behavior and provides the information needed for setting realistic goals (these are variously called action goals, subgoals, or proximal goals). We then set specific behavioral change or action goals and learn the food and nutrition skills needed to achieve them. We monitor our progress toward achieving these action goals, and reward ourselves when we meet them. This reward may be our satisfaction in doing the right thing for our health.

Goal setting. The process just described is called *goal setting* (Bandura, 1986; Cullen, Baranowski, & Smith, 2001; Shilts, Horowitz, & Townsend, 2004). Setting action goals or action plans increases our motivation to act through anticipation of self-satisfaction in achieving our goals, builds our perceptions of our self-efficacy and mastery, creates self-satisfaction and a sense of fulfillment from having achieved our goals, and contributes to the cultivation of intrinsic interest through active involvement in the process. Goal setting is similar to implementation or action plans in other self-regulation theories. These theories point out that such planning ahead means the behavior is decided ahead of time and will not require a new decision to be made in each new situation, thus reducing stress and effort (Gollwitzer, 1999). In the self-regulation process, when we do not attain our action goals, we engage in problem solving and decision making to find more effective ways to attain the goals we set or set new ones that are more attainable. Evidence shows that those who are successful at self-directed change are highly skilled at enlisting these self-regulatory skills to work for them. Maintenance

of personal change requires not only a set of behavioral and self-regulation skills but a resilient sense of efficacy. If we are not convinced of our sense of personal efficacy, we may abandon the skills we have been taught when we experience difficult situations or do not get quick results.

In general, social cognitive theory places great importance on mastery experiences for individuals. There is a difference between self-efficacy and actual skills, and we must have opportunity to learn and practice the behavioral skills to achieve our goals.

Environmental Factors
Social cognitive theory distinguishes between *situation*, which is our perception or cognitive representation of the environment, and *environment*, which represents the objective factors affecting our behavior that are external to us. Numerous environmental factors influence behavior, as we saw in Chapter 2. Social cognitive theory describes the environment as taking three different forms: imposed, selected, and created (Bandura, 1997). *Imposed environments* are the physical and sociostructural environments over which we have no control. These have an impact on us whether we like it or not. Examples in the area of food-related behaviors are the physical availability of food, such as the availability of fruits and vegetables at home and school, at the workplace, or in the local grocery store and the social environment, such as whether family or friends eat fruits and vegetables. The only control we have is how we react to them, act within them, or work to change them.

Selected environments are based on the notion of *potential* and *actual* environments. The environment is not a fixed entity. The potential environment becomes actual depending on how we act in that environment. The actual environment is different for any given individual depending on whether he or she takes advantage of the opportunities in the potential environment.

Created environments are those that were not even potentially there waiting to be selected. They are created by individuals. These might include creating nutrition committees within workplaces or schools that would recommend actions to improve nutrition at the site. We are thus constantly interacting with our environments, selecting them, negotiating with them, or changing them, so that we influence our environments even as our environments influence us. Nutrition education thus seeks to create environments that are supportive.

Observational learning from the environment. The environment is also the source for *modeling* of the behavior. We can learn from other people, or models, through observational learning, a very important construct in social cognitive theory. Trial-and-error learning from our own experiences—that is, feedback from the consequences of our own behavior—is one source of learning. However, observational learning enables us to more quickly learn about the rules of behavior by observing the behavior of others and the consequences that follow for their behavior. For example, children, who are trying to figure out the world, learn from observing their parents. Teenagers learn from observing the food-related behaviors of their peers, valued adults, or relevant celebrities and public figures. Modeling can be used as a strategy in nutrition education to teach people food-related skills, such as through cooking demonstrations. In interventions, individuals are often also provided the opportunity to practice making the recipes that have been demonstrated. This process is then called *guided mastery experience*, which enables individuals to gain the needed physical behavioral skills. The role of environment is described in greater detail in the next chapter.

Relationship to Biological Variables
In the area of food choice and dietary behaviors, biological variables are also important, as we saw in Chapter 2, and interact reciprocally with the social psychological variables that we have examined. Food choice may be influenced by biology, just as foods eaten have an impact on physiological systems or biology. Clearly, physiological processes such as hunger and satiety are crucial in influencing the quantity of foods eaten, and different kinds of foods have varying effects on physiological systems. Research suggests there is also a genetic component to taste, especially in the ability to taste the bitter substance PROP and in the preference for sweet substances (Keller, Peitrobelli, & Faith, 2002; Mennella, Pepino, & Reed, 2005). Thus, genetic factors may also influence the kinds of food we eat. Researchers in the food and health area have therefore suggested that biology should be added as another set of influences in reciprocal determinism (Thoresen, 1984; Baranowski et al., 2003) to yield interacting influences of person, behavior, biology, and environment. The importance of a psychobiological perspective on health and the role of physiological processes has been noted in social cognitive theory (Bandura, 1997).

Evidence from Research and Intervention Studies

Research Studies Using the Theory
Although social cognitive theory has become widely used in interventions, few studies have tested the relative contributions of various components of the theory in predicting eating behavior. One study examined the three social cognitive theory components for their usefulness in predicting fruit and vegetable consumption in elementary school children (Reynolds et al., 1999). It is summarized in Nutrition Education in Action 5-1. As you can see from the information in the feature, the study found that availability and motivation each had a significant direct effect on consumption, but

knowledge did not. Motivation had a significant relationship to knowledge.

A study conducted with those participating in a weight control course examined the relationships among self-efficacy, social environmental factors, and behavior (Shannon et al., 1990). Behavior was divided into two categories—choosing appropriate foods and avoiding overeating—because it has been suggested that avoidance behaviors are different from prescriptive behaviors and may be more difficult to carry out. The researchers found that self-efficacy did contribute significantly to the explanation of eating behavior, and that family and friend support generally influenced eating behavior through self-efficacy. The contributions of outcome expectations were inconsistent and weak, not surprising given that the study subjects were already motivated and participating in a program.

Social cognitive theory was used in a study examining the relationships of the constructs of social environment, reinforcement, commitment, modeling, knowledge, and attitude to the consumption of four beverages: whole milk, low-fat/skim milk, regular soda, and diet soda (Lewis, Sims, & Shannon, 1989). They found that the factors influencing consumption varied by forms of the beverage and by the two age groups they studied, students and adults. Clearly, then, both the behavior and the intended audience are important considerations when the theory is applied.

Theory can also be used in descriptive studies as the basis of questions to ask in open-ended interviews or as the basis of questionnaires. Table 5-2 gives an example of how social cognitive theory was used to construct questions to determine the influences on fruit and vegetable consumption by low-income black American adolescents (Molaison et al., 2005).

Intervention Studies Using the Theory
Numerous intervention studies in the domain of food and diet have been conducted using social cognitive theory, although the full model is not usually used in all studies. A few studies are described here to illustrate the theory.

Children. The Child and Adolescent Trial for Cardiovascular Health (CATCH) program was a large randomized controlled trial with third to fifth graders designed to reduce risk for cardiovascular disease (Luepker et al., 1996). The educational activities were based on social cognitive theory constructs and emphasized reduction in fat intake and increase in physical activity. The program resulted in a significant reduction in fat intake and increased physical activity compared with controls. It also resulted in changes in behavior, measured as usual food choice and dietary intention; in social reinforcement by parents, friends, and teachers; and in self efficacy for diet and physical activity (Edmundson et al., 1996).

Gimme 5! was a program, also with fourth and fifth graders, that used social cognitive theory at every stage of the program development and evaluation (Baranowski et al., 1993;

NUTRITION EDUCATION IN ACTION 5-1

Using Social Cognitive Theory to Understand Fruit and Vegetable Consumption by Elementary School Children

This study used social cognitive theory to examine factors that would explain why third-grade children did or did not eat fruits and vegetables. The constructs of the theory, how they were measured, and the results of the study are summarized here.

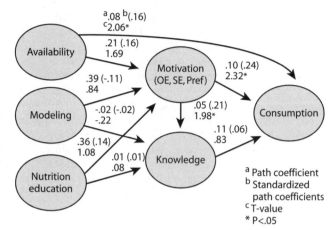

Using social cognitive theory to understand fruit and vegetable consumption in elementary school children.

Behavior: 24-hour recalls, analyzed for fruits and vegetables.

Environmental component: The environmental component was measured by three constructs:

- Availability of fruits and vegetables at home, measured by parents' response about the presence of 31 items in the home
- Social modeling, measured as the sum of the number of people that the child indicated he or she saw eating fruits and vegetables (e.g., friends their age, teacher)
- Nutrition education, measured as the number of sources that the children said taught them about fruits and vegetables from a choice of six persons (e.g., teachers, parent) and four sources (e.g., poster, TV)

Person-related component: This component consisted to two constructs: motivation and knowledge.

- *Motivation* was measured as a composite, latent construct made up of three constructs put together:
  — Outcome expectancies (OE), measured with items such as "eating fruits and vegetables will make me smarter"
  — Self-efficacy (SE), measured with items such as "I can drink a glass of my favorite juice with my dinner"
  — Preference (Pref), measured as liking for 20 items
- *Knowledge* was measured with 10 true-false and multiple choice questions related to fruits and vegetables.

Results: Results are shown in the accompanying diagram, which depicts the relationship between theory constructs in environmental and personal components and the behavior—consumption of fruits and vegetables. You can see that availability and motivation each had a significant direct effect on consumption, but knowledge did not. Motivation had a significant relationship to knowledge.

Source: Reynolds, K.D., A.W. Hinton, R. Shewchuk, et al. 1999. A social cognitive model of fruit and vegetable consumption in elementary school children. *Journal of Nutrition Education* 31(1): 23–30. Figure used with permission of the Society for Nutrition Education.

Kirby et al., 1995). Gimme 5! activities addressed issues identified through focus groups and other needs assessment activities. The program taught students to ask their parents to buy more fruits and vegetables (environmental factor: to increase availability and accessibility), attempted to increase children's preference for fruits and vegetables through taste tests and other fun activities (personal factors: outcome expectancies), and taught the self-regulation skills of goal setting and self-monitoring (behavioral factors). The program resulted in modest increases in vegetable intake that did not last, most likely because the program was not fully implemented in the classroom as it was designed (Baranowski et al., 2000). To overcome the problem of implementation by classroom teachers, the program was redesigned and deliv-

ered through a 10-session interactive multimedia computer game (*Squire's Quest*). This time the program resulted in significant increases in fruit, juice, and vegetable consumption (Baranowski et al., 2003).

Adolescents. An intervention with adolescents in middle school (TEENS) that was based on social cognitive theory focused on eating a lower-fat diet high in fruits and vegetables (Lytle et al., 2004). Individual, behavioral, and environmental factors that were associated with teenage dietary intake were identified from existing studies and confirmed by focus group studies of the particular teens. Nutrition education was then directed at these factors. A classroom component, through a series of hands-on activities, focused on awareness of outcomes of behavior, such as the benefits of eating fruits and

TABLE 5-2 Using Social Cognitive Theory (SCT) to Guide Questions About Influences on Fruit and Vegetable Consumption in a Sample of Low-Income Black American Adolescents

Open-Ended Questions	SCT Construct
Home	
If you looked in the refrigerator or the kitchen cabinet of your home right now, what kinds of fruits (vegetables) would you find?	Environmental
Do you ever eat fruits (vegetables) away from home? What are some other places that you eat fruit (vegetables)?	Environmental
Behavior	
Do you help prepare the meals and snacks in your home?	Behavior
Personal beliefs	
What do you think would happen if you don't eat fruit (vegetables)?	Outcome expectancies
What would make you want to eat more fruit (vegetables)?	Outcome expectancies
If you wanted to eat more fruit or vegetables, would you be able to? Why or why not? How would you get them?	Self-efficacy
Family and friends	
Do you think your friends (family members) would help you eat more fruits and vegetables?	Social support
What would you do if no one is eating fruits (vegetables), but you would like to eat fruit (vegetables)?	Social expectations
What are some reasons you and your friends eat fruit (vegetables)?	Social expectations

Source: Molaison, E.F, C.L. Connell, J.E. Stuff, M.K. Yadrick, and M. Bogle. 2005. Influences on fruit and vegetable consumption by low-income black American adolescents. *Journal of Nutrition Education and Behavior* 37(5): 246–251. Used with permission of the Society for Nutrition Education.

vegetables and a lower-fat diet, and enhancement of self-efficacy through behavioral skills in snack preparation, selecting healthful foods, and overcoming barriers. The program also had an environmental component, including making school lunches lower in fat and adding salad bars, and activities for parents. It resulted in desired changes during the first year of implementation that was not sustained in the second year.

EatFit, another intervention with middle school students, was directed at both dietary and physical activity behaviors (Horowitz, Shilts, & Townsend, 2004). Nutrition Education in Action 5-2 shows how theory was used in practice. The program focused on goal setting. It had been found that adolescents are often not yet at a stage of development to be able to set appropriate goals. Hence the teens were given choices among major goals, such as healthy eating habits, and intakes of calcium, iron, fruits and vegetables, sugar, and fat. The curriculum included experiential lessons that motivated; taught skills, including goal-setting skills; provided goal performance feedback; and involved practice of behaviors. You can see from Nutrition Education in Action 5-2 how the educational strategies of the curriculum were designed to address specific social cognitive theory constructs. For example, students completed contracts for their goals. The program addressed self-efficacy by providing opportunities

for students to learn how to read food labels and to practice those skills by answering questions on foods that were specific to their chosen goal. Self-assessment tools were developed so that students could self-monitor their eating and fitness practices. Relapse prevention was operationalized by worksheets in the student workbook that helped students maintain, set, and achieve new goals. The intervention had a positive impact on dietary behavior but not dietary self-efficacy, and on physical activity self-efficacy but not physical activity behavior.

In another study with EatFit, the effectiveness of the process of guided goal setting was specifically examined (Shilts, Horowitz, & Townsend, 2004). It was found that adding a guided goal-setting component to the intervention improved students' dietary behaviors, physical self-efficacy, and behaviors compared with the same intervention without goal setting.

Worksites. Nutrition educators undertaking interventions at worksites have also used social cognitive theory to plan their programs. An example is the Treatwell Trial (Sorensen et al., 1990, 1999). Here the activities were directed at both the individual and the environment. Activities directed at the individuals focused on promotional activities to increase awareness and motivation, skills training, and activities to encourage maintenance of the dietary changes. Environ-

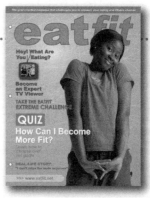

NUTRITION EDUCATION IN ACTION 5-2

EatFit: A Goal-Oriented Intervention That Challenges Adolescents to Improve Their Eating and Fitness Choices

Surveys show that the diets of youth do not meet those recommended by the *Dietary Guidelines*, nor do they engage in recommended amounts of physical activity. This program was designed to improve the dietary and physical activity behaviors of middle school students. It consisted of a classroom for the teacher or leader; a workbook for each student, a Web-based interactive program in which students received personalized assessment based on a 24-hour diet record that they had completed, personalized dietary feedback, goal-setting, and a contract. The program was based on social cognitive theory:

Outcome expectancies: Motivators identified from focus groups were as follows: improved appearance, increased energy, and increased independence. These were used in the lessons.

Self-efficacy: Students were provided opportunity to practice skills (recipe preparation and tasting, physical activities), receive encouragement, and develop social support among the group.

Self-regulation:
- Self-monitoring of their own diets and physical activity patterns
- Setting goals
- Monitoring their progress towards the goals
- Problem-solving activities to overcome perceived barriers (e.g. how to select fast foods that support their goals)
- Rewards or positive reinforcements for attaining goals.

Details of how the food choice determinants or theory constructs were operationalized in the program are shown in the table below.

Examples of Use of Social Cognitive Theory in EatFit

Theory Construct/Strategy	Theory-Based Activities
Self-efficacy/skills mastery	Students increase their self-efficacy in choosing foods that meet their selected dietary goals. They learn ho to read food labels and practice those skills by answering questions on dozens fo food that are specific to their goals.
Modeling	Students interview a parent or guardian about their goal-setting experiences.
Barriers counseling	During the parent interview, students ask about barriers/hurdles encountered during parent's goal progress and the resolution of those hurdles.
Self-monitoring	Students complete self-assessments of current dietary and fitness practices.
Goal setting	Students set physical activity goals using results from the self-assessments.
Contracting	Students complete contracts for their dietary and fitness goals. This contract specifies the goal and the motivation for attainment, and has space for signatures from student, a friend, and a parent.
Cue management	A teacher-led discussion asks "What are some negative cues that may prevent you from reaching your fitness goal?"
Social support	To strengthen social support networks, students are placed into groups based on chosen goals.
Reinforcement	Students receive raffle tickets for goal attainment.
Cognitive restructuring	By restructuring the way students think about breakfast, options open up for their morning meal such as leftover pizza, or a microwaveable burrito, thus making breakfast easier to obtain.
Relapse prevention	The student workbook includes a section devoted to helping students maintain, set, and achieve new goals after the completion of the intervention.
Environment/reciprocal determinism	Homework assignment focus on the role of the environment on behavior change. For example, students identify five locations where they could exercise after school, the hours of operation, and cost. Students find one food from an on-campus source that meets their dietary goals.

Source: Horowitz M., M.K. Shilts, and M.S. Townsend. EatFit: A goal-oriented intervention that challenges adolescents to improve their eating and fitness choices. *Journal of Nutrition Education and Behavior* 36:43–44. Used with permission of the Society for Nutrition Education. Photo used courtesy of the authors.

mental activities included social support at the worksite and involvement of families, as well as changes in the foods offered in the cafeterias. Such a combination of activities led to significant increases in fruit and vegetable consumption. The worksite-plus-family intervention was more successful than the worksite intervention alone.

Summary of Social Cognitive Theory

In summary, the primary motivating force for change in social cognitive theory, according to Baranowski and colleagues (2003), is the construct of outcome expectancies or beliefs about the outcomes to be achieved by a given action or behavior. We desire to achieve positive outcomes and avoid negative outcomes. These are reasons *why to* change. In addition to being convinced that taking a given behavior will be effective in leading to the outcome we desire, we must also believe that we can carry out the behavior even in the face of difficulties and setbacks. Therefore skills and self-efficacy are the major resources for making change. These represent resources for *how to* change. Bandura (1997) contends that when it comes to health, most of us already understand why we need to make changes (that is, outcome expectations are already present) but we just can't seem to do so. Thus, self-efficacy is paramount, making it possible for us to act on our outcome expectations. Bandura suggests that there are three basic processes or phases of health-promoting behavior change: adoption of new behavior patterns, their generalized use under different circumstances, and maintenance over time.

Social cognitive theory has several strengths that make it attractive in the fields of health education and nutrition education: it is a comprehensive theory that not only explains health-related behavior but also describes strategies for changing behavior. It thus provides a framework that can be used to design and implement nutrition education programs. Its major strengths also present a dilemma. Its very comprehensiveness means that it has numerous constructs, too numerous to include in every intervention. The relationships among them are not clearly specified, and their relative importance has not been determined. Those who use social cognitive theory to design interventions often selectively use only one or two constructs, such as self-efficacy or goal setting. In addition, because social cognitive theory emphasizes skills and self-efficacy, many nutrition education interventions that claim to be based on social cognitive theory are sometimes in reality "knowledge and skills" interventions—which have not been shown to be effective in behavior change except among those already motivated. Finally, although outcome expectations are an important construct in social cognitive theory, this mediator of behavior change is common to all the theories we have examined so far. What social cognitive theory adds is an emphasis on self-efficacy and self-regulation skills and the role of our cognitions in controlling our behavior (or self-control). It can thus

provide a good framework for the development of activities that help to bridge the intention–behavior gap and to facilitate the ability to maintain change over time. In addition, its emphasis on the importance of environment in influencing behavior suggests that nutrition education should also create a supportive environment.

Practice examples. Many programs in community settings focus on outcome expectations plus skill building. An example is the "Just say yes to fruits and vegetables" (JSY) program for food stamp populations, discussed in Nutrition Education in Action 5-3. Another is the *Little by Little* CD-ROM discussed in Nutrition Education in Action 5-4. The usefulness of a one-time interactive experience with the latter program was examined for low-income women. The CD-ROM included a self-assessment with immediate feedback to make the need for change individually relevant. This was followed by suggestions on how to add fruits and vegetables to the diet, and finally goal setting and individual commitment.

Self-Regulation Models

Many other researchers have found from research that self-regulation is a key process in initiating and maintaining health behavior change (Bagozzi, 1992; Gollwitzer, 1999; Gollwitzer & Oettingen, 2000; Rothman, 2000). The processes described are similar to those in social cognitive theory. However, these models note that becoming motivated to initiate a behavior requires a different mind-set and different tasks from maintaining a behavior once we have started taking action. In the motivation phase, a deliberative—or thinking—mind-set predominates, and in the action phase an implementation—or doing—mind-set predominates (Abraham, Sheeran, & Johnson, 1998; Gollwitzer & Oettingen, 2000).

Health Action Process Approach Model

We describe the health action process approach model here because it is a simple model that integrates several theories and models and adds a time dimension (Schwarzer & Fuchs, 1995; Sniehotta, Scholz, & Schwarzer. 2005). It is shown in Figure 5-2. The model proposes two phases—a preaction phase and an action phase—and focuses on the important role of self-efficacy at various points in the dietary change process, as shown in the figure.

Motivational phase. The focus in the motivational phase is on beliefs and affect or feelings, and a deliberative mind-set prevails. In this model, the motivational phase involves the relationships among potential mediators of behavior change, as shown in Figure 5-2. Our intention to adopt a valued health behavior, (such as eating a low-fat, high-fiber diet), depends on three sets of beliefs:

1. *Risk perceptions:* The belief that we are at risk for disease (e.g., heart disease). This is the perceived risk or threat construct from the health belief model.

NUTRITION EDUCATION IN ACTION 5-3

Just Say Yes to Fruits and Vegetables

The Just Say Yes to Fruits and Vegetables Project (JSY), in partnership with organizations that serve the food insecure, is dedicated to improving the health and nutritional status of food stamp populations in New York State. The project accomplishes this by providing comprehensive nutrition education programs for food stamp populations in a variety of community settings.

About JSY: Nutrition Education Sessions
- Does your organization work with food stamp eligibles, recipients, or applicants?
- Is your organization interested in offering free nutrition education programs to your clients?
- Do your clients want to know what to do with some of the produce you give them?
- Do your clients need help with preparing healthy meals on a budget?

If you said "Yes" to these questions, then the Just Say Yes to Fruits and Vegetables Project would love to visit your site!

How does the Just Say Yes to Fruits and Vegetables program work with food pantries and other communities?
Nutritionists from this program provide nutrition education sessions at local food pantries and agencies that provide services to the emergency feeding network. Sessions emphasize the use of frozen, canned, and dried products as well as fresh in-season fruits and vegetables. Each session offers the following:
- Easy, low-cost recipes
- A taste sample of a recipe made with the featured fruit or vegetable
- Tips and ideas for planning and preparing delicious, healthy meals
- Information on stretching food dollars
- Food safety information
- Food and nutrition resource information

What is the purpose of a nutrition education session?
Nutritionists from the JSY program provide nutrition education sessions at a variety of sites across the state of New York. The purpose of this program is to
- Empower low-income New Yorkers to make healthier food choices
- Convey the message that consumption of fruits and vegetables may reduce the risk of chronic diseases (such as heart disease, diabetes, and cancer)
- Enhance nutrition knowledge and skills in purchasing and preparing the best-quality fruits and vegetables
- Improve food safety skills

Source: New York State Department of Health. 2005. Just say yes to fruits and vegetables. http://www.jsyfruitveggies.org. Logo used with permission.

2. *Outcome expectancies:* The belief that a change in behavior would reduce the health threat ("If I eat healthful foods, I will reduce my risk for heart disease"). This is the perceived benefits construct of the health belief model or the outcome expectations of the theory of planned behavior and social cognitive theory.
3. *Perceived Self-efficacy:* The belief that we are sufficiently capable of exercising control over a difficult behavior, such as "I am capable of controlling my diet to make it healthful in spite of temptations to eat sweets." This may be called "motivational self-efficacy."

Risk perceptions serve predominantly to set the stage for a thinking process early in the motivation phase but do not extend beyond this phase. Similarly, outcome expectancies or anticipations about potential future outcomes are mostly important in the motivation phase, when individuals are balancing the perceived benefits and barriers of the behavior. These anticipations would be expected to lose their predictive power after a personal decision has been made. Lack of perceived self-efficacy, however, will limit motivation as well as the ability to initiate a behavior and is important in both phases of behavior change, as is posited in social cognitive theory. This has been demonstrated in many studies, including a study that found that risk perceptions, outcome expectancies, and self-efficacy were predictors of intention to initiate a low-fat, high-fiber diet, particularly for those over

NUTRITION EDUCATION IN ACTION 5-4

The *Little by Little* CD-ROM: Eat Better for a Better You

People find it hard to change dietary behavior. So asking them to eat five to nine servings of fruits and vegetables per day may be overwhelming, and many may be afraid to undertake any change at all if they believe it will be too difficult. The *Little by Little* CD-ROM program encourages small dietary changes to move people in the right direction toward a better diet. It is brief and easy, and takes only about 12 to 15 minutes.

Program

The program has three components:

- *Self-assessment and feedback.* Participants complete a 10-item survey on their usual intake of fruits and vegetables and get immediate feedback on their intake so as to make the need for change personally meaningful.
- *Modules on suggestions for specific situations.* Individuals click on only those modules that are relevant to them. The program is thus very flexible. For example, those who think that time is the issue can go to the Time section. Those who eat out a lot can find hints on getting more fruits and vegetables when eating out. If money is an issue, they can go to that section. If they pack lunches for themselves or their children, the program offers ideas. The whole point is giving people something easy that they can do to improve their diets.
- *Goal setting and individual commitment.* To facilitate goal setting, the program suggests several goals to work toward, guided by options that the participant had chosen throughout the program, and the participant is asked to choose one or two of them.

Evaluation

The program was evaluated though a randomized trial in which one group used the interactive CD-ROM program, a second group used the CD-ROM program and also received reminder phone calls, and a third (control) group received a stress management CD-ROM. The study participants were low-income African American and white women, mean age 50.1 years (SD 7.22, range 39–65).

Results

Two months after the one-time experience with the CD-ROMs, both intervention groups reported significantly higher intakes of fruits and vegetables than the control group. The *Little by Little* group with reminder calls increased daily intake by 1.32 fruits/vegetables, an 86% greater increase than the control group ($P = .016$). The *Little by Little* group without reminder calls increased daily intake by 1.20 fruits/vegetables, a 69% greater increase than the control group ($P = .052$). Significantly greater movement in stage of readiness for change also occurred in the *Little by Little* groups compared with the control group.

Source: Block, G., P. Wakimoto, D. Metz, et al. 2004, July. A randomized trial of the *Little by Little* CD-ROM: Demonstrated effectiveness in increasing fruit and vegetable intake in a low-income population. *Preventing Chronic Disease* [online serial] 1(3); available at www.cdc.gov/pcd/issues/2004/jul/04_0016.htm.

age 30. Six months later, however, intention and the belief in one's ability to cope with the diet were important during the maintenance phase (Schwarzer & Renner, 2000).

Planning. Strategic planning has been found to greatly enhance the translation of intentions into action. Here people begin to make plans to carry out the behavior and confidence in being able to make plans becomes important.

Action phase. In the action phase, the mind-set is one of implementation (or doing), and the focus is on self-regulatory processes (Gollwitzer & Oettingen, 2000). Studies suggest that initiating a behavior and maintaining it involve somewhat different tasks. In the health action process approach, these constitute the action initiation and the action maintenance subphases.

The *action initiation* subphase is a planning phase in which we first convert intentions (e.g., eating five fruits and vegetables a day) into *action plans* or *implementation intentions, specifying when, where, and how we will take action* ("I will add orange juice at breakfast each day next week; I will have a fruit for a snack three days this coming week"). Making very specific action plans has been shown to be effective in assisting individuals to initiate action (Gollwitzer, 1999; Armitage, 2004; de Nooijer et al., 2006).

Implementation intentions or action plans are effective in bridging the intention–behavior gap because the decision is made ahead of time and they link the specific actions to a given situation, so that when the situation arises, such as when

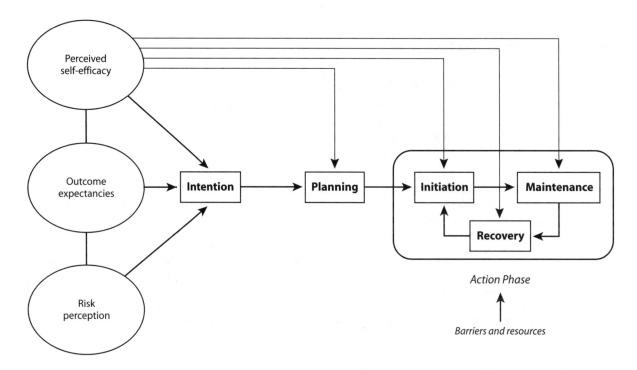

FIGURE 5-2 The health action process approach.

Source: R. Schwarzer, Freie Universitat Berlin, Germany. Used with permission.

breakfast time comes, we do not have to think and make a new decision each time. By having made anticipatory decisions, the behavior is also on our minds and so the plan is easily accessible. Such *planning ahead* means the behavior will require less mental effort each time (Gollwitzer, 1999). After making clear implementation intentions or action goals, we also need to learn new knowledge and skills in food and nutrition (e.g., what constitutes a serving of fruits and vegetables), strengthen our self-efficacy through practicing goal-setting skills.

The *action maintenance* subphase is a behavioral maintenance phase in which we gain control over our behaviors. It requires self-regulatory skills by which we develop the ability to influence and take charge of our own actions or behavior through our own efforts (Box 5-2). A major challenge for us at this stage—indeed, an ongoing challenge in maintaining healthful practices—is setting priorities between conflicting goals or desires, such as between the goal to eat more healthfully and our personal agenda, which may involve work-related aspirations that do not leave much mental and physical time for planning and eating healthfully. At this time, the chosen behavioral goal, such as to eat healthful lunches at work, needs to be protected from being interrupted or given up prematurely due to competing intentions, such as the desire to be a productive worker and hence to

work through lunch. Higher-order thinking or metacognitive activity is needed for us to stick with our chosen behavior and ignore the distracting action imperatives.

Self-regulatory skill development thus relies on conscious control and attention. It also relies on strategies for coping with emotions, such as the ability to ignore feelings of worry or of disappointment in not meeting the goals we set. These skills are important because many desirable food- and nutrition-related practices require effort, for example, seeking out farmers' markets in order to eat locally, or learning to cook so as to gain control over what ingredients are in the food we eat. We should also remember that implementing a new, more healthful behavior, such as adding fruit to the diet, does not automatically reduce less healthful habits such as eating high-fat, high-sugar snacks (Verplanken & Faes, 1999). Optimistic beliefs about our ability to deal with barriers, although a major hindrance in getting us motivated, may be helpful here because a new behavior may turn out to be much more difficult to adhere to than we had anticipated. These beliefs are sometimes referred to as *coping self-efficacy*. An example is "I can stick with a healthful diet even if I have to try several times until it works" or "even if I need a long time to develop the necessary routines" (Schwarzer & Renner, 2000). The aim here is for the new behavior to become habitual and routine.

Just as initiation of a behavior is based on our *anticipation* of the satisfaction we will obtain from a behavior, so maintenance of the new behavior is based on our experience of the satisfaction of the *actual outcomes* we obtain from the new behavior (Rothman, 2000).

We may not be able to maintain our goal behaviors at all times. Recovery self-efficacy now becomes important–the conviction that we are able to get back on track after being derailed from our goal, or after we experience setbacks. High recovery self-efficacy enables individuals to get back on track.

Evidence for the Model from Research Studies
The model is an integration of theories that we have examined before, for which there is already a body of evidence. Additional studies have examined the importance of these variables in relation to diet (Sheeshka, Woolcott, & MacKinnon, 1993; Schwarzer & Fuchs, 1995). A study to test the self-regulation theory (Bagozzi, 1992), and the model of action phases in relation to weight loss or maintenance did indeed confirm the essential features and sequence of phases (Bagozzi & Edwards, 1999). Important pre-action factors were expectations about the goal, social norms, attitudes toward success and failure, and attitudes toward the process itself. These contributed to desire to take action and goal intention (or the decision to take action). Subsequently, implementation intentions in the form of mental and physical "trying" led to the dieting and exercise behaviors that resulted in goal attainment. Studies on physical activity behavior have also provided support for this model (Ziegelmann, Lippke, & Schwarzer, 2006). An implementation mind-set is important in the action and maintenance phases because it triggers cognitive processes, such as our attention and perceptions, and mobilizes effort to pursue the decision we have made or the goal we have set.

Personal Food Policies: Findings from Interpretative Studies

As noted before, we hold many different and often conflicting motivations or values for the same foods: we want the food to be inexpensive or "good value for our money," but we also want it to be convenient; we want it to be nutritious, but we also want it to be something that our families will eat. Studies using an interpretative approach or grounded theory approach have found that individuals develop personal food policies or systems to manage, over the long term, the numerous and conflicting values they hold about their food choices (Connors et al., 2001; Bisogni et al., 2005; Contento et al., 2006). They attempt to simplify decisions by various strategies. They can choose one value and use it predominantly, such as choosing the least expensive option, the one that tastes the best, or the healthiest, regardless of other criteria. Or they can prioritize by various values or criteria, such as using cost as the crite-

---

▶ BOX 5-1 Action Plans/Goal Setting: Why They Help Us Translate Intentions into Action

Action plans (or implementation intentions) are highly effective in bridging the intention to behavior gap for many reasons:

- Stating a clear action plan is usually understood by individuals as committing themselves to an action, resulting in a sense of control, of determination, and also obligation to realize the action or behavior.
- The decision is made ahead of time, linking specific actions to a given situation, so that when the situation arises we do not have to think and make a new decision each time. Such *planning ahead* means the behavior will require less mental effort each time.
- Because the decision about a behavior is made in advance, it is also on our minds and so the action plan is easily accessible.
- Developing action plans contributes to the cultivation of intrinsic interest through our active involvement in the process.
- Action plans increase motivation through anticipation of self-satisfaction in achieving our goals.

---

rion for home meals, but relaxing this criterion when guests are coming for dinner; using health as the main criterion, but building in occasions (e.g., eating out) when health will be relaxed in favor of taste; or accommodating the needs of others rather than their personal values in order to manage social relationships, such as when invited out to dinner. A study with adolescents obtained similar kinds of personal policies: they balanced "unhealthy foods" with "healthy foods" within a meal, between meals (less-healthy lunches with peers and healthful dinners at home), and between weekdays and weekends (Contento et al., 2006).

Managing healthy eating for a sample of adults meant being concerned about balance, low fat, weight control, whether foods were natural, disease management, or disease prevention (Falk et al., 2001). Strategies to ensure healthful eating were avoidance or limitation of foods that were less healthful, substitution with others, and using appropriate food preparation methods. For those experiencing food insecurity, the personal food policies were chosen to cope with the lack of sufficient quantity of wholesome, nutritious food. Here the personal food policies included substituting less expensive foods for more expensive (e.g., dried beans instead of canned beans, or canned fruits instead of fresh), reducing or omitting unaffordable ingredients, looking for foods from atypical sources such as food pantries, and putting children's food needs first (Hoisington, Shultz, & Butkus, 2002).

People who are diagnosed with type 2 diabetes as adults need long-term maintenance of behavior change. Diabetics are required to adopt and maintain a number of dietary patterns and self-care behaviors in order to achieve and sustain control of their blood sugar. They use many of the strategies described previously: making action plans and protecting their action plans from competing goals, being mindful about their eating so that they are not distracted by alternative intentions, and making personal food policies. A study that examined diabetics' beliefs and perceptions about their diets and how to manage them is described in Nutrition Education in Action 5-5.

▶ BOX 5-2 Meeting the Challenge of Maintaining Healthful Behaviors

Maintaining chosen behaviors over the long term requires self-regulatory skills by which individuals develop the ability to influence and take charge of their own actions through their own efforts. Some of the strategies that are helpful are listed here.

Maintaining Goals
- *Prioritizing competing goals.* Individuals all have competing goals at any one time. To maintain their chosen behavioral goal, they need to protect it from being interrupted or given up prematurely due to competing intentions. They can also seek ways of satisfying both their health goal and other goals at the same time.
- *Mindful eating: protecting action goals from distractions.* Individuals can become busy and distracted by the presence of friends or colleagues or of nonhealthful foods, and, without thinking, they fail to follow their action plan. Sticking with their plan is not about being rigid or about denial. It is about being mindful about their eating and thinking about whether this is what they really want to be doing. In our current food environment, eating healthfully requires conscious attention.
- *Focusing on the big picture in the achievement of action goals.* Individuals can remember that if they eat foods they had not planned to on one occasion, they can always compensate for it at the next, so that overall they achieve their goal.
- *Linking action goals to their self-identity.* Sometimes it can help for individuals to remember that they now have a new identity—for example, as individuals who want to take care of themselves, or as active people.
- *Correctly attributing their successes and failures.* This allows individuals to claim successes and feel good about them, and recognize that failures may be due to circumstances beyond their control.

Developing Routines and Habits
- Sticking with action plans can make the chosen behavior become more routine; new habits are developed.

Countering
- Individuals can substitute alternative thoughts and behaviors for less healthful eating behaviors.

Coping Self-Efficacy
- Optimistic beliefs about their ability to deal with barriers—the conviction that they can carry out their intentions even under difficult circumstances—can be very helpful at this stage.

Creating Personal Environments to Achieve Goals
- *Stimulus control.* Individuals can restructure their personal environment to make it more supportive by removing cues to less healthful eating and adding cues for more healthful eating.
- *Seeking social support.* Individuals can seek the help of those around them.

Enjoying Healthful Food: Coming to Like What One Eats
- Eating healthfully becomes enjoyable as healthful foods become familiar and when individuals learn the skills to make them tasty.

Developing Personal Policies: Expressing Agency
- Individuals can develop personal food policies or systems to manage, over the long term, the numerous and conflicting values they hold about their food choices. For example, they may have a policy that they will always have breakfast before leaving the house, even if it is modest.

The Transtheoretical Model and the Stages of Change Construct

The transtheoretical model has become one of the most widely used models in the study of health behaviors, including dietary behaviors (Prochaska & DiClemente, 1984; Prochaska & Velicer, 1997). It originated from an analysis of 18 systems of psychotherapy that identified common processes that individuals use to make changes in their own behavior (Prochaska & DiClemente, 1984), hence the name *transtheoretical*. During this analysis, Prochaska and DiClemente found that behavior change seemed to occur through a series of stages. When the model was originally used in the area of

---

NUTRITION EDUCATION IN ACTION 5-5

Food Selection and Eating Patterns Among People with Type 2 Diabetes

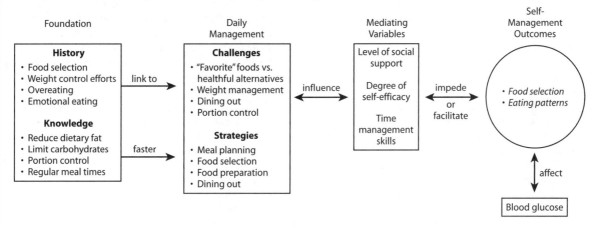

Elements influencing food selection and eating patterns among people with type 2 diabetes.

People with type 2 diabetes are required to adopt and maintain for the long term many dietary and self-care behaviors to achieve and sustain control of their blood sugar. This study used semistructured, in-depth interviews to explore the beliefs and perspective of those with type 2 diabetes about dietary requirements, food selection and eating patterns, and their attitudes about self-management practices. These interviews were analyzed for themes, which are captured in the accompanying diagram.

Prior history with food selection and weight control efforts are linked to current challenges involving avoiding favorite foods and choosing more healthful alternatives, managing weight, dining out, and exercising restraint in terms of portions. Their prior knowledge was helpful in using strategies to manage their diets.

The mediators that facilitated or impeded their food selection behaviors and eating patterns were as follows:

- Level of social support, particularly support of spouse.
- Degree of self-efficacy or confidence that they would be able to stay with their eating plans even in difficult situations, such as when eating with coworkers who were eating fast foods they liked, or resisting rich baked goods at family gatherings.
- Time management, which was a problem because they always had to plan ahead of time what they were going to eat and stick with a schedule. They had to time their insulin or oral medication to food intake.

In general, they developed specific practices, routines, or personal policies to support their self-management efforts.

Source: Savoca, M., and C. Miller. 2001. Food selection and eating patterns: Themes found among people with type 2 diabetes mellitus. *Journal of Nutrition Education* 33:224–233. Figure used with permission of the Society for Nutrition Education.

health, it was applied to smoking and other addictive behaviors. It has now been applied to a range of health behaviors, including safer sex practices, mammography screening, weight control, and diet and physical activity behaviors.

The transtheoretical model proposes that self-change in behavior is a process that occurs through five stages. It also proposes that there are two mediators of change (decisional balance based on pros and cons of change, and self-efficacy) and ten processes of change. The transtheoretical model is a model of behavior *change*, not a model predicting behavior. Like social cognitive theory, it provides guidance on actual strategies for bringing about behavior change. Unlike social cognitive theory, it adds a time dimension to the behavior change process: it proposes that behavior change occurs through a series of stages; social cognitive theory does not.

The Stages of Change Construct

The transtheoretical model proposes that health behavior change is a gradual, continuous, and dynamic process that can be seen as occurring through a series of five stages or phases, as described in this section. Stages are thus a way of categorizing people according to their readiness to adopt healthful behaviors. Knowledge of the stage or readiness of individuals and groups can be used to inform intervention design. The stages of change construct has been used in dozens of studies in the health area, including many in the areas of diet and physical activity. Many such studies use the stages of change construct without using transtheoretical model "processes of change," described later in this chapter, making the underlying theory a stages of change model. Often such a stages of change model is combined with the psychosocial constructs of the other theories we have discussed, such as perceived benefits and barriers or outcome expectations. In addition, the stages in many studies are collapsed into pre-action and action/maintenance stages, resulting in a stage structure similar to some of the theories described earlier in this and previous chapters.

A major contribution of the stages of change construct is a reminder that most nutrition education programs are "action centered," assuming a certain degree of readiness to take action on the part of program participants. They thus fail to address the needs of those who are not yet emotionally prepared to act. The stages as are follows:

1. *Precontemplation* (PC) is the time during which individuals are not aware of, or not interested in, a behavior or practice that might enhance their own health or that of the natural environment (such as eating less saturated fat or buying local foods). This may be because they are uninformed or underinformed about the impacts of such behavior. Also included in this category are those who have tried and failed to make the behavior change, perhaps many times, and no longer want to think about it.

2. *Contemplation* (C) is the stage in which individuals are considering making a change sometime in the near future, usually defined as within the next six months. They are more aware of the pros of changing but are especially aware of the costs of changing. They struggle between thinking about the positive outcomes of the behavior and the amount of time, energy, and other resources that will be needed to change. This can cause enormous ambivalence, resulting in "chronic contemplation" or procrastination (Prochaska, DiClemente, & Norcross, 1992). Individuals at this stage need motivational activities rather than action-oriented, behavioral change strategies.

3. *Preparation* (P) is the stage in which individuals intend to make a change in the immediate future, usually defined as one month, and may have already taken some steps in that direction. This stage is similar to the behavioral intention stage of the theory of planned behavior and the health action process approach. Individuals in this stage are ready for action-oriented strategies that will help them initiate action.

4. *Action* (A) is the stage in which individuals have started to engage in the new behavior or practice (often defined as within the previous six months). They may adopt the practice (e.g., eat less fat) on a small scale at first or try out alternative practices, such as eating less meat rather than using low-fat milk in place of whole milk, to find one at which they can be successful and that fits into their usual routine. Action-oriented strategies are particularly helpful here.

5. *Maintenance* (M) refers to the period in which people have performed the new behavior or practice for long enough (usually defined as longer than six months) to be comfortable with incorporating it as part of their way of life (e.g., they now routinely buy and use nonfat milk or eat five fruits and vegetables a day). Individuals may need to continue to exert effort in order to maintain the behavior and avoid relapse.

For addictive behaviors, a sixth stage, *termination*, is included, during which individuals no longer succumb to any temptation and feel total self-efficacy. For dietary behaviors, this stage may not be practical or applicable because we all have to eat; hence, a more realistic goal is a lifetime of maintenance.

Specifying Behavior and Identifying Stage of Change in Individuals

To use the stages of change construct, the behavior of interest must be clearly specified. The early studies in the health area involved smoking, an easily observable behavior. In the dietary behavior area, eating fruits and vegetables may be seen as similarly easily observed and specified. However, even here, eating fruits and eating vegetables are often seen by the public as different behaviors. Classifying individuals in terms of whether they are eating less fat or more fiber becomes more complicated because more categories of foods contribute to fat and fiber in the diet. When the goal of dietary improvement is even more general, such as to eat according to the *Dietary Guidelines*, multiple changes are necessary in several behavioral categories, and hence identifying the stage of change is more difficult.

Staging individuals. There is some debate on how best to place individuals into stages (Richards et al., 1997; Green & Rossi, 1998; Greene et al., 1999; Kristal et al., 1999). Generally speaking, placement into stages is based on individuals' *perceptions* about their dietary behaviors. A variety of instruments have been developed, most of them quite short (five or six questions) and easily administered orally or through a brief questionnaire. An algorithm or formula is then applied to classify people. For example, the simplest is as follows: "I am not (eating five fruits and vegetables [F&V] daily) and do not intend to start in the next six months" will place a person in the precontemplation stage. "I am not (eating five F&V daily) but intend to start in the next six months" places a person in the contemplation stage. "I am not (eating five F&V daily) but intend to do so within the next month" places the person in the preparation stage. "I have been eating five F&V daily, but for less than six months" places the person in the action stage. "I have been eating five F&V daily for more than six months" places the person in the maintenance stage. Instruments like this have been used in various studies (Campbell et al., 1998; Cullen et al., 1998; Ma et al., 2002). Placing people into stages with respect to fat and fiber intake is more complicated, but instruments have been developed and validated in which the questions are made quite general. For example, assigning people into stages of change for a low-fat diet can be based on a series of questions about eating "less fat," such as "Are you seriously thinking about eating less fat over the next six months?" Other time frames have also been used (Sporny & Contento, 1995; Povey et al., 1999).

Some instruments use the criterion of *actual* behavior or nutrient intake, such as eating less than 30% calories from fat, to place individuals into action/maintenance stages (Green et al., 1994), rather than *perception* of fat intake. This approach is based on the observation that there is often a discrepancy between self-perceived and actual diet, particularly with respect to fat because it is difficult for people to judge the fat content of their diets (Glanz & van Assema, 1997; Lechner, Brug, & De Vries, 1997). Other classification schemes have been proposed, based on both perceived *and* actual diet (Auld et al., 1998). Using a behavioral or nutrient criterion makes it more likely to assign a stage accurately, so that those who think they are in the maintenance stage and are not will receive the right kind of nutrition education. On the other hand, using self-reported diet tells us about what a person is thinking and tells us the extent to which individuals

are *engaged* with the dietary change process, which also provide us with important information for designing appropriate nutrition education activities.

It should be noted that individuals can be, and usually are, at different stages of change for different diet-related behaviors. For example, individuals wanting to "eat more healthfully" may be at the action stage in terms of adding fruits and vegetables to their diets but still contemplating cutting down on high-fat, high-sugar food products. Or people may have started adding fruits to their diets but have not yet been able to increase the amount of vegetables they eat. There are also considerable spontaneous changes in stages among people over time, both forward and backward (Kristal et al., 2000; de Nooijer et al., 2005).

Decisional Balance: The Pros and Cons of Change
Decisional balance, or the weighing of the pros and cons of change, is an important construct in the transtheoretical model. Pros are our beliefs about the anticipated benefits of changing, and cons are the costs of changing. Decisional balance is based on a model of decision making that proposes that behavior change emerges when the pros, or anticipated benefits, outweigh the cons, or costs, of the behavior. The pros and cons of change are similar to the perceived benefits and barriers constructs of the health belief model and the outcome expectations construct of the theory of planned behavior and social cognitive theory. Examples of pros of change are "Eating healthy food is helpful in preventing cancer" and "Eating healthful food will improve the way I look." Examples of cons of change include "I would find it hard to give up some of my favorite foods to follow a healthier diet" and "It is too expensive to eat organic foods."

In the pre-action stages, the cons of change have been found to be higher than the pros. Cons might include unacceptable changes in taste, difficulty in thinking of recipes and preparing new foods, or increased length of time in preparing food. In the action stages, the pros of change are higher than the cons (Steptoe et al., 1996; Prochaska & Velicer, 1997). The crossover point in the diet and physical activity areas is generally between the contemplation and the preparation and action stages. Thus it can be concluded that only when perceived benefits outweigh perceived barriers will contemplators move into preparation and action. Some studies indicate that the pros of change have to increase twice as much as the cons must decrease for action to be initiated. This suggests that considerable emphasis may need to be paid to raising the benefits of change in order to overcome the barriers to change.

Self-Efficacy
The self-efficacy construct was integrated into the stages of change model from social cognitive theory. It is the confidence that people have that they can carry out the behav-

ior across different challenging situations and not relapse to their previous, less healthy behavior. Self-efficacy tends to decrease between the precontemplation stage and contemplation stage, probably because in the precontemplation stage individuals have an optimistic bias about what they can do, and it is during the contemplation stage that they first realize how difficult the new behavior may be. Self-efficacy then steadily increases through the action and maintenance stages (Sporny & Contento, 1995; Steptoe et al., 1996; Campbell et al., 1998; Ma et al., 2002)

Temptation is a construct that reflects the urge to engage in a less healthful behavior in difficult situations, such as we might experience at a party laden with high-fat, high-sugar foods when we are watching our weight. Temptation is low in precontemplation, as would be expected; we would only perceive temptation as a problem if we have become concerned about eating high-fat, high-sugar foods and are trying to avoid them. Temptation is especially strong during the contemplation and preparation stages and declines substantially in the maintenance stage.

The Processes of Change
The processes of change are overt and convert strategies that individuals use to move themselves through the stages of change. Each of the change processes is a category of similar activities and experiences that facilitate individuals' progress through the stages. Ten processes have been proposed. These include *experiential* or *cognitive processes* that focus on thoughts, feelings, and experiences and *behavioral processes* that focus on behaviors and reinforcement. The transtheoretical model proposes that behavior change is facilitated if interventions focus on change processes that are matched to the stage of change of individuals.

The processes associated with change are as follows:

Experiential

- *Consciousness-raising*: Increasing one's awareness about the causes, consequences, and cures for a health issue and seeking new information about healthy behaviors. For example, "I seek out magazine articles to learn more about how eating fruits and vegetables can affect health." This process is somewhat similar to the *perceived benefits* of the health belief model and the *outcome expectations* of the theory of planned behavior and social cognitive theory.
- *Dramatic relief or emotional arousal*: Experiencing and expressing the negative emotions or feelings (fear, anxiety, worry, sense of threat) about our problems, followed by reduced emotion if appropriate action is seen as possible. For example, "Warnings about how diet can contribute to the risk of developing heart disease make me anxious." (Thus it is similar to *perceived threat* in the health belief model.)

- *Self-reevaluation*: Reassessing our beliefs, knowledge, feelings, or self-image about a particular unhealthy food-related behavior or practice in relation to ourselves (e.g., an image of self as a junk food eater). For example, "I think about how I would be a healthier person if I ate more fruits and vegetables."
- *Environmental reevaluation*: Examining our positive and negative beliefs and feelings about the impact of our personal diet-related behaviors on others. This could also include our evaluation of ourselves as a role model to others, positive or negative. For example, "I realize that I may be able to keep local farmers in business if I join a community-supported agriculture farm" or "I realize that I would be a role model to my children if I ate more fruits and vegetables daily."
- *Self-liberation or commitment*: Believing that we can change, and making a conscious choice and firm commitment to make the change. For example, "I am committed to eating more fruits and vegetables each day." (This is similar to *behavioral intention* of the theory of planned behavior, or *goal intention* of social cognitive theory.)

Behavioral

- *Helping relationships*: Enlisting the trust, caring, and acceptance in our relationships with others to help us change (such as making pacts with coworkers not to eat donuts for snacks). (This is similar to *social support* in social cognitive theory.)
- *Counterconditioning*: Learning to replace less healthful behaviors with more healthful ones, such as eating fruit instead of high-fat, high-sugar desserts.
- *Managing rewards*: Reevaluating the way in which we use food as a reward or punishment. Evidence suggests that self-changers use rewards more than punishment to manage their behaviors.
- *Stimulus or environmental control*: Removing cues or triggers for undesirable behavior (e.g., avoiding walking past a bakery with one's favorite pastries) and adding cues or prompts for more healthful alternatives, such as putting on one's office calendar a reminder to walk during lunch hour.
- *Social liberation*: Becoming aware of environmental factors that influence our dietary patterns and using the external environment to help us get started or to stay with a change. For example, if we are trying to eat more vegetables, we will choose a restaurant that offers salads and vegetable entrées for lunch. This process also involves the notion of advocacy, for example, to increase the availability of more healthful foods in schools and communities. This might mean advocating for increasing the availability of salad bars in the school cafeteria as an alternative to fast food.

Integrating Stages and Processes of Change

Studies have provided evidence that individuals use these processes in self-change to different extents as they move through the stages (Prochaska & Velicer, 1997). In the area of diet, it has been found that experiential and behavioral processes increased together through the stages (Greene et al., 1999; Rosen, 2000).

More specifically, the transtheoretical model proposes, and research evidence confirms, that when we are in the precontemplation stage, we use all of these processes significantly less than in all the other stages. In the contemplation stage we become open to consciousness-raising strategies, such as observations, self-assessments, and other strategies to raise awareness about our behavior, such as self-assessments of our fruit and vegetable intakes per day, combined with information about the benefits of fruits and vegetables for health or disease risk. During contemplation we are also open to emotionally arousing experiences, such as stories about the impact of diabetes on given individuals, which can lead to dramatic relief as we make changes (e.g., based on information about the efficacy of fruits and vegetables for reducing disease risk). As we become more conscious of ourselves and the nature of our food-related issues, we are more likely to reevaluate ourselves, our values, and our problems both cognitively and affectively. We also evaluate the effects of our behaviors on those around us and on the physical environment. Movement through the contemplation stage involves increased use of the cognitive, affective, and evaluative processes of change.

We begin to take action when we believe that we have the autonomy to make changes through a self-liberation process, and make a firm commitment to change. As we take action, we call on skills in counterconditioning (substituting more healthful foods for those less healthful) as well as environmental or stimulus control such as making sure not to keep large supplies of energy-dense foods in the house to help us maintain our weight. Successful maintenance of change involves the use of behavioral processes to prevent relapse to less healthy patterns of behavior. Here nutrition education can assist us to acquire and practice these skills. Social support can be important, as well as rewards given by others or by ourselves. Most important to maintenance is the sense we have that we are becoming who we want to be.

Research and Intervention Examples

Support for the stages of change construct in the area of diet has been seen from a number of studies. For example, those individuals in the action and maintenance stages have lower intakes of fat and higher intakes of fiber and of fruits and vegetables compared with those in the pre-action stages (Brug et al., 1994; Glanz et al., 1994; Sporny & Contento, 1995; Steptoe et al, 1996; Glanz et al., 1998). In studies, the stage of change is useful as a predictor of health behavior change, as

a way to stratify people so as to match interventions to individuals on the basis of their readiness to change, and as an intermediate outcome measure to indicate progress toward health behavior change.

Mediators and stages. The motivating force for movement through the stages according to the transtheoretical model is the balance of pros and cons of change (perceived benefits and barriers), and the major resource for change is self-efficacy.

Many cross-sectional studies have examined the relationship between these variables and stages of change in the area of diet. Psychosocial constructs from the other theories are often also included (Sporny & Contento, 1995; Steptoe et al., 1996; Glanz, & Kok, 1997; Campbell et al., 1998, 1999b; BrugKristal et al., 2000; Horacek et al., 2002; de Nooijer et al., 2005). Taken together, these and other studies suggest that although there is considerable moving back and forth among stages, perceived benefits or pros are especially important in the early stages, where they serve a motivational role, and must become greater than cons if change is to take place. Self-efficacy has been found to influence movement through the stages (O'Hea et al., 2004).

Stage-matched interventions tailored to individuals. One of the main implications of the stages of change model is that different kinds of nutrition education activities should be used with individuals at different stages of psychological readiness to change. Extensive research in the area of smoking has found that the use of a stage-matched approach to intervention is more effective than a one-size-fits-all traditional action-oriented approach (Velicer & Prochaska, 1999). Here the stages of change construct is used to design interventions that are specifically tailored to *individuals* at different stages of change (Prochaska et al., 1993). Tailoring differs from targeting in that *targeted* interventions are directed at groups or populations with similar characteristics, whereas *tailored* interventions are directed at individuals within target populations. Here individuals complete a questionnaire by phone, paper, or computer to assess their pros and cons and self-efficacy, and are then provided with individualized feedback reports based on their responses. They are then provided with information (e.g., through newsletters or self-help manuals) on the processes of change that they can use, appropriate to their stage.

In the area of diet, tailored interventions have been conducted in a variety of settings, such as primary care settings (Campbell et al., 1994), health departments (Jacobs et al., 2004), worksites (Brug et al., 1996; Campbell et al., 2002; Brug, Oenema, & Campbell, 2003) and families (De Bourdeaudhuij et al., 2002). Other channels have also been used, such as the Web (Oenema, Tan, & Brug, 2005), CD-ROM (Campbell et al., 2004), and multimedia programs (tailored soap opera and interactive infomercials) (Campbell et al., 1999a). These studies suggest that tailoring the intervention to a given individual's stage of psychological readiness to take action can enhance the effectiveness of nutrition education.

Stage-matched interventions with groups. In a group or population-wide setting, we cannot provide interventions that are specific to each individual's stage of readiness to change. However, assuming that there will be people at all stages of change in a group, we can sequence activities in a stepwise fashion:

1. Promotional activities to promote awareness and enhance motivation, targeting those in the pre-action stages
2. Action and skills training, targeting those in the action stage
3. Social support and maintenance of behavior
4. Environmental supports

> **▶ BOX 5-3   Using the Transtheoretical Model Processes of Change to Promote Dietary Fat Reduction**
>
> A study with college students focused on the pre-action, stage-oriented change processes to foster motivation to change. The sessions focused on the following:
>
> - A high-fat diet increases blood lipid levels and promotes abnormal blood clotting, which in turn increase risk for heart disease. *Change processes emphasized:* consciousness raising and emotional arousal.
> - A high-fat diet can increase risk for certain types of cancer. *Change processes emphasized:* consciousness raising and emotional arousal.
> - Personal risks come from fat intake as well as biology; analysis of self. *Change processes emphasized:* consciousness raising and self-evaluation.
> - Low-fat eating can taste good, and low-fat cooking can be used to decrease fat in home-cooked foods. *Change processes emphasized:* self-evaluation and social liberation.
> - Strategies can be used to control fat intake when dining out. *Change processes emphasized:* self-evaluation and social liberation.
>
> This intervention produced a significant increase in movement of those in the pre-action stage into action, and a significant reduction in fat intake that persisted for at least one year.

Such strategies, if effective, should accelerate movement from pre-action stages into the action and maintenance stages. Consequently, intervention outcomes can be measured in two ways: change in the targeted behavior, such as reduction in fat intake or increase in fruit and vegetable intake, or progression to a later stage of change (Glanz et al., 1998; Kristal et al., 2000). Use of stage-matched group activities in these studies did indeed find that those in pre-action stages at baseline were much more likely to move into action and maintenance stages than controls. Changes in stage were associated with decreases in fat intake and increases in fiber, fruit, and vegetable intake.

Interventions have also been conducted in which the activities have been specifically based on the 10 processes of change specified by the transtheoretical model. One study with college students (Box 5-3) was delivered in a group setting and focused on pre-action, stage-oriented change processes of the model (Finckenor & Byrd-Bredbenner, 2000). The rationale was that much of nutrition education tends to focus on providing knowledge and skills—that is, it is action-oriented, how-to knowledge. Although such information is useful for those in the later stages of change, it may not facilitate the movement of those in pre-action stages to take action. The first half of the sessions focused on the processes of consciousness raising and emotional arousal, which are very similar to the mediating variable of perceived risk and perceived benefits from other theories. The later sessions focused on self-evaluation and social liberation, which included some skill building.

In another study, the transtheoretical model processes of change were used in a clinic-based program that focused on a healthy lifestyle approach to weight management that also included exercise. It was successful in promoting changes in exercise and dietary behaviors, weight loss, increased cardiorespiratory fitness, and improved lipid profiles (Riebe et al., 2003).

Summary of the Transtheoretical Model

In summary, the transtheoretical model emphasizes that self-directed behavior change is a dynamic process that unfolds over time through a series of stages in terms of readiness to change. The pros and cons of change are the motivational force for change in the transtheoretical model, according to Velicer and Prochaska (1999) and Baranowski and colleagues (2003), and represent beliefs about why to change. Individuals seek to engage in behaviors to achieve positive ends and to avoid negative ones. The personal resource needed for change (or "how to" change) within the transtheoretical model is self-efficacy, that is, the confidence that we can engage in the behavior even in the face of difficulties. The processes by which change is likely to occur are described in the model. Procedures that can be used by nutrition education interventions to encourage change are based on these processes.

A major strength of the transtheoretical model is its emphasis that individuals are at different stages in terms of their readiness to engage in a health- or food-related behavior and that consequently, health promotion interventions must be designed to meet the needs of individuals at each stage of change. Indeed, the transtheoretical model argues that the majority of people are not ready for action in terms of healthy behaviors and that they will not be well served by traditional action-oriented programs, which generally assume that people are ready for action and need only factual and procedural knowledge and skills. People can be categorized fairly easily into the different stages or states of readiness to change. Activities appropriate for each stage are shown in Table 5-3.

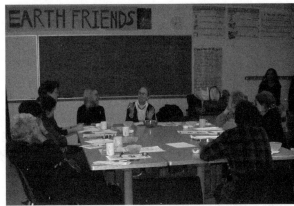

Learning to set action plans for healthy living.

TABLE 5-3 Transtheoretical Model: Application to Nutrition Education Interventions

Stage of Readiness to Change	Important Processes for Moving to Next Stage	Nutrition Education Intervention Strategies
Precontemplation	Increased awareness, sense of risk, understanding, and recognition of emotional adjustments needed for change	Provide personalized information on own eating pattern (e.g., fruit and vegetable intake) through self-assessment and feedback (e.g., group 24-hour recall); personalize risk; help individuals understand and express emotions about the need for change Media: trigger films, personal testimonies, media campaigns to address feelings and personalized risks
Contemplation	Recognition of ambivalence but increased appreciation for benefits of behavior, and confidence in one's ability to enact the recommended behavior	Messages or strategies in groups to enhance people's pros/benefits of change (taste, health benefits, convenience); discuss barriers to change; assist individuals to recognize own ambivalence; provide positive feedback about individuals' current abilities and assets
Preparation	Making a commitment to change; resolving ambivalence	Have individuals state goal intention (e.g., to eat more fruits and vegetables), develop specific action plans, start taking small steps toward goal; reinforce attempts to change
Action	Building skills and seeking social support	Teach food- and nutrition-specific knowledge and skills needed for behavior change; goal setting and self monitoring skills; provide encouragement and support; encourage seeking of social support network
Maintenance	Self-management and relapse prevention skills creating social and environmental support	Teach new ways of thinking about behavior, restructuring environment, rewarding themselves; anticipate and plan for potential difficult situations; create buddy systems; problem-solving if they lapse; strengthen skills to advocate for environments that support healthful food practices

Comparing Social Cognitive Theory and the Transtheoretical Model: Change as a Process

The theories and models reviewed in this chapter provide understandings for both motivations for behavior and the process of behavior change. In summary, the theories and the research based on them suggest that outcome expectations—also labeled perceived benefits or barriers and the pros and cons of change—are important motivators of change, that self-efficacy beliefs are important resources for making changes, and that behavioral and self-regulatory skills are essential for the ability to act on our motivations. These theories thus provide guidance for how to design nutrition education intervention strategies to assist individuals to take action in a way that the theories and the models described in the previous chapter did not.

Social cognitive theory emphasizes the reciprocal nature of these potential mediators of change acting at all times, whereas the transtheoretical model emphasizes that behavior change is a process, with individuals being at different stages in terms of their readiness to take action, so that the relative importance of these mediators of behavior change differs depending on the individual's state of readiness to take action. However, these two approaches are not so different from each other. Bandura himself has noted the special importance of outcome expectations and self-efficacy beliefs for motivating individuals to form goal intentions to initiate behavior and the importance of self-regulation processes for maintaining behavior, referring to these as phases of behavioral change (Bandura 1997, 2000). At the same time, he transtheoretical model acknowledges that change is more like a spiral than a straight line, with a great deal of back and forth movement and recycling between the stages. Research studies are also finding that in the area of diet, the stages are often not clearly delineated. Both social cognitive theory and the transtheoretical model provide guidance on procedures that can be used to design nutrition education activities for assisting individuals to take action. In social cognitive theory, these procedures involve goal setting and self-monitoring. In the transtheoretical model, practical procedures are based on the processes of change. Thus it would appear that both theories are consistent with the emerging evidence from research based on the extended behavioral intention models (described in the last chapter) and the health action process approach that although dietary behavior change is very complex, it can be seen as involving a motivational, deliberative phase (or component) with an emphasis on thoughts, beliefs, and affect that are important for *why to* initiate action, and an action and maintenance phase (or component) with an emphasis on self-regulation skills that are important for *how-to* take action.

The Case of Ray

How can we apply what we have learned to Ray? Let's say the doctor sends Ray and others like him to you for nutrition education. They are motivated at that moment to reduce their risk of diabetes. What can you do to help Ray and the others translate intentions into action? You could start with reviewing with them some reasons to make some changes so as to reinvigorate their motivation—emphasizing that perhaps they want to be healthy at their children's graduation or wedding, or to enjoy their retirement. Then ask them to choose one healthy behavior that they will start with, such as their eating habits at work.

Ask Ray to think of specific actions he could take, for example, bringing food such as apples or bananas from home to keep at his desk instead of packaged snacks. Develop an action plan or pledge form for him to complete and sign. Have someone from the group or, better yet, from his place of work witness the pledge. You can teach him about being mindful about his eating and about protecting his commitment from competing priorities and distractions. As he develops this new routine and is confident that he can maintain it, ask him to select further actions he can take to improve his health, such as taking a walk during his lunch hour or bringing lunch from home. Draw attention to the fact that he is now taking care of himself and taking control of his eating.

Implications for How-to Nutrition Education to Facilitate the Ability to Take Action

We have examined some of the key theories or models for understanding how individuals translate motivation and intention to act into action. What are the implications for nutrition education practice? How can we use this information to design nutrition education that emphasizes how to take action?

Integrative Conceptual Framework for Nutrition Education

Influencing Factors That Are Potential Mediators of Behavior Change

Figures 5-3 and 5-4 summarize the processes of change going on within individuals as they seek to take action and maintain the food choices and dietary changes they have voluntarily chosen on the basis of personal health or other criteria.

Educational goal. For those initiating a behavior, the educational goal is to facilitate the development of implementation plans or action plans and to build skills in both the food and nutrition areas and increase their sense of self-efficacy.

For those who are seeking to maintain behaviors they have chosen, the educational goal is to assist these individuals to strengthen their self-regulation skills and adopt personal food policies that will sustain them.

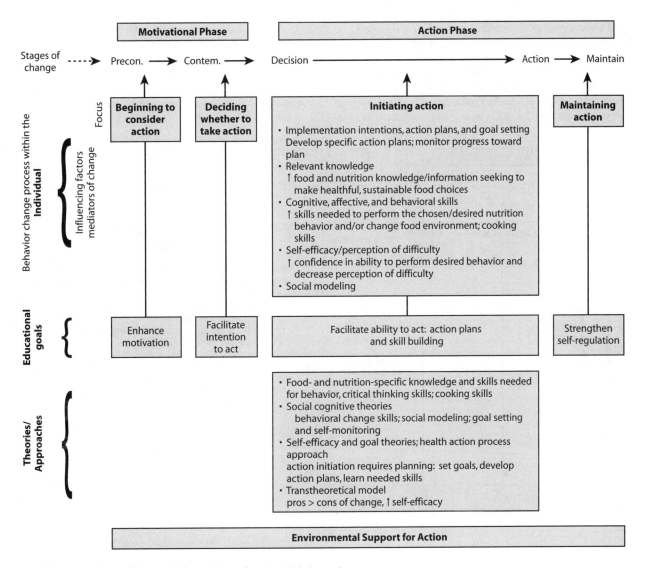

FIGURE 5-3 Conceptual framework for nutrition education: Initiating action.

Useful theories. The most helpful theories are social cognitive theory, self-regulation theories, the health action process approach, the transtheoretical model, and findings from grounded theory. If theory is seen as summarized and interpreted evidence, we can see that there is considerable agreement among the theories about how to assist individuals to initiate and maintain diet-related change.

Nutrition Education Strategies to Facilitate the Ability to Take Action

Appropriate translation of information about determinants that can mediate the targeted behavior changes into practical theory-based strategies for addressing them in an inter-

vention, whatever the channel used, is a crucial process for assuring the effectiveness of nutrition education interventions. Potential practical strategies are suggested only briefly here. They are described more fully within the nutrition education design model described in Part II.

The strategies listed here are the practical operationalizations of theory constructs for mediators of behavior change.

Action Plans

In the postdecision action phase, nutrition education activities should assist individuals to construct specific detailed implementation intentions (Gollwitzer, 1999) or action plans to bridge the intention/decision-to-behavior gap, such as "I will add one fruit to my breakfast each morning this week" or "I will eat two servings of vegetables each dinner this week."

Food- and Nutrition-Related Knowledge and Cognitive Skills
After individuals become motivated to take a nutrition-related action, they will need specific knowledge and skills in order to act on their decision. For example, individuals will need to know

how to select foods for optimal health from the 50,000-item supermarket; evaluate the nutrition information that bombards them from magazines, newspapers, advertising, and friends; and interpret personal medical information provided by their physicians. Food and nutrition education must therefore provide information and opportunity to develop the cognitive skills that will enhance people's power to act on their desire to change.

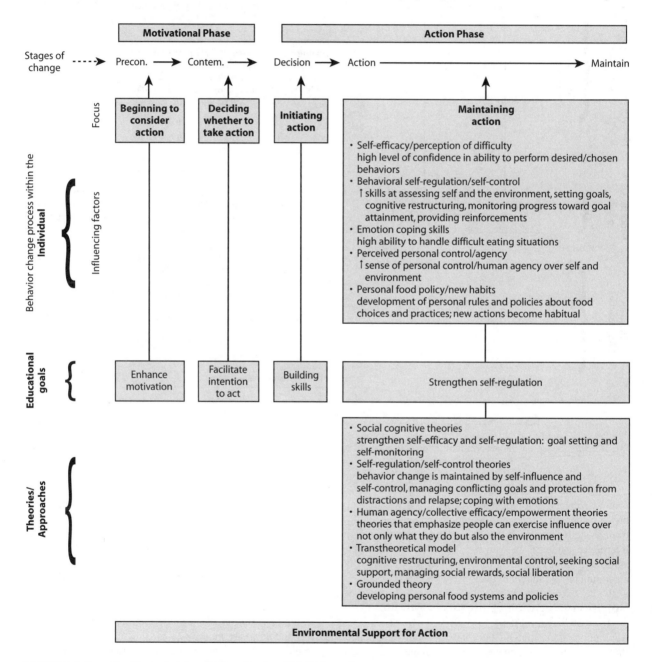

FIGURE 5-4　Conceptual framework for nutrition education: Maintaining action.

Now is the time to provide how-to information (factual knowledge) about foods, nutrients, dietary guidelines, label reading, or MyPyramid and ways to apply this information in people's daily eating plans (procedural knowledge). If a low-fat diet is the focus of the program, the fact that chicken eaten with skin is three times the calories as chicken without skin, and five to ten times as caloric (due to fat) if it is also battered and deep fried, is important knowledge. As nutrition educators, we are very good at designing these kinds of activities! Lectures, handouts, tip sheets, newsletters, flyers, and Web-based programs are all suitable here, depending on the behavior or practice and the channel chosen (e.g., mass media or in person).

Critical Thinking Skills
Food and nutrition issues are often complex. The nutrition research findings are sometimes contradictory. Individuals need the ability to evaluate evidence and understand reasoned arguments for different options, such as whether to reduce dietary fat or carbohydrate to lose weight. They need critical thinking skills in order to evaluate controversial issues or to understand complex issues related to health and food policies Nutrition education activities such as written or oral critiques, debates, and trigger films for discussion can be useful here.

Building Behavioral Skills in Foods and Nutrition and Self-Efficacy
Beliefs about the anticipated consequences of behavior (outcome expectations) are less important in the action phase while self-efficacy is more important. Self-efficacy may increase with increased levels of skills, but self-efficacy is not the same thing as physical skills such as food preparation or safe food handling. Self-efficacy involves both skills and the confidence that individuals can consistently use them even in the face of impediments or barriers. To develop food- and nutrition-related behavioral skills, the behavior should be modeled, such as through food demonstrations accompanied by clear instructions. However, individuals must also be provided with opportunities to practice the behavior, such as cooking. Verbal encouragement by the nutrition educator can overcome self-doubts.

Cooking skills. Social cognitive theory emphasizes that it requires actual experience to develop physical skills, such as cooking, safe food preparation practices, and other food-related skills. Research has shown that cooking experiences, as part of nutrition education, are likely to enhance behavior change (Liquori et al., 1998; Ammerman et al., 2002).

Goal Setting
Behavior change requires not only behavioral skills but also the ability of individuals to exercise self-influence or self-control over their own behavior. This ability does not involve

willpower so much as a set of self-regulation skills, including goal setting (Bandura, 1986; Cullen, Baranowski, & Smith, 2001; Shilts, Horowitz, & Townsend, 2004). Nutrition education interventions need to teach individuals the skills of goal setting and provide opportunities to practice them, with guidance. Goal setting is a process involving the following steps (Shilts, Horowitz, & Townsend, 2004):

- *Performing self-assessment or observation.* The purpose is to identify ways in which individuals' current actions or behaviors contribute to the issue or problem they are concerned about.
- *Setting action goals.* Individuals then need to set action goals to address their concern or problem, for example, to eat more fruits and vegetables.
- *Contracting.* Commitment to the action goal is strengthened by believing in the value of the behavior, perceiving that the goal is attainable, and making binding pledges, often called *contracts.* Such pledges have motivational impact because there are consequences or costs to not following through on an agreement. These consequences may be personal, such as self-reproof, or social, if the commitments were made in public or involve others, where the costs may include embarrassment or social disapproval.
- *Acquiring relevant knowledge and skills.* Information and skills to attain the goal are needed next.
- *Monitoring of progress toward the goal.* The focus should be on positive accomplishments rather than failures.
- *Attaining goals.* Attaining a goal can result in a sense of self-efficacy, self-satisfaction, and accomplishment that sustains effort or leads to the setting of increasingly more difficult behavior change goals.
- *Using problem-solving and decision-making strategies.* These strategies are mobilized if the goal is not achieved. The goal can be modified, or a new, more achievable one can be set.

The use of contracting has been studied. In one study it was shown to increase the effectiveness of nutrition education in a pilot program with low-income women (Heneman et al., 2005). They significantly increased their fruit intake, and in terms of stages of change, they moved toward acceptance of vegetable consumption. The "Contract for Change" that was used in the study is shown in Figure 5-5.

Self-Regulation Skills and Personal Food Policies for Maintenance of Change
Nutrition education activities designed to assist individuals to maintain their chosen action should focus on other aspects of self-regulation in addition to goal setting. In particular, the nutrition educator needs to teach individuals how to handle competing goals, such as whether to go out and eat a health-

ful lunch or work through lunch with what is available; competing distractions, such as having the TV on at dinner; and how to plan for potential difficulties, such as maintaining dietary changes while on vacation.

Teaching individuals many of the behavioral processes of the transtheoretical model can be helpful here to prevent relapse to less healthful ways of eating—for example, removing cues or triggers for undesirable behavior (stimulus control), helping individuals reevaluate how they use food in their lives (e.g., as rewards) and to replace less helpful

ways with more helpful ways, and discussing how to select places to eat that support the new behavior. In general, it means assisting individuals to develop their own personal food policies that facilitate healthful eating patterns. The nutrition education intervention can also provide individuals with social support or assist them in seeking social support; assist individuals to enjoy healthful food through a variety of activities involving tasting or cooking food in a pleasant atmosphere; and teach skills in advocating for more healthful options at work, school, or in the community.

The aim of this is to help you make and keep healthy eating habits.

1. Goals: List two ways you can eat more fruits and vegetables.

1) _____

2) _____

2. Setting a goal: Choose one goal from the above two lines and make it into something you can do.

Action goal: _____

What will you do differently? _____

_____

How often?_____

How much?_____

Where?_____

With whom?_____

3. Make a plan: List two reasons why this change may be hard.

1) _____

2) _____

What will you do to beat these problems?

1) _____

2) _____

Let's Try to Make This Change!

FIGURE 5-5 Example of a contract for setting goals. *Source:* Heneman, K., A. Block-Jay, S. Zidenberg-Cherr, et al. 2005. A "contract for change" increases produce consumption in low-income women: A pilot study. *Journal of the American Dietetic Association* 105:1793–1796. Used with permission of the authors.

Questions and Activities

1. Describe in your own words the following theory constructs. How are the terms related to behavior change?
   a. Outcome expectations
   b. Self-efficacy
   c. Modeling
   d. Behavioral capability
   e. Reinforcement
   f. Pros and cons of change
2. Describe what is meant by the "processes of change" in the transtheoretical model.
3. Compare social cognitive theory, the transtheoretical model, and the health action process approach in terms of (a) what motivates behavior, (b) what facilitates the ability to change one's behavior, and (c) how change occurs. In what ways are the constructs similar or different in the three theories?
4. What strategies can be used to increase self-efficacy in individuals?
5. Why is goal setting (developing action plans) so important as a process? What does it accomplish? What are some key steps?

6. Think about the food-related behavior changes that those you interviewed attempted to make. Now that you have read the chapter:
   a. How would you now describe the factors involved in the failures and successes, using the language of the theory constructs described in this chapter?

Reasons Given for Being Successful/ Not Successful	Name of Construct of Theory	Justification for Assignment

   b. Can you now explain why one was successful whereas the other was not?
   c. For the person who was not successful, what five tips can you give him or her to help that individual be more successful in the future?

REFERENCES

Abraham, C., P. Sheeran, and M. Johnson. 1998. From health beliefs to self-regulation: Theoretical advances in the psychology of action control. *Psychology and Health* 13:569–591.

Ammerman, A.S., C.H. Lindquist, K.N. Lohr, and J. Hersey. 2002. The efficacy of behavioral interventions to modify dietary fat and fruit and vegetable intake: A review of the evidence. *Preventive Medicine* 35(1): 25–41.

Armitage, C. 2004. Evidence that implementation intentions reduce dietary fat intake: A randomized trial. *Health Psychology* 23:319–323.

Auld, G.W., S.A. Nitzke, J. McNulty, et al. 1998. A stage-of-change classification system based on actions and beliefs regarding dietary fat and fiber. *American Journal of Health Promotion* 12(3):192–201.

Bagozzi, R.P. 1992. The self-regulation of attitudes, intentions, and behavior. *Social Psychology Quarterly* 55:178–204.

Bagozzi, R.P., and E.A. Edwards. 1999. Goal striving and the implementation of goal intentions in the regulation of body weight. *Psychology and Health* 13:593–621.

Bandura, A. 1977. *Social learning theory*. Englewood Cliffs, NJ: Prentice Hall.

———. 1986. *Foundations of thought and action: A social cognitive theory*. Englewood Cliffs, NJ: Prentice-Hall.

———. 1997. *Self-efficacy: The exercise of control*. New York: WH Freeman.

———. 2000. Health promotion from the perspective of social cognitive theory. In *Understanding and changing health behavior: From health beliefs to self-regulation*, edited by P. Norman, C. Abraham, and M. Conner. Amsterdam: Harwood Academic Publishers.

Baranowski, T., J. Baranowski, K.W. Cullen, et al. 2003. *Squire's Quest!* Dietary outcome evaluation of a multimedia game. *American Journal of Preventive Medicine* 24(1):52–61.

Baranowski, T., K.W. Cullen, T. Nicklas, D. Thompson, and J. Baranowski. 2003. Are current health behavioral change models helpful in guiding prevention of weight gain efforts? *Obesity Research* 11(Suppl.):23S–43S.

Baronowski, T., M. Davis, K. Resnicow, et al. 2000. Gimme 5 fruit, juice, and vegetables for fun and health: Outcome evaluation. *Health Education and Behavior* 27(1):96–111.

Baranowski, T., S. Domel, R. Gould, et al. 1993. Increasing fruit and vegetable consumption among 4th and 5th grade students: Results from focus groups using reciprocal determinism. *Journal of Nutrition Education* 25(3):114.

Bisogni, C.A., M. Jastran, L. Shen, and C.M. Devine. 2005. A biographical study of food choice capacity: standards, circumstances, and food management skills. *Journal of Nutrition Education and Behavior* 37(6):284-291.

Brug, J., K. Glanz, and G. Kok. 1997. The relationship between self-efficacy, attitudes, intake compared to others, consumption, and stages of change related to fruit and vegetables. *American Journal of Health Promotion* 12(1):25-30.

Brug, J., A. Oenema, and M. Campbell. 2003. Past, present, and future of computer-tailored nutrition education. *American Journal of Clinical Nutrition* 77(Suppl):1028S–1034S.

Brug, J., I. Steenhuis, P. van Assema, and H. de Vries. 1996. The impact of a computer-tailored nutrition intervention. *Preventive Medicine* 25:236–242.

Brug, J., P. van Assema, G. Kok, T. Lenderink, and K. Glanz. 1994. Self-rated dietary fat intake: Associations with objectively assessed intake, psychosocial factors and intention to change. *Journal of Nutrition Education* 26:218–223.

Campbell, M.K., E. Carbone, L. Honess-Morreale, J. Heisler-Mackinnon, S. Demissie, and D. Farrell. 2004. Randomized trial of a tailored nutrition education CD-ROM program for women receiving food assistance. *Journal of Nutrition Education* 36:58–66.

Campbell, M.K., B.M. DeVillis, V.J. Strecher, A.S. Ammerman, R. DeVellis, and R.S. Sandler. 1994. Improving dietary behavior: The effectiveness of tailored messages in primary care settings. *American Journal of Public Health* 84:783–787.

Campbell, M., L. Hones-Morreale, D. Farrell, E. Carbone, and M. Brasure. 1999a. A tailored multimedia nutrition education pilot program for low-income women receiving food assistance. *Health Education Research* 14:257–267.

Campbell, M.K., K.D. Reynolds, S. Havas, et al. 1999b. Stages of change for increasing fruit and vegetable consumption among adults and young adults participating in the national 5-a-Day for Better Health community studies. *Health Education and Behavior* 26(4):513–534.

Campbell, M.K., M. Symons, W. Demark-Wahnefried, et al. 1998. Stages of change and psychosocial correlates of fruit and vegetable consumption among rural African-American church members. *American Journal of Health Promotion* 12(3):185–191.

Campbell, M.K., I. Tessaro, B. DeVellis, et al. 2002. Effects of a tailored health promotion program for female blue-collar workers: Health Works for Women. *Preventive Medicine* 34(3):313–323.

Chang, M.W., S. Nitzke, R.L. Brown, L.C. Bauman, and L. Oakley. 2003. Development and validation of a self-ef-ficacy measure for fat intake behaviors of low-income women. *Journal of Nutrition Education and Behavior* 35:302–307.

Connors, M., C.A. Bisogni, J. Sobal, and C.M. Devine. 2001. Managing values in personal food systems. *Appetite* 36:189–200.

Contento, I.R., S.S. Williams, J.L. Michela, and A. Franklin. 2006. Understanding the food choice process of adolescents in the context of family and friends. *Journal of Adolescent Health* 38:575–582.

Cullen, K.W., T. Baranowski, and S.P. Smith. 2001. Using goal setting as a strategy for dietary behavior change. *Journal of the American Dietetic Association* 101:562-566.

Cullen, K.W., L.K. Bartholomew, G.S. Parcel, and L. Koehly. 1998. Measuring stage of change for fruit and vegetable consumption in 9- to 12-year-old girls. *Journal of Behavioral Medicine* 21(3):241–254.

De Bourdeaudhuij, I., J. Brug, C. Vandelanotte, and P. Van Oost. 2002. Differences in impact between a family- versus an individual-based tailored intervention to reduce fat intake. *Health Education Research* 17(4):435–449.

de Nooijer, J., E. de Vet, J. Brug, and N.K. de Vries. 2006. Do implementation intentions help to turn good intention into high fruit intakes? *Journal of Nutrition Education and Behavior* 38:25–29.

de Nooijer, J., P. van Assema, E. de Vet, and J. Brug. 2005. How stable are stages of change for nutrition behaviors in the Netherlands? *Health Promotion International* 20:27–32.

Edmundson, E., G.S. Parcel, H.A. Feldman, et al. 1996. The effects of the Child and Adolescent Trial for Cardiovascular Health upon psychosocial determinants of diet and physical activity behavior. *Preventive Medicine* 25(4):442–454.

Falk, L.W., J. Sobal, C.A. Bisogni, M. Connors, C.M. Devine. 2001. Managing healthy eating: Definitions, classifications, and strategies. *Health Education and Behavior* 28:425–439.

Finckenor, M., and C. Byrd-Bredbenner. 2000. The development and long-term effectiveness of a nutrition intervention program for lowering dietary fat intake based on the transtheoretical (stages of change) model. *Journal of the American Dietetic Association* 100(3):335–342.

Glanz, K., A.R. Kristal, B.C. Tilley, and K. Hirst. 1998. Psychosocial correlates of healthful diets among male auto workers. *Cancer Epidemiology, Biomarkers and Prevention* 7(2):119–126.

Glanz, K., R.E. Patterson, A.R. Kristal, et al. 1994. Stages of change in adopting healthy diets: Fat, fiber, and correlates of nutrient intake. *Health Education Quarterly* 21:499–519.

Glanz, K., R.E. Patterson, A.R. Kristal, Z. Feng, L. Linnan, and J. Hebert. 1998. Impact of worksite health promotion on stages of dietary change: The Working Well Trial. *Health Education and Behavior* 25:448–463.

Glanz, K., and P. van Assema. 1997. Are awareness of dietary fat intake and actual fat consumption associated? A Dutch-American comparison. *European Journal of Clinical Nutrition* 51:542–547.

Gollwitzer, P.M., 1999. Implementation intentions—strong effects of simple plans. *American Psychologist* 54:493–503.

Gollwitzer, P.M., and G. Oettingen. 2000. The emergence and implementation of health goals. In *Understanding and changing health behaviour from health beliefs to self-regulation*, edited by P. Norman, C. Abraham, and M. Conner. Amsterdam: Harwood Academic Publishers.

Greene, G.W., and S.R. Rossi. 1998. Stages of change for reducing dietary fat intake over 18 months. *Journal of the American Dietetic Association* 98:529–534.

Greene, G.W., S.R. Rossi, G.R. Reed, C. Willey, and J.O. Prochaska. 1994. Stages of change for reducing dietary fat to 30% of energy or less. *Journal of the American Dietetic Association* 94:1105–1110.

Greene, G.W., J.S. Rossi, S.R. Rossi, et al. 1999. Dietary applications of the stages of change model. *Journal of the American Dietetic Association* 99:673–678.

Heneman, K., A. Block-Joy, S. Zidenberg-Cherr, et al. 2005. A "Contract for Change" increases produce consumption in low-income women: A pilot study. *Journal of the American Dietetic Association* 105:1793–1796.

Hoisington, A., J. Armstrong Shultz, and S. Butkus. 2002. Coping strategies and nutrition education needs among food pantry users. *Journal of Nutrition Education and Behavior* 34:326–333.

Horacek, T.M., A. White, N.M. Betts, S. Hoerr, et al. 2002. Self-efficacy, perceived benefits, and weight satisfaction discriminate among stages of change for fruit and vegetable intakes for young men and women. *Journal of the American Dietetic Association* 102(10):1466–1471.

Horowitz, M., M.K. Shilts, and M.S. Townsend. 2004. EatFit: A goal-oriented intervention that challenges adolescents to improve their eating and fitness choices. *Journal of Nutrition Education and Behavior* 36(1):43–44.

Jacobs, A.D., A.S. Ammerman, S.T. Ennett, et al. 2004. Effects of a tailored follow-up intervention on health behaviors, beliefs, and attitudes. *Journal of Women's Health* 13:557.

Keller, K.L., A. Peitrobelli, and M.S. Faith. 2002. Genetics of eating and its relation to obesity. *Current Atherosclerosis Reports* 4:176–182.

Kirby, S.D., T. Baranowski, K.D. Reynolds, G. Taylor, and D. Binkley. 1995. Children's fruit and vegetable intake: Socioeconomic, adult-child, regional, and urban-rural influences. *Journal of Nutrition Education* 27(5):261.

Kristal, A.R., K. Glanz, S.J. Curry, and R.E. Patterson. 1999. How can stages of change be best used in dietary interventions? *Journal of the American Dietetic Association* 99:679–684.

Kristal, A.R., K. Glanz, B.C. Tilley, and S. Li. 2000. Mediating factors in dietary change: Understanding the impact of a worksite nutrition intervention. *Health Education and Behavior* 27:112–125.

Lechner, L., J. Brug, and H. De Vries. 1997. Misconceptions of fruit and vegetable consumption: Differences between objective and subjective estimation of intake. *Journal of Nutrition Education* 29:313–320.

Leupker, R.V., C.L. Perry, S.M. McKinlay, et al. 1996. Outcomes of a field trial to improve children's dietary patterns and physical activity: The Child and Adolescent Trial for Cardiovascular Health (CATCH). *Journal of the American Medical Association* 275:768–776.

Lewis, C.J., L.S. Sims, and B. Shannon. 1989. Examination of specific nutrition/health behaviors using a social cognitive model. *Journal of the American Dietetic Association* 89(2):194-202.

Liquori, T., P.D. Koch, I.R. Contento, and J. Castle. 1998. The Cookshop Program: Outcome evaluation of a nutrition education program linking lunchroom food experiences with classroom cooking experiences. *Journal of Nutrition Education* 30(5):302–313.

Lytle, L.A., D.M. Murray, C.L. Perry, et al. 2004. School-based approaches to affect adolescents' diets: Results from the TEENS study. *Health Education and Research* 31:270–287.

Ma, J., N.M. Betts, T. Horacek, C. Georgiou, A. White, and S. Nitzke. 2002. The importance of decisional balance and self-efficacy in relation to stages of change for fruit and vegetable intakes by young adults. *American Journal of Health Promotion* 16(3):157–166.

Mennella, J.A., M.Y. Pepino, and D.R. Reed. 2005. Genetic and environmental determinants of bitter perception and sweet preferences. *Pediatrics* 115(2):216–222.

Molaison, E.F., C.L. Connell, J.E. Stuff, M.K. Yadrick, and M. Bogle. 2005. Influences on fruit and vegetable consumption by low-income black American adolescents. *Journal of Nutrition Education and Behavior* 37(5):246–251.

Oenema, A., F. Tan, and J. Brug. 2005. Short-term efficacy of a Web-based computer-tailored nutrition intervention: Main effects and mediators. *Annals of Behavioral Medicine* 29:54–63.

O'Hea, E.L., E.D. Boudreaux, S.K. Jeffries, et al. 2004. Stage of change movement across three health behaviors: The role of self-efficacy. *American Journal of Health Promotion* 19:94–102.

Ounpuu, S., D.M. Woolcott, S.R. Rossi. 1999. Self-efficacy as an intermediate outcome variable in the transtheoretical model: Validation of a measurement model for applications to dietary fat reduction. *Journal of Nutrition Education* 31:16–22.

Povey, R., M. Conner, P. Sparks, R. James, and R. Shepherd. 1999. Critical examination of the application of the transtheoretical model's stages of change to dietary behaviors. *Health Education Research* 14:641–651.

Prochaska, J.O., and C.C. DiClemente. 1984. *The transtheoretical approach: Crossing the traditional boundaries of therapy*. Homewood, IL: Dow Jones-Irwin.

Prochaska, J.O., C.C. DiClemente, and J.C. Norcross. 1992. In search of how people change: Applications to addictive behaviors. *American Psychologist* 47(9):1102–1114.

Prochaska, J. O., C.C. DiClemente, W.F. Velicer, and J.S. Rossi. 1993. Standardized, individualized, interactive and personalized self-help programs for smoking cessation. *Health Psychology* 12:399–405.

Prochaska, J.O., and W.F. Velicer. 1997. The transtheoretical model of health behavior change. *American Journal of Health Promotion* 12:38–48.

Reynolds, K.D., A.W. Hinton, R. Shewchuk, et al. 1999. A social cognitive model of fruit and vegetable consumption in elementary school children. *Journal of Nutrition Education* 31(1):23–30.

Richards, G., W.F. Velicer, J.O. Prochaska, J.S. Rossi, and B.H. Marcus. 1997. What makes a good staging algorithm: Examples for regular exercise. *American Journal of Health Promotion* 12:57–66.

Riebe, D., G. Greene, L. Ruggiero, et al. 2003. Evaluation of a healthy-lifestyle approach to weight management. *Preventive Medicine* 36:45–54.

Rosen, C.S. 2000. Is the sequencing of change processes by stage consistent across health problems? A metaanalysis. *Health Psychology* 19:593–604.

Rothman, A.J. 2000. Toward a theory-based analysis of behavioral maintenance. *Health Psychology* 19:64–69.

Schwarzer, R., and R. Fuchs. 1995. Self-efficacy and health behaviors. In *Predicting health behavior*, edited by M. Conner and P. Norman. Buckingham, UK: Open University Press.

Schwarzer, R., and B. Renner. 2000. Social-cognitive predictors of health behaviour: Action self-efficacy and coping self-efficacy. *Health Psychology* 19:487–495.

Shannon, B., R. Bagby, M.Q. Wang, and L. Trenkner. 1990. Self-efficacy: A contributor to the explanation of eating behavior. *Health Education Research* 5:395–407.

Sheeshka, J.D., D.M. Woolcott, and N.J. MacKinnon. 1993. Social cognitive theory as a framework to explain intentions to practice health eating behaviors. *Journal of Applied Social Psychology* 23:1547–1573.

Shilts, M.K., M. Horowitz, and M. Townsend. 2004. An innovative approach to goal setting for adolescents: Guided goal setting. *Journal of Nutrition Education and Behavior* 36:155–156.

Sniehotta, F.F., U.R. Scholz, and R. Schwarzer. 2005. Bridging the intention-behaviour gap: Planning, self-efficacy, and action control in the adoption and maintenance of physical exercise. *Psychology and Health* 20: 143-160

Sorensen, G., M.K. Hunt, D.H. Morris, et al. 1990. Promoting healthy eating patterns in the worksite: The Treatwell intervention model. *Health Education Research* 5(4):505–515.

Sorensen, G., A. Stoddard, K. Peterson, et al. 1999. Increasing fruit and vegetable consumption through worksites and families in the Treatwell 5-a-day study. *American Journal of Public Health* 89(1):54–60.

Sporny, L.A., and I.R. Contento. 1995. Stages of change in dietary fat reduction: Social psychological correlates. *Journal of Nutrition Education* 27:191–199.

Steptoe, A., S. Wijetunge, S. Doherty, and J. Wardle. 1996. Stages of change for dietary fat reduction: Associations with food intake, decisional balance, and motives for food choice. *Health Education Journal* 55:108–122.

Thoresen, C.E. 1984. Strategies for health enhancement overview. In *Behavioral health: A handbook of health enhancement and disease prevention*, edited by J.D. Matarazzo, S.M. Weiss, J.A. Herd, and N.E. Miller. New York: John Wiley & Sons.

Velicer, W.F., and J.O. Prochaska. 1999. An expert system intervention for smoking cessation. *Patient Education and Counseling* 36:119–129.

Verplanken, B., and S. Faes. 1999. Good intentions, bad habits, and effects of forming implementation intentions on healthy eating. *European Journal of Social Psychology* 29:591–604.

Ziegelmann, J.P., S. Lippke, and R. Schwarzer. 2006. Adoption and maintenance of physical activity: Planning interventions in young, middle-aged, and older adults. *Psychology and Health* 21: 145-163

CHAPTER 6

Foundation in Theory and Research:
Promoting Environmental Supports for Action

OVERVIEW This chapter describes key issues and educational approaches that can be used to address environmental determinants that can mediate healthful food and nutrition actions. The focus of this chapter is on providing social support and educating key decision makers and policy makers in order to increase support for action.

OBJECTIVES At the end of the chapter, you will be able to

- Identify approaches to address environmental determinants that can mediate healthful food and nutrition actions
- Appreciate the importance of social support for the initiation and maintenance of healthful food- and nutrition-related actions
- Appreciate the importance of educating key decision makers and policy makers in order to address environmental determinants that mediate healthful action
- Describe interventions that have addressed interpersonal, organizational, and community influences on behavior to make them more supportive of healthful eating
- Recognize the importance of collaborations and partnerships for promoting environmental supports for action
- Define the concepts of social networks, social support, collaboration, partnership, empowerment, and collective efficacy and describe how they have been used in nutrition education
- Describe how nutrition education can address several levels of influence to support people's willingness and ability to take action
- Understand that nutrition education occurs through multiple venues and involves policy and environmental activities as well as individual-level educational activities

SCENARIO

Before you begin, think about one or two dietary changes you have tried to make. What factors in the environment have been helpful in supporting your change, and what factors have not been helpful? List five of each. As you read through this chapter, link your factors with those described in the text.

What would the ideal healthful food environment look like to you—at work or school or in the community? What role do you think nutrition educators should play in promoting an environment that is supportive of healthful eating?

Introduction: Addressing Environmental Factors Influencing People's Health Actions

Often individuals are willing and able to take action and have the intention to do so but find that whether they will actually take action is very much influenced by environmental factors—by whether the desired foods are available at a price they can afford or accessible when they need them, by what other members of their families do, by policies at their schools or places of work, and by the structure of their communities. Thus, helping individuals bridge the intention–behavior gap requires that nutrition educators also seek to make the healthful actions the easy ones. This chapter focuses on environmental determinants that mediate behavior change by facilitating or hindering us from being able to act on a need, problem, or issue of concern to us. It examines approaches and recent studies that suggest strategies for how nutrition education interventions can work toward promoting environments that are supportive of action.

What Do We Mean by Environment?

The terms *environment* and *ecology* can have varying meanings. The term *ecology* is derived from the biology literature, where it refers to the relationship between organisms and their environments, and so the term *ecological factors* refers to those relating to the natural environment. In the social sciences, environments, or the context in which we live, are often also called ecologies. Those aspects of the environment that are physical are called ecological factors, and those that include people are called social ecological factors.

In this text, *environment* refers to factors that are external to the individual. Thus, a social norm is a perception that influences behavior but is not classified as an environmental determinant of behavior because it is our *perception* of the environment and is not external to us. Social networks and social support, on the other hand, are external to us and so are considered potential environmental mediators of behavior. Culturally based institutional practices and social structures such as family meals or community holiday practices are also considered part of the environment.

In this text, the term *ecological* refers to issues within the field of food and nutrition related to the natural environment. Ecological concerns are thus concerns about the impact of food production, marketing, and consumption practices on the natural environment, and hence the ability of the food system to produce wholesome food in a way that remains sustainable. Examples are issues related to the availability and accessibility of foods produced using sustainable practices or to the vibrancy of local farms.

In the health promotion field, *social ecological models* refer to approaches that address several social ecologies or levels of influence on behavior at once. These levels are labeled intrapersonal factors, interpersonal processes and primary groups, institutional factors, community factors, and public policy and legislation (McLeroy et al., 1988; Green & Kreuter, 1999). In the social ecological model, activities and initiatives are designed to change institutions, communities, policy, and legislation in order to foster individual and community health. Such social ecological approaches to intervention thus address both environmental and personal determinants of behaviors.

Changes in environments, however, most often result from changes in the behaviors of those who have the power and authority to modify the environment—decision makers and policy makers and role actors at the various levels of influence, ranging from the interpersonal to organizational, from community to societal. Thus, to bring about food-related changes in the environment to make it more supportive of behaviors targeted by a program usually requires that we educate these decision makers or policy makers, such as school food service personnel, school principals, worksite managers, community leaders, and local, state, or national agencies. We may also work in collaboration with them to seek changes. Addressing environmental determinants that mediate individual action therefore takes many different approaches and involves a variety of activities.

Why Address Environmental Mediators of Action in Nutrition Education?

There are many reasons why a nutrition education program should, to the extent possible, address environmental mediators of behavior change. Even with motivation, knowledge, and skills, we can often still face difficulties in taking action because of environmental obstacles. As we have seen, health behavior and nutrition education research, particularly that based on social cognitive theory, has demonstrated that biological predispositions, behaviors, personal factors such as outcome expectations and self-efficacy, and the environment are intimately linked and reciprocally related to each other. All must be addressed if nutrition education is to be effective. However, social cognitive theory points out that although environments influence our perceptions and behaviors, we also influence our environments. There is a dynamic relationship between person and environment. Individuals are producers as well as products of social systems. Enhancement of environmental support for healthful practices can be initiated by nutrition educators but also by the individuals themselves, individually, as a group, or as a community. Personal and collective agency becomes a possibility.

Environmental supports help to bridge the intention–behavior gap and are particularly important during the action/maintenance phase, when we start taking action. For example, after we become concerned and motivated, healthful food must be available and accessible if we are to act on our motivation. A supportive environment seeks to make the healthful choice the easy choice. Indeed, in many instances a supportive environment is what makes it possible for those with limited incomes to adopt healthful food-related behaviors.

A focus on the environment also provides recognition that environments can impede or enable healthful behaviors, so that people are not held responsible for choices that were not theirs to make; or the converse, that good health, which may be attributed to healthful choices, was in fact due to a positive environment that enhanced the likelihood of good health.

Addressing Potential Environmental Mediators of Action or Behavior Change: Approaches and Studies

Many of our activities as nutrition educators involve *direct, in-person* activities directed at individual intrapersonal mediators of behavior change through group sessions, discussion groups, or workshops as well as *indirect, non-personal* methods such as newsletters, curricula, or social marketing, the subjects of later chapters in the book . However, nutrition education programs also address potential environmental mediators of behavior, as shown in our logic model framework for the design of nutrition education, Figure 6-1.

Addressing potential environmental mediators for the behaviors that are the focus of our programs involves two major approaches: a direct role with the intended audience and an indirect, educative and collaborative role with others in the environment. A direct role includes strategies that nutrition educators can use to address interpersonal factors that are external to the individuals to make them more

supportive of behavior by creating informational and social supports for their intended audience. These strategies might include creating support groups for the program participants, working with peer educators, developing a family component to support school- and worksite-based programs, and creating informational environments that reinforce behavior and change social norms.

An indirect role is one in which we educate and work with decision makers and others to bring about changes in the environment to support actions by our intended audience. Creating supportive environments often requires that we educate a new audience—for example, those who provide food and services (such as those in food assistance programs and public health departments) and those who have decision-making power and authority in other fields that affect the lives of our participants, such as decision makers in the home, or policy makers in organizations and at the city, state, and national levels. These people can also be considered to be gatekeepers. Our role here is to educate these individuals and groups about the importance of issues that are the focus of our program, and to develop collaborations with them in order to bring about changes in the relevant food environments.

In many instances, such as with food service directors in schools and workplaces, or leaders in the community, the "education" will be collegial and quite informal, through activities such as individual meetings, presentations to poten-

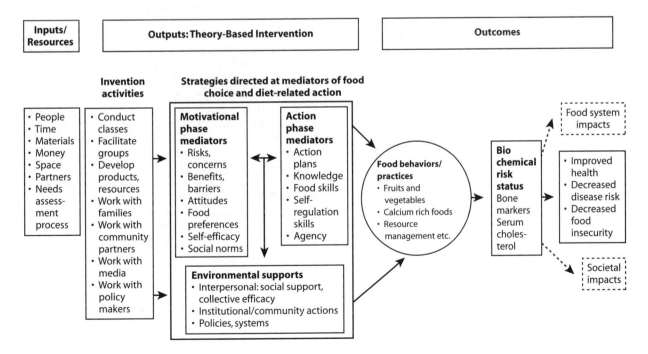

FIGURE 6-1 A logic model framework for theory-based nutrition education

tial coalition members, or task force meetings. If these individuals or organizations are convinced of the importance of your program goals, you will then work in collaboration with them to provide professional development to their staffs and other activities as needed. In other cases the education may be quite formal, in the sense that these individuals become a new, secondary audience for us, and we need to conduct separate theory-based nutrition education activities such as workshops, group sessions, or professional development to increase awareness, enhance motivation, and provide skills just as we do for our primary audience. This means that you will write educational goals and objectives and develop learning or lesson plans for this audience. A prime example is the development of a parent component for a school-based nutrition education program. At the same time, you may find yourself also working in collaboration with parents as members of the school health policy council.

Interpersonal Environment: Social Support, Collective Efficacy, and Empowerment

Social Networks and Social Support
We all live within a network of social relationships. These networks involve family, peers, coworkers, and those in various organizations to which we belong. These social relationships greatly influence individuals' food choices and dietary behaviors. Thus, strategies to promote supportive environments usually address these social networks and social support.

Researchers characterize social networks as follows (Israel & Rounds, 1987):

- *Structure:* The size and number of members in the network
- *Density:* The extent to which members know and interact with each other
- *Proximity:* The degree to which individuals in the network are similar to each other or located in close proximity
- *Interaction:* The frequency of contact, the variety of functions that the network serves (complexity), and how close members are emotionally (intensity)
- *Reciprocity:* The extent to which individuals help each other with resources and support

Some individuals are within very extensive social networks of family and friends who are in frequent contact with each other, whereas others have few friends and family with whom they interact.

Social support refers to the support that individuals in social networks provide each other in various areas:

- *Emotional support:* Involves empathy, trust, caring, and esteem

- *Instrumental support:* Involves money or other tangible resources and help, such as with babysitting or shopping
- *Informational support:* Involves advice and information useful in solving problems
- *Appraisal support:* Involves constructive feedback and self-evaluation

Again, individuals differ in the degree to which they receive social support for their eating patterns.

It has been shown that social relationships influence health status, probably both through direct effects and through their ability to buffer the negative effects of life stressors on health (Berkman & Glass, 2000). In particular, emotional support is related to good health and to reduced all-cause mortality.

In the area of diet, food choices and eating patterns are directly influenced by our social networks. The resemblances of food choices within the family are significantly greater than between family members and their friends. On the other hand, family members and others who live together may not all like or want to eat the same foods. Thus, there is a need to negotiate with the family or others about what to buy or eat (Furst et al., 1996; Feuenekes et al., 1998; Contento et al., 2006). Relationships with peers and those with whom we work also have an impact on our day-to-day choices.

Nutrition education interventions can seek to strengthen existing social networks to make them more supportive of health (such as involving the family in the intervention), provide structured social support groups, or initiate new social networks in which individuals participating in the intervention can help each other (such as regular meetings of participants, walking groups, or buddy systems). Social support is incorporated into many health interventions and indeed was identified in a review of nutrition education as one of the elements that contributed to effectiveness (Ammerman et al., 2002). Weight loss interventions routinely incorporate social support groups (e.g., Weight Watchers). Interventions in schools and workplaces have also incorporated social support in various forms. A few illustrations are provided here.

Parental support. Many interventions in schools have focused on *family involvement* as a way to work with existing social networks to make them more supportive of health. Although youth frequently eat outside the home, they still eat many of their meals with the family, particularly when they are younger. Surveys show that about three quarters of those aged 12 to 14 still eat five meals a week with their families, declining to about 60% for those aged 15 to 16, and about 40% for those aged 17 to 19 (Council of Economic Advisers, 2000). Another study found that the resemblance between food choices of teens and their parents was 76% to 87% depending on the food, whereas between teens and their peers it was 19% (Feuenekes et al., 1998). Thus, family eating patterns are very important and can be addressed

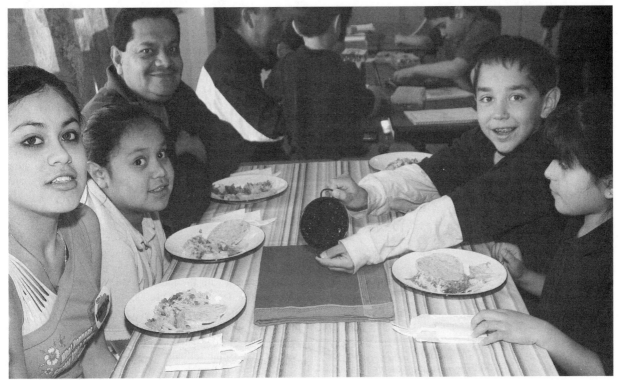

Parents and their kids enjoy a meal they have cooked together at one school's "Family Night."

by nutrition education. However, nutrition educators often find that parents are busy and cannot attend regular classes designed for them. Likewise, newsletters sent home have not been found to be effective. Hence the strategies described in the following paragraphs have been found to be more effective. In each of these examples, the parents were considered a new audience for which a separate set of educational goals and objectives, educational strategies, and evaluation measures had to be designed.

In a large study with third graders, school and school-plus-family interventions were compared (Edmundson et al., 1996). Packets containing games and activities that required parental or adult involvement to complete were sent home to families each week for five weeks. Rewards were given for completed lessons that were returned. There were also two family fun nights. Results showed that there was a greater improvement in dietary intentions and usual food choices for lower-fat and lower-sodium foods for those who had the additional family interventions. The family component of a different study, this time with middle school students, consisted of three newsletters and a set of 10 behavioral coupons with simple messages such as "Serve a fruit or vegetable with dinner tonight" (Lytle et al., 2004). About 30% of parents completed at least one set of behavioral coupons.

A more intense family component was Family Fun Nights, in which families actually came together over a meal for a food-and-game experience (Harrington et al., 2005). Each of the seven sessions offered a game, new recipe choices, intervention messages to parents, a children's fun page that reinforced program themes, optional conversation topics, and menu suggestions.

Social support in workplaces. In worksite interventions, social support has been operationalized as peer support at the worksite and involvement of family. The interventions have attempted to make these existing social networks more supportive of health. Most of the interventions have used group education classes along with other strategies. When intervention components were compared in one study, it was found that interactive strategies such as group education classes and contests were more effective in terms of nutritional outcomes (e.g., eating more fruits and vegetables) than one-time activities such as kickoffs or more passive efforts such as use of printed materials (Patterson et al., 1997).

In a study in which a family component was included (the Treatwell 5 A Day study), results showed that total fruit and vegetable intake increased by 19% in the worksite-plus-family group, 7% in the worksite intervention-only group, and 0%

in the control group, suggesting that including a family component can be an effective strategy (Sorensen et al., 1999). This study also measured coworker support for healthful eating, asking questions such as how often coworkers "encourage you to eat vegetables," "complement your attempts to eat a healthy diet," or "bring fruit to work for you to try." Coworker support increased significantly in both intervention conditions compared with the control condition. Taken together, these studies suggest that incorporating social support into nutrition education interventions is an important strategy to increase effectiveness.

Peer educators as social support. Peer educators have served an important role in nutrition education in several settings. In schools, the use of peers has been found to be very accepted and popular among the peer leaders themselves, their classmates, and teachers (Story et al., 2002). Their role is not only to teach sessions and serve as models, but also to provide social support to classmates. The Expanded Food and Nutrition Education Program of the U.S. Department of Agriculture (USDA) serves several hundred thousand low-income youth and families each year and is based on the use of paraprofessionals and peers, many of whom are indigenous to the target population. These peer educators work with small groups, often in their homes, thus providing modeling and social support as well. Results show that this approach is effective in improving eating patterns (USDA, 2003). Use of peer counselors also increased breastfeeding duration, as did support at home (Kistin, Abramson, & Dublin,1994; Sciacca et al., 1995). Peer educators were also effective among older adults (Ness, Elliott, & Wilbur, 1992).

Support groups. Often nutrition educators have the opportunity to provide individuals with social support by the creation of a new support group as part of the intervention. Many of the facilitated discussion groups in the Women, Infants, and Children (WIC) program and other programs serve this function. Weight management groups that meet over a long period can also provide support to each other. The social support approach is especially useful for those who have been diagnosed with type 2 diabetes. Controlling blood sugar and preventing complications are unending challenges and require changes in diet for a lifetime. Consequently, the impact of receiving a diagnosis can devastating. Nutrition educators can provide group members an opportunity to process their feelings with others like them through a series of structured activities. Nutrition educators can also help individuals develop action plans, and group members can meet to share challenges and successes. Such groups can provide emotional support, involving empathy and caring; informational support in the form of advice and information useful in solving problems; and appraisal support in terms of accurate feedback. They do not usually provide instrumental support.

Collective Efficacy

Nutrition education interventions can also focus on enhancing collective efficacy in groups, by facilitating the process or providing technical assistance. *Collective efficacy* is the belief of groups and community members that they have the capacity to take collective action to create change in their environment. Bandura (2001) notes that because human functioning is rooted in social systems, personal agency operates within a broad network of social structures, which individuals, in turn, also help to create. Thus personal agency and social structures operate interdependently. According to Bandura (2001), personal agency is not about self-centered individualism; rather, studies show that a high sense of efficacy tends to promote a prosocial orientation, involving cooperativeness and an interest in each other's welfare.

According to social cognitive theory, collective efficacy can be enhanced by "equipping people with a firm belief that they can produce valued effects by their collective action and providing them with the means to do so" (Bandura, 1997). This is a group enablement process. Group efficacy becomes more than the sum of the personal efficacies of group members because there is an interaction among members and a coordination of their skills, competencies, and activities. In parallel to personal self-efficacy, the strength of individuals' belief in their collective efficacy determines the goals they are willing to set, how much effort they put into the group's endeavors, how much they are willing to persist in the face of difficulties, their morale and resilience, and their level of performance.

Just as perceived personal efficacy involves the power to produce personal effects and not just to understand them, so too collective efficacy involves the power to produce change in the social or political environment. Social cognitive theory suggests that to build collective efficacy, individuals need to learn how to exert influence over community practices that affect their lives. The process for building collective efficacy is rather like a group goal-setting process: group members identify the issue of concern, set small goals to address the concern, and, when these produce tangible results, come to believe that they have the capability to change the social and political environment in which they live. This leads them to believe they can overcome even more difficult problems and hence to set more ambitious goals. Other processes are also used. However, they all work, in part, by enhancing individuals' sense of efficacy that they can bring about tangible changes in their lives. There is evidence that skills in advocacy and community building raise both personal and collective efficacy, which can result in collective actions that may in turn change community practices and policies.

Empowerment

The process of group enablement of social cognitive theory is somewhat similar to *empowerment*—a term that is used loosely and has many definitions. Many see it as largely a personal process in which individuals develop and use needed knowledge, competence, or confidence for making their own decisions (somewhat like personal efficacy). Some may even refer to learning to read food labels as empowerment. However, empowerment is generally described as "a social process through which individuals, communities, and organizations gain mastery over their lives, in the context of changing their social and political environment to improve quality of life" (Wallerstein, 1992). That is, it is a social process of recognizing and enhancing people's abilities as a group to meet their own needs and to mobilize the necessary resources to take more control of their environment. It is about political and social power, not just personal power.

The concept of empowerment education was originally developed by Paolo Freiere of Brazil as a "pedagogy of the oppressed," or education for critical consciousness, that involves developing an understanding of root causes of problems. The central method for empowerment is *conscientizacion*, or group consciousness-raising (Freiere, 1970, 1973). Empowerment education is a process whereby the group members develop identity and social support for each other, specify the problems in their lives, reflect on the root causes of these problems, and develop plans of social or political action. It is thus education for social change. It emphasizes the importance of social context in food- and nutrition-related practices, and shifts the viewpoint away from victim blame and toward system blame. However, the social context is not to be seen as a structural barrier to good health that needs to be changed by health promotion interventions much the way a wall needs to be torn down, but as something to be understood and transformed by people and communities through the process of empowerment (Travers, 1997b).

Nutrition educators may facilitate this educational process, when appropriate, or provide technical assistance. More specifically, in this consciousness-raising process, the educator poses problems to the group participants, who draw upon their own knowledge and experiences to try to understand their lives in relation to the problem. Group members, through dialogue, come to a collective understanding of the root causes of the problem and begin to see how they can make changes in their situation. They become empowered to transform their reality through change in the social or political condition of their lives. Such an empowerment process can bring about not only *personal empowerment* but also empowerment at the *organizational level,* where the influence of the organization in broader society is enhanced, and at the *community level,* where individuals and organizations work together to bring about desired outcomes in the community (Israel et al., 1994). As the word *power* in the term *empowerment* suggests, the process is ultimately about changed power relationships between individuals within groups and between groups and social structures. Such an

approach has been advocated for nutrition education (Kent, 1988; Rody, 1988; Travers 1997b; Arnold et al., 2001).

Several examples from the food and nutrition field illustrate this approach. The Tenderloin Senior Organizing Project (TSOP) involved seniors who lived isolated lives in hotel residences in a crime-ridden neighborhood (Minkler, 1997). Health educators used a combination of educational and organizing approaches to assist residents to identify issues of importance to them, understand the root causes of these issues in the political and social structures of the community, and develop social support and a sense of community through group discussions and tasks. The hotel residents recognized the need to work with other hotels and community groups on shared problems, such as crime. As they achieved success on this issue, including convincing the mayor to put more beat patrol officers in the neighborhood, they took on the issue of poor food availability. They established mini-markets in three hotels, a cooperative breakfast program in another, and a no-cook cookbook for those not allowed to cook in their hotels. As they developed more collective efficacy and became more empowered, they took more control of the project and the health education staff decreased their roles, serving primarily as resource persons.

Another nutrition education program for social change involved low-income women who met weekly informally over coffee at a Parent Center (Travers, 1997a). The issue of common concern to them was feeding their families on a low income. The nutrition educator posed questions that led to group dialogue and discussion, out of which emerged the group's perception that foods cost more in low-income neighborhoods. This led them to make a structured comparison study of prices for foods in their local stores and prices in stores of the same chain in middle-income neighborhoods. The nutrition educator provided technical assistance on this task. When their findings showed that prices in inner-city stores were consistently higher than in middle-income neighborhoods, the women came to realize that the difficulty they had in getting adequate nutrition was partly due to social inequities. They came to the decision to write to the stores to express their concern about inequities in pricing and quality. This resulted in the chain store lowering the prices within the low-income neighborhoods. The nutrition educator facilitated the process by obtaining a word processor and writing the letter with them. This success led to a sense of empowerment. The activity also led them to recognize that their welfare allowances were not adequate to meet their needs. The impact of this information on them personally was a relief from self-blame as they realized that their inability to purchase enough food for their families was not due to their personal inadequacies but due to government policy. This then led them to decide to take action toward change. They wrote letters to political leaders and worked with other community groups, resulting in some increase in the welfare allowances.

Finally, when some time later there was an attempt to close the Parent Center because of budget cuts, the women organized a march on city hall and got media attention, which prevented closure.

In a more formal setting of a school, an empowerment process was used in a curriculum development project (da Cunha, Contento, & Morin, 2000). In this process, the nutrition educator first met with the teachers, school food personnel, and administrators in several high-poverty schools to raise questions about the problem of poor nutrition among the students. The school staff were concerned. The schools nominated a small group, made up of teachers, school food service personnel, and a parent, to meet with the nutrition educator to address their concerns. They realized that they needed to find out more about the problem, so they designed and conducted a comprehensive needs assessment among the students and their families. From this needs assessment they then designed a nutrition education curriculum to address the needs identified and helped each other in the implementation of the curriculum. The group met weekly after school on their own time for seven months. The nutrition educator used a consciousness-raising and empowerment process throughout, helping the group, through dialogue and interpretations based on their own experience and knowledge, to make their own decisions. The nutrition educator acted as a facilitator and provided technical assistance in conducting the needs assessment and developing the curriculum.

Youth empowerment was the basis of a project in which youth operated farm stands in low-income communities (Hughes, Blalock, & Streiter, 2005). High school youth made changes in their communities by creating affordable, locally grown food and supporting local farmers and growers. At the same time, youth learned important skills in business, finance, and working together in mature and productive ways, preparing them for the workforce.

In all the food-related cases just described, it can be seen that the specific issues of concern are identified by the people in the community rather than the intervention staff, that the process aims to bring about social change through the empowerment of individuals and groups, that the role of the nutrition educator is to facilitate and advocate rather than to be the expert who provides all the information, and that forming collaborations may enhance effectiveness of action. It should also be noted that collective efficacy and empowerment approaches work on a long time frame, often involving months and years, but the environmental changes brought about are more likely to be long-lasting.

Educating and Working with Organizational-Level Decision Makers and Policy Makers

To make the food environment in organizations more supportive of healthful action, nutrition education interventions generally focus on educating and working with those who have power and authority to make healthful foods more available and accessible in the given setting, such as in schools and workplaces. After decision makers support making changes in the food environment, nutrition educators often assist in providing professional development to those who prepare the food.

Educating and Working with Decision Makers in School Settings

The school food environment can have a large impact on the quality of children s food choices and intakes because they eat a large proportion of their daily calories at school. For example, foods eaten at lunch constitute 35% to 40% of students daily calorie intake, through eating foods obtained from the school meals program, à la carte offerings, vending machines, and school stores. Participation in the National School Lunch Program (NSLP) declines with age, with about two thirds of elementary school children participating, down to about half in middle school, and then to one third in high school. Foods available in venues that are alternatives to the NSLP, called *competitive foods,* tend to be higher in fat and sugar and less nutritious. For example, the availability of vending machines and snack bars lowers the level of participation in the NSLP, and at the same time, these venues tend to stock high-fat, high-sugar items such as snack chips, candy, and soda and are low in fruits and vegetables. Because it has been shown that the availability and accessibility of fruits and vegetables increases consumption of such foods (Hearn et al., 1998), it is not surprising that when students move from an elementary school, where only the NSLP was available, to a middle school with à la carte and snack bar meals, their intakes of fruit, vegetable, and milk decrease and their consumption of sweetened beverages and high-fat, high-sugar foods increases (Cullen & Zakeri, 2004).

Many nutrition education interventions with school-aged youth have worked with school staff to increase the availability and accessibility of targeted foods in the school meals program, such as lower-fat foods, fruits, and vegetables (French & Stables, 2003; French & Wechsler, 2004). The interventions share many features, and so only a few are described here to illustrate. Three categories are described here briefly: interventions that focused on increasing fruit and vegetable intake, those that aimed to improve several behaviors at once, and those that made environmental changes only. For all of them, the outcomes were improved intake of the targeted foods or nutrients by students.

Fruit and vegetable interventions. Some interventions have focused on increasing fruit and vegetable intake. For example, two studies based on social cognitive theory and conducted with fourth and fifth graders involved not only a classroom component but also a number of changes in the school environment: improved variety and attractiveness of the fruits and vegetables served at lunch, availability of an extra fruit item at lunch when a dessert was served, and point-of-purchase signs in the cafeteria (Perry et al., 1998; Reynolds et al., 2000). Results showed that the intervention increased the intake of fruits and vegetables combined. In one study, the intervention was equally effective with boys and girls and by ethnicity, whereas in the other, changes occurred more readily for fruits than for vegetables, and girls were more responsive than boys.

Interventions directed at several dietary behaviors. Other interventions have addressed several dietary behaviors at once. The Child and Adolescent Trial for Cardiovascular Health (CATCH) was a large randomized study with third to fifth graders based on social cognitive theory and designed to lessen cardiovascular disease risk factors by focusing on decreasing fat intake, increasing intake of higher-fiber foods, and increasing physical activity (Luepker et al., 1996). It consisted of a classroom education component, physical education intervention, food service cafeteria intervention, and a parent/home component. The food service intervention (the environmental component) focused on decreasing total fat, saturated fat, and sodium in the school meals through training of staff in the areas of menu planning, food purchasing, food preparation methods, and program promotion (posters, taste tests, table tests). The food service intervention successfully reduced the fat, sodium, and calories and increased the content of fiber and vitamins A and C in meals. The success was due to methods that were used to change the staff's food preparation behaviors, a finding that has made this intervention a model for school cafeteria interventions. The intervention was able to achieve a significant reduction in fat intake in the children and an increase in targeted mediators of behavior: behavior-relevant knowledge, behavioral intention, food choices, and perceived support from teachers and parents (Edmundson et al., 1996; Lytle et al., 1996).

In the TEENS study with middle school teens, also based on social cognitive theory, nutrition educators worked with food service staff to provide greater offerings and promotion of fruits and vegetables and healthier, lower-fat snacks à la carte, in addition to a classroom component that focused on goal setting and skill development (Lytle et al., 2004). Intakes improved in the first year but not in the second, partly because many teachers did not implement the program completely. There was a dose effect, in that the classroom-plus-environment intervention was more effective than environment alone, and adding a peer leader component improved effectiveness further (Birnbaum, Lytle, & Story, 2002).

An intervention study with children in kindergarten to the sixth grade, called Cookshop, was designed to increase preferences for and consumption of minimally processed whole grains and fresh vegetables; it combined cooking these foods in the classroom with multiple exposures to these same foods in the same recipes in the cafeteria (Liquori et al., 1998). Using fresh vegetables meant that children were actively involved in

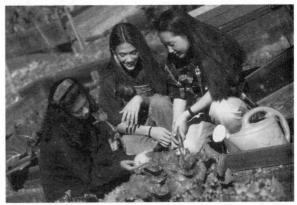

Students learn about more than growing produce when they create local farm stands—they also provide fresh grown vegetables for their community.

the food preparation process, such as cutting and chopping. Nutrition educators worked with school food service directors to provide training to the staff to also cook these same recipes from scratch. The study compared cooking as an educational strategy with the more usual educational methods, but both groups received the environmental cafeteria component. The intervention was based on social cognitive theory and emphasized that eating a plant-based diet was not only important for personal health but also encouraged a more resource-conserving and sustainable food system. The results showed that actual cooking experiences and eating with peers in the classroom resulted in increased consumption of targeted foods as measured by plate waste observations in the lunchroom. Control classes, receiving the environmental intervention only, did not increase their intake of these foods, suggesting that increased awareness and motivation through education are needed along with environmental opportunities for action.

Environmental-change-only interventions. Several studies have focused on changes in the food environment only. One study designed to increase fruits and vegetables intake among first- and third-grade students used as its intervention strategy increasing the availability and attractiveness of fruits and vegetables and having the school food service and staff daily encourage students to eat them. The intervention included special events, such as kickoffs, samplings, challenge weeks, a theater production, and a final meal (Perry et al., 2004). Students in the intervention schools significantly increased their total fruit intake. Researchers concluded that although this intervention was partly successful, multicomponent interventions are more powerful than cafeteria programs alone. Studies that focused on increasing the availability or offerings of lower-fat entrées in the school lunch, with and without promotional activities, were able to moderately increase consumption of lower-fat entrées, but researchers concluded that including promotional activities was more effective (Whitaker et al., 1994).

An environmental intervention in middle schools was directed at increasing physical activity and at providing and marketing low-fat food items in all school food sources, including à la carte sources, school stores, and bag lunches (Sallis et al., 2003). It was successful in increasing physical activity in boys, but was not able to reduce fat intake of students at the schools, due in part to barriers to full implementation of the program. These findings, along with those of the Cookshop and TEENS programs described earlier, suggest that interventions involving the cafeteria and competitive foods are difficult to implement and, even when implemented, are more likely to be successful in improving student intakes of targeted foods if they are accompanied by promotional or educational activities that draw attention to the importance and availability of healthier options.

Use of multiple channels. Many interventions are able to use multiple channels to address food and nutrition issues. This requires considerable effort and coordination on the part of nutrition educators because they have to work with multiple decision makers within the school setting. A high school intervention called Gimme 5 focused on increasing the intake of fruits and vegetables. There was minimal classroom exposure beyond some workshops. Instead the intervention provided extensive education to school food service personnel to increase the availability, portion size, variety, and taste of fruit and vegetables served in the cafeteria; provided recipes; and conducted monthly marketing activities to promote eating fruits and vegetables. Nutrition educators also provided education to the parent–teacher organization. The intervention components are described in Nutrition Education in Action 6-1. Gimme 5

NUTRITION EDUCATION IN ACTION 6-1

Gimme 5 High School Intervention Activities by Levels of Influence on Behavior Change

Components	Awareness Development/Interest Stimulation	Information Transfer/Skills (How-to Knowledge)	Reinforcement	Application/Maintenance
Classroom		Workshops; supplemental subject activities; school staff training		
Cafeteria	Taste testing of Gimme 5 recipes and food giveaways	Menu/recipe modification; food purchasing; food preparation; food service staff training	Taste testings of Gimme 5 recipes and food giveaways	
Media	Marketing stations; posters; table-tents; public service announcements; point-of-service signs; faculty fruit/vegetable baskets; Power lotto	Faculty tip sheets	Faculty fruit/vegetable baskets; incentives; coupons	Student recipes
Parents	PTO meetings; media displays and activities	PTO meetings; media displays and activities; Gimme 5 column in school newspapers		Newsletter; PTO meetings; media displays and activities

PTO = parent–teacher organization.

Source: Nicklas, T.A., C.C. Johnson, R. Farris, et al. 1997. Development of a school-based nutrition intervention for high school students: Gimme 5. *American Journal of Health Promotion* 11:315–322. Used with permission.

resulted in an increase in fruit and vegetables intake during two years, although in this case, consumption in the control school caught up in the third year (Nicklas et al., 1997, 1998).

Farm to School programs. Farm to School programs connect schools with local farms (Center for Food and Justice, 2004). Schools buy and feature foods such as fruits, vegetables, eggs, honey, meat, and beans on their menus or offer farm-fresh salad bars as part of the National School Lunch Program. These programs also provide students experiential learning opportunities through farm visits, classroom visits by farmers, cooking demonstrations, school gardens, and recycling and composting programs. Through these programs, farmers have access to a new market and participate in a program designed to educate children about local food and agriculture. Such programs require the participation of a wide variety of people and organizations, and nutrition educators can have a key role. Other participants include parents, school principals, school board members, school food service staff, and students. In the United States, legislation now makes some funds available for such projects.

Food Pricing and Promotions in Schools

To educate decision makers about the importance of healthful food in their organizations, nutrition educators have to convince them that making the food environment more healthful is feasible financially. To do so, several nutrition education interventions have explored the role of changing pricing structure and promotions on sales of targeted foods in high schools and workplaces as a way to create an enabling environment. One short-term study of three weeks found that when prices on fresh fruit, carrots, and salad were reduced 50%, sales of fruit went up 400% and carrots 200%. Salad sales did not change (French et al., 1997). Contextual factors were important—where the items were placed in the cafeteria area and how the items were presented (e.g., whether the baby carrots were prepackaged with an accompanying low-fat dip or were unlabeled in plastic cups with plastic wrap). A longer-term study of one school year found that increasing prices slightly on three popular high-fat foods as a way to subsidize lower prices on more healthful foods resulted in stable food service revenues and more nutritious foods being sold (Hannan et al., 2002). Another one-year study with both high schools and workplaces found that lower prices were effective in promoting choices of targeted food items in vending machines and that signage had a smaller but significant independent effect on sales (French et al., 2001). By providing such information to school administrators or school food service mangers, nutrition educators can help them in their decisions.

One study focused on promoting low-fat milk consumption in elementary schools because schools were concerned that if they switched to low-fat milk, students would not drink it. Health educators developed a campaign that featured Low-Fat

Lucy the Cow, a volunteer dressed up as a Holstein cow, whose appearance at educational school assemblies to promote 2% white milk instead of whole milk was preceded and accompanied by posters, puzzles, handouts, and other promotional activities. The campaign increased the choice of low-fat milk from 25% to 57% (and 70% among first and second graders), with no net decrease in milk consumption. The effect remained even after three to four months (Wechsler et al., 1998). This program is described in Nutrition Education in Action 6-2.

Another study that focused on implementing a large number of school-wide promotional activities rather than pricing, this time in high schools, found that over a two-year period, the number of promotions was associated with the increase in percentage of sales of lower-fat foods in à la carte areas of school cafeterias (Fulkerson et al., 2004). These results suggest that intense promotion can be an effective strategy in both elementary and secondary schools.

Educating and Working with Decision Makers in Workplaces

A number of health promotion interventions in workplaces have similarly attempted to make changes in the food environment by increasing the number of low-fat and high-fiber foods and fruits and vegetables available in the employee cafeteria and other sources of food at work, such as vending machines (e.g., Sorensen et al., 1990, 1996). Nutrition and health professionals educate and work with worksite decision makers and policy makers to develop a variety of activities for the worksite. Along with other educational, promotional, organizational, and policy activities, these interventions have had a positive impact on eating patterns (Sorensen et al., 1999).

An example of a worksite program to increase fruit and vegetable consumption that addressed multiple levels of influence is summarized in Nutrition Education in Action 6-3. The Treatwell program randomly assigned 22 worksites into three groups: minimal intervention controls, worksite intervention, and worksite plus family (Sorensen et al., 1998, 1999). The worksites were community health centers with racially and ethnically diverse employees, providing services to low-income community residents. The behavioral goal of the program and hence the expected outcome of the intervention was that the employees in these worksites would increase their consumption of fruits and vegetables. The table in Nutrition Education in Action 6-3 lists the theoretical models that were used. The study also tested whether the intervention had an impact on the potential mediators of behavior change. These are shown in the table, along with how the changes were measured. (The results were described earlier, in the section "Social Support in the Workplace.")

Increasing the purchase of locally grown produce through worksite sales was the objective of another intervention (Ross et al., 2000). Here workers were given the opportunity to order local produce, which was then delivered to the

---

NUTRITION EDUCATION IN ACTION 6-2

Celebrity Cow Promotes Low-Fat Milk to Elementary Schoolers

When studies revealed that children in New York City were eating too much saturated fat, the state health department and a university decided to do something about it: they launched a Low-Fat Milk Education Project. The problem was how to encourage children to make the switch from whole milk to low-fat milk, usually thought as being low in taste too. The solution was Low-Fat Lucy the Cow. Lucy became the celebrity "spokes-cow," played by a volunteer dressed in a black-and-white Holstein costume. Lucy put in live appearances in school assemblies. The message was "Choose low-fat milk in the school cafeteria and urge your parents to buy it at home." For two weeks prior to the assemblies, Lucy was promoted as a "mystery guest" via posters and announcements. On the day of her debut, students in the assemblies were primed for her appearance with a participatory game of Fat-BUSTERS, in which they were challenged to identify high- and low-fat foods from slides.

Lucy entered the school auditorium to the lively accompaniment of dance music. She carried two cartons of low-fat milk, which she displayed to the children as she danced down the aisle. Lucy then explained how changing to low-fat milk can help students keep their diets healthy and how, most of all, low-fat milk tastes great. In the auditorium after Lucy's presentation, the students were given low-fat milk, a low-fat cookie, and a pencil with Lucy's picture and the message "Drink Low-Fat Milk" in English and Spanish. This tasting helped to surmount a large obstacle to children switching milks: they do not like to try unfamiliar foods.

The children were then given handouts, refrigerator magnets to take home, and a simple puzzle. A week later, Lucy returned for a ceremony to select winners from students who had solved the puzzle. A second tasting took place, this one at school dismissal time, for both students and parents. Lucy also visited a parent association meeting about the same time.

Here we can see theory being used to design the program:

- Students were told that low-fat milk was good for their health and tasted great (outcome expectations).
- Children tasted low-fat milk to increase the liking for it (social-affective experience) and to create familiarity (food-related factor).
- Lucy the Cow was a celebrity (social norms and social modeling).
- School assembly setting indicated that the school was setting a social norm.
- Handouts, magnets, and puzzle (reinforcements).
- Ceremony to select winners and give prizes (incentives and a reinforcement).
- Parental support (promoting a supportive environment).
- School support: school now displayed low-fat milk prominently (promoting a supportive environment).

Did Lucy succeed? Before the project, 25% of the students who drank milk selected low-fat milk. That increased to 57%, whereas the control-school students did not change.

Source: Wechsler, H., C.E. Basch, P. Zybert, and S. Shea. 1998. Promoting the selection of low-fat milk in elementary school cafeterias in an inner-city Latino community: Evaluation of an intervention. *American Journal of Public Health* 88:427–433.

---

worksite. This environmental change was accompanied by promotional materials about the farms that grew the produce, and an opportunity to sample the produce. The delivery was very public so that friends' ordering and satisfaction could be observed to provide a social normative influence. Results showed that workers who ordered local foods at the worksite were motivated to purchase locally grown produce outside the worksite as well.

Emergency Food Programs

The quality of foods offered at emergency food programs such as food banks or soup kitchens is dependent on what

is available to these institutions. Nutrition professionals have worked with many of these to investigate opportunities for improving the quality of the foods offered by incorporating foods from local farmers or using the soup kitchens as a training program for chefs.

Organizational Policy Activities

Organizational policies regarding school, worksite, and community food environments influence people's food choices and eating patterns. Thus, an important venue for nutrition education is working with policy makers to develop or modify policies.

NUTRITION EDUCATION IN ACTION 6-3

Theories Used and Hypothesis About Potential Mediators of Behavior Change in the Treatwell 5 A Day Worksite Program

Level of influence	Intervention audience	Theoretical models	Hypotheses about mediators of behavior change	Measures
Intrapersonal	• Worker	• Transtheoretical stages of change • Social cognitive theory • Health belief model	• Higher readiness to change is associated with increased fruit and vegetable consumption. • Higher self-efficacy about dietary change is associated with increased fruit and vegetable consumption. • Knowledge of the diet–cancer link (outcome expectations) is associated with increased fruit and vegetable consumption.	• Readiness for change • Self-efficacy • Knowledge (outcome expectations)
Interpersonal	• Family • Coworkers	• Social support • Social networks and ties • Social cognitive theory	• High family and coworker support for dietary change is associated with increased fruit and vegetable consumption. • High family support for dietary change is associated with increased availability of fruits and vegetables in the home. • The type of family ties will influence the strength of the relationships between family support and changing eating habits.	• Family support • Coworker support • Social norms • Availability of fruits and vegetables in the home • Type of family ties
Organizational	• Worksite	• Organizational change and development • Policy	• Worksite mean increases in fruit and vegetable consumption will be greatest where fruits and vegetables are most available and a catering policy supports the purchase of healthy foods. • Program implementation and participation will be highest where effective communication channels exist and policies permit employee change agents to participate. • Coworker support for dietary changes will be highest in worksites with high coworker cohesion and positive labor–management relations.	• Worksite characteristics
Community	• Media • Grocery store (national campaign)	• Diffusion of innovation • Social marketing	• Workers reporting awareness of the national campaign are more likely to increase consumption of fruits and vegetables. • Workers reporting participating in grocery store programs are more likely to report increased consumption of fruits and vegetables.	• Awareness of grocery store campaign • Participation in grocery store campaign

Source: Sorensen, G., M.K. Hunt, N. Cohen, et al. 1998. Worksite and family education for dietary change: The Treatwell 5 A Day program. *Health Education Research* 13:577–591. Used with permission.

School Policies

Many food-related environmental issues that influence youth food intake in schools need to be addressed by institutional policy action rather than, or in addition to, classroom education

- Food used in school fundraising. Short of funds, many schools sell food products to raise money; these products are usually high-fat or high-sugar items such as candy, chips, or sweetened beverages.
- Food is often used in the classroom as a reward or incentive. Again, most often such foods tend to be high-fat and high-sugar, largely because these are liked by students.
- Food advertising in schools occurs directly on vending machines, book covers, wall boards, hallways, sports scoreboards, and in student publications and yearbooks, and indirectly through coupons to fast food outlets given for academic achievement.
- Contracts for beverage sales in schools, usually soft drinks, have become more common in exchange for signing bonuses and a percentage of the profits. They present a nutrition education challenge because the schools must urge students to consume these beverages to guarantee contracted minimum purchases, yet nutrition guidelines would advocate for healthier options on a regular basis.

Local wellness policies. Over the years, nutrition educators have advocated that schools form school nutrition advisory councils or health councils made up of teachers, administrators, parents, students, and intervention staff to assess the overall school food environment, consider and discuss issues, and advance school-level policy that promotes a healthful food environment so as to make the healthful choice the easy choice (Kubik, Lytle, & Story, 2001; Lytle et al., 2004). In the United States, such an approach has become reality. The Child Nutrition and WIC Reauthorization Act of 2004 required each local educational agency participating in a program authorized by the National School Lunch Act or the Child Nutrition Act to establish a local school wellness policy. The policy at a minimum has to include the following (USDA, n.d.):

- Goals for nutrition education, physical activity, and other school-based activities that are designed to promote student wellness
- Nutrition guidelines selected by the local school for all foods available on campus during the school day, with the objectives of promoting student health and reducing childhood obesity
- Guidelines for reimbursable school meals that are no less restrictive than regulations and guidance of the USDA for program requirements and nutrition standards
- A plan for measuring implementation of the local wellness policy

Anyone can initiate a process to create a new policy or adopt an existing policy, but the law requires the following to be involved in the process: parents, students, representatives of the school food authority, the school board, school administrators, and the public. A nutrition educator is not specifically required to be part of the team, but can offer his or her services as a member of the public or as a parent. Many schools have initiated actions that address all these policy concerns (USDA, 2005).

Workplace Policies

Many interventions in the worksite have tested a comprehensive, multilevel approach to creating an environment supportive of healthy eating by addressing organizational issues as well as the physical and social environments (Sorenson et al., 1998; Beresford et al., 2001). Health professionals are very important for educating decision makers and management about the importance of food and health issues and convincing them to take action. They also can initiate programs and provide services and technical support. However, they need to work in collaboration with both employees and management to develop policies and procedures so as to implement and institutionalize programs.

A review of such studies finds that a number of organizational factors are related to program effectiveness (Sorensen, Linnan, & Hunt, 2002). Management commitment and supervisory support is essential. Policies need to be modified. Just as important, however, is worker involvement in planning and implementation, through such mechanisms as an "employee advisory board" at each site and through delivery of the intervention by peers. The employee advisory board chooses the intervention components to be implemented in the individual worksite setting, disseminates program messages and information throughout the worksite, and encourages long-term incorporation of the program into the worksite (Sorensen et al., 1990, 1992). The more that employees are involved, the greater are the number of activities implemented (Hunt et al., 2000). Worksite management must put in place policies to permit and encourage employees to take work time to participate in these health promotion activities.

Community-Level Activities: Building Coalitions and Collaborations

We have seen that in organizational-level interventions, working in collaboration with decision makers and policy makers is vital. This is even more true at the community level. Here, nutrition educators in most cases must develop partnerships and participate in coalitions with other groups who have similar goals in order to bring about community changes that are supportive of the behavioral goals of the nutrition education program. Nutrition educators participate in numerous coalitions. In some cases, nutrition educators initiate activities by educating decision makers. In other cases, nutrition educators provide technical support to community groups who want to take action and need food and nutrition information. The following text describes a few examples to illustrate the types of collaborations in which individual nutrition educators or programs can participate.

Community Coalitions and Partnerships: Examples

An example in the United States of a collaboration regarding a very specific behavior is a program wherein WIC nutritionists worked with other food assistance programs and a variety of community partners to build breastfeeding-friendly communities (Singleton et al., 2005). The aim was to increase public awareness, acceptance, and community support for breastfeeding. The program in one state included a public forum with 145 key community stakeholders to develop a blueprint for action to assist communities, families, schools and childcare centers, health care systems, policy makers, and worksites in their efforts to make breastfeeding the norm for infant feeding. The partnership also initiated a public awareness campaign and activities to advocate for changes in health care systems, the insurance industry, the business community, and educational systems to encourage breastfeeding, and advocacy for changes in the availability of resources for community organizations and families.

Another example is a partnership between two organizations—Share our Strength and Head Start—to improve the diets of low-income community members. Share our Strength is a national organization with presence in many communities that seeks to inspire and organize individuals and businesses to share their strengths to help end hunger. Its national nutrition education program, Operation Frontline, mobilizes volunteer chefs, nutritionists, and financial planners to teach nutrition, healthy cooking, and food budgeting classes to individuals at risk of hunger. Head Start provides education and meals to low-income preschool children. Operation Frontline teaches its six-week curriculum to Head Start program parents, providing an example of a partnership between a government program and a community program to enhance the reach and effectiveness of both organizations (Jones, 2005). The program has resulted in increased parental knowledge and skills.

Nutrition Education Networks

Nutrition education networks have also come into existence in many states in the United States, with funding from the USDA and other sources. These networks are partnerships and coalitions among the Food Stamp program, the Cooperative Extension Service, private volunteer organizations such as the American Cancer Society or American Heart Association, grocery stores, universities, and others with the aim of fostering collaboration among food assistance programs and developing and delivering consistent nutrition messages across network partnerships to low-income, food stamp audi-

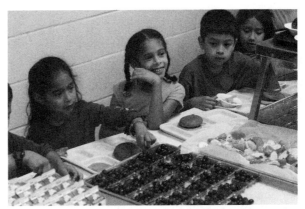

Local school wellness policies have improved the nutritional value of school lunches.

ences. These partnerships have used a variety of channels to reach these audiences—direct and indirect nutrition education as well as social marketing.

Nutrition education networks often work with physicians, health departments, school districts, and community-based organizations to promote healthy eating and physical activity habits in school-aged children and their parents. They have also initiated a wide range of activities to promote policy initiatives and to empower people to be advocates for healthier food and activity environments in their schools and communities. They have often worked to change organizational policies and the physical environment to help low-income families eat healthier diets, be more active, and participate in USDA nutrition assistance programs. An example is the California Nutrition Network, which sponsors a wide range of nutrition education activities (California Nutrition Network, 2004).

Community-Level Food Policy Activities

Many community organizations focus on food policy. For example, the food policy council is composed of stakeholders from various segments of a state or local food system. Councils can be officially sanctioned through a government action such as an executive order or can be grassroot efforts. The primary goal of many food policy councils is to examine the operation of a local food system and provide ideas or recommendations for how it can be improved. Nutrition educators are often members of such councils to broaden the scope of the councils, in which members may be more concerned with emergency food assistance or agriculture policy in the most traditional sense (see www.statefoodpolicy.org).

Various food security coalitions and farm and food projects also work to analyze and develop policy initiatives to link local farmers and communities so as to rebuild and restore regional food and agriculture systems to enhance the economic livelihoods of family farms and rural communities and at the same time provide healthy and affordable food for the community (e.g., see www.foodsecurity.org)

Working in Coalitions: Benefits and Costs

The attempts of any given group to bring about social change are greatly enhanced by building coalitions with other groups who have similar goals. Coalitions and collaborations can mobilize material resources and peoples' knowledge, skills, and enthusiasms to achieve desired goals in a way that is not possible for small groups alone. There are costs as well, however. Collaborative efforts are complex, and leadership roles, decision making, social support, and social network concerns are issues that must be addressed satisfactorily for all collaborating groups involved; working these out may take time and effort. Even when coalition members are satisfied and actively involved, this does not guarantee that the coalition will be effective in achieving agreed-upon goals. Leadership and management must also be effective.

Factors that are likely to enhance successful collaboration include the following: a shared and agreed-upon vision and mission, reached by consensus through open dialogue, negotiation, and problem solving; a unique purpose that is meaningful to members; tasks that are clear and empowering; a sense of productivity and efficiency; a skilled convener and facilitator of team building and conflict resolution; broad-based involvement in decision making; open, frequent communication, with communication feedback loops; benefits that accrue to members for participation; relationships that are based on trust, openness, and respect; power sharing; and adequate resources (Rosenthal, 1998).

Policy Activities

We have seen that policy activities are extremely important. Policy complements education (Rothschild, 1999). *Educa-*

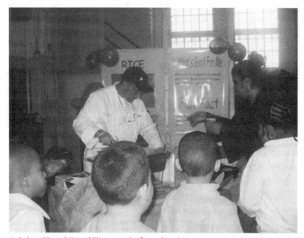

A SchoolFood/FoodChange chef teaches how to prepare an easy and nutritious meal.

tion, as we have seen, involves a combination of strategies to inform, persuade, and facilitate the voluntary adoption or maintenance of behavior that is considered important. It does not provide, on its own, direct or immediate reward or punishment. Indeed, the anticipated outcomes are often far into the future, such as "If you drink milk now, you are less likely to develop osteoporosis when you are old."

Environmental changes, such as social marketing, attempt to make the environment favorable for the new behavior. They promote voluntary changes in behavior by offering audiences the benefits they want and reducing the barriers they are concerned about, accompanied, in social marketing, by effective communications or persuasion to enhance motivation. Environmental changes reduce barriers by providing the products or services that would make enacting the behavior easier, for example, by increasing the availability of fruits and vegetables in grocery stores in the audience's community and making them more accessible through pricing incentives or the use of coupons. In this case, the anticipated outcomes or rewards are more immediate. However, *policy* complements these approaches, and can also have an important and positive role. Policies and regulations can ensure the performance of a desirable behavior when it would be difficult to do because of social pressure to conform to a different standard. For example, food policies or nutrition standards for all foods available in school would make it easier for students to eat more fruits and vegetables or drink fewer sweetened beverages, even though less healthy options might be more appealing to students and financially desirable to schools. Nutrition educators need to participate in relevant food policy decisions. This may require them to serve as advocates for healthy policies to policy makers and even lawmakers at the local or national level.

Implications for Addressing Potential Environmental Mediators of Action or Behavior Change

Based on the considerations just discussed, many different kinds of activities can be used to address environmental determinants of health actions or behavior change. In most of these activities, nutrition educators will need to work in collaboration with others, such as food or service providers and decision makers. This usually involves educating decision makers or policy makers in organizations and communities about the importance of food and nutrition issues and then building coalitions with them to develop and implement plans to enhance the opportunities for individuals to engage in identified health-promoting actions. It also means collaborating with program participants and other like-minded community groups to work toward developing or revising public policies, or even legislation, to support the behaviors or issues that are of concern to the program.

Figure 6-2 shows how nutrition education can be directed at various levels of influence: the individual and household level; the interpersonal level; the institutional, organizational, and community level; and the social structures, policies, and practices level. The educational activities at both the individual and interpersonal levels address personal mediators of action or behavior change, such as beliefs, attitudes, affect, and skills, with short-, medium-, and long-term outcomes for individuals. The activities at the other levels are directed at environmental mediators of behavior change and are also designed to affect individuals, but in this case by making the healthy action also the easy action through changes in policy and social structures.

Nutrition Education Activities Directed at the Interpersonal Level

Social Networks and Social Support

Enchancing existing social networks. To enhance social support for the key food- and nutrition-related behavior or

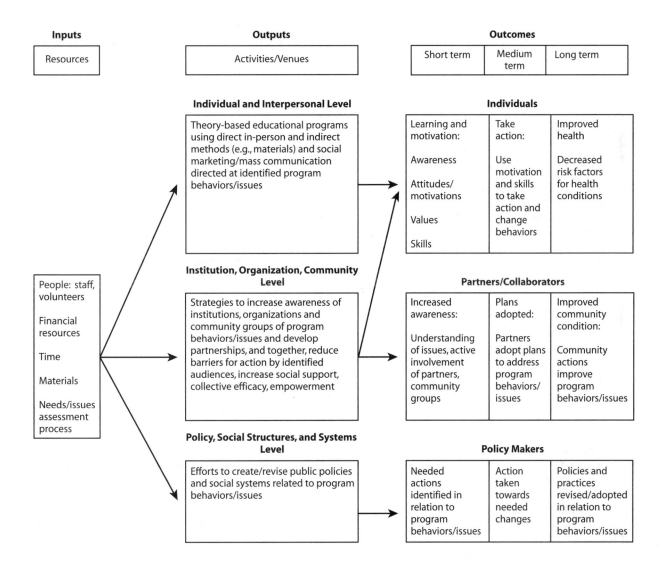

FIGURE 6-2 A nutrition education logic model framework addressing multiple levels of intervention

Source: Based on Community Nutrition Education (CNE) Logic Model, Version 2 — Overview 2006, January. Helen Chipman, National Coordinator, Food Stamp Nutrition Education, CSREES/USDA, and Land Grant University System Partnership. http://www.csrees.usda.gov/nea/food/fsne/fsne.html. Used with permission.

behaviors that have been identified as of concern to the program (e.g., increasing breastfeeding rates or increasing the consumption of fruits and vegetables), existing social networks can be called upon and expanded. For example, parent associations in schools, employee associations at workplaces, and groups that meet regularly in communities and organizations may be interested in nutrition issues. Nutrition education programs can work with these groups to make them more supportive of the behavior.

Developing new social network linkages. Programs frequently create social support for program participants through creating a social support group through which new social network linkages are built. For example, a group can be developed for those in a workplace who are interested in weight control or weight acceptance. Support groups can be developed at a health center for those with HIV/AIDS, or cooking classes and behavioral change sessions can be created for participants in a program.

Facilitating Collective Efficacy and Empowerment

The processes of enhancing collective efficacy and empowerment are somewhat similar. In the process of enhancing collective efficacy, group members, with the assistance of the nutrition educator, identify the issue of concern to them in the social and political environment. They can start out by setting small goals that will help to address the concern. When these are accomplished, the group members can pose even more difficult problems and set more ambitious goals. Such an approach can be effective with many age groups, particularly youth.

Empowerment strategies generally involve some sort of consciousness-raising process, whereby the educator poses problems to the group participants and asks them to draw on their own knowledge and experiences to try to understand their lives in relation to the problem. Group members, through dialogue, come to a collective understanding of the root causes of the problems and begin to see how they can make changes in their situation. They then set goals for actions that they will take to transform their reality through making changes in the social or political condition of their lives. In these settings, the role of the nutrition educator is to facilitate the process at the beginning, if needed, until the group has developed its own agendas and procedures and no longer needs the nutrition educator. Another possibility is that a group has already initiated community action and needs the nutrition educator as a resource person.

Educating and Working with Organizational-Level Decision Makers and Policy Makers

Changing the Food Environment

Foods offered at nutrition education program sites, such as schools, workplaces, communities, soup kitchens, or food banks, can be modified to make them more supportive of the healthful behaviors identified as important by nutrition educators or by participants. In schools, this means making changes in the school meals offerings, vending machines, à la carte offerings, and food items sold in school stores.

Bringing about changes at such sites may require the use of both motivational- and action-phase activities, this time directed at the providers of food as the audience, so that they will be motivated to make changes in the foods offered. Professional development workshops and incentives are important here. Changes in the food offered may require changes in organizational policy and union rules so that food service staff can make the changes, which will require negotiations and advocacy. Making such food changes possible may also require changes in physical facilities at sites such as schools or other locations, so that foods can actually be cooked or prepared on site. All of these actions require coalition building with groups that have authority in the relevant areas.

Pricing and Promotional Activities

Changes in the pricing of food items can be helpful in supporting healthful eating. As we have seen, large price changes are effective in increasing the sales of healthy items in organizations, but are not financially sustainable over the long term. A more sustainable strategy is to raise prices slightly (5% to 10%) on more popular, high-fat, high-sugar foods in order to subsidize more healthful, but higher-priced, foods such as fruits and vegetables or lower-fat alternatives (sold at, say, 15% lower than otherwise) in such a way as to be revenue neutral to the organization in which the food sales occur. Attractive presentation of the foods and promotional activities can further increase the choice of these foods. Again, nutrition educators need to work with food providers to bring about such changes.

Organizational Food Policy

Nutrition educators can assist organizations to develop appropriate policies with respect to foods offered on site. Thus, in schools, they can work with local wellness councils made up of teachers, school food service staff, administrators, community members, and students. They can provide technical assistance to these councils to review and help evaluate the effectiveness of policies to encourage healthful food environments which address the following issues: food used in school fundraising or in the classroom as a reward or incentive, food advertising in schools, and beverage sales in schools. The Centers for Disease Control and Prevention (CDC) has developed a monitoring tool that schools can use to assess the school health environment and evaluate how they are doing (CDC, 2004a, 2004b). Within workplaces and other settings, vendors are usually for-profit operations. However, even here food policies can be developed so that healthful foods are more available and accessible.

Informational Environment

Information provided in public forums serves several purposes. It can provide motivational (why-to) or instrumental (how-to) information on an important issue. However, the information can also help to establish social and community norms that are supportive of dietary change. For example, numerous posters in a setting about breastfeeding or eating fruits and vegetables can encourage people to see these behaviors as the social norm. They can also serve as cues to action. In addition to posters in schools, at work, or in community centers, billboards in the community can help establish norms and serve as cues to action. Promotions through other media, such as radio and magazines, can be supportive of the behavior change that is targeted by the intervention.

Policy Activities at the Community and National Level

As we have seen, there are many community organizations and national organizations that focus on food policy. There are also many food assistance programs and public health agencies where nutrition educators can provide technical assistance as well as influence so as to advocate for, create, or revise policies that will be supportive of the behaviors or issues that are important for nutritional health. We need to stay informed about policies and issues as they come up and participate, where possible and appropriate, in order to have a voice in how they will be developed and implemented. Some of these policy activities are described in Chapter 18 of this book.

Summary

Environmental interventions seek to enhance opportunities for people to engage in healthful nutrition- and food-related behaviors. We have seen that addressing environmental mediators of individual action takes many different approaches and involves a variety of activities. Nutrition educators inform, educate, and form partnerships with others—food and service providers, decision makers with authority and power, and policy makers—to address the environmental determinants that mediate the behaviors or practices targeted by nutrition programs. Thus, nutrition educators work with schools, Head Start programs, workplaces, and congregate meals sites for older adults to make healthful foods available and accessible and to develop policies that encourage and reinforce healthful eating practices.

In schools, school-wide food-related policies about beverage availability, vending machines, and school stores, as well as school cafeteria policies, should provide students the opportunity to have easy access to healthful food choices and to see healthful food practices modeled. In workplaces, healthful alternatives should be made available in the cafeteria and in vending machines and should be promoted. In all settings, the healthful choice should be an easy choice. Active participation of community members and worksite employees as well as leaders must be incorporated into any interventions. Indeed, community empowerment and collective efficacy are high priorities. Adopting these comprehensive approaches enhances the likelihood of improving the effectiveness of nutrition education interventions for individual and environmental change.

Questions and Activities

1. Define the following terms:
    a. Social networks
    b. Social support
    c. Collective efficacy
    d. Empowerment
    e. Collaboration
    f. Partnership
2. Look over your answer to the question posed at the beginning of the chapter about the role nutrition educators should play in creating an environment that is supportive of healthful eating. Has your thinking on that question changed? How?
3. What skills do you think nutrition educators should have to be able to work in collaboration with others to bring about more healthful environments? What role would you like to see yourself play in these activities?

REFERENCES

Ammerman, A.S., C.H. Lindquist, K.N. Lohr, and J. Hersey. 2002. The efficacy of behavioral interventions to modify dietary fat and fruit and vegetable intake: A review of the evidence. *Preventive Medicine* 35(1):25–41.

Arnold, C.G., P. Ladipo, C.H. Nguyen, P. Nkinda-Chaiban, and C.M. Olson. 2001. New concepts for nutrition education in an era of welfare reform. *Journal of Nutrition Education and Behavior* 33(6):341–346.

Bandura, A. 1997. *Self-efficacy: The exercise of control.* New York: WH Freeman.

———. 2001. Social cognitive theory: An agentic perspective. *Annual Review of Psychology* 52:1–26.

Beresford, S.A.A., B. Thompson, Z. Feng, A. Christianson, D. McLerron, and D.L. Patrick. 2001. Seattle 5 A Day worksite program to increase fruit and vegetable consumption. *Preventive Medicine* 32:230–238.

Berkman, L.F., and T. Glass. 2000. Social integration, social networks, social support, and health. In *Social epidemiology,* edited by L.F. Berkman and I. Kawachi. New York: Oxford Press.

Birnbaum, A.S., L.A. Lytle, and M. Story. 2002. Are differences in exposure to a multicomponent school-based intervention associated with varying dietary outcomes in adolescents? *Health Education Behavior* 29(4):427–443.

California Nutrition Network. 200. Program description. http://www.dhs.ca.gov/ps/cdic/cpns/network/.

Center for Food and Justice. 2004. About the national Farm to School program. http://www.farmtoschool.org/about.htm.

Centers for Disease Control and Prevention. 2004a. *School Health Index: A self-assessment and planning guide. Elementary school version.* Atlanta, GA: Author.

———. 2004b. *School Health Index: A self-assessment and planning guide. Middle school/high school version.* Atlanta, GA: Author.

Contento, I.R., S.S. Williams, J.L. Michela, and A. Franklin. 2006. Understanding the food choice process of adolescents in the context of family and friends. *Journal of Adolescent Health* 38:575–582.

Council of Economic Advisers. 2000. *Teens and their parents in the 21st century: An examination of trends in teen behavior and the role of parental involvement.* Washington, DC: Author.

Cullen, K.W., and I. Zakeri. 2004. Fruits, vegetables, milk and sweetened beverages consumption and access to a la carte/snack bar meals at school. *American Journal of Public Health* 94:463–467.

da Cunha, Z., I.R. Contento, and K. Morin. 2000. A case study of a curriculum development process in nutrition education using empowerment as organizational policy. *Ecology of Food and Nutrition* 39:417–435.

Edmundson, E., G.S. Parcel, C.L. Perry, et al. 1996. The effects of the Child and Adolescent Trial for Cardiovascular Health Intervention on psychosocial determinants of cardiovascular disease risk behavior among third-grade students. *American Journal of Health Promotion* 10(3):217–225.

Feuenekes, G.I.J., C. De Graff, S. Meyboom, and W.A. Van Staveren. 1998. Food choice and fat intake of adolescents and adults: Association of intakes within social networks. *Preventive Medicine* 26:645–656.

French, S.A., R.W. Jeffrey, M. Story, et al. 2001. Pricing and promotion effects on low-fat vending machines purchases: The CHIPS study. *American Journal of Public Health* 91:112–117.

French, S.A., and G. Stables. 2003. Environmental interventions to promote fruit and vegetable consumption among youth in school settings. *Preventive Medicine* 37(6):593–610.

French, S.A., M. Story, R.W. Jeffrey, et al. 1997. Pricing structure to promote fruit and vegetable purchase in high school cafeterias. *Journal of the American Dietetic Association* 97:1008–1010.

French, S.A., and H. Wechsler. 2004. School-based research and initiatives: Fruit and vegetable environment, policy and pricing workshop. *Preventive Medicine* 39(Suppl. 2): S101–107.

Friere, P. 1970. *Pedagogy of the oppressed.* New York: Continuum.

———. 1973. *Education for critical consciousness.* New York: Continuum.

Fulkerson, J.A., S.A. French, M. Story, H. Nelson, and P.J. Hannan. 2004. Promotions to increase lower-fat food choices among students in secondary schools: Description and outcomes of TACOS (Trying Alternative Cafeteria Options in Schools). *Public Health Nutrition* 7:665–674.

Furst, T., M. Connors, C.A. Bisogni, J. Sobal, and L.W. Falk. 1996. Food choice: A conceptual model of the process. *Appetite* 26:247–266.

Green, L.W., and M.M. Kreuter. 1999. *Health promotion planning: An educational and ecological approach.* 3rd ed. Mountain View, CA: Mayfield Publishing.

Hannan, P., S.A. French, M. Story, and J.A. Fulkerson. 2002. A pricing strategy to promote sales of lower fat foods in high school cafeterias: Acceptability and sensitivity analysis. *American Journal of Health Promotion* 17:1–6.

Harrington, K.F., F.A. Franklin, S.L. Davies, R.M. Schewchuk, and M. Brown Binns. 2005. Implementation of a family intervention to increase fruit and vegetable intake: The Hi5 + experience. *Health Promotion Practice* 6:180–189.

Hearn, D.M., T. Baranowski, J. Baranowski, et al. 1998. Environmental influences on dietary behavior among children: Availability and accessibility of fruits and vegetables enable consumption. *Journal of Health Education* 29:26–32.

Hughes, L.J., L. Blalock, and L. Strieter. 2005. Youth-oriented farm stands as a vehicle for improving food security in targeted low-income communities. *Journal of Nutrition Education and Behavior* 37(Suppl. 1):S36.

Hunt, M.K., R. Lederman, S. Potter, A. Stoddard, and G. Sorensen. 2000. Results of employee involvement in planning and implementing the Treatwell 5 A Day worksite study. *Health Education Behavior* 27:223–231.

Israel, B., B. Checkoway, A. Schulz, and M. Zimmerman. 1994. Health education and community empowerment: Conceptualizing and measuring perceptions of individual, organizational, and community control. *Health Education Quarterly* 21(2):149–170.

Israel, B.A., and K.A. Rounds. 1987. Social networks and social support: A synthesis for health educators. *Advances in Health Education and Promotion* 2:311–351.

Jones, A.S. 2005. Start by eating right: Promoting healthy eating in young children through partnerships between Share our Strength and Head Start and other community agencies. In *National nutrition education conference.* Washington, DC: USDA Food and Nutrition Service.

Kent, G. 1988. Nutrition education as an instrument of empowerment. *Journal of Nutrition Education* 20:193–195.

Kistin, N., M.S. Abramson, and P. Dublin. 1994. Effect of peer counselors on breastfeeding initiation, exclusivity, and duration among low-income urban women. *Journal of Human Lactation* 10:11–16.

Kubik, M.Y., L.A. Lytle, and M. Story. 2001. A practical, theory-based approach to establishing school nutrition advisory councils. *Journal of the American Dietetic Association* 101:223–228.

Leupker, R.V., C.L. Perry, S.M. McKinlay, et al. 1996. Outcomes of a field trial to improve children's dietary patterns and physical activity: The Child and Adolescent Trial for Cardiovascular Health (CATCH). *Journal of the American Medical Association* 275:768–776.

Liquori, T., P.D. Koch, I.R. Contento, and J. Castle. 1998. The Cookshop Program: Outcome evaluation of a nutrition education program linking lunchroom food experiences with classroom cooking experiences. *Journal of Nutrition Education* 30(5):302.

Lytle, L.A., D.M. Murray, C.L. Perry, et al. 2004. School-based approaches to affect adolescents' diets: Results from the TEENS study. *Health Education and Research* 31:270–287.

Lytle, L.A., E.J. Stone, M.Z. Nichman, and C.L. Perry. 1996. Changes in nutrient intakes of elementary school children following a school-based intervention: Results from the CATCH study. *Preventive Medicine* 25:465–477.

McLeroy, K., D. Bibeau, A. Steckler, and K. Glanz. 1988. An ecological perspective on health promotion programs. *Health Education Quarterly* 15:351–377.

Minkler, M. 1997. Community organizing among the elderly poor in San Francisco's Tenderloin district. In *Community organizing and community building for health*, edited by M. Minkler. New Brunswick, NJ: Rutgers Press.

Ness, K., P. Elliott, and V. Wilbur. 1992. A peer educator nutrition program for seniors in a community development context. *Journal of Nutrition Education* 24:91–94.

Nicklas, T.A., C.C. Johnson, R. Farris, et al. 1997. Development of a school-based nutrition intervention for high school students: Gimme 5. *American Journal of Health Promotion* 11:315–322.

Nicklas, T.A., C.C. Johnson, L. Myers, R.P. Farris, and A. Cunningham. 1998. Outcomes of a high school program to increase fruit and vegetable consumption: Gimme 5—a fresh nutrition concept for students. *Journal of School Health* 68:248–253.

Patterson, R.E., A.R. Kristal, K. Glanz, et al. 1997. Components of the Working Well Trial intervention associated with adoption of healthful diets. *American Journal of Preventive Medicine* 13(4):271–276.

Perry, C.L., D.B. Bishop, G. Taylor, D.M. Murray, and R.W. Mays. 1998. Changing fruit and vegetable consumption among children: The 5 A Day Power Plus Program. *American Journal of Public Health* 88:603–609.

Perry, C.L., D.B. Bishop, G.L. Taylor, et al. 2004. A randomized school trial of environmental strategies to encourage fruit and vegetable consumption among children. *Health Education and Behavior* 31(1):65–76.

Reynolds, K.D., F.A. Franklin, and D. Binley, et al. 2000. Increasing fruit and vegetable consumption of fourth-graders: Results from the High 5 Project. *Preventive Medicine* 30:309–319.

Rody, N. 1988. Empowerment as organizational policy in nutrition intervention program: A case study from the Pacific Islands. *Journal of Nutrition Education* 20:133–141.

Rosenthal, B.B. 1998. Collaboration for the nutrition field: Synthesis of selected literature. *Journal of Nutrition Education* 30(5):246–267.

Ross, N.J., M.D. Anderson, J.P. Goldberg, and B.L. Rogers. 2000. Increasing purchases of locally grown produce through worksite sales: An ecological model. *Journal of Nutrition Education* 32(6):304–313.

Rothschild, M.L. 1999. Carrots, sticks, and promises: A conceptual framework for the management of public health and social issue behaviors. *Journal of Marketing* 63:24–37.

Sallis, J.F., T.L. McKenzie, T.L. Conway, et al. 2003. Environmental interventions for eating and physical activity: A randomized controlled trial in middle schools. *American Journal of Preventive Medicine* 24:209–217.

Sciacca, J.P., B.L. Phipps, D.A. Dube, and M.I. Ratliff. 1995. Influences on breast-feeding by lower-income women: An incentive-based, partner-supported educational program. *Journal of the American Dietetic Association* 95:323–328.

Singleton, U., A. Williams, C. Harris, and G.G. Mason. 2005. Building breastfeeding friendly communities with community partners. In *National nutrition education conference*. Washington, DC: USDA Food and Nutrition Service.

Sorensen, G., J. Hsieh, M.K. Hunt, D.H. Morris, D.R. Harris, and G. Fitzgerald. 1992. Employee advisory boards as a vehicle for organizing worksite health promotion programs. *American Journal of Health Promotion* 6(6):443–450, 464.

Sorensen, G., M.K. Hunt, N. Cohen, et al. 1998. Worksite and family education for dietary change: The Treatwell 5 A Day program. *Health Education Research* 13:577–591.

Sorensen, G., M.K. Hunt, D. Morris, et al. 1990. Promoting healthy eating patterns in the worksite: The Treatwell intervention model. *Health Education and Research* 5(4):505–515.

Sorensen, G., L. Linnan, and M.K. Hunt. 2002. Worksite-based research and initiatives to increase fruit and vegetable consumption. *Preventive Medicine* 39(Suppl. 2):S94–100.

Sorensen, G., A. Stoddard, K. Peterson, et al. 1999. Increasing fruit and vegetable consumption through worksites and families in the Treatwell 5 A Day study. *American Journal of Public Health* 89:54–60.

Sorensen, G., B. Thompson, K. Glanz, et al. 1996. Worksite based cancer prevention: Primary results from the Working Well Trial. *American Journal of Public Health* 86:939–947.

Story, M., L.A. Lytle, A.S. Birnbaum, and C.L. Perry. 2002. Peer-led, school-based nutrition education for young adolescents: Feasibility and process evaluation of the TEENS study. *Journal of School Health* 72:121–127.

Travers, K.D. 1997a. Nutrition education for social change: Critical perspective. *Journal of Nutrition Education* 29(2):57–62.

———. 1997b. Reducing inequities through participatory research and community empowerment. *Health Education and Behavior* 24:344–356.

U.S. Department of Agriculture. 2003. *Expanded food and nutrition education program, national impact data.* Washington, DC: Author.

———. n.d. Healthy Schools: Local wellness policy requirements. http://teamnutrition.usda.gov/tn/Healthy/wellness_policyrequirements.html).

———. 2005, January. *Making it happen! School nutrition success stories* (Food and Nutrition Service FNS-374). Alexandria: Food and Nutrition Service, USDA; Centers for Disease Control and Prevention; U.S. Department of Health and Human Services; and U.S. Department of Education.

Wallerstein, N. 1992. Powerlessness, empowerment and health: Implications for health promotion programs. *American Journal of Health Promotion* 6:197–205.

Wechsler, H., C.E. Basch, P. Zybert, and S. Shea. 1998. Promoting the selection of low-fat milk in elementary school cafeterias in an inner-city Latino community: Evaluation of an intervention. *American Journal of Public Health* 88:427–433.

Whitaker, R.C., J.A. Wright, T.D. Koepsell, A.J. Finch, and B.M. Patsy. 1994. Randomized intervention to increase children's selection of low-fat foods in school lunches. *Journal of Pediatrics* 125:535–540.

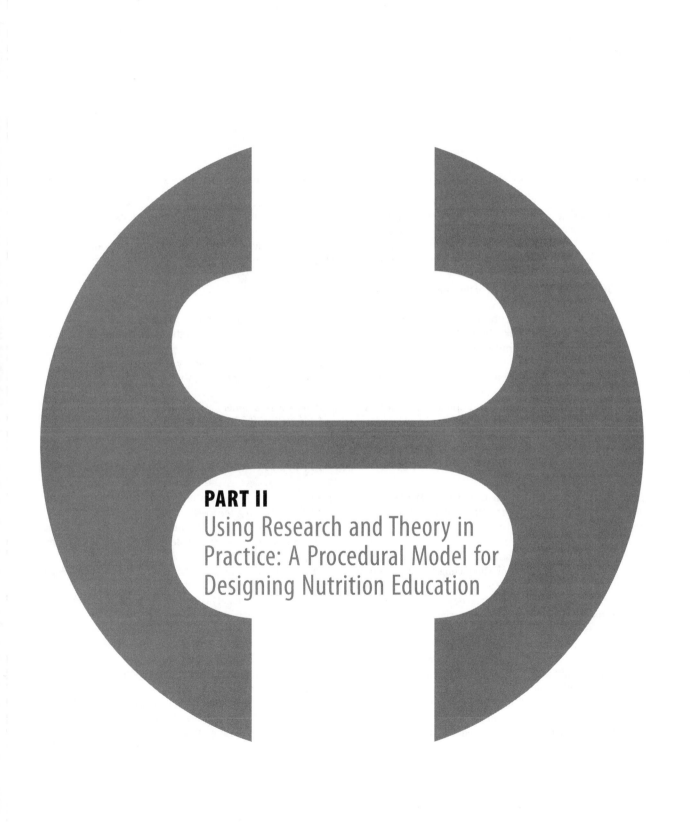

PART II
Using Research and Theory in
Practice: A Procedural Model for
Designing Nutrition Education

CHAPTER 7

Step 1: Analyze Needs and Behaviors: Specify the Behavior or Action Focus of the Program

OVERVIEW   This chapter provides an overview of a systematic process for designing nutrition education that integrates theory, research, and practice. It also describes Step 1: how to conduct an assessment of needs and issues of concern, identify contributing behaviors or practices for given audiences, and specify the behaviors or actions that will be the focus of the program.

OBJECTIVES   At the end of the chapter, you will be able to

- Describe a six-step procedural model for designing theory-based nutrition education
- State why it is important to go through a systematic process to identify the focus and targets for nutrition education
- Develop skills in conducting a needs assessment: identifying the primary intended audience and high-priority food or health needs and the behaviors or practices that contribute to the needs or issues
- Identify appropriate information sources for these assessments
- Compare advantages and disadvantages of different methods for obtaining the assessment information

Introduction: A Theory-Based Procedural Model for Designing Nutrition Education

This chapter begins a new section of the book. So far, we have learned about the research that has been going on in nutrition education, the theories and evidence it has generated, and the implications for conducting nutrition education. We are now ready for the task that is the central concern of this book: using this information to design nutrition education for the typical practice settings in which most nutrition educators work.

The first part of the book used a simple logic model to integrate theory and research evidence from a variety of studies into a conceptual framework for theory-based nutrition education. This section describes how to design the components of the simple logic model—the inputs, the outputs, and the outcomes, with a focus on the outputs. More specifically, this section of the book presents a systematic step-by-step procedure for designing behavior-focused and evidence-based nutrition education that integrates theory and research with

practice at each step. This process is called the *procedural model for designing theory-based nutrition education* (abbreviated sometimes as the *design model*). It consists of six steps, which are shown in a logic model format in the accompanying figure.

This part of the book describes each of the six steps, beginning with an overview of the design model and discussion of Step 1 in this chapter. This part of the book aims to be very practical so that you will be able to apply the six-step process to any program of your choosing. Worksheets are provided for you to use for each step. This chapter introduces a case study that we will follow throughout the six steps as an example. Clearly, how we translate theory into appropriate educational practice in real-world situations is crucial for success. In the design model shown here, the process starts when a food- or nutrition-related need or issue of concern is considered serious and prevalent enough to justify the expenditure of time and resources. We also identify for whom this need or issue is of greatest concern. This first step is extremely important

A Procedural Model For Designing Theory-Based Nutrition Education

INPUTS: COLLECTING ASSESSMENT DATA		DESIGNING THE OUTPUTS			DESIGNING OUTCOMES EVALUATION
STEP 1 ←→ **Analyze needs and behaviors: Specify the behavior or action focus of the program** • Assess needs and identify audience: select need(s) or issue(s) to address • Identify behaviors of concern that contribute to need(s) or issue(s) • Select core behaviors or practices to address	**STEP 2** ←→ **Identify relevant potential mediators of program behaviors** • Identify potential personal psychosocial mediators • Identify potential environmental mediators	**STEP 3** ←→ **Select theory, philosophy, and components** • Select theory and/or create appropriate model • Articulate educational philosophy • Clarify perspectives on content • Determine program components	**STEP 4** ←→ **State educational objectives for potential mediators** • Select relevant mediators to address • State educational objectives for each selected mediator: —Personal psychosocial mediators —Environmental mediators	**STEP 5** ←→ **Design theory-based educational strategies and activities to address potential mediators** • Design strategies and activities for each selected mediator: —Personal psychosocial mediators —Environmental mediators	**STEP 6** **Design evaluation** • Design evaluation of program's impact on behaviors and mediators • Design process evaluation

for designing an effective program. This step is often called a *needs assessment, needs analysis,* or *formative research.*

In the second step, we identify the behaviors or practices that contribute to the need, problem, or issue for the given audience and prioritize them. From these, we select one or a few major behaviors or practices for the program to address. These are called the *core behaviors, target behaviors, or core practices.* Examples are breastfeeding, safe food handling behaviors, and eating more fruits and vegetables. These behaviors or practices are stated in terms of changes the program seeks to achieve. Then we identify the personal psychosocial determinants of behavior (such as perceived benefits or sense of self-efficacy) that are relevant and of high priority for the selected core behavior or behaviors in a given group and setting. We also identify modifiable environmental determinants that facilitate or impede the core behaviors. Because these identified determinants are those that can be modified by educational means and can thus mediate changes in the core behaviors, we call them *potential mediators of behavior change* in the context of nutrition education.

In Step 3, we need to clarify the theory to be used and the educational philosophy that will guide the session or intervention and to select program components. In Step 4, we state appropriate educational objectives for each mediator. In Step 5, we select theory-based strategies and practical learning experiences for each mediator. Designing educational strategies and practical learning experiences matched to behavioral theory constructs is at the heart of effective nutrition education. Finally, we design the evaluation.

The process may at first glance seem very structured. You may have conducted nutrition education before and did not use such a systematic or structured approach—and the sessions went well, so you wonder about the necessity for going through these steps so systematically. The best way to view this section of the book is to see it as guidance from research and evidence on refining the practice of nutrition education to enhance its effectiveness. An analogy may be useful here. A young girl is an excellent baseball player and seems to have natural talent as a pitcher. The coach carefully analyzes her moves as she pitches, giving her specific guidance on making her moves more precise and effective. He gives her specific moves to practice, which do not come naturally at first, but she practices these moves until they become second nature, making her a formidable pitcher.

In the same way a pitcher can have natural talent, you already have skills in nutrition education. This book offers coaching based on research evidence. Designing effective nutrition education sessions takes work and requires a systematic process. The process described here may be new to you or similar to a process you have used before. Try it out and use it a few times. With practice, this systematic process will become second nature and you will adapt it to your own style to design lessons with ease.

The terms *behaviors* and *practices* are here used interchangeably, although *practices* has a connotation of long-standing behaviors or commonly practiced behaviors in the community, such as safe food handling practices or buying produce in a farmers' market. The term *intended audience* is used rather than *target population* to refer to the individuals or specific subgroup of the population with whom you will be working, to convey the sense that the group members are not a "target" of our activities so much as partners with whom we work so that together we can address needs and issues of importance.

The term *nutrition education intervention* is here used to denote any set of systematically planned educational activities or learning experiences that is provided to a group in a variety of settings, along with relevant environmental supports where appropriate. The term *intervention* is problematic to some educators because it can seem to imply that nutrition educators are intervening in people's lives, possibly against their will. It is not used in that sense here; rather, it is a convenient way to describe a range of planned activities of varying scope. Thus, the term encompasses both nutrition education of several sessions delivered by one person and programs involving many components and perhaps several media and delivered by many nutrition educators over a long time span.

The steps of the design model are summarized as follows:

Step 1. Analyze needs and specify the behaviors or actions to be the focus of the program for a given audience.
- Assess needs or issues and audience(s) for whom these needs or issues are relevant and important.
- Identify behaviors of concern that contribute to the identified needs, problems, or issues.
- Select core behaviors or practices as the focus of the session or program.

Step 2. Identify potential mediators of action or behavior change targeted by the program.
- Identify potential personal psychosocial mediators of the program's target behaviors or practices.
- Identify environmental factors that may mediate the target behavior or practices.

Step 3. Select theory, philosophy, and components.
- Select a theory or create a relevant theoretical model.
- Articulate the educational philosophy underlying the intervention.
- Determine the channels and components for the program.

Step 4. State educational objectives for mediators.
- State educational objectives for the personal psychosocial mediators of core behaviors of the program.
- State educational objectives for the environmental mediators of core behaviors of the program.

Step 5. Design theory-based educational strategies and practical activities to address mediators.
- Design educational strategies and activities for the personal psychosocial mediators of core behaviors of the program.
- Design educational strategies and activities for the environmental mediators of core behaviors of the program.

Step 6. Design the theory-based evaluation.
- Design the outcome evaluation.
- Design the process evaluation.

The procedural steps for designing nutrition education activities are laid out sequentially, but in reality they are closely interrelated, so you must go back and forth between steps when designing nutrition education (Box 7-1). This is graphically indicated by the arrows that go in both directions in Design Model 7-1. In addition, at each step you will need

SCENARIO

A nutrition educator has been asked to design a three-session program on "nutrition" to a group of women at the local Y. She decides that she will talk about the new food pyramid and healthful eating. She chooses as her first session a lecture on the different components of food—carbohydrates, protein, and fat, and MyPyramid—with an emphasis on healthful eating. She is in the middle of it when a member of the audience blurts out, "Do you have any recipes for making healthy snacks for my kids?" Another asks, "What is the best diet to lose weight?" This is followed by an avalanche of questions from others on how to select and pre-

pare healthful foods—and *none* on the topic of the lecture.

What is going on here? The nutrition educator believes that her talk is appropriately directed at what the audience should know about nutrition. How did she come to that conclusion? Newly graduated, she did an informal "needs assessment" in her head, which probably went something like this: "People need to become more knowledgeable about the principles of nutrition science and MyPyramid if they are to be able to make wise food choices, and a lecture is the quickest way to get a lot of information to the audience."

COMMENT

The nutrition educator doesn't have a clear focus on an issue of importance to the audience and a specific behavior

or action that the audience can take. Clearly, the audience did not find this kind of general information very helpful.

to check to see if what you are doing is on track and appropriate. This may mean conducting focus groups or interviews, pilot testing intervention components, rewriting material, seeking new information, and so forth.

Step 1: Analyze Needs or Issues and Specify the Behaviors to Be the Focus of the Program for a Given Audience

A nutrition education activity, whether it is one session or a program of several months with many components, is initiated when someone, some group, or some organization expresses an interest or a concern about some food- or nutrition-related issue. The interest may be expressed quite informally: the leader of an after-school program for high school students may think that it would be a good idea for the group to learn about eating more healthfully because she has observed that they skip lunch and grab some less than healthful snacks or fast food on the way to the program. She invites you to come provide a couple of sessions. Or the concern may be based on extensive national data about the health concerns of a particular group, such as overweight in children. Our tendency is to rush to design activities for our sessions or program based on what we know. After all, designing and implementing exciting learning experiences, seeing the group gain new insights and respond with enthusiasm, and making a difference in people's lives are what drew us to the profession in the first place. Indeed, many of us have made career changes to become nutrition educators.

However, for nutrition education to be effective and of value to the audience, we must clarify a few questions: What exactly are the needs or issues that any given nutrition education activity should address? For whom are these issues or concerns? Are they concerns of the nutrition educator or nutrition agency or are they concerns of the audience? Why are they of concern? What are the possible causes? It is extremely important to understand the intended audience as thoroughly as possible given practical and resource constraints.

Although informal judgments of needs and issues of concern can sometimes suffice, a more systematic or formal assessment of issues and problems has the following advantages:

- Helps us better understand our audience and the context of their lives
- Takes much of the guesswork out of nutrition education design
- Provides a basis for selecting behaviors and practices that are of concern and the development of appropriate educational goals and objectives to address them
- Makes clear the rationale for choosing particular priorities
- Makes it easier to use scarce resources appropriately
- Documents the need for funding or justifies expenditure of resources
- Provides a basis for measuring results

> **BOX 7-1 Using the Procedural Model for Designing Theory-Based Nutrition Education**
>
> The procedure laid out here can be used to develop a detailed plan for nutrition education, whether it is several sessions or a larger enterprise. If the agency or organization for which you are designing the sessions or program already has determined the issues you should address or the audience, or both, and has a history of lesson plans and activities, you can go through the process more quickly. After you have used this process a few times and are comfortable with it, or if you are already an experienced facilitator of behavior-focused nutrition education groups, you may use the process more informally. It is still important, however, to address *all* steps in the process, and to link theory, research, and practice at each step.

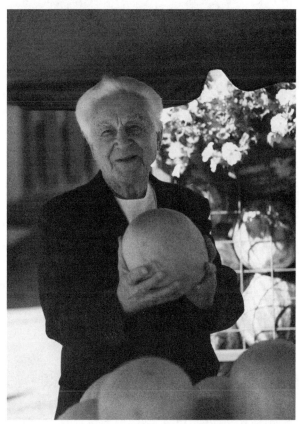

In many communities, buying produce at a local market is a common practice.

Such an assessment ensures that our food and nutrition education sessions or programs are directed at issues, needs, or problems that have been identified as important national or local priorities or that are perceived to be of concern or interest to the community or intended audience.

This systematic assessment process is called by different names in different arenas. Educators talk about identifying the "sources of the curriculum"—how to select what they will teach. Program planners talk about "needs assessments" or "formative assessments." Included here are identification of the needs and assets of the group or community. Social marketers talk about "market research," "formative research," or "front-end assessment" and consider this activity to be of crucial importance to the social marketing process. The term *needs assessment* is frequently used across many fields. This book uses the term *needs analysis*. However, the term is used in a broader sense, encompassing the notion of analysis

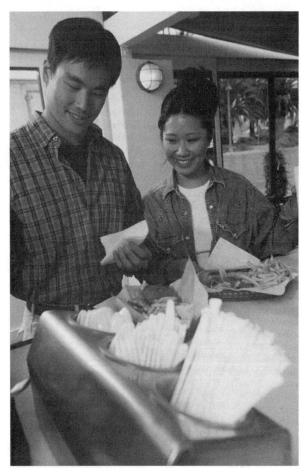

Helping teenagers learn to substitute french fries and chips for healthier snack alternatives is just one example of a nutrition education activity.

beyond identifying needs and problems to include issues of concern or interest in the food and nutrition areas.

Identification of needs, problems, and issues is only one step in a series of processes that must be repeated in the life of any food and nutrition education program, as shown in the design model. Together, these processes form the cycle of educational design, implementation, and evaluation that functions continuously throughout the duration of the program. For a new program, the first identification of issues and analysis of needs sets the cycle in motion. For an ongoing program, evaluations will provide this sort of information for future program planning.

Who Will Participate in Identifying and Analyzing Issues or Needs?

In many situations, you as the nutrition educator will be the person identifying the issues or conducting the needs analysis. You may have been asked to conduct short-term nutrition education with a group such as a seniors' lunch program, a program with people with AIDS, or an after-school program with adolescents. With few resources, the responsibility rests with one person: you. In other situations, a department, community group, or an agency will be charged with providing nutrition education services, and several staff members may be involved. Examples might be a community program or other long-term project, such as a school curriculum or nutrition education activities and programs sponsored or funded by a government agency. Here staff, along with an advisory group made up of some key individuals from the setting or community in which the nutrition education will be conducted, may suffice.

However, as noted earlier, in a comprehensive review of nutrition education programs conducted around the world from 1900 to 1970, Whitehead (1973) found that the programs that were more successful in changing behavior were those that did two things: they explicitly made behavior change a goal of the program, and they involved community stakeholders in all phases of the program, including the issues identification and needs analysis process, program planning, implementation, and evaluation. Thus, even in the previously described situations, involving others in the needs analysis process may be beneficial.

The initiative for a new nutrition education program or for modifying an existing one can come from the top (such as the national, state, or local government, or agency and program directors), from the grass roots (such as community members or parents of school children), or from anywhere in between (such as the nutrition educator in a community organization, government agency, or corporation). Regardless of the level at which the program idea originates, it is important to involve in the needs analysis process appropriate levels of people who have a stake in the program, such as community members, citizen groups or students, nutrition education staff, teachers, agency heads, or school principals. The decision who to include is an important one. Researchers have found that the more individuals or groups are involved in the decision making, the greater their acceptance of, and their sense of satisfaction with, decisions made (Rogers & Shoemaker, 1971).

The functions and roles to be played by the people selected then need to be clarified. Will their role be informal? Will they constitute a committee or a task force that will actually do some of the work, or will they serve as an advisory board, with staff members of an organization, nutrition educators, or others doing the actual assessment? Some members of this group may also serve later as knowledgeable informants about the needs of the intended audience. We refer to any of these configurations as the *nutrition education team*.

Identifying the Focus and Targets of Nutrition Education: General Considerations

Reliable information forms the basis for designing nutrition education. Many different kinds of information need to be collected, and many different methods for collecting data are available. It is important to gather more than one category of information and to use several methods to collect information in each category. The questions that should guide this process are as follows:

1. What is the food or health issue or need that the program will address, and for whom is it an issue or problem? Why?
   Objective data: Gathered from research and monitoring data
   Subjective data: What are the views of the intended audience or community about what they see as issues, concerns, and assets?
2a. What are the individual behaviors or community practices that may have contributed to the nutritional need or food-related issue and hence are of concern?
2b. What, then, should be the behaviors that the program should target, stated in terms of desired outcomes or program behavioral goals?
3a. What are the potential personal psychosocial mediators of the program's selected actions or behavioral goals?
3b. What are the potential environmental mediators for the achievement of these selected behaviors?
4. What are the administrative and resource issues that need to be considered?
5. What are some audience characteristics that are important to consider?

The end product of the needs analysis process is the establishment of one or more behaviors or practices that the intervention will seek to address and, depending on the intensity and duration of the intervention, the identification of several or many factors contributing to those behaviors and practices

(i.e., mediators) that can become the target of educational strategies. This chapter explores methods to collect data for questions 1 and 2. Chapter 8 describes methods to collect information for questions 3 through 5. Use the worksheets at the end of this chapter and the next to identify and analyze issues and needs and to record findings from the different components of the process.

Step 1a: Identify Target Food or Health Issue and Intended Audience

The first decision you have to make is who you want to reach and about what issue. In many cases, the intended audience or the food or health issue to be addressed will already be determined by others, such as by the mission of the agency or organization in which the nutrition education will be conducted, or by some funding source. For example, the audience will already be determined if the setting is an adolescent health clinic, a school, a Women, Infants and Children (WIC) clinic, or a senior center. Or the issue may be determined if the setting is a heart association, a cancer society, or an HIV clinic.

Alternatively, it may be that a community expresses the desire for something of importance to them, such as a community vegetable garden and nutrition education to go with it. Or you may have been asked to provide a series of sessions to some intended audience, such as adolescent girls, or in a specific location, such as the local Y. Yet, even in these settings there are both subpopulations and a variety of issues that can be addressed. In addition, often organizations are looking for new directions. It may also be that an organization needs data to provide a rationale for selection of a new focus. Because there are obviously many populations that experience numerous issues of concern, and resources are usually limited so that you cannot address them all, it is very important to carefully identify a primary audience and to focus on a specifically defined health, nutrition, or food issue. Use Worksheet 7-1 to record your findings in Step 1a.

Sources of Concern About Issues and Needs

Expert Inputs: Issues or Problems from the Point of View of the Food and Nutrition Profession

One good place to start in identifying critical food and nutrition issues and a primary audience is to examine the nutrition science, epidemiology, and food systems literature. What does the latest scientific research suggest are important health issues facing the nation or a particular group? What are some key concerns about ecological or community issues with respect to the food system? For which populations or groups are these nutritional and food concerns most urgent?

Although the choice of focus of nutrition education is usually based on considerations of health problems in which dietary behaviors and practices play a role, the choice of focus can also be based on concerns about the food system in which we make our choices and its impact on the natural environment. Choice of focus can also be based on social concerns arising from food production, marketing, and consumption practices. These are shown in Figure 7-1, and described in the following paragraphs.

Health concerns. Health concerns can be described in terms of food-related issues or nutritional problems identified through national mortality and morbidity data, including indicators of health or rates of disease, or through data about specific populations, such as rates of cardiovascular disease, cancer, hypertension, or diabetes, malnutrition in infants, breastfeeding, childhood obesity, or bone health. Health concerns can also be described in terms of physiological risk status within the potential primary audience—for example, in terms of serum lipid levels, blood pressure, blood glucose level, or body mass index.

Nutrition science research based on experimental, clinical, epidemiological, or field studies is constantly generating data on the relationship between food and health. Consequently, the nutrition profession has expectations about what

nutrition education should address. For example, scientific research or expert panels may have determined that a nutrition-related issue is of national concern, such as childhood obesity, bone health in adolescents, or cancer in the public at large. Epidemiological data may indicate that the mortality or morbidity due to disease is high in a particular population (e.g., a community is known to have a high rate of hypertension or diabetes). Or data may show that the nutritional status of a given group is considered to place them at risk (e.g., their serum cholesterol values are high or their vitamin A status is low). These data can cause concern for health professionals or nutrition experts and engender a sense of need for action.

Food system concerns. For some nutrition education programs that focus on food education, the choice of focus of an intervention may be based on concern about food system issues, such as a desire that children grow up knowing how food is produced, or concern whether our current food system is sustainable in the long term. For these programs, needs analysis information might include scientific research data on the impact of genetically engineered foods on health

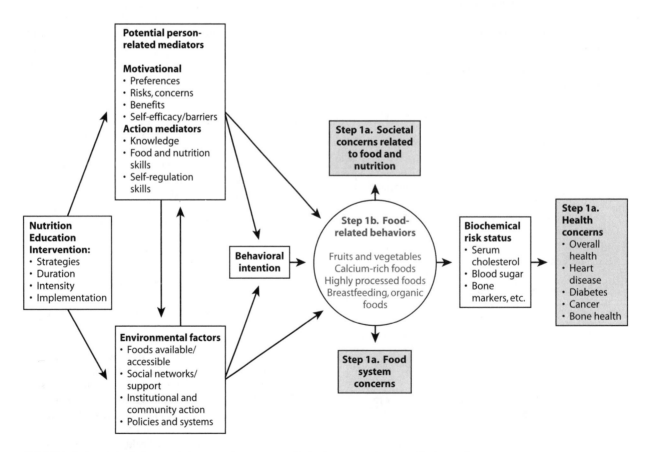

FIGURE 7-1 Step 1. Analyzing needs, issues, and concerns, and behaviors or practices contributing to them.

or on the natural environment, pesticides in the food supply, or food safety. Epidemiological data may provide information on rate of loss of farmland, or on the prevalence of farmer's markets, small and medium-sized farms, and community-supported agriculture farms in the local area.

Societal concerns related to food. For some nutrition education programs, a choice of focus might be based on a concern about the impact of food system practices on social systems in communities or whether food production labor and trade practices are fair, described in terms of impacts on farmers and local communities (so-called fair trade foods). Assessment data might include information about the availability of foods produced through fair trade practices and institutional policies with respect to purchasing and serving such foods.

Information sources. Information on all these issues can be obtained from literature reviews, national and local food and nutrition surveillance and monitoring data, health surveys, policy documents, local food and nutrition data, existing records, and communications with other researchers, program developers, or nutrition education practitioners through national or local professional meetings, annual meetings of professional associations, e-mail professional listservs, or telephone conversations.

Societal Inputs: Issues and Concerns Identified by National Food and Nutrition Goals and Policy Documents

What does the nation need in terms of the nutritional health of its citizenry? What are the stated national education, health, and nutrition goals of the country? Each country has developed nutrition, health, and food policy documents to guide government programs and provide information to the public. The choice of issues to address in a nutrition education intervention can be based on such policy initiatives. The specific health needs of the population are identified in various government surveys, such as the National Health and Nutrition Examination Survey (NHANES) or Continuing Survey of Food Intake of Individuals (CSFII). In the United States, nutrition recommendations based on the results of these and other surveys are spelled out from time to time in various government documents such as the surgeon general's *Report on Nutrition and Health*, the *Dietary Guidelines for Americans*, MyPyramid, and so forth. Private voluntary health organizations, such as cancer societies or heart associations, also publish guidelines for the public that can be used as a basis for choice of issue for an intervention program.

To national health goals, many food and nutrition professionals would add a need for a food system that is sustainable for the long term. Concerns about the food system becoming and remaining sustainable are described in various government documents, policy documents of food system research institutes and organizations, and publications of world health

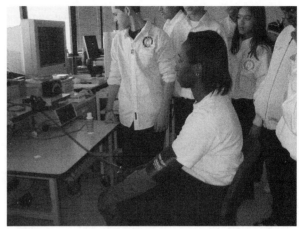

Students learn about their blood pressure and how it relates to their diet.

and agricultural organizations. You should consult these and other documents as you design your nutrition education sessions or program.

Audience Inputs: Concerns About, and From, the Intended Audience

Information about the audience can come from objective or subjective data sources.

Epidemiological and empirical information (objective data). If the intended audience or primary group has already been selected based on specific requests or on the mission of an agency or organization, you may be able to obtain information about the health conditions or nutritional status of a specific intended audience directly from previously collected data in local databases (e.g., city or county health data), existing records, in-depth interviews, focus groups, or direct observation. In many situations, however, the information will be inferred either from general surveys or from indirect indicators. For example, the seniors who are likely to participate in your program may have diets high in fat and low in fruits and vegetables and calcium because national surveys indicate that such nutritional problems are common among older adults in general.

Perceptions and desires of the intended audience (subjective data). Just as important as the actual, objective food and nutritional needs identified by science research or national policy documents are the issues and needs as perceived by the intended audience or primary group. Individuals are the experts on their own lives, so it is important to understand what they perceive as issues and dilemmas. What food- or nutrition-related issues are they concerned about? What other health concerns or competing, non-health-related interests do they have? What is the group interested in learning about? Such information can be obtained from national or regional opinion polls of the intended audience (such as adolescents) or from surveys of consumer practices and eating styles. If at all possible, the nutrition educator should obtain information directly from the intended audience through focus group discussions, in-depth interviews of key informants, or surveys.

The needs as seen from the point of view of the group or intended audience may or may not be the same as the objective nutritional problem or issue of concern. Given the health status data, the community may be as concerned as nutrition experts about the high rate of diet-related diseases such as heart disease or hypertension. An example is the town of Kerelia in Finland, where the heart disease rate was one of the highest in the world. In this case, when the citizens heard the statistics, they were very concerned and requested the government to do something about it. Here objective data and subjective perceptions converged. But sometimes a community or group may have concerns that are different from those of the nutrition professional. For example, parents of a child in a child-care facility may be mostly concerned about the cost and hours of the facility, whereas a nutritionist may be mostly concerned that the facility provide tasty and healthful food for the children.

Sometimes programs are initiated in the absence of a current pressing need. For example, a group of pregnant women may want a nutritionist to speak to them because they are interested in having healthy babies. Another group may be interested in eating more healthfully and would like a cooking class. Nutrition educators must keep this in mind as they conduct the process of identifying and analyzing issues and needs. Indeed, nutrition education programs often fail because they do not pay enough attention to the participants' *own* perception of their concerns and interests (and existing strengths). In conducting assessments, then, whether formally or informally, with individuals or with small groups, you need to *listen carefully*. You may find that potential participants have important insights into their condition and

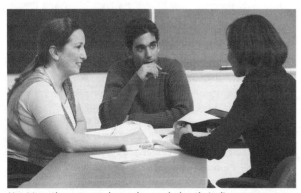

Nutrition educators need to understand what their clients want to achieve and what food-related issues concern them.

useful ideas about possible solutions if they are encouraged to share them with you.

Administrative Inputs: Issues and Concerns of the Sponsoring Organization or Funding Source

There are some administrative issues that you may need to consider as you choose the nutrition education focus. You may work for an agency or organization, or the nutrition education sessions you have been asked to design will be conducted in, or for, an agency or organization , such as an after-school program, extension program, public health department, or senior center. Thus, information on the general administrative needs of the sponsoring agency or agencies may also be necessary before you plan and implement a nutrition education program.

For example, in order to receive further funding, the agency may need to design a really successful program, regardless of the area of concern, rather than to come up with a program in an area of specific need if the program addressing that need might be less successful. It may also be that, because of the funding source, the program must be focused on a given issue or primary population and must conform to specified expectations about outcomes. Perhaps agency staff members may need to implement a program primarily to maintain their jobs or the existence of the agency or organization. Or staff may want to design a program using materials they already have on hand.

What is the expectation of your funding source? These organizational needs and wants should be aired at the time that the needs analysis is being conducted so that program expectations are realistic. You can ask questions such as the following:

- What is the overall mission of the organization, agency, or funding source?
- In what way will the program to be designed enhance the overall mission of the organization or funder?
- What are the expectations of the agency, organization, or funding source about the nutrition education component? What factors within the organization will facilitate or hinder the design and implementation of your nutrition education program? For example, will the nutrition education component compete with other components for funds? For facilities?
- How much do other personnel expect to become involved with the nutrition education sessions or program you design?

Prioritize Food or Health Issues and Choose Primary Audience

Whether the needs analysis has been comprehensive or brief, you, or the nutrition education committee, will probably have gathered information on more issues than you have the time or resources to address. Thus you will have to prioritize and focus. In addition, the information from all the various sources should be balanced with each other. For example, the perceptions of the intended audience may be at odds with the issues of professional concern based on scientific findings and epidemiological data. These differing interests have to be balanced as you select an issue or need to address that is appropriate to a given nutrition education sessions or program.

Choice of *issue or need* to address can be based on the following (as suggested by Green and Kreuter, 1999):

- Which of these issues or problems are ranked as local, regional, or national priorities?
- Which issues, if appropriately addressed, are likely to have the greatest impact on the outcomes desired?
- Which issues or problems are most amenable to intervention by educational means?
- Which issues or problems are considered by the intended audience to be most important?
- Which issues or problems are considered by the sponsoring agency or funding source to be most important?

Choice of *primary audience* can be based on greatest need or interest using criteria such as the following:

- Size of the population for whom the issues are a problem or of concern
- The severity or incidence of the nutritional condition or food system situation
- Those who are most ready for change
- Those with the greatest influence on others

Conclusion for Step 1a: Select the Food or Health Issues and Intended Audience

Using the criteria listed in this chapter, you, or the nutrition education team, should now be in the position to prioritize health conditions, food-related concerns, and group interests to identify the major issues and the intended audience that the intervention will address. Use Worksheet 7-1 to help you in this process. You may discuss competing priorities as a team and come to consensus, or use some more formal process. Examples of issues and audiences are childhood overweight prevention, osteoporosis prevention among community adults, increased breastfeeding among women, or eating more local foods among adult low-income urban families. See Nutrition Education in Action 7-1 for some specific examples.

Step 1b: Identify the Behaviors and Practices of Concern That Contribute to the Need or Issue

Information about the health status or the food-related concerns of a group does not provide a sufficient basis for an educational intervention. As discussed in some detail in Part

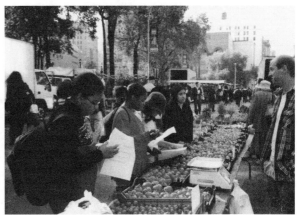

Students can find out the cost of tomatoes as part of a scavenger hunt.

I of this book and as indicated in our overall conceptual framework, we need to know the diet-related behaviors and practices contributing to the food- and nutrition-related problems because *these behaviors* will be the focus of nutrition education. The extensiveness of the information you want, as well as the degree of accuracy you need, depends very much on the nature and duration of your intervention. If you will be providing only one or two sessions with a given audience, it is still important to collect behavioral information, but a simple questionnaire that you design may be sufficient. If the intervention is with a group that you will be working with for some time, and formal evaluation data will be needed for the agency or funder, you will want to use some more formal instruments that are available or adapt them for your use.

Identify Behaviors and Practices of Concern

The next step, then, is to identify which behaviors or dietary practices may have contributed to the nutritional problems or food-related issues that are of concern to the intended audience. This is shown in Figure 7-1 as Step 1b. The choice of which behaviors or practices to assess will depend on the issues and primary audience you have selected. Worksheet 7-2 can help you with this process. A review of measures is provided by Contento, Randell, and Basch (2002).

Review of the Relevant Nutrition Research Literature

The nutrition research literature is a good place to start for information regarding the primary audience you have selected and the key needs or issues that you have identified. Here you are seeking data on food-related behaviors that have been shown to have impacts on the specific health or food system outcomes you identified. The degree of specificity of the information may vary for each issue and population. We know that diet is related to chronic disease, and that both diet and physical activity are related to overweight. But it is important to have more specific information if it is available.

NUTRITION EDUCATION IN ACTION 7-1

Choice of Focus for Nutrition Education: Examples of Issues, Audiences, and Behaviors

A diabetes education program for community adults (audience) with type 2 diabetes (issue), delivered in a community setting (*JNEB* 2004, O11)
  • *Behavioral focus:* Diet, exercise, medications, blood glucose monitoring, and foot care

Promoting healthy eating and physical activity behaviors (issue) among middle school students (audience)
  • *Behavioral focus:* Fruit and vegetable intake and physical activity

Increasing healthy eating (issue) among men, ages 18 to 44, at a sawmill worksite (audience) (*JNEB* 2004, P11)
  • *Behavioral focus:* Fruit and vegetable intake

Garden-based learning experiences for sixth-grade students (audience) to increase vegetable intake (issue) (*JNEB* 2005, O25)
  • *Behavioral focus:* Frequency and variety of vegetables consumed

Promotion of the healthy traditional Latino diet (issue) among youth aged 8 to 12 years (audience) (*JNEB* 2005, O23).
  • *Behavioral focus:* More beans, fruits, and vegetables and fewer high-sugar and high-fat foods

Overcoming "picky eating" (issue) in preschoolers (audience) (*JNEB* 2005, O17)
  • *Behavioral focus:* Increasing familiarity with 13 novel foods

Promoting healthful eating through youth-operated farm stands (issue) in low-income communities (audience) (*JNEB* 2005, O26, O27)
  • *Behavioral focus:* Increased access to affordable, high-quality, locally grown produce (environmental support), and increased redemption of food stamps and consumption of local produce

Improving the school food environment with the use of local foods (issue) by food service directors (audience)
  • *Behavioral focus:* Use of foods from local producers through a Farm to School program

Improving child feeding practices and physical activity behaviors of preschoolers (issue) (*JNEB* 2005, O75) through a newsletter intervention with parents (audience)
  • *Behavioral focus:* Child feeding practices of parents (pressure to eat, restriction, perceived responsibility, and monitoring of child's eating) and physical activity behaviors in children (time spent playing outdoors, active play, and watching television)

Food safety education (issue) for persons living with HIV/AIDS (audience)
  • *Behavioral focus:* Appropriate food handling and cooking behaviors; personal behaviors such as handwashing

A health-centered curriculum (issue) for community adults (audience) (*JNEB* 2004, O47)
  • *Behavioral focus:* Increased pleasurable and healthy eating, enjoyment of physically active living, and body-size acceptance of self and others

Journal for Nutrition Education and Behavior 2004;36(Suppl.1).
Journal for Nutrition Education and Behavior 2005;37(Suppl. 1).

For example, which food practices of the family or social environment contribute to the high incidence of overweight in this particular group of school-aged children? Too many sweetened beverages? Too little physical activity? Or both? Which behaviors of the identified primary audience lead to the audience's high serum cholesterol levels? Do people eat high-fat foods too often or do the food preparation methods add fat to foods (e.g. frying foods), or both? Which behaviors contribute to the low vitamin C status? Are people eating too few vegetables and fruits in their diets or are they cooking vegetables in such a way as to destroy the vitamin C, or both? Which healthful behaviors and practices are already being practiced by the group (i.e., what are the group's assets)?

Perhaps they already practice a number of behaviors that are healthful, such as a high consumption of beans and whole grains, and can be encouraged to do more.

Review of Monitoring Data or Consumer Surveys

Reviewing the monitoring data or consumer surveys on the primary audience you have selected and the key issues that you have identified can also provide valuable information. For example, if adolescents are the primary audience that you have selected and overweight prevention is the key issue identified for the focus of the nutrition education program or sessions, then you will want to review existing consumer surveys, national or local monitoring data, or surveys of food purchasing practices for information on behaviors that might contribute to the issue of overweight. Even if it is not possible to obtain information directly from the group, knowledge about the food practices and habits of people similar to the primary group is extremely helpful. This information search may yield the finding, for example, that frequent consumption of high-fat fast foods and sweetened drinks and low intakes of fruits and vegetables are contributing behaviors to overweight in adolescents.

Survey Information from the Intended Audience

If it is possible to survey the primary audience, you should do so, because questionnaires that ask about specific dietary practices provide you with specific information that is extremely useful. For example, people often have misconceptions about the amount of fat or amount of fruits and vegetables in their diets (Bogers, Brug, van Assema, Dagnelie, 2004).

Informal surveys using short checklists to find out about behaviors and practices of your audience may be sufficient for your purposes. If you need to be more systematic, you may need to use more formal instruments. The terms *behaviors* and *practices* can have many meanings in the context of food and nutrition. Some of these are listed here, along with methods for assessing them. Examples of some instruments that you might use are given in Tables 7-1 and 7-2.

- *Food purchasing behaviors or practices.* Specific shopping practices, such as using a shopping list, doing comparison shopping, or using coupons can be obtained from surveys and interviews (Hersey et al., 2001).The behavior of purchasing local or organic foods can be measured with sales data for a community or with specifically designed instruments.

- *Intake of specific foods or food items.* A very useful survey method is for the group to record what they eat and then compare their intakes to the recommended MyPyramid servings for their age and sex (www.mypyramid.gov).

  More formal assessments of intakes of specific foods can be measured using 24-hour dietary recalls, one- or three-day food records, or food frequency questionnaires. For the recalls, the participants are asked to recall all the foods and beverages that they consumed during the previous 24-hour period. You can do this individually or in a group setting. The recalled foods can be scored for the quantity of intakes of the foods targeted by the program, such as fruits and vegetables or calcium-rich foods. In the case of food records, participants keep a record of their intakes of food and drinks over a one- or three-day period. The foods recorded can then be analyzed for the targeted foods.

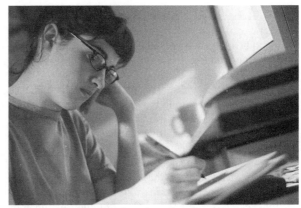

Nutrition education research can be gathered at places such as local town or university libraries.

Food frequency questionnaires can be comprehensive (Willett et al., 1987; Block et al., 1992) or can be short and targeted to the behaviors of interest, in which case they are often called *checklists* or *screeners* (such as screeners for fruits and vegetables, high-fat foods, or local foods) (Thompson & Byers, 1994; Block et al., 2000; Yaroch, Resnicow, & Khan, 2000; Townsend et al., 2003; McPherson et al., 2000; McClelland et al., 2001). For nutrition education in most practice settings, short food intake checklists will be sufficient. An example is shown in Table 7-2. It can be scored manually and given back to the participants. Table 7-1 shows an instrument that has been validated for low-income audiences.

- *Specific observable behaviors.* Examples are using skim milk instead of whole milk, taking the skin off chicken when eating chicken, or eating whole-grain bread instead of white bread. These behaviors can be assessed using questionnaires such as the Kristal Food Habits Questionnaire (Shannon et al., 1997) (see Table 7-2). In this questionnaire the behaviors related to reducing fat in the diet are categorized into (1) exclusion, which refers to avoiding high-fat foods through elimination of items or preparation techniques; (2) modification, which refers to modifying commonly available foods to make them lower in fat; (3) substitution, which refers to maintaining one's usual dietary pattern but using specially formulated or processed lower-fat versions of high-fat foods; and (4) replacement, which refers to changing one's diet by replacing high-fat foods with fruits and vegetables or with low-fat foods other than fruits and vegetables. Those behaviors related to fiber are: eating cereals and grains, eating fruits and vegetables, and substituting high-fiber for low-fiber foods.

Food safety behaviors belong in this category and can also be assessed; examples are cooking foods adequately, practicing personal hygiene, and keeping foods at a safe temperature (Meideros et al., 2001).

● *Eating patterns.* Examples are whether the audience eats breakfast, or fruit as a snack, or three meals a day. You can devise an instrument to fit your purposes.

● *Quality of diet.* Sometimes a single question can be used, such as "How would you describe the quality of your diet?" Alternatively, it can be judged from analysis of MyPyramid servings or other instruments.

● *Sub-behaviors or actions that are necessary for the behaviors to be enacted.* For example, eating four or more cups of fruits and vegetables each day requires the sub-behaviors or actions of purchasing fruits and vegetables, preparing them for consumption, storing fruits and vegetables properly, and adding them to the daily diet at specified times or occasions (e.g., orange juice at breakfast, fruit as a mid-morning snack). Identifying the specific actions that the intended audience does or does not undertake will help with the writing of specific educational objectives and the design of educational activities.

Interviews

If at all possible, talk to the intended audience about their behaviors and practices. Behavioral data can be obtained through individual interviews, focus groups, or intercept interviews as people leave a food store. Pay special attention to culture-specific foods and practices. Twenty-four-hour dietary recalls, conducted in person or by phone, can also yield valuable information.

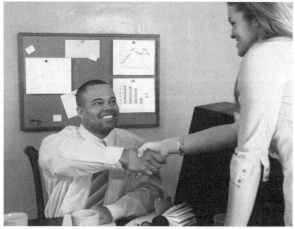

Behavioral data can be gathered in formal and informal interviews.

TABLE 7-1 Food Behavior Checklist for Limited-Resources Audiences

Scores of 1 to 4 = Never, Sometimes, Often, Usually, Always. Scores for those items with yes/no responses are shown in parentheses.

Fruit and vegetable items

Do you eat more than one kind of fruit daily? _____

During the past week, did you have citrus fruit (such as orange or grapefruit) or citrus juice? (yes = 2; no = 1) _____

How many servings of vegetables do you eat each day? _____

Do you eat two or more servings of vegetables at your main meal? _____

Do you eat fruits or vegetables as snacks? _____

How many servings of fruit do you eat each day? _____

Milk items

Do you drink milk daily? _____

During the past week, did you have milk as a beverage or on cereal? _____

Fat and cholesterol items

During the past week, did you have fish? (yes = 2; no = 1) _____

Do you take the skin off chicken? _____

Diet quality

When shopping, do you use the Nutrition Facts label to choose foods? _____

Do you drink regular soft drinks? _____

Do you buy Kool-Aid, Gatorade, Sunny Delight, or other fruit drink/punch? _____

Would you describe your diet as excellent (5), very good (4), good (3), fair (2), or poor (1)? _____

Food security

Do you run out of food before the end of the month? _____

Source: Townsend, M.S., L.L. Kaiser, L.H. Allen, A. Block Joy, and S.P. Murphy. 2003. Selecting items for a food behavior checklist for a limited-resources audience. *Journal of Nutrition Education and Behavior* 35:69–82. Used with permission of the Society for Nutrition Education.

TABLE 7-2 Food Habits Questionnaire: Measuring Fat- and Fiber-Related Diet Behaviors

Circle *one answer* each for each question below. If the question does not apply to you, circle "N/A" for "not applicable." For example, if you do not eat chicken, circle "N/A" for questions 1 and 2.

Fat-Related Behavior Questionnaire

In the *PAST MONTH*, how often did you . . .	Usually or Always	Often	Sometimes	Rarely or Never	Not Applicable
Meat, fish, and eggs	1	2	3	4	N/A
1. When eating chicken, have it baked or broiled (versus fried)?	1	2	3	4	N/A
2. When eating chicken, take off the skin before eating it?	1	2	3	4	N/A
3. Use a meatless sauce on spaghetti or noodles?	1	2	3	4	N/A
4. When eating red meat, eat only small portions?	1	2	3	4	N/A
5. When eating red meat, cut away all visible fat?	1	2	3	4	N/A
6. Have a vegetarian dinner?	1	2	3	4	N/A
7. Eat fish or chicken instead of red meat?	1	2	3	4	N/A
Milk and cheese	1	2	3	4	N/A
8. Have low-fat (1%) or nonfat milk?	1	2	3	4	N/A
9. Eat special low-fat diet cheeses?	1	2	3	4	N/A
10. Eat ice milk, frozen yogurt, or sherbet instead of ice cream?	1	2	3	4	N/A
Fruits, vegetables, and salads	1	2	3	4	N/A
11. Put butter or margarine on cooked vegetables? (R)	1	2	3	4	N/A
12. Eat boiled or baked potatoes without butter?	1	2	3	4	N/A
13. Use low-calorie instead of regular salad dressing?	1	2	3	4	N/A
14. Put sour cream, cheese, or other sauces on vegetables and potatoes? (R)	1	2	3	4	N/A
15. Have only fruit for dessert?	1	2	3	4	N/A
16. Eat at least two vegetables (not green salad) at dinner?	1	2	3	4	N/A
17. Snack on raw vegetables instead of potato chips, corn chips, or taco chips?	1	2	3	4	N/A
18. Eat bread, rolls, or muffins without butter or margarine?	1	2	3	4	N/A
19. Use yogurt instead of sour cream?	1	2	3	4	N/A
20. Use PAM or other nonstick spray when cooking?	1	2	3	4	N/A

Add up the scores for each individual and then for the group. For the items labeled R, you need first to reverse the scoring—that is, change 4 to 1, 3 to 2, 2 to 3, and 1 to 4. The higher the score, the greater the number of high-fat behaviors, and the higher the amount of fat in the diet. High scores for individual foods or food groups tell you which specific low-fat behaviors are being rarely practiced and can be addressed in nutrition education.

Fiber-Related Behavior Questionnaire

In the *PAST MONTH*, how often did you . . .	Usually or Always	Often	Sometimes	Rarely or Never	Not Applicable
Grains and cereals	1	2	3	4	N/A
1. Eat high-fiber cereals?	1	2	3	4	N/A
2. Eat cereal (hot or cold) for breakfast?	1	2	3	4	N/A
3. Eat whole-grain bread or crackers?	1	2	3	4	N/A
4. Add bran to cereal or casseroles?	1	2	3	4	N/A
Fruits and vegetables	1	2	3	4	N/A
5 Eat fruit for dessert?	1	2	3	4	N/A
6. Eat vegetables for snacks instead of chips?	1	2	3	4	N/A
7. Eat fruit for breakfast?	1	2	3	4	N/A
8. Eat a vegetable for lunch?	1	2	3	4	N/A
9. Eat two or more vegetables at dinner?	1	2	3	4	N/A
Substituting high-fiber for low-fiber foods	1	2	3	4	N/A
10. Eat whole-wheat pasta instead of regular pasta?	1	2	3	4	N/A
11. Eat brown rice instead of white rice?	1	2	3	4	N/A
12. Eat a vegetarian dinner?	1	2	3	4	N/A

Add up the scores for each individual and then for the group. The higher the score, the fewer are the number of high-fiber behaviors, and the lower the fiber intake in the diet. High scores for individual foods or food groups tell you which specific high-fiber behaviors are being rarely practiced and can be addressed in nutrition education.

Source: Shannon, J., A.R. Kristal, S.J. Curry, and S.A. Beresford. 1997. Application of a behavioral approach to measuring dietary change: The fat and fiber-related diet behavior questionnaire. *Cancer Epidemiology, Biomarkers and Prevention* 6:355–361. Used with permission of American Association for Cancer Research and the authors.

Observations

Observations are difficult to do but can be very informative. They can be quite informal, such as observing what children eat in school or what teenagers purchase in the school neighborhood after school.

Prioritize the Behaviors or Practices of Concern That Contribute to the Selected Needs, Problems, or Issues

Again, you or the nutrition education team will probably have gathered information on more behaviors or practices than you have the time or resources to address, so you will have to prioritize and focus. For example, the behaviors could be as follows: eating few fruits and vegetables, high intake of high-fat foods and snacks, sedentary behaviors, and high consumption of sweetened drinks and low consumption of milk and dairy products. These are probably more behaviors than you can address in your program, given time and resource constraints, if you wish to have a meaningful impact on behavior. (You could provide informational talks on all of these topics to raise awareness of the issues, but that does not mean the lectures will have an impact on attitudes or action.) Rate the behaviors or practices on the basis of the criteria described in the following subsections (Rogers, 1995; Green & Kreuter, 1999) and use Worksheet 7-2 to record your ratings.

Importance of Engaging in This Action or Changing This Behavior

Each of the behaviors or practices you have identified should be rated in terms of importance based on its *prevalence* in the population and the *strength of its contribution* to the health condition or food-related issue identified. This can be done by asking the following questions: Do these behaviors occur frequently in the population identified? Do these behaviors clearly and significantly contribute to the health condition or food-related issue that you have identified as of concern for your selected group or population?

Prevalence information can be obtained from national or local monitoring data. The strength of the evidence linking the behaviors to the health condition or food issue can be evaluated based on a review of the relevant nutrition science literature. For example, several behaviors have been shown to be of high prevalence and to be strongly linked to cardiovascular risk: a diet high in saturated fat and a diet low in fruits and vegetables. Sedentary behavior is also highly prevalent and highly linked to risk of overweight, but only moderately related to cardiovascular and cancer risk. Breastfeeding is of low prevalence but is highly linked with healthy outcomes for the baby.

Modifiability of the Behavior or Practice by Educational Methods

For each of the behaviors identified, ask: How amenable to change or modification is the behavior? A given behavior may be a very important contributor to the health or food system issue identified, but it will not be a suitable target for a nutrition education intervention unless there is reasonable evidence that it is changeable by educational means. This judgment can be based on evidence from the scientific and professional nutrition education, health education, and health promotion literature that such behaviors have responded previously to interventions.

You can also select the behaviors to focus on based on criteria from the Diffusion of Innovations literature (Rogers & Shoemaker, 1971; Rogers, 1995). Studies in this area have found that the likelihood of people accepting or adopting an innovation (in our case, a diet-related behavior) is influenced by a number of features of the innovation or behavior. We can use these findings as criteria for the changeability of the behaviors you have identified as potential targets of the program:

- *Relative advantage:* Is the new behavior seen by the intended audience as better than the one it will replace?
- *Complexity:* Is the new behavior easy to understand, act on, and adopt? How many substeps may be involved?
- *Compatibility:* How compatible is the new behavior with existing practices, values, and cultural norms of the primary group or intended audience?
- *Trialability:* Can the behavior be tried out before making a long-term commitment to act upon it or to adopt it?
- *Observability:* Are the positive results of the behavior change easily visible to the intended audience?

Feasibility

How feasible will it be to design an intervention that can address the behavior or practice, based on considerations of available resources and the potential duration and intensity possible for the intended nutrition education intervention? How much time and resources will you be able to devote to the intervention? How long a program can you offer? Will that be sufficient to show change?

Desirability by the Primary Group or Intended Audience

It is extremely important to obtain more subjective information from the intended audience. How desirable is it to the intended audience to take action or to adopt this particular dietary behavior? Do they see the behavior as realistic? Effective? Practical? Easy to do?

Conclusion for Step 1b

The information that you have collected so far should now permit you to identify the specific food- and diet-related behaviors or practices of concern or risk that will be the focus of your nutrition education intervention or program. Some kind of rating system can be devised to evaluate each behavior on all of these criteria. See Worksheet 7-2 as an example.

Filling out this worksheet can help you systematically review the data and make a judgment about choice of behavioral focus. If a team is involved, it may be most useful if each member first completes such a rating scheme and then the team meets to discuss the choices. This process encourages an informed and reasoned discussion of the evidence in order to make a sound decision.

Worksheet 7-2 asks you to identify up to five behaviors or practices that are of concern or of importance. From these you will select one to three behaviors that will be the focus of your nutrition education program. How many and which behaviors you select will depend largely on the intensity and duration possible for the program; that is, how many sessions or components comprise the program and how long each session or component lasts, as well as the resources and personnel available. Sometimes one or two behaviors may be closely related to each other and can be

addressed together. For example, eating more fruits and vegetables and eating fewer high-fat foods might be addressed together because an increase in fruits and vegetables in the diet may substitute for high-fat foods (e.g., fruits instead of high-fat desserts). For the issue of childhood overweight prevention, the behaviors identified as relevant may be eating more fruits and vegetables, eating more low-fat foods, drinking fewer sodas, and decreasing sedentary behavior. For the issue of eating more local foods, the behaviors may be buying more local foods and cooking more local foods. For each example, you may not have the time and resources to address all the behaviors, so select those that you *can* address.

Nutrition Education in Action 7-2 provides some examples of how the nutrition education focus and issues, audiences, and behaviors have been stated for the Food Stamp Nutrition Education program and the Team Nutrition program.

NUTRITION EDUCATION IN ACTION 7-2

Examples of Core Behavior Goals of Nutrition Education Programs and Their Rationales

Food Stamp Nutrition Education

Although there are many important nutrition-related issues that affect the food stamp–eligible audience, the Food and Nutrition Service of the U.S. Department of Agriculture (USDA) encourages states to focus their Food Stamp Nutrition Education (FSNE) program efforts on the following behavior outcomes:

- Eat fruits and vegetables, whole grains, and nonfat or low-fat milk or milk products every day.
- Be physically active every day as part of a healthy lifestyle.
- Balance calorie intake from foods and beverages with calories expended.

These behaviors are associated with a reduced risk of some forms of cancer, type 2 diabetes, and coronary heart disease. It is appropriate to focus on these behavior outcomes for FSNE because low-income individuals often experience a disproportionate share of diet-related problems that are risk factors for the major diseases contributing to poor health, disability, and premature death.

Team Nutrition

The USDA's Team Nutrition promotes comprehensive, behavior-based nutrition education to enable children to make healthy eating and physical activity choices. Social cognitive theory is the foundation of efforts to help children understand how eating and physical activity affect the way they grow, learn, play, and feel today as well as the relationship of their choices to lifelong health. These efforts are designed to increase their understanding that healthy eating and physical activity are fun and that skills developed today will assist them in enjoying healthy eating and physical activity in later years.

All program materials encourage students to make food and physical activity choices for a healthy lifestyle. The focus is on five behavior outcomes:

- Eat a variety of foods.
- Eat more fruits, vegetables, and grains.
- Eat lower-fat foods more often.
- Get your calcium-rich foods.
- Be physically active.

Sources: Food and Nutrition Service, U.S. Department of Agriculture. 2005. *Food stamp nutrition education guiding principles.* http://www.fns.usda.gov/oane/menu/FSNE/FSNE.htm; and Food and Nutrition Service, U.S. Department of Agriculture. n.d. About Team Nutrition. http://www.fns.usda.gov/tn/about.

Step 1c: Choose Behaviors to Be the Focus of the Sessions (Program Behavioral Goals)

From the set of identified behaviors or practices of concern, select and finalize those that the program or sessions will address and state them in terms of targeted core behaviors or program behavioral goals. These goals should describe the purpose or desired *behavioral outcomes* for the program, whether the program is a few sessions or a multicomponent intervention. As we have noted many times before, evidence suggests that nutrition education is more likely to be effective if it focuses on *specific* behaviors or community practices. Thus, the program goals should be stated in terms of behaviors or practices. The scope of the behavioral goal or goals will reflect the duration, intensity, and extensiveness of the program. Examples of behavioral goals are to increase fruit and vegetable consumption among adolescents, increase calcium-rich foods among women in the WIC program, increase participation in the food stamp farmers' market program, increase the choice of more healthful snacks and beverages by elementary school students, increase the proportion of women with type 2 diabetes who practice effective food management skills, and increase the number of people who participate in community-supported agriculture.

Some nutrition educators like to state program behavioral goals in terms of specific behavioral objectives, specifying the exact changes desired, such as the following: adolescents will eat two or more cups of fruits and vegetables a day, or the proportion of women breastfeeding for at least four weeks will increase from 20% to 40%. We will refer to both levels of specificity as *behavioral goals* for two reasons. First, writing "behavioral objectives" in addition to "behavioral goals" adds another step in an already long process. Second, the term *behavioral objectives* has other meanings in the educational field, as we shall see in Chapter 10; thus, there may be confusion about what the term means. The choice of specificity depends on the purposes of your program. If you will be measuring specific behavioral outcomes in your evaluation, you will need to state your behavioral outcomes in specific terms.

For example, a behavioral goal can be stated generally as follows: to increase fruit and vegetable intake among adolescents. To state the goal more specifically, you can considering the following:

- Who is the primary audience for the intervention? *Answer:* Seventh and eighth graders.
- What is the exact action or change in behavior or practice to be achieved? *Answer:* Increase daily fruit and vegetable intake.
- How much change is expected? *Answer:* Increase to 2.5 or more cups of fruits and vegetables a day.

The program behavioral goal can thus be stated as follows: Adolescents in seventh and eighth grade in program schools will increase their fruit and vegetable intake to 2.5

cups or more a day. In a nutrition education research intervention study, these outcomes would generally be considered the primary outcomes.

Nutrition Education in Action 7-3 provides some examples of how the nutrition education focus and issues, audiences, and behaviors have been stated for some social marketing and Web-based programs.

It is important at this point to resist a strong desire to launch into designing the food and nutrition education program given what you already know about the participants. Even knowledge about the specific behaviors leading to a given condition may not be sufficient. In one study, the diets of low-income families in Brazil were found to be deficient in protein (the nutritional status problem), and the families were not using soybeans as part of the diet. Since soybeans are produced in Brazil and are a good source of protein, a nutrition education campaign was developed directed at increasing consumption of these beans (Wright, Horner, & Charini, 1982). When it met with very little success, families were then interviewed about *why* they did not eat soybeans. Among the reasons were dislike of the taste of soybeans, unfamiliarity, lack of interest, unavailability of soybeans, and lack of knowledge about preparation methods. Only when such information was available was it possible to design and test several more appropriate approaches. Such considerations, then, lead to another set of factors that must be assessed when we wish our nutrition education efforts to be successful; these are described in the next chapter.

Your Turn

The worksheets that have been described throughout the chapter can be found at the end of the chapter. Use them as you start the design process for a hypothetical or real nutrition education program.

Case Study

A case study is presented after the worksheets to illustrate the design process. This case study is used throughout the next several chapters for each of the steps. Here we begin with Step 1 of the nutrition education design process.

Our case involves a university-affiliated organization that works with children and youth. Thus, the general audience is already determined. The mission of the organization is to provide health services, including nutrition services, to youth and their families in the community. The community is ethnically and economically diverse. The agency has provided health and nutrition services, but it has not developed a nutrition education program before. Agency directors think that it will be important to use some of its funds to develop a nutrition education program for youth in the area it serves, because they believe, from their experience, that the diets of youth need improving. However, they do not have any specific data on their youth or what kind of program should

---

NUTRITION EDUCATION IN ACTION **7-3**

Examples of Goals and Objectives of Nutrition Education Programs

Sisters Together: Move More, Eat Better

Sisters Together is a national initiative of the Weight-control Information Network (WIN) designed to encourage black women aged 18 and older to maintain a healthy weight by becoming more physically active and eating healthier foods.

Sisters Together works with national and local newspapers, magazines, radio stations, schools, and consumer and professional organizations to raise awareness among black women about the health benefits of regular physical activity and healthy eating. This effort is timely, because recent statistics indicate that nearly 80% of black women are overweight or obese.

Pick a Better Snack

Pick a Better Snack is a social marketing campaign in Iowa directed at low-income families and children. The objectives are to

- Increase awareness of the campaign's logo and supporting messages
- Improve attitudes about eating fruits and vegetables as snacks
- Increase fruit and vegetable consumption among low-income children and their families

We Can!

We Can! (Ways to Enhance Children's Activity and Nutrition) is a national education program designed for parents and caregivers to help children 8 to 13 years old stay at a healthy weight. Parents and caregivers are the primary influencers for this age group. We Can! offers parents and families tips and fun activities to

- Encourage healthy eating
- Increase physical activity
- Reduce sedentary or screen time

Sources: Weight-control Information Network. Sisters Together: Move More, Eat Better. http://win.niddk.nih.gov/sisters/index.htm; Iowa Department of Public Health and Iowa Department of Education. Pick a better snack and act. http://www.idph.state.ia.us/Pickabettersnack; and Department of Health and Human Services, National Institutes of Health. We Can! http://www.nhlbi.nih.gov/health/public/heart/obesity/wecan/.

---

be developed. Thus, the organization needs to find out the major nutrition-related health issues and problems that face the youth in their community and to develop a nutrition education program that addresses these issues.

In Step 1 of the design model, we first analyze the health issues, problems, and needs of this audience, and then the behaviors or practices that youth engage in that contribute to these health issues or concerns. From this analysis we can identify the few behaviors or practices that the program will encourage in order to address these concerns. These recommended practices or behaviors will become the behavioral focus of the program.

In the case study, we conduct all the steps described in this chapter:

Step 1a. Analyze the food and nutrition-related needs, issues, or concerns of the audience.

Step 1b. Identify the high-priority behaviors or practices that are of concern because they contribute to the needs and issues.

Step 1c. State the program's core behavioral goals for the audience, or the recommended practices. These behavioral goals describe the desired behavioral outcomes for the program.

Questions and Activities

1. What do you see as the advantages and disadvantages of using a systematic process for designing theory- and evidence-based nutrition education?

2. Why is it important to do a thorough assessment of the needs, interests, and concerns of the intended audience?

3. On what basis would you select the issues or problems you would address in a nutrition education program?

4. We have said earlier in the book that nutrition education is more likely to be effective if it focuses on behaviors and practices. What does that mean for the needs analysis process?

5. How would you select which behaviors or practices your program should address for your intended audience? That is, what criteria would you use and why?

STEP 1 WORKSHEETS　**Identify Focus of the Program: Analyze Needs and Intended Audience, and Specify Target Behaviors**

Before you design any nutrition education intervention, whether it is a few sessions or a larger program with several components, it is important to determine your intervention focus and identify your intended primary audience. When those have been determined, you will need detailed information on the behaviors that contribute to the issue or problem you have selected as your focus and the determinants or mediators of these behaviors. These worksheets or outlines will help you conduct the assessments to obtain the information you will need.

Think of yourself as a detective as you work through this assignment. You are trying to find out as much as you can in order to determine the core behaviors or behavioral goals that will be the targets for your educational sessions. On the worksheets, indicate the source of each piece of information. Was it from a review of the literature or from existing data? From information in the earlier chapters of this book? A discussion with members of your intended audience? Focus groups with your intended audience? A walk around the neighborhood where the intervention will be conducted?

Use the printed worksheets as outlines. Create a needs assessment document in which you record your findings for the following categories of information. The information may be quite extensive and will vary with category. Record the information and your information sources as shown in the worksheets.

At the end of Worksheets 7-1, 7-2, and 7-3, you should have statements for Steps 1a, 1b, and 1c as follows:

1. Step 1a. *Health or food needs or problems (one or two) and primary intended audience for the nutrition education intervention.* Examples are "overweight in teenagers" or "low rates of breastfeeding in a low-resources audience."
2. Step 1b. *High-priority behaviors or actions that are of concern.* A set of one to three related behaviors or community practices that contribute to the health or food issue(s) that will be the intervention focus of your sessions or program.
3. Step 1c. *Statement of the program's core behavioral or action goals.* The core behavioral or action goals describe the purpose or desired behavioral outcomes for the program.

WORKSHEET 7-1   **Step 1a: Identify Issue or Problem and Primary Group or Intended Audience**

ASSESSMENT INFORMATION *(RECORD FINDINGS ON SEPARATE SHEETS.)*	INFORMATION SOURCES
A. Expert inputs: Science research findings and inputs of food and nutrition experts	Examples:
• *Health issues:* Issues of concern in terms of personal health (e.g., anemia, eating disorders, high serum cholesterol level, heart disease, diabetes, obesity) and populations for whom these are issues	*Review of literature, monitoring data, etc.*
• *Food system issues:* Food practices that contribute to sustainable food systems (e.g., eating locally grown or organic foods, foods with less packaging)	
• *Social issues related to food:* Impacts of food production labor and trade practices on communities and farmers	
Findings:	

B. Societal inputs: National food and nutrition policy goals and documents	*Government policy documents, etc.*
Findings:	

C. Audience inputs: Concerns about and from the intended audience/group	• *National, state, and county data; research studies*
• Epidemiological and empirical data (objective data)	
• Perceptions and desires of intended audience (subjective data)	• *Interviews, surveys*
Findings:	

D. Administrative inputs: Concerns of the agency or organization sponsoring the intervention	• *Organizational or agency documents, mission statements*
• What is the overall mission of the agency?	
• In what way will the program to be designed enhance the overall mission of the agency?	
• What are the agency's expectations about the nutrition education component?	• *Interviews*
Findings:	

Prioritize issues
1. Which of these issues or problems are ranked as regional or national priorities?
2. Which issues, if appropriately addressed, are likely to have the greatest impact on the outcomes desired?
3. Which issues or problems are most amenable to being addressed by educational means?
4. Which issues or problems are considered by the intended audience to be the most important?
5. Which issues or problems are considered priorities by the agency or organization?

Prioritize audience
1. Size of the population for whom the issues are a problem or of concern
2. The severity or incidence of the nutritional conditions or food system situations

Conclusion 1: Priority needs or health or food issues that are of concern, and primary population or audience for whom these are concerns (one or two major issues) and rationale.

WORKSHEET 7-2 **Step 1b: Identify Behaviors or Practices of Intended Audience That Are of Concern and Contribute to the Problems or Issues**

ASSESSMENT INFORMATION	INFORMATION SOURCES
Describe the group's food-related behaviors and practices as they are relevant to the issues and problems identified in Worksheet 7-1. • Intakes of specific foods • Behavioral practices • Eating patterns **Findings:**	*Literature reviews, food frequency questionnaires, food behavior checklists, interviews, etc.*

If applicable: Describe your group's physical activity behaviors. Are they active in their daily lives; if so, how so? Do they engage in formal exercise? If so, how often and what type? Do they like to exercise?
Findings:

Prioritize and Select Behaviors That Will Be the Focus of the Nutrition Education Program

Realize that you will not be able to address, in one program, all the behaviors that could be appropriate for your intended audience with respect to the high-priority issues you have identified. You, or the nutrition education committee, will need to prioritize and select one or two behaviors or sets of behaviors as the target of the intervention. These behaviors will be the focus of the program. This is what is meant by behavior-focused nutrition education.

From everything you have learned so far, write up to five behaviors or practices that your program could potentially address with your audience. These can be related to personal health, food system issues, or societal food concerns.

Here are four criteria you can use, and a rating scale for each. Use these criteria to rate *each* of the behaviors you have selected. In the needs assessment document that you have created, include the accompanying table and enter the information as shown.

CRITERIA	NOT AT ALL		MODERATELY		EXTREMELY
1. How *important* is taking action or changing this behavior or practice or addressing this issue? Base judgments on • Its prevalence in the population • Strength of its contribution to health conditions or to food-related issues	1	2	3	4	5
2. How *changeable or modifiable* is this behavior or practice by educational methods?	1	2	3	4	5
3. How *feasible* is it, in terms of time and resources, to develop a program that will achieve change?	1	2	3	4	5
4. How *desirable* is it to the intended audience to take this action or achieve this target behavior?	1	2	3	4	5

Rate each of the issues or behaviors you have identified, using the scale above.

| | CRITERIA | | | |
BEHAVIORS OR PRACTICES OF CONCERN*	IMPORTANCE (1–5)	MODIFIABILITY (1–5)	FEASIBILITY (1–5)	DESIRABILITY (1–5)
1.				
2.				
3.				
4.				
5.				

* Remember, behaviors are specific, such as the following: low intake of fruits and vegetables, sedentary behaviors, high consumption of sweetened drinks, and no purchases of fresh produce from a farmers' market.

Interpretation of the Behavioral Assessment Data for Designing the Intervention

Now choose one to three of the behaviors or practices of concern you have just listed to become the focus of your sessions or program. We will call these the program-specified or target behaviors or practices for the program. Write a short paragraph to justify why you selected this/these target behavior(s). Be sure to pull in what you found in your assessment and the results of the above table as you justify your choice of target behaviors.

WORKSHEET 7-3   **Step 1c: State the Behavioral Goals of the Sessions or Program**

Programs seek to address the behaviors and practices that are of concern. So state the behavioral goals in positive terms. For example, if the group does not eat enough calcium-rich foods, state your behavioral goal as "to increase the intake of calcium-rich foods." If the group does not breastfeed or only for a short duration, the behavioral goal may the "to increase the rate and duration of breastfeeding in this group." Limit the number of behaviors you can address given the duration and intensity of your program. You are more likely be effective if you focus on a few behaviors or practices and address them thoroughly than to address many superficially.

Step 1c: State the behavioral goals of the sessions or program or the outcomes to be achieved

1.

2.

3.

CASE STUDY 7-1   **Step 1: Identify Focus of the Program: Analyze Needs and Intended Audience, and Identify Behaviors of Concern**

Worksheet 7-1: Step 1a: Identify Issue or Need and Primary Intended Audience
Our organization is a university-affiliated agency that works with children and youth. Thus, the general audience is already determined. However, setting and location are not determined.

ASSESSMENT INFORMATION	INFORMATION SOURCES
A. Expert inputs: Science research findings and food and nutrition experts **Findings:**	Based on review of the literature and monitoring data
Health issues: A key health issue for youth today is overweight prevention.	Surgeon General's Call to Action (DHHS, 2001); other studies
• Overweight has doubled in U.S. children in the past two decades, so that about 14% of 6- to 19-year olds are now estimated to be overweight, and another 14% are "at risk for overweight" (85th to 95th percentile) (Troiano & Flegal, 1998; Ogden et al., 2002; U.S. Department of Health and Human Services [DHHS], 2001).	
• Childhood overweight is a public health concern because it is associated with immediate consequences such as increased cholesterol levels and risk of type 2 diabetes. Risk factors for cardiovascular disease, such as high serum cholesterol levels and high blood pressure, occur with increased frequency in overweight children and adolescents compared with children with a healthy weight (DHHS, 2001). Type 2 diabetes, previously considered an adult disease, has increased dramatically in children and adolescents and is related to body fatness (DHHS, 2001; Gutin et al., 1994). For example, data from the third National Health and Nutrition Examination Survey found that the overall prevalence of metabolic syndrome among adolescents aged 12 to 19 years was 4.2%, but the syndrome was present in 28.7% of overweight adolescents, compared with 6.8% in at-risk adolescents and 0.1% of those with a body mass index (BMI) below the 85th percentile ($p < .001$), suggesting that approximately 910,000 adolescents may have metabolic syndrome (Cook et al., 2003).	
• Childhood overweight is also a public health concern because it is associated with long-term consequences. Overweight adolescents have a 70% chance of becoming overweight or obese adults, who in turn are at risk for a number of health problems, including heart disease, type 2 diabetes, high blood pressure, and some forms of cancer (DHHS, 2001).	
• Costs associated with childhood obesity have risen 263% between 1979 and 1999.	
• Childhood overweight also carries with it immediate social consequences because overweight children often experience rejection by peers, psychological distress, dissatisfaction with their bodies, and low self-esteem (DHHS, 2001).	
• Prevention of weight gain in youth is more effective than weight loss efforts in adulthood. Studies have shown weight loss success rates to be low.	
Ecological and food system issues: Food practices that contribute to sustainable food systems.	
• The food production, processing, and marketing system provides numerous tasty, highly processed, high-fat, high-sugar food products that are also convenient and cheap. Youth could be made aware of less highly processed, locally produced foods and their benefits, and provided skills to access them.	
Social issues related to food: Impacts of food production labor and trade practices on communities and farmers.	
Local mid-sized farms can supply selected foods for school meals programs.	

B. Societal inputs: National food and nutrition policy goals and documents

Government policy documents, etc.

Findings: (Based on review of government policy documents)

Surgeon general's *Call to Action:* The surgeon general and others have called for action to stem this rapid increase in obesity (DHHS, 2001). The *Call to Action* includes the following goals:

- Build awareness among students, teachers, and parent about the contribution of proper nutrition and physical activity to the maintenance of lifelong healthy weight.
- Educate students, teachers, and parents about the importance of body-size acceptance and the dangers of unhealthy weight control practices.
- Provide age-appropriate and culturally sensitive instruction in health education that helps students develop the knowledge, attitudes, skills, and behaviors to adopt, maintain, and enjoy healthy eating habits and a physically active lifestyle.

Many other nongovernmental organizations have stated similar policy goals.

C. Audience inputs: Concerns about and from the intended audience/group

National, state, and county data; research studies

Findings:

Epidemiological and empirical data (objective data): Children in urban settings present a special challenge to the surgeon general's call: a survey of students in New York City (Perez-Pena, 2003), for example, found that 14% to 16 % of white and Asian students were overweight, and about one quarter of black and one third of Hispanic students. There are no specific data for the community served by the organization. However, informal review of city and public health department records suggests the statistics are similar.

In the area of food choice, Contento and Michela (1998) have shown that although preferences are the primary determinants of food choices for young children and remain important for people of all ages, as children become older they become increasingly able to align their food choice behaviors with their goals. By middle school, children are able to integrate motivations and cognitions in a self-regulatory process for a variety of food choice criteria, including not only taste and convenience but also health and weight concern issues. In terms of opportunity, by adolescence children are spending $4 billion per year on foods and snacks for themselves and are receiving an additional $19 billion from their families to spend for family shopping (McNeal, 1992). Thus, middle school youth would be a good audience for an appropriately designed overweight prevention program.

Perceptions and desires of intended audience (subjective data): Interviews with youth in this community indicate that they are interested in being healthy and would welcome nutrition education, but the program has to be interesting, cool, and useful to them *now*—they are busy and have lots of friends and do not want to be lectured about being healthy. Parents are also very concerned; they express that they would like to help, and want to know the best way to do so.

Interviews, surveys

D. Administrative inputs: Concerns of the agency or organization sponsoring the intervention

Agency documents, mission statements
Interviews

Findings: The mission of our university-affiliated organization is to provide health and nutrition services to the pediatric population and their families in the community. The community is ethnically and economically diverse.

Designing an educational program to address overweight prevention in youth would fulfill, and indeed enhance, the mission of the organization. Addressing overweight prevention has been selected by the agency as one of its priority areas for education and service.

It is expected that the nutrition education program would be able to be delivered by existing staff with existing resources.

Prioritize issues and audience

Conclusion 1: Priority health or food issues (one or two major issues), primary population or intended audience, and rationale. *(Record information on separate sheets)*

A number of sources have identified prevention of childhood overweight or weight gain as the most pressing nutritional issue facing youth. Overweight prevention is not only a national priority issue but also one of interest to the local community. The organization has also made the issue one of its priority areas for education and service.

Overweight is an issue for a large segment of the youth population. As has been shown, overweight has severe immediate and long-term consequences.

Worksheet 7-2: Step 1b: Identify Behaviors or Practices of Intended Primary Audience That Contribute to the Issues or Problems

ASSESSMENT INFORMATION	INFORMATION SOURCES
Describe the group's food-related behaviors and practices as they are relevant to the issues and problems identified in Worksheet 7-1.	*Literature reviews; monitoring data*

Findings:

General: Trends in intakes among children aged 6 to 11 years using data from the Nationwide Food Consumption Survey 1977–1978, the Continuing Survey of Food Intakes by Individuals (CSFII) 1994–1996 (Agricultural Research Service [ARS], 2000), and the CSFII 1989–1991 (Enns, Mickle, & Goldman, 2002) show increases in intakes of soft drinks, total grain products, grain mixtures, crackers/popcorn/pretzels/corn chips/, fried potatoes, noncitrus juices/nectars, low-fat milk, skim milk, cheese, candy, and fruit drinks/ades; and decreases in whole milk and total milk, yeast breads and rolls, green beans, corn/green peas/lima beans, beef, pork, and eggs. Intakes of discretionary fat and added sugars were much higher than recommended.

Fruits and vegetables: Surveys show that only 30% of youth are eating the recommended amount of fruit and about 36% are eating the recommended servings of vegetables, which included fried potatoes (Munoz et al., 1997). In their natural state, fruits and vegetables have high water and fiber content, which increase volume, and are low in calories and energy density. Eating fruits and vegetables can contribute a sense of fullness and help people maintain their weight (Centers for Disease Control and Prevention, 2000).

Beverages: Between 1977–1978 and 1994–1996, milk consumption by adolescents aged 12 to19 dropped by a third, and the proportion of those drinking carbonated soft drinks increased by 52% (Borrud, Enns, & Mickle, 1997; Guthrie & Morton, 2000). Adolescents aged 12 to 17 get, on average, 11% of all their calories from carbonated beverages, fruit-flavored and part-juice drinks, and sports drinks; they consume, on average, 15 teaspoons of sugar per day from these drinks, or 48% of their total intake of refined sugar (ARS, 2000). High intakes of added sweeteners make it difficult for all but the most active people to maintain their weight. Ludwig, Peterson, and Gortmaker (2001) show that consumption of sugar-sweetened beverages is an independent risk factor for obesity in children aged 11 to 12 years. For every additional serving of sugar-sweetened drink consumed, the odds of becoming obese increase by 60%. Another study links soft drink consumption to excess energy intake and weight gain among adolescents. (Harnack, Stang, & Story, 1999). Carbonated beverages may also contribute to increased bone fractures (Wyshak, 2000).

Fast food meals away from home: From 1977 to 1996, consumption of home meals dropped from 83% to 70%, and snacks away from home increased from 13% to 20%. In the CSFII surveys of 1994–1996 and 1998, 42% of children had eaten at fast food restaurants on the two days of the survey. Those who ate there had higher intakes of calories, fat, saturated fat, sodium, and carbonated soft drinks, and lower intakes of vitamins A and C, milk, and fruits and vegetables (Paeratakul et al., 2003).

Portion sizes: Portion sizes of foods served in a variety of settings have increased, and these increases are related to the increased prevalence of overweight and obesity (Young & Nestle, 2003; Nielsen & Popkin, 2003).

Specifics on intended audience These students eat on average only two servings of fruits and vegetables each day—mostly fruits. They drink two 12-ounce bottles of sugar-sweetened beverages each day; they eat packaged sweet and salty snacks every day, such as cookies, baked goods, or potato chips, averaging three 150-calorie packages a day; and they eat at fast food places four times a week.	*Food behavior checklists; interviews*

If applicable: Describe your group's physical activity behaviors.   *Survey data; research studies*

Findings:

Increased sedentary activity

According to the Kaiser Family Foundation (1999), 6% of households had three or more TVs in the home in 1970; this figure increased to 60% in 1999. In 1970, 6% of sixth graders had TVs in their bedroom; this figure increased to 77% in 1999.

Young people aged 2 to 18 spend on average over 4 hours per day watching television or videotapes, playing video games, or using a computer. Most of the time is TV viewing, with 2 hours 46 minutes of TV per day. One third of children and adolescents watch TV more than 3 hours a day, and nearly one fifth (17%) watch more than 5 hours of TV daily.

Watching TV and using computers increase the odds of being overweight by 4.5 times if an individual watches more than five hours of TV daily (Gortmaker et al., 1996). Time watching TV correlated with children's requests for and parent's purchase of foods shown on TV, as well as overall intake (Taras et al., 1989).

Decreased physical education in schools   *Survey data*

Only a handful of states require daily physical education (PE) for all students. In a span of eight years (1991–1999), PE participation dropped from 42% to 29%. Walking and bicycling by children aged 5 to 15 dropped 40% between 1977 and 1995. More than one in three students (35%) do not participate regularly in vigorous physical activity. Regular participation in vigorous activity drops from 73% of ninth graders to 61% of twelfth-grade students. Almost half (45%) do not play on any sports teams during the year. Nearly half (44%) are not even enrolled in a physical education class; enrollment in PE drops from 79% in ninth grade to 37% in twelfth grade (DHHS, 2001).

Specifics on intended audience   *Interviews, survey*

Students all live close to school and thus walk to school (a few blocks). But they do not walk much otherwise. Some go to the park and play basketball with friends. They watch TV about two to three hours a day. Those who have computers at home average an hour each day, and play video games as well as doing homework.

Rate each of the issues or behaviors you have identified, using a scale of 1 (not important) to 5 (extremely important).

	CRITERIA			
BEHAVIORS OR PRACTICES OF CONCERN	**IMPORTANCE** **(1–5)**	**MODIFIABILITY** **(1–5)**	**FEASIBILITY** **(1–5)**	**DESIRABILITY** **(1–5)**
1. Eating too few fruits and vegetables	5	5	4	3
2. Drinking too many sweetened drinks	5	4	5	2
3. Eating too many high-fat, high-sugar, highly processed snacks	5	4	5	3
4. Eating out at fast-food restaurants	5	4	4	3
5. Sedentary behavior	5	4	5	3

Interpretation of the Behavioral Assessment Data for Designing the Intervention

Now choose one to three of the behaviors or practices you listed previously to become the focus of your sessions or program. We will call these the target behaviors or practices for the program. Write a short paragraph to justify why you selected this/these target behavior(s).

Four of the previously determined behaviors that contribute to childhood overweight will be addressed by this program:

1. Insufficient intake of fruits and vegetables
2. High consumption of sweetened beverages each day
3. Large number of high-fat, high-sugar snacks
4. Lack of physical activity

These behaviors are the highest priority in terms of importance, modifiability, and feasibility. Youth expressed interest in a nutrition education program that would address issues that were pressing for them and was not based on lecturing about health in general. Addressing these specific behaviors would fit that criterion. The rationales for these behaviors have been adequately given earlier. High frequency of eating at fast food restaurants is also of high concern. However, one nutrition education program cannot address so many behaviors. Therefore, the four behaviors listed above are chosen as feasible for this program. A school-based program is selected as most appropriate.

Worksheet 7-3: Step 1c: State the Behavioral Goals of the Sessions or Program

The title of the program will be "Taking Control: Eating Well and Being Fit"
The behavioral goals of the program are for youth to
1. Increase intake of fruits and vegetables (youth to aim for 2.5 cups or more a day)
2. Decrease amount of sweetened beverages consumed each day (aim for no more than 8 ounces a day)
3. Decrease number of packaged high-fat, high-sugar snacks so that they contribute no more than 150 calories a day (targets for drinks and snacks are based on the discretionary calories allowance for this age group)
4. Increase physical activity to 10,000 steps a day and participate actively, when possible, in gym or other school-sponsored physical activities

Assessment Instrument for "Taking Control: Eating Well and Being Fit"

We are developing a program about food and physical activity for youth like you. We would really like your help by telling us what interests you, what you do, and some of your opinions about food and physical activity. So we ask you to participate in taking this survey. You are not required to answer all of the questions, but complete questionnaires will be greatly appreciated. In order to respect your privacy and anonymity, please do not write your name on the questionnaire. Please feel free to ask if you have any questions. We thank you in advance for your participation.

Questions 1 to 5 are designed to provide us with information regarding your typical or usual eating pattern. For each meal, please indicate if it was prepared at home or was purchased outside of the home. If the meal was purchased outside the home, please mention the brand name of the restaurant from which you purchased the food.

1. Do you usually eat breakfast? Please circle YES or NO. If yes, what does it usually consist of?

2. Do you usually eat lunch? Please circle YES or NO. If yes, what does it usually consist of?

3. Do you usually eat dinner? Please circle YES or NO. If yes, what does it usually consist of?

4. Do you usually eat snacks? Please circle YES or NO. If yes, please indicate how many snacks each day and what these snacks usually consist of.

   Home-made snacks: How many each day? _____ What _____

   Prepackaged snacks (such as cookies, donuts, sweet baked goods, potato or corn chips, etc): How many each day? _____

   What _____

5. If you eat prepackaged snacks, why? _____

6. What is your favorite food?

7. What is your least favorite food?

8. How many days a week do you eat at fast food restaurants (e.g., McDonald's, Burger King, Popeye, KFC) _____

9. If you typically eat at fast food restaurants, circle the reasons that most apply.

   a. It is less expensive than preparing food at home.

   b. It is faster than preparing food or a snack at home.

   c. It tastes better than home-cooked meals.

   d. It is convenient—right near the school and/or my house.

   e. I like to go with my friends after school.

10. How many days each week do you drink regular soda or other sugar-sweetened beverages? _____

How much do you typically drink each time? _____12 or less ounces;

_____13–20 ounces; 20–39 ounces; _____more than 40 ounces (two large 20-oz bottles)

11. Do you eat fresh fruits and vegetables on a daily basis? Please circle YES or NO.

If yes, how many servings a day? _____ Fruits; _____ Vegetables

12. How many servings of fruits and vegetables do you think we should be eating each day?

_____

13. Do you like to try new kinds of fruits and vegetables?

Definitely like___; somewhat like ___; somewhat don't like ___; definitely don't like ____

Why? _____

14. If you typically do not eat a lot of fruits and vegetables, circle the reasons that most apply.

a. Lack of time.

b. Fresh fruits and vegetables are not available in my grocery store.

c. Fresh fruits and vegetables are too expensive.

d. Fresh fruits do not taste good.

e. Fresh vegetables do not taste good.

f. It takes too much effort to prepare fruits and vegetables.

g. Fruits and vegetables go bad quickly.

h. My friends do not eat fruits and vegetables.

15. Circle the diseases that members of your family have.

a. Diabetes

b. Heart disease

c. Obesity

d. High blood pressure

e. Cancer

f. Macular degeneration (eyes cannot see well in the middle of the view)

16. How concerned are you that you might develop one of these diseases?

     _____Not at all concerned; _____Somewhat concerned; _____Very concerned

17. What you think are features of a healthy diet?

18. Based on your description of a healthy diet, do you think you eat healthfully?

     _____ Not very healthy; _____ Somewhat healthy; _____Very healthy

     Why?_____

19. How important to you is it to eat healthfully?

     _____ Not very important; _____ Somewhat important; _____Very important

     Why?_____

20. How confident are you that if you wanted to, you could prepare your favorite *home-made*

     Snack: _____Not very confident; _____ Somewhat confident; _____Very confident

     Why?_____

     Meal: _____ Not very confident; _____ Somewhat confident; _____Very confident

     Why?_____

21. On average, how many city blocks do you walk in a day? _____

22. If you watch television, on average, how many hours do you sit and watch on a typical workday? _____

     Weekend day?_____

23. What are your favorite shows or commercials? _____

24. Do you currently make a point to exercise on a daily or weekly basis outside of school gym? Please circle YES or NO.

     If yes, what do you do for exercise? _____

     How many times a week? _____

     If no, circle the reasons that most apply:

     a. Lack of time

     b. No access to fitness facilities

     c. Lack of desire

     d. Other _____

25. Any other comments: _____

Once again, thank you for your time.

REFERENCES

Agricultural Research Service, U.S. Department of Agriculture. 2000. *Continuing survey of food intakes by individuals 1994–1996 (CSFII 1994–1996)*. Washington, DC: Author.

Block, G., C. Gillespie, E.H. Rosenbaum, and C. Jenson. 2000. A rapid food screener to assess fat and fruit and vegetable intake. *American Journal of Preventive Medicine* 18:284–288.

Block, G., F.E. Thompson, A.M. Hartman, F.A. Larkin, and K.E. Guire. 1992. Comparison of two dietary questionnaires validated against multiple dietary records collected during a 1-year period. *Journal of the American Dietetic Association* 92:686–693.

Bogers R.P., J. Brug, P. van Assema, and P.C. Dagnelie. 2004. Explaining fruit and vegetable consumption: the theory of planned behavior and misconception of personal intake levels. Appetite 42: 157-166.

Borrud, L., C.W. Enns, and S. Mickle. 1997, April. What we eat: USDA surveys food consumption changes. *Community Nutrition Instruction* 18:4–5.

Centers for Disease Control and Prevention. 2000. *Can eating fruits and vegetables help people to manage their weight?* (Research to Practice Series, No. 1). Washington, DC: Author.

Contento, I.R., and J.L. Michela. 1998. Nutrition and food choice behavior among children and adolescents. In *Handbook of pediatric and adolescent health psychology*. Boston: Allyn and Bacon.

Contento, I.R., J.S. Randell, and C.E. Basch. 2002. Review and analysis evaluation measures used in nutrition education intervention research. Journal of Nutrition Education and Behavior 34:2-25.

Cook, S., M. Weitzman, P. Auinger, M. Nguyen, and W. Dietz. 2003. Prevalence of a metabolic syndrome phenotype in adolescents: Findings from the third National Health and Nutrition Examination Survey, 1988–1994. *Archives of Pediatric and Adolescent Medicine* 157:821–827.

Enns, C.W, S.J. Mickle, and J.D. Goldman. 2002. Trends in food and nutrient intakes by children in the United States. *Family Economics and Nutrition Review* 14:56–68.

Gortmaker, S.L., A. Must, A.M. Sobol, K. Peterson, G.A. Colditz, and W.H. Dietz. 1996. Television viewing as a cause of increasing obesity among children in the United States, 1986–1990. *Archives of Pediatric and Adolescent Medicine* 150:356–362.

Green, L.W., and M.M. Kreuter. 1999. *Health promotion planning: An educational and ecological approach*. 3rd ed. Mountain View, CA: Mayfield Publishing.

Guthrie, J.F., and J.F. Morton. 2000. Food sources of added sweeteners in the diets of Americans. *Journal of the American Dietetic Association* 100(43):48–51.

Gutin, B., S. Islam, T. Manos, N. Cucuzzo, C. Smith, and M.E. Stachura. 1994. Relation of percentage of body fat and maximal aerobic capacity to risk factors for atherosclerosis and diabetes in black and white seven- to eleven-year-old children. 125(6 Pt .1) *Journal of Pediatrics*: 847–852.

Harnak, L., J. Stang, and M. Story. 1999. Soft drink consumption among US children and adolescents: Nutritional consequences. *Journal of the American Dietetic Association* 99:436–441.

Hersey, J., J. Anliker, C. Miller, R.M. Mullis, et al. 2001. Food shopping practices are associated with dietary quality in low-income households. *Journal of Nutrition Education and Behavior* 33:S16–S26.

Kaiser Family Foundation. 1999. *Kids and media @ the new millennium*. Menlo Park, CA: Kaiser Family Foundation.

Ludwig, D.S., K.E. Peterson, and S.L. Gortmaker. 2001. Relation between consumption of sugar-sweetened drinks and childhood obesity: A prospective, observational analysis. *Lancet* 357:505–508.

McClelland, J.W., D.P. Keenan, J. Lewis, et al. 2001. Review of evaluation tools used to assess the impact of nutrition education on dietary intake and quality, weight management practices, and physical activity of low-income audiences. *Journal of Nutrition Education* 33:S35–S48.

McNeal, J.U. 1992. *Kids as customers: A handbook of marketing to children*. New York: Lexington Books.

McPherson, R.C., D.M. Hoelscher, M. Alexander, K.S. Scanlon, and M.K. Serdula. 2000. Dietary assessment methods among school-aged children. *Preventive Medicine* 31: S11–S33.

Medeiros, L., V. Hillers, P. Kendall, and A. Mason. 2001. Evaluation of food safety education for consumers. *Journal of Nutrition Education* 33:S27–S34.

Munoz, K.A., S.M. Krebs-Smith, R. Ballard-Barbash, et al. 1997. Food intakes of US children and adolescents compared with recommendations. *Pediatrics* 100:323–329.

Nielsen, S.J., and B.M. Popkin. 2003. Patterns and trends in food portion sizes, 1977–1998. *Journal of the American Medical Association* 289(4):450–453.

Ogden, C.L., K.M. Flegal, M.D. Carroll, and C.L. Johnson. 2002. Prevalence and trends in overweight among US children and adolescents, 1999–2000. *Journal of the American Medical Association* 288:1728–1732.

Paeratakul, S., D.P. Ferdinand, C.M. Champagne, D.H. Ryan, and G.A. Bray. 2003. Fast-food consumption among US adults and children: Dietary and nutrient intake profile. *Journal of the American Dietetic Association* 103:1322–1338.

Parham, E. 1990. Applying a philosophy of nutrition education to weight control. *Journal of Nutrition Education* 22:194–197.

Perez-Pena, R. 2003, July 9. Obesity on the rise in New York public schools. *New York Times.*

Rogers, E.M. 1995. *Diffusion of innovations.* 4th ed. New York: Free Press.

Rogers, E.M., and F.F. Shoemaker. 1971. *Communication of innovations: A cross-cultural approach.* New York: Free Press.

Shannon, J., A.R. Kristal, S.J. Curry, and S.A. Beresford. 1997. Application of a behavioral approach to measuring dietary change: The fat and fiber-related diet behavior questionnaire. *Cancer Epidemiology, Biomarkers and Prevention* 6:355–361.

Taras, H.L., J.F. Sallis, T.L. Patterson, P.R. Nader, and J.A. Nelson. 1989. Television's influence on children's diet and physical activity. *Journal of Developmental and Behavioral Pediatrics* 10(4):176–179.

Thompson, F.E., and T. Byers. 1994. Dietary assessment resource manual. *Journal of Nutrition* 124(11 Suppl.):2245S–2317S.

Townsend, M.S., L.L. Kaiser, L.H. Allen, A. Block Joy, and S.P. Murphy. 2003. Selecting items for a food behavior checklist for a limited-resources audience. *Journal of Nutrition Education and Behavior* 35:69–82.

Troiano, R.P., and K.M. Flegal. 1998. Overweight children and adolescents: Description, epidemiology, and demographics. *Pediatrics* 101:497–504.

U.S. Department of Health and Human Services. 2001. *Surgeon general's call to action to prevent and decrease overweight and obesity.* Washington, DC: Author.

Whitehead, F. 1973. Nutrition education research. *World Review of Nutrition and Dietetics* 17:91–149.

Willett, W.C., R.D. Reynolds, S. Cottrell-Hoehner, L. Sampson, and M.L. Browne. 1987. Validation of a semi-quantitative food frequency questionnaire: comparison with a 1-year diet record. *Journal of the American Dietetic Association* 87:43–47.

Wright, M., M.R. Horner, and L.H. Charini. 1982. Approaches for increasing soybean use by low-income Brazilian families. *Journal of Nutrition Education* 14(3):105–107.

Wyshak, G. 2000. Teenaged girls, carbonated beverage consumption, and bone fractures. *Archives of Pediatric and Adolescent Medicine* 154:610–613.

Yaroch, A.L., K. Resnicow, and L.K. Khan. 2000. Validity and reliability of qualitative dietary fat index questionnaires: A review. *Journal of the American Dietetic Association* 100(2):240–244.

Young, L.R., and M. Nestle. 2003. Expanding portion sizes in the US marketplace: Implications for nutrition counseling. *Journal of the American Dietetic Association* 103(2):231–234.

Step 2: Identify Potential Mediators of Program Behaviors and Actions

OVERVIEW This chapter describes how to use theory and research to identify personal psychosocial determinants and environmental factors that are potential mediators of the actions or behavior changes targeted by the program.

OBJECTIVES At the end of the chapter, you will be able to

- Appreciate the importance of thoroughly understanding the intended audience
- Develop skills in identifying the personal psychosocial factors that are potential mediators of the program's targeted core behaviors, as well as the environmental factors that impede or facilitate these behaviors for this audience
- Compare the advantages and disadvantages of different methods for obtaining the assessment information

SCENARIO

A nutrition educator in a Women, Infants and Children clinic wanted to plan several sessions on breastfeeding. She had decided on a discussion of the nutritional advantages of breastfeeding followed by a demonstration of how to do it when she realized that she should first survey the participating pregnant women regarding what they already knew about breastfeeding versus bottle-feeding and regarding what might motivate them to breastfeed. She based her survey on the theory of planned behavior. She was surprised to discover that the greatest barriers to breast-feeding as perceived by the pregnant women were their embarrassment about doing it (social norm) and their concern about its effect on their breasts (attitudes). They were already quite knowledgeable about the nutritional and medical advantages of breastfeeding and knew how to do it. The nutrition educator then changed her plans entirely to direct the learning experiences at these concerns.

Introduction: Identifying the Potential Mediators of the Target Behaviors

We have seen that the procedural model for designing theory-based nutrition education provides a systematic way to design nutrition education. In Step 1 we identified the health-promoting actions or behavior changes that the program should aim for, our *program behaviors* or *target behaviors,* such as increased consumption of calcium-rich foods or increased healthy snacks for children. These represent the behavioral goals or desired outcomes for the program.

Now in Step 2 of the process, we identify the determinants of behavior that can potentially mediate the actions or behavior changes that are the focus of the intervention. Step 2 is highlighted in the design model. A worksheet is provided at the end of the chapter for you to use as you proceed through this chapter. The case study is continued.

A Procedural Model For Designing Theory-Based Nutrition Education

INPUTS: COLLECTING ASSESSMENT DATA		DESIGNING THE OUTPUTS			DESIGNING OUTCOMES EVALUATION
STEP 1 ←——→ **Analyze needs and behaviors: Specify the behavior or action focus of the program** • Assess needs and identify audience: select need(s) or issue(s) to address • Identify behaviors of concern that contribute to need(s) or issue(s) • Select core behaviors or practices to address	**STEP 2** ←——→ **Identify relevant potential mediators of program behaviors** • Identify potential personal psychosocial mediators • Identify potential environmental mediators	**STEP 3** ←——→ **Select theory, philosophy, and components** • Select theory and/or create appropriate model • Articulate educational philosophy • Clarify perspectives on content • Determine program components	**STEP 4** ←——→ **State educational objectives for potential mediators** • Select relevant mediators to address • State educational objectives for each selected mediator: —Personal psychosocial mediators —Environmental mediators	**STEP 5** ←——→ **Design theory-based educational strategies and activities to address potential mediators** • Design strategies and activities for each selected mediator: —Personal psychosocial mediators —Environmental mediators	**STEP 6** **Design evaluation** • Design evaluation of program's impact on behaviors and mediators • Design process evaluation

The theory and research presented in the conceptual framework discussed in the first part of the book indicate that potential mediators of behavior change can be placed into two major categories: person-related psychosocial mediators (often referred to as individual-level mediators) and environment-related factors. These potential personal and environmental mediators are the primary targets of nutrition education. Theory provides guidance as to which mediators of behavior to assess. This is important because the specific personal and environmental mediators that you identify will become the primary targets of the educational strategies and learning experiences that you will design. Theory can thus provide an important and efficient framework for conducting the needs analysis, just as it does for conducting the nutrition education intervention itself. Knowledge of theory will enable you to conduct a more thorough, accurate, and complete analysis.

If you have identified more than one behavior, practice, or issue, the potential mediators of each of these may have to be assessed separately. For example, there is evidence that the motivations and barriers may be different for actions involving *adding* foods to the diet (such as fruits and vegetables) compared with those of *reducing* the amount in the diet, such as eating fewer high-fat foods or drinking fewer sodas. The kinds of mediators may also differ between food-related behaviors and physical activity behaviors. Thus, the determinants that may mediate behaviors may be quite different for each of the following target behaviors if they are chosen: eating more fruits and vegetables, drinking fewer sodas, and reducing sedentary behaviors. Clearly, limiting the number of behaviors or practices to address makes the nutrition educa-

tion sessions or program easier to conduct and more likely to be effective.

Step 2a: Identify the Potential Person-Related Mediators of the Target Behaviors

It is important to ask the intended audience about determinants of their *current* behavior as well as about *potential* motivators, barriers, and skills needed to adopt the targeted behaviors. Social marketing places a high priority on this component of assessment, calling it *formative research*. The answers will be crucial for determining educational objectives in Step 3 and for designing educational strategies in Step 4. Record your answers in Worksheet 8-1 at the end of the chapter.

We saw in earlier chapters that theories and research evidence to date suggest that behavior change can be seen as occurring in two phases: a motivational, pre-action phase, where the emphasis is on beliefs and feelings, and an action phase, where the emphasis is on knowledge and skills. Some mediating determinants are more important in each phase. In the following we discuss in greater detail how to find out more about the intended audience's perceptions of their interest, motivations, and skills.

Identify Potential Mediators Relevant to Decision Making and Motivation to Act

Understanding the interests, motivations, cultural values, and concerns of a given audience is very challenging because individuals' food and physical activity behaviors involve many complex, and often conflicting, beliefs and emotions that are embedded in many aspects of their life histories and current life situations. But understand these we must if we are to design learning experiences that are meaningful and useful to the intended audience. Our questions should help us understand the audience's perceptions about what's in it for them (or their families or community) if they take action or change. The questions should also help us understand the group's stage of motivational readiness to take action.

Where then to begin? What shall we ask about? This is where theory and prior research can be of assistance: they provide a framework for asking questions. You might want to consider assessing some or all of the items in the following lists, depending on which theory you use to structure the intervention. If you have already chosen an existing theory or have created an intervention model based on theory and evidence, then you need to assess only those mediators or constructs that are part of your model. If you are not yet sure which model will be appropriate, then you should collect the information on a variety of mediators of behavior or theory constructs such as those listed here. Information on them will be usable for whatever model you will create for the intervention. Ask about determinants of the audience's cur-

rent behaviors as well as about potential motivators to take action. Table 8-1 is an example of an instrument to assess determinants that are potential mediators of behavior change. It has been validated for use with low-income audiences and assesses motivational readiness to take action as well as various mediators. Table 8-2 is an example of an instrument that was used with children. Table 8-3 is an example of an instrument to measure self-efficacy in relation to fat intake of low-income women.

- *Motivating factors or determinants of current behavior of concern.* What are some factors motivating your intended audience to engage in their current practices? For example, if they eat very few fruits and vegetables, ask them what they see as the consequences of this behavior; ask them about their attitudes, values, social norms, emotions, self-perceptions, or self-efficacy that result in their current eating patterns. Do they see their current behaviors as a risk or threat?
- *Potential motivating factors.* What do they think will help them become more interested in or willing to take

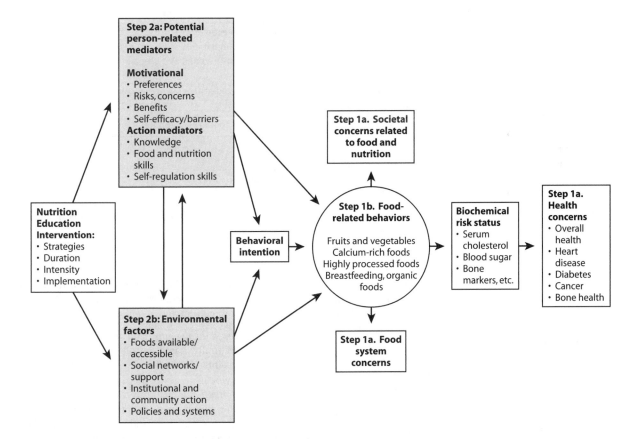

FIGURE 8-1 Step 2. Identifying determinants of behavior or practices that may mediate dietary change.

TABLE 8-1 Tool to Assess Psychosocial Indicators of Fruit and Vegetables Intake in Limited-Resources Audiences

Mediator/Theory Construct	Items
Perceived benefits[a]	I feel that I am helping my body by eating more fruits and vegetables.
	I may develop health problems if I do not eat fruits and vegetables.
Perceived barriers	I feel that fruit is too expensive.
	I feel that fruit is not always available.
	I feel that fruit is time-consuming to prepare.
	I feel that fruit is not liked by my family.
	I feel that fruit is not tasty.
	(Similar items for vegetables)
Perceived control[a]	In your household, who is in charge of what foods to buy?
	In your household, who is in charge of how to prepare the food?
Self-efficacy[a]	I feel that I can plan meals or snacks with more fruit during the next week.
	I feel that I can eat fruits or vegetables as snacks.
	I feel that I can add extra vegetables to casseroles and stews.
	I can eat two or more servings of vegetables at dinner.
Social support[b]	Are there other people encouraging you to buy, prepare, and eat fruits and vegetables?
	My children, partner, mother, father, other
Perceived norms[a]	People in my family think I should eat more fruits and vegetables.
	My doctor (or WIC nutritionist) tells me to eat more fruits and vegetables.
Intention: readiness to eat more fruits and vegetables[c]	I am not thinking about eating more fruit (coded as 1; precontemplation).
	I am thinking about eating more fruit (coded as 2; contemplation).
	I am definitely planning to eat more fruit in the next month (coded as 3; preparation).
	I am trying to eat more fruit now (coded as 4; action).
	I am already eating two or more servings of fruit a day (coded as 5; maintenance).
	(Similar items for vegetables)
Diet quality	How would you describe your diet? (5-point scale: Very poor to very good)

Only selected items of this assessment tool are shown.

[a] Scores of 1 to 3 range from disagree (1), neither agree or disagree (2) to agree (5).

[b] Instructions to client: "Check as many as apply." Coding: no = 0= no support; yes = 1 =support by one person; yes = 2 = support by > 2 persons.

[c] Instructions to client: "Check one."

Source: Townsend, M.S., and L.L. Kaiser. 2005. Development of a tool to assess psychosocial indicators of fruit and vegetables intake for two federal programs. *Journal of Nutrition Education and Behavior* 37:170–184. Used with permission of the Society for Nutrition Education.

action? Would increasing their awareness of actual risk or vulnerability be useful? What are their values in relation to making a dietary change? What are their attitudes to the recommended behavior? What would motivate them to change? What do they see as the barriers to healthful behaviors, and how could you decrease these barriers and help them see increased benefits to healthful actions? Do they feel self-efficacious in regard to taking action on the targeted food-related health behaviors? Also, remember that all behavior occurs within a cultural context, so try to understand cultural influences on behavior.

Here is a list of potential motivation-related mediators of behavior change or health actions to assess (be sure to include perceptions of both current and potential motivators):

- *Culture-specific health and food beliefs.* What are the specific culturally based beliefs that will influence whether the intended audience will engage in the identified behaviors?
- *Stage of motivational readiness to take action.* At what stage are they with respect to motivational readiness to take action—pre-action or ready to take action? More specifically, are they in the precontemplation, contemplation, preparation, action, or maintenance stage?

TABLE 8-2 Assessing Mediating Variables in a School-Based Nutrition Education Program for Fourth Graders and Their Parents, Designed to Increase Fruit and Vegetable Consumption

Mediator/Theory Construct	Items
Positive outcome expectancies	Children respond using a 3-point scale ranging from *disagree* to *agree*. I will have healthier skin if I eat fruits and vegetables. I will be better at sports if I eat fruits and vegetables. I will get sick more often if I do not eat fruits and vegetables. Eating fruits and vegetables will keep me from getting cavities.
Self-efficacy	Children respond using a 3-point scale ranging from *not sure* to *very sure*. I can eat fruits I like (such as bananas or raisins) at breakfast. I can eat fruits I like (such as applesauce or fruit cocktail) at lunch. I can eat vegetables I like (such as salad) at lunch. I can eat vegetables I like (such as corn or beans) at dinner. I can snack on fruits I like (such as grapes or bananas) instead of on foods like cake or cookies. I can snack on vegetables I like (such as carrot or celery sticks) instead of foods like potato or corn chips. I can ask my mom or dad to buy fruits for snacks. I can help my mom or dad fix a fruit or vegetables snack. I can eat at least five servings of fruit and vegetables each day.

Norms
  Family norms
 	
  Peer norms
  Teacher norms
	
	Most people in my family think that eating five servings of fruit and vegetables each day is a good thing for me to do.
	Most kids my age think that eating five servings of fruit and vegetables each day is a good thing to do.
	My teacher will be proud of me if I eat five servings of fruit and vegetables each day.

Knowledge	Children answered using true/false and multiple choice responses. Eating ¼ cup of dried fruit (like raisins) counts as a *whole* serving. How many servings of fruits and vegetables do you think a person should eat *each day* for good health? Which of these would be the best example of a short-term goal to help you begin to eat more fruits and vegetables? Which of the following would be the best way to add a serving of fruit or vegetables to your meal at a fast food restaurant?
Availability	Parents indicate whether a list of 22 fruits and vegetables are present in the home.
Eating meals together	How often do all the people in your home sit down together to eat a meal?
Parent consumption	Parents report quantity and frequency of eating a list of fruits and vegetables.

Only selected items of this assessment tool are shown.

Source: Reynolds, K.D., A.L. Yaroch, F.A. Franklin, and J. Maloy. 2002. Testing mediating variables in a school-based nutrition intervention program. *Health Psychology* 21:51–60. Used with permission of the American Psychological Society and the authors.

- *Attitudes.* What are the intended audience's attitudes toward (1) the health problem or other issue of concern (e.g., cardiovascular health), (2) behaviors that contribute to the nutritional problem, such as excess consumption of high-fat foods, and (3) the behaviors that may be advocated by the program as a solution to the problem (e.g., increased intake of foods low in fat)? Attitudes depend on beliefs and outcome expectations (see the next two items in this list).

- *Beliefs or risk perceptions.* What are their beliefs regarding the severity of the nutritional or food-related problem identified and their perception of their personal vulnerability to it? For example, how likely do they think it is that they will develop heart disease?
- *Outcome expectations.* What expectations do participants have about how certain behaviors relate to the condition? For example, do they believe that eating dark green vegetables will improve their health and well-being and/or

reduce risk of cancer or macular degeneration? To what extent do they value the outcomes of the behavior (e.g., overall health, or decreased risk of blindness)?

TABLE 8-3 A Self-Efficacy Measure for Fat Intake Behaviors of Low-Income Women

Item	Domain
I can stick to low-fat foods on a regular basis . . .	
When nervous	Negative
When angry	affect/feelings
When upset about events in my life	
When happy	Positive
At a party	affect/feelings
When eating out at a restaurant with others	
When lots of high-fat foods are available	Availability
When someone offers me high-fat foods	

Source: Chang, M.W., S. Nitzke, R.L. Brown, L.C. Baumann, and L. Oakley. 2003. Development and validation of a self-efficacy measure for fat intake behaviors of low-income women. *Journal of Nutrition Education and Behavior* 35:302–307. Used with permission of the Society for Nutrition Education.

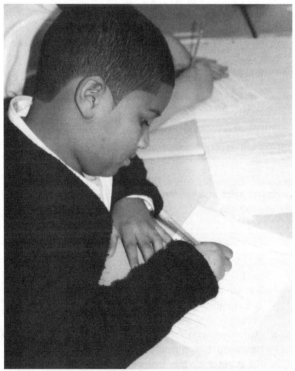

Questionnaires provide an excellent window into motivations and barriers for nutritious eating.

- *Barriers.* What barriers do the intended audience see for engaging in the behavior? What costs? In social marketing language, what must they exchange or sacrifice for the benefits they will experience?
- *Values.* What state of affairs is considered to be of worth or desirable? Examples are being a vegetarian for health, ecological, or religious reasons or eating whatever one is served so as not to waste food and resources. What values do the intended audience have that might influence whether they will consider taking action on the needs or issues identified?
- *Food preferences and enjoyment (sensory-affective factors related to food).* What are the participants' food preferences, likes, and dislikes? We know that taste is one of the most important mediators of food choices. How do they judge the recommended behavior in terms of foods they will eat? Will these foods be enjoyable? Satisfying? Filling?
- *Feelings or affect.* What feelings do they anticipate they will have about engaging in the targeted behavior? Will they have anticipated regret about not taking action?
- *Social norms or felt group pressure.* Do participants believe that their culture or specific individuals or groups important to them think they should or should not perform a particular behavior (either their current behavior or one recommended in the educational intervention to solve the nutritional problem identified)? How much are they motivated to comply with these expectations of how they should behave?
- *Roles.* What are participants' conceptions of behaviors that are appropriate or desirable for people holding their particular position in their group or society? For example, what is the perception a group of women have about whether women in their station in life should breastfeed or bottle-feed?
- *Cultural and ethnic identities.* What are participants' ethnic and cultural identities? If they are immigrants, what is their degree of acculturation? It has been found that degree of acculturation is a better gauge of attitudes and practices in terms of diet than length of stay (Lion & Contento, 2001).
- *Self-identities.* What are their self-identities? For example, do they see themselves as health-conscious consumers, "green" consumers, vegetarians, or other identities?
- *Personal sense of control or agency or perceived behavioral control.* To what extent do participants believe that they have some control over their behaviors, their health, and their environment?
- *Perceived self-efficacy.* What are the participants' perceptions of their ability to carry out desirable health actions? For example, although participants may believe that eating fewer rich desserts will lead to the weight loss they desire, they may not feel confident that they can resist eating rich desserts.

- *Life stage and life trajectories.* What life stage are they in at this time? How does that influence their perceptions and behaviors? What previous life experiences, life trajectories, or life stage considerations are important to them at this point?
- *Media messages.* What are the media they watch? What media images are important to them?
- *Others.*

Information on the motivations of the target group is vital for effective nutrition education. Such information will be important for developing sessions, programs, and media campaigns to assist the intended audience to understand and appreciate why to take action. However, such information may not be enough to plan a successful program. Participants must have access to both the resources and the skills needed to carry out the advocated behaviors. Determining whether they do is the next step.

Identify Potential Mediators That Facilitate Action or Behavior Change: Behavioral Capabilities and Self-Regulation Skills

Behavioral capabilities are the food- and nutrition-specific knowledge and cognitive, affective, and behavioral skills that people need in order to be able to act on their motivations to eat healthfully. For example, during earlier decades in the United States, many people thought that eating large quantities of red meat was vital to getting enough protein in the diet. They were motivated to eat healthfully, but their knowledge about what constitutes healthful eating was not correct. Thus, before conducting an educational intervention, we must find out what the intended audience already knows about the selected health or food system issues. This is also the time to probe for misconceptions they may have. In addition, do the participants have the necessary nutrition information and food-related skills to act upon their motivations? For example, do they have the skills to prepare or cook targeted foods in a way that is more healthful and at the same time results in something they will enjoy eating? It is important to find out their perceptions: what skills do *they* think they will need in order to take action?

What self-regulation skills do they currently have to take control of their behaviors, such as goal-setting and self-monitoring skills? Do they have the skills to refuse offers of food items that they deem inappropriate or not healthful, or the emotion-coping skills to handle stress more appropriately so as not to use food as a stress reducer? What are the reward structures for people's behaviors? In what stage of change are most members of the intended audience? Do they have the group organizing skills needed so that they can work with others in the community to develop collective efficacy to change the food environment or gain access to food?

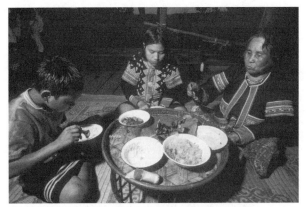

Cultural identity and acculturation are factors in food choices.

As you can see, it is important to ask the intended audience not only about *current* barriers and skills but also about *potential* skills they think they will need to overcome barriers and enact the targeted behaviors. For example, if they are currently not eating enough fruits and vegetables a day, ask them whether they know how to cook vegetables or prepare fruits as snacks, and also what the barriers are to preparing fruits and vegetables, what they are willing and able to do given their life situations, which skills they would need, and what would motivate them to learn the needed skills.

Summary of Assessment Methods for Potential Personal Mediators of Behavior Change

You can find out about the attitudes, beliefs, and other person-related variables listed earlier indirectly through a review of the relevant literature from behavioral nutrition, nutrition education, and health education studies on motivation to act and the dietary change process; monitoring and research data for the primary population or target audience or similar population (e.g., adolescents, postmenopausal women, African American men); government and industry opinion surveys of people's beliefs and attitudes; food marking surveys; studies of population segmentation by psychographic variables; or existing records for the group. A review of measures used in nutrition education programs for various population groups is provided by Contento, Randell, and Basch (2002).

It is best to obtain information directly from the intended audience, if possible. You can administer surveys or brief questionnaires, using existing instruments or intervention-specific instruments that you design. Talking personally with the group is highly desirable. You can conduct focus group interviews, in-depth individual interviews of individuals from the intended audience or key informants, or intercept interviews as individuals leave stores, clinics, or service centers. Use Worksheet 8-1 as a guide and record your answers on it.

Nutrition Education in Action 8-1 contains examples of open-ended questions for use with young adults, and Nutrition Education in Action 8-2 describes the outcomes of in-depth interviews with community members. Table 8-4 summarizes the advantages and disadvantages of a variety of methods to gather assessment data.

Step 2b: Identify Environmental Factors That Can Potentially Mediate the Target Behaviors

Identifying the environmental conditions that either facilitate or impede healthful dietary practices by a given group is very important. It will ground your educational activities in the real world of your audience. You can use the information in two major ways: (1) to plan educational activities that take into account the realities of the participants' lives, for example, in terms of their time and resources; or (2) to embark on partnerships with providers of food or services or with community organizations to facilitate and enlarge the audience's opportunities for action. See Chapter 6 for more details.

Information About Environments for Planning Appropriate Educational Activities

In order to design appropriate educational activities, you will need information about various aspects of the environment such as the following.

- *Social environment.* What is the general life situation of members of the target group? Find out about the family or household structures of the group; for example, are they mostly single parents? Who is responsible for buying food and for preparing it? Do they eat with others whose needs must be considered, such as children or partners? What is the size and quality of their social networks? Do they have the social and cultural supports necessary to maintain the desired behavior after it has been adopted? Are work arrangements conducive to the new behaviors being enacted on a long-term basis? Also inquire about *potential* social supports: how could you, or the nutrition education program, help them develop better social supports for enacting the

---

NUTRITION EDUCATION IN ACTION 8-1

Open-Ended Questions

The following questions were used for assessing the opinions on fruits and vegetables of ethnically diverse, young adults (aged 16–25) in a community program.

- *How many fruits and vegetables do you believe you need to eat each day? Why or why not?* Responses varied, with a majority indicating between two and five servings a day. "Good for the body" or health-related answers were the top reasons to eat fruits and vegetables each day.
- *If you learned the following facts (list provided) about fruits and vegetables, which would most likely cause you to eat more fruits and vegetables?* The top two facts selected from the list were "eating fruits and vegetables gives me healthy and beautiful teeth, gums, skin, and hair" and "eating fruits and vegetables helps reduce my risk of developing a chronic disease such as cancer, heart disease, or stroke."
- *What would encourage you to eat more fruits and vegetables?* Freshness, increased availability and selection, and health were the top reasons mentioned.
- *How important is it to you to eat fruits and vegetables?* Seventy-one percent said that it was "very important," and 21% said it was "somewhat important."
- *Do you eat fruits and vegetables in the cafeteria? Why or why not?* Seventy-five percent indicated that they ate fruits and vegetables in the cafeteria for reasons of taste or health. Those who did not cited the lack of freshness and availability.
- *When you buy beverages from vending machines, which ones do you usually choose?* Cola, water, and non-cola-flavored soda were the more frequent choices. Only 5% indicated usually purchasing fruit juice. Thirty-nine percent indicated that they would purchase 100% fruit juice if it were available in the vending machine.
- *When are you most willing to eat more fruits and vegetables? Breakfast, lunch, between meals, dinner, or dessert?* Responses were divided between all times, with slightly more respondents favoring fruits and vegetables for lunch.
- *How would you prefer to receive nutrition information?* Taste tests, brochures, posters, classes, staff at the campus health clinic, radio, and television were the top preferred methods for the target audience to receive nutrition information.

Source: California Project LEAN, California Department of Health Services. 2004. *Community-based social marketing: The California Project LEAN experience.* Sacramento, CA: Author. http://www.californiaprojectlean.org/resourcelibrary/. Accessed 3/15/06.

targeted healthful behaviors? Is the intended audience interested in working with others in order to change their food environment? If so, what exactly would they like to do? Does the group have collective efficacy skills in order to advocate for themselves?

- *Physical food environment.* Find out whether the foods the intended audience need to enact the targeted behaviors are available and accessible to them. Are these foods available and accessible in their workplaces or school cafeteria or the local grocery store? For example, are fruits and vegetables or local or minimally processed and packaged foods easily accessible? You or your team can draw a map of the community showing the location and type of grocery stores, fast food outlets, restaurants, or farmers' markets. If that is not possible, at least walk around the neighborhood

and see what is there. Is good-quality, fresh produce available? What kind of restaurants and food vendors are around? Where do most people seem to be eating? If it is a school, college, or workplace, what is available in the cafeteria?

- *Resources.* Do members of the intended audience have enough money to afford the foods targeted in the intervention? Do they have cooking facilities or refrigerators? Do they have access to food assistance programs? Are prices of foods in their neighborhood supportive of the targeted behaviors? Do they have transportation to and from stores? What are the causes of the "problems behind the problems" in terms of the social and economic realities of people's lives? What are the time constraints of the intended audience? Such information will assist you to develop a nutrition education

---

NUTRITION EDUCATION IN ACTION 8-2

Wellness IN the Rockies (WIN the Rockies): A Research, Education, and Outreach Project That Seeks to Address Obesity Innovatively and Effectively

The Focus of the Program
Overall project goals are to enhance the well-being of individuals by improving their attitudes and behaviors related to food, physical activity, and body image; and to help build communities' capacities to foster and sustain these changes.

Assessment
Prior to developing the various nutrition education programs of this project, program staff gathered narratives or life stories related to physical activity, food and eating, and body image from extensive interviews and focus group discussions with 103 adults. The narratives were tape recorded. Key quotations were identified and grouped into 146 narrative thematic codes using grounded theory.

Values
Values emerged as an important theme. A major finding of relevance here is that being productive, working hard, and not wasting resources were important values. Thus, physical activity should be productive or serve some purpose, such as mowing the lawn or doing other chores. Going to the gym to exercise or just going for a walk was not seen as productive. These activities were a "waste" of time compared with activities in which work was being accomplished, or compared with other things that they might be doing with their families or communities.

In the same way, wasting food was seen as violating an important value of not wasting resources. That value led to the importance of cleaning one's plate and not squandering food.

The Power of Others
The study also found that other people have profound and often lifelong impacts on individuals' feelings about their body and physical abilities. These feelings in turn can contribute to their sense of identity and influence their lifestyles and their long-term health. Thus, individuals need to create social environments that nurture others, particularly youth, rather than be critical and hurtful. Respecting diverse body sizes becomes highly important.

Sources: Pelican, S., F. Vanden Heede, B. Holmes, et al. 2005. The power of others to shape our identity: Body image, physical abilities, and body weight. *Family and Consumer Sciences Research Journal* 34:57–80; Wardlaw, M.K. 2005. New You: Health for Every Body: Helping adults adopt a health-centered approach to well-being. *Journal of Nutrition Education and Behavior* 37:S103–106; and Pelican, S., F. Vanden Heeds, and B. Holmes. 2005. *Let their voices be heard: Quotations from life stories related to physical activity, food and eating, and body image.* Chicago, IL: Discovery Association Publishing House.

TABLE 8-4 Advantages and Disadvantages of Various Methods of Issue Identification and Needs Analysis

	Advantages	Disadvantages
Review of research or survey literature	Quick, inexpensive, nonthreatening	Information not specific to intended audience
National survey and monitoring data, opinion polls	Quick, inexpensive, nonthreatening	Information not specific to intended audience
Review of existing records of intended audience	Information specific to intended audience; quick, inexpensive, nonthreatening to intended group	Limited to quality of data, scope of data
Surveys of intended audience		
Telephone	Information specific to group; chance for detailed insight into perceived and real needs	Expensive; extensive training needed for interviewers; leaves out people with no phones or unlisted numbers
Group administered	Quick, inexpensive; information specific to intended audience	Survey instrument must be designed and tested
Mailed survey	Information specific to intended audience; chance for more honest answers	Eliminates low-literacy individuals; responses less open-ended than in-person interviews; moderately expensive; time delay in getting information; may get low response rate
Individual interviews		
Informal	Information specific to intended audience; inexpensive	Not systematic
Formal in-person interviews	Information specific to intended audience; comprehensive insight into intended audience	Expensive; extensive training needed for interviewers; time-consuming
Group meetings		
Group discussion	Relatively low cost, quick	People attending may not be representative; not enough time for people to express their thoughts or needs publicly
Focus groups	Provides detailed information on beliefs, emotions, and attitudes	Expensive; training needed for interviewers
Observation	Accurate information on behaviors	Expensive; can be intrusive; can alter the behavior being observed if observation is known

program that is realistic for the intended audience. For example, if they work two jobs and have little time to prepare food, educational activities will need to take this into consideration. You may also need to direct them to other nutrition services and resources that may be available to them.

- *Information environment.* Ask about what media they use, and the frequency and intensity of their use of these media (such as viewing TV or reading magazines). What is the information environment of the setting in which the intervention itself will take place (such as the school or workplace)? How may it be changed to be more supportive of the targeted behaviors?

Information About Environments so as to Educate Decision Makers and Policy Makers to Promote Environmental Supports for Action

Promoting environmental supports for action is important where it is possible, given the resources and the goals, duration, and scope of the program. You will most likely need first to educate others who are the direct providers of foods or services and those who have decision-making roles in various settings. When such people or groups are convinced of the importance of your program goals, you can then work in coalition with them to bring about environmental supports for action.

Identify Decision Makers and Policy Makers in Organizations and Communities

In this substep, you will first want to identify the potential organizations or agencies with whom you can partner in order to increase opportunities for taking the actions that are the focus of the program. Here are some potential partners:

- Principals and school superintendents
- Food service providers in schools and workplaces
- Public health agencies (local, state, and national)
- Hospitals and school health services personnel
- State and local Cooperative Extension Service personnel
- Chefs and restaurant owners
- Supermarkets and local grocery stores
- Farmers and farmers' markets
- Gardening associations
- Sustainable food systems organizations
- Community organizations related to food and nutrition, such as food recovery programs, food banks, soup kitchens, and food security and hunger organizations
- Grocery stores

Conduct Environmental Assessments with Coalition Partners

With partnerships or coalitions in place, you and the partners can list assessment activities you will conduct. These might include the availability and accessibility of food and food-related services in communities. If you are working in schools and have formed a partnership with the school principal and the school food service director, you may all decide that a first step is to survey the school food and policy environments. It is best to include other stakeholders in this process as well: teachers, parents, and students. In this survey, you could ask about the following: Does the school have a written food policy? Is nutrition addressed in it? Does the school have a nutrition advisory council? Does the school have a soft drink policy? Do teachers/faculty use food as a reward or incentive? Does the school permit food promotion and advertising? If your program will be quite extensive, you may consider using some of the food environment assessment tools that are available, such as the School Health Index (SHI) from the Centers for Disease Prevention and Control (CDC, 2000); the Changing the Scene assessment tools from the U.S. Department of Agriculture's Team Nutrition program (USDA, 2000); and the Healthy Schools Action Tool (HSAT) from the Michigan Department of Community Health (2005).

Some of the same assessment questions may be applicable for other organizational settings, such as workplaces or health care facilities in relation to employees, if your program will be in these settings. If you are working in coalition with others about food sustainability issues, you might want to survey how many farmers' markets are available and accessible to your intended audience and whether they accept food stamps.

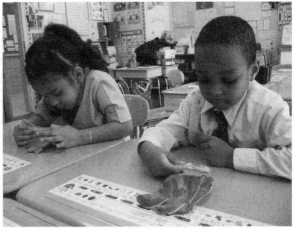

Children can examine different foods in a scientific way in order to become familiar with them.

Summary of Assessment Methods for Potential Environmental Mediators of Behavior Change

Data concerning potential environmental mediators can be obtained from quantitative and qualitative methods such as the following: literature review of similar settings; available data; surveys, checklists, and environmental health index assessments; observation of availability of food in the setting (grocery stores, farmers' markets, workplace, school, and so forth); focus group discussions; and interviews of key informants.

Step 2c: Identify Relevant Individual and Community Strengths or Assets

What is the intended audience already doing that is healthy? For example, what current diet-related practices are health enhancing? What personal or cultural beliefs and attitudes do the intended audience possess that make positive contributions to nutritional health or the sustainability of the food system? What do they already know about the issues of concern? What knowledge and skills do they already possess to address the concerns? What are the strengths of the community in terms of environmental infrastructure or activities that are conducive to health? What resources are available, such as healthy food stores, farmers' markets, or food pantries? What nutrition education services are already available? What do audience members say they would like their environments to be like?

Table 8-5 provides a summary of what might be found from an assessment process. The worksheets in Case Study 8-1 show the details.

Program Resource Considerations

Practical and resource considerations may dictate the duration and intensity of the program that are possible, whatever

TABLE 8-5 Summary of Identification of Potential Mediators of the Targeted Behavior for the Case Study Example: Increase Intake of Fruits and Vegetables Among Middle-School Adolescents

Food Practices or Behaviors to Be Targeted	Potential Personal Mediators of Targeted Behaviors		Potential Environmental Mediators of Targeted Behaviors
	Motivational Mediators	**Behavior Change Mediators**	
Current practice: Low intake of F&V	*Sense of threat/awareness of risk* *Current:* Low *Potential motivators:* Personalizing the risks	*Self-efficacy* *Current:* Not familiar with different F&V; unwilling to venture *Potential:* Exposure to new foods	*Barriers* *Current:* Not easily available; expensive *Potential:* Learn skills to decrease cost
Targeted behavior: Intake of five or more F&V servings per day	*Outcome expectancies/barriers* *Current:* Taste bad, inconvenient, go bad quickly *Potential motivators:* If taste good, etc.; immediate benefits for health (skin, eyes), for performance of activities they value	*Food/nutrition skills* *Current:* Need skills to choose and prepare F&V snacks *Potential:* Making learning skills fun and convenient	*Social support* *Current:* No support for F&V among teens *Potential:* Train peer educators; find celebrity role models
	Social norm *Current:* Friends do not eat vegetables; unaware of media influence *Potential motivators:* Make veggies cool; make aware of media influence on food choices	*Self-regulation skills* *Current:* Impulse eating; low SR *Potential:* Learn goal setting and self-monitoring	*Information environment* *Current:* No role models of teens eating F&V; few ads *Potential:* Provide posters, newsletters, etc.
			Availability and accessibility *Current:* Students do not eat F&V offered *Potential:* In partnership with school food service, develop salad bars at reasonable cost to students

F&V = fruits and vegetables; SR = self-regulation.

the merits of nutrition education identified in the previous assessments. Ask questions such as the following: What resources will be available for the nutrition education intervention in monetary terms? How long a program is possible or considered desirable? One session or many? One component or many? What space and equipment are available? What other resources will be available? What is the nature of the facilities and the setting? What channels are possible given these constraints? Will the program involve group sessions, audiovisual or print media, health fairs, media campaigns, all of them, or other channels?

If the nutrition education you are planning involves group sessions, here are some practical details to consider:

- *Time.* How much time do you have for your sessions? How much time will you have for setup and cleanup?

- *Space available and its arrangement.* What is the physical space like? How can you change the space to meet your needs? What space restrictions are you working within?
- *Equipment available.* What equipment (audiovisual, cooking, etc.) is available to you? What could you bring if you needed to?
- *General administrative/facilities support.* How helpful are your key contact persons in terms of troubleshooting, providing supplies, helping with promotion, and providing technical assistance during your sessions? For example, will the classroom teacher remain in the room and help with classroom control? Will the senior center director remain in the room and help with technical problems if they come up?

Identify Relevant Audience Characteristics

This is the time to find out some relevant specifics about the audience or primary group: cultural background considerations, educational level, academic skills, the physical and cognitive developmental level of children, preferred learning styles and instructional formats, and special needs. More specifically, find out about the following (if relevant):

- *Demographics.* What are the age, sex, race, socioeconomic status, and ethnic backgrounds of the intended audience?
- *Specific cultural practices of the community.* What are the typical meal patterns? What is the community's sense of time and space?
- *Educational level.* What grade are they in (for children)? How much schooling have they completed (for adults)? Where?
- *Physical and cognitive developmental levels/abilities (children only).* At what stage is their physical and cognitive development?
- *Academic skills.* How well can your audience read? What are their math skills?
- *Preferred learning styles or instructional formats.* Which do they prefer: lectures, reading, discussion, activities, group work, or field projects?
- *Special needs.* Are there learning disabilities or physical disabilities that you should consider? If you will be working with an adult group, will children be present? Can child care be provided?
- *Emotional needs.* What is going on emotionally in the lives of your audience? How will this influence their ability to hear your message?
- *Social needs.* How well does your group know each other? Does the intended audience have high community cohesion?

Your Turn

In Step 1 you selected one or two high-priority food and/or health issues and a high-priority primary audience. You also identified some key behavioral outcomes that will be the focus of the intervention. During this chapter, you recorded your assessment results on Worksheet 8-1, and identified key relevant potential mediators of the actions or behaviors that are the focus of the program. These key mediators of behavior change will be the targets of your educational strategies.

At the end of Step 2 you should have statements regarding the following:

- *Health or food issues and intended audience for the program.* For example, overweight prevention in middle school youth, or increased fruit and vegetable intakes among pregnant women.

- *High-priority target health-promoting actions or changes in behavior* (one or two) or a set of related behaviors or community practices that will be the focus of the intervention or program. These are the behavioral goal(s) or targeted behaviors or practices of the program.
- *Personal and environmental determinants that are potential mediators of the target behavior changes or practices.* This list can, and indeed should, be quite long (e.g., 10 to 20 items). You will prioritize them later, in Step 3, when they become the basis for writing general educational objectives that will guide the development of strategies over several sessions of the intervention or across several components, and for writing specific educational objectives for the learning experiences *within* the individual sessions or individual components of the program.

Although a comprehensive process of selecting the behavioral focus of the intervention and identifying the specific mediators that will be the targets of educational strategies may seem time-consuming and even tedious, it is probably the most critical step in creating effective nutrition education learning experiences in a community. Besides providing you with helpful data, an audience assessment can be a useful tool in establishing a rapport with audience participants. If done thoughtfully, a good assessment of issues and their causes for an audience may even reveal preconceptions you may have had about the participants, as well as your own attitudes about teaching and learning. Nutrition education is most successful when both group participants and educators can communicate openly, honestly, and with respect for each other as individuals. A comprehensive assessment process helps to establish this relationship.

Case Study

From our Step 1 assessment in the last chapter for our case study, we chose "Taking Control: Eating Well and Being Fit" as the title of the program and identified four goal behaviors for our audience. For reasons of space, we focus on only one of the four behaviors—eating more fruits and vegetables—and seek to identify only those determinants of behavior that can potentially mediate an increase in the behavior of eating more fruits and vegetables.

Questions and Activities

1. In the last chapter you identified food and nutrition issues of concern for a given audience and the behaviors or practices that contribute to them. You also identified the behaviors or practices that will be the focus of your program. Why is it important to identify the potential mediators of these behaviors and practices?

2. Name and briefly describe the two major categories of potential mediators of healthful action or behavior change.

3. Summarize some methods for assessing potential personal mediators of behavior change. Which methods for which potential mediators do you think will be useful for an audience you have in mind or will be working with? Why? Give their relative advantages and disadvantages.

4. How can we use information about potential environmental influences on behavior in our nutrition education programs? How shall we assess such influences for a given audience? Describe several methods of assessment and their relative advantages and disadvantages.

5. List five audience characteristics that are important to know before you embark on your nutrition education program.

STEP 2 WORKSHEET Identify the Potential Personal and Environmental Mediators of the Program-Specified Behavioral Goals Identified in Step 1

The potential personal and environmental mediators of the program-specified goal behaviors or practices that you identified in Worksheet 7-3 now need to be identified and prioritized. The list of determinants that can be potential mediators can, and indeed should, be quite long (10 to 20 items). You will prioritize them later, in Step 3, when they become the basis for writing general and specific educational objectives that will guide the development of the educational activities within the individual sessions or individual components of the program.

Use the worksheet printed here as an outline. Enter the information you collect into the needs assessment document that you created in the last chapter. Include both the information and the information sources.

WORKSHEET 8-1

Step 2a: Identify the person-related psychosocial determinants that are potential mediators of the target behaviors

---

Identify determinants of behavior or potential mediators of action or behavior change

ASSESSMENT INFORMATION (*Record findings in your needs assessment document.*)	INFORMATION SOURCES
Identify potential mediators motivating the behavior, based on theory variables or constructs. Use those determinants that research evidence suggests are important for the identified issue and audience. For each of these determinants, assess motivating factors for *current* behavior(s) as well as *potential* motivations for engaging in the program-specified behavior(s). The latter are the potential mediators of behavior change. (*Record findings for the relevant variables listed below.*)	*Review of behavioral nutrition and nutrition education studies and opinion polls; questionnaires, interviews, focus groups, etc.*

- *Motivational readiness to change.* At what motivational stage are the group members?
- *Outcome expectations or beliefs.* What are their beliefs about the outcomes of their current behavior? What are some potential motivators for engaging in the program-specified behaviors or practices?
- *Barriers.* What are the barriers to engaging in the program behaviors or practices?
- *Values.* What are some of the larger values that might influence their relationship to food?
- *Awareness of risk.* Do they see their current behaviors or practices as a risk? In what way? If not, what would increase their perception of realistic risk?
- *Attitudes and feelings.* What are their attitudes or feelings about engaging in the behavior(s) identified?
- *Sensory-affective food-related factors.* Which foods do they like or prefer? What would make the targeted foods taste better to them?
- *Self-efficacy.* How confident are they in taking the actions identified?
- *Social norms or peer pressure.* What are the participants' social norms? What do they see as useful ways to resist social pressure?
- *Cultural beliefs and identities.* What cultural beliefs and identities are relevant to the actions targeted by the program? How strong are the cultural influences?
- *Life stage.* Are they in their child-rearing stage? Retired? How does that affect their food choices and other dietary behaviors?
- *Others.*

Identify behavioral capabilities and self-regulation skills: factors that facilitate taking action or behavior change

ASSESSMENT INFORMATION (*Record findings for the relevant variables listed below in your needs assessment document.*)	INFORMATION SOURCES
Identify potential mediators that facilitate action based on theory variables. For each variable, assess *current* knowledge and skills and *potential* knowledge and skills.	*Review nutrition education studies; conduct surveys, interviews, focus groups, etc.*

Behavioral capabilities
- *Food- and nutrition related knowledge to carry out targeted behavior (how-to knowledge).* For example, do they know how many servings of fruit and vegetables they should eat? Which foods are high in saturated fat? The nutritional value of favorite snacks? What information would they like to learn about?
- *Food- and nutrition-related skills.* Examples are label reading, food safety practices, cooking skills, menu modification skills, breastfeeding, and choosing local foods. What skills would they like to acquire?
- *Critical thinking skills.* Can they discuss what the advantages and disadvantages of different kinds of foods and food practices (e.g., traditional, organic, local, or genetically modified) are?
- *Misconceptions.* What are their misconceptions?

Self-regulation skills
- *Ability to make action plans; goal-setting and self-monitoring skills.* How do they usually make changes? Have they made action plans before? How useful were they for them?
- *Emotion-coping skills.* Do they cope with stress by eating food? Do they have specific difficulties in certain situations?

Collective efficacy, empowerment skills

- *Skills in organizing groups, building coalitions, and advocacy.* What experiences have they had before in working with groups to change their environment? What skills would they like to acquire?

Step 2b: Identify environmental factors that might mediate the program-specified behaviors or practices

ASSESSMENT INFORMATION (*For each of the categories, assess both the current situation and potential changes that are possible and desired. Record findings for the relevant variables listed below in your needs assessment document.*)	INFORMATION SOURCES
Information about environments to plan appropriate educational activities **Social environment** • *Social networks.* What size and quality are the participants' social networks? How can they be changed? • *Social and cultural support.* What degree of family and community support is there for the targeted behaviors? How could support be increased? • *Collective efficacy activities.* Is the group interested in advocacy to improve their food environment? If so, what skills do they have or want?	*Review literature and existing data; conduct surveys, observations, and interviews*
Food environment • *Availability and accessibility of food needed to enact the target behaviors.* Are the foods they need in their stores, workplaces, or schools?	
Resources: What resources (time, money, etc.) does the group have for healthful eating?	
Informational environment: Posters, media at site.	
Information about environments so as to educate decision makers and policy makers **Food environment** • *Potential food availability and accessibility.* How feasible will it be to make changes in food in the intervention setting? What will be required? With whom will you need to collaborate to make these changes?	
Organizational policy environment • *Policies related to food at school or work that might impede or facilitate healthful behaviors.* What policies need to be enacted?	
Other	

Step 2c: Identify individual and community strengths or assets

ASSESSMENT INFORMATION (*Record findings for relevant variables below in your needs assessment document.*)	INFORMATION SOURCES

Assets
• Behaviors
• Person-related determinants that already mediate behaviors targeted by program
• Environmental factors in the environment that already facilitate the targeted actions or behaviors
   – Social networks and support
   – Physical resources: stores, services
   – Informational support
   – Supportive policies
	Review existing data; conduct surveys, observations, and interviews

Other	

CASE STUDY 8-1 **Step 2: Identify the Potential Personal and Environmental Mediators of the Target Behaviors Identified for the Program**

From Step 1, the behavioral goals of the program identified for youth are to

- Increase intake of fruits and vegetables (youth to aim for 2.5 cups or more a day)
- Decrease amount of sweetened beverages consumed each day (aim for no more than 8 ounces a day)
- Decrease number of packaged high-fat, high-sugar snacks so that they contribute no more than 150 calories a day (targets for drinks and snacks are based on the discretionary calories allowance for this age group)
- Increase physical activity to 10,000 steps a day and participate actively, when possible, in gym or other school-sponsored physical activities

The title chosen for the program is "Taking Control: Eating Well and Being Fit." The setting is the school.

Worksheet 8-1: Identify the Potential Personal and Environmental Mediators of the Target Behaviors
The potential personal and environmental mediators of the specified behavior changes need to be identified for each of the four behaviors. For reasons of space, only the potential mediators of the behavior change of eating more fruits and vegetables are explored in this case study.

Step 2a: Identify the potential person-related mediators of the target behaviors

---

Identify determinants of behavior or potential mediators of action or behavior change

ASSESSMENT INFORMATION	INFORMATION SOURCES
Identify potential mediators motivating the behavior, based on theory constructs.	*Reviews, opinion polls, surveys, or interviews*
Outcome expectations or beliefs/barriers: What are their beliefs about the outcomes of their current behavior? What are the barriers? • *Current motivation:* Middle school youth understand that fruits and vegetables have health benefits. But they also think that most fruits and vegetables don't taste as good as the other foods they eat, are inconvenient to carry around and eat, go bad quickly, and are very uneven in quality. • *Potential motivators:* Good taste; provide immediate benefits for health (skin, eyes); help them look good; provide energy; build strong bones and muscles for athletic performance.	*A survey questionnaire; group discussion*
Awareness of risk: Do they see their current behaviors or practices as a risk? • *Current motivation:* They have no sense of urgency about eating fruits and vegetables. They know it is good for them, but see no risk to not eating them. • *Potential motivators:* Personalized risk through a self-assessment process.	
Attitudes and feelings: What are their attitudes toward engaging in the behavior(s)? • *Current motivation:* Their attitude toward eating fruits was positive, but not toward eating vegetables.	
Sensory-affective food-related factors: Which foods do they like or prefer? • *Current motivation:* Most youth like the taste of fruit but do not like most vegetables. They feel that most fruits and vegetables don't taste as good as the other foods they eat and are very uneven in quality—sometimes delicious and other times having no flavor or having blemishes. • *Potential motivators:* Will eat fruits and vegetables if they smell and taste good and look attractive.	
Self-efficacy: How confident are they in taking the action identified? • *Current motivation:* They are not familiar with different fruits and vegetables and are unwilling to try them. They are not confident that fruits and vegetables will taste good or that they will know what to do with them. • *Potential motivators:* Exposure to new fruits and vegetables and preparation methods.	
Social norms or peer pressure • *Current motivation:* Friends do not eat vegetables; unaware of media influence. • *Potential motivators:* Make fruit and veggies cool; make audience aware of the lack of media attention to fruits and vegetables.	

Cultural beliefs and identities
- *Current motivation:* For most, fruits are very much part of their ethnic heritage and cultural practice, but vegetables less so.
- *Potential motivators:* Emphasize that eating fruits and vegetables is expressing their cultural heritage.

Stage of readiness to change: This was not specifically assessed, but most are in a pre-action stage of readiness. Many are contemplating change and will eat fruits and vegetables if they are provided cues to action and if barriers are reduced.

Life stage: Students in middle school.

Identify behavioral capabilities and self-regulation skills: factors that facilitate taking action or behavior change

ASSESSMENT INFORMATION	INFORMATION SOURCES
Identify mediators facilitating action based on theory variables.	*Survey, informal group discussion, and interviews*
For each variable, assess *current* knowledge and skills and *potential* knowledge and skills.	

Behavioral capabilities (food- and nutrition-related knowledge and skills)
- *Current skills:* They do not have the needed skills to choose and prepare fruits and vegetables as snacks; have misconception that they need only two servings of fruits and vegetables a day.
- *Potential motivators for skills:* Expressed interest in learning if the program could make learning skills fun and convenient.

Self-regulation skills
- *Current skills:* Impulse eating of high-fat, high-sugar snacks and beverages; weak intentions to eat fruits and vegetables; low self-regulation skills.
- *Potential motivators for skills:* Action plans and tips to help them actually do what they would like to do—eat more fruits and vegetables.

Step 2b: Identify environmental factors that can potentially mediate the target behaviors or practices

ASSESSMENT INFORMATION	INFORMATION SOURCES
For each of the categories, assess both the current situation and potential changes that are possible and desired.	
Social environment	*Interviews*

- *Parents:* Parents are very interested in helping their children eat more fruits and vegetables but don't know how to get their children to do so. They say their children are reluctant to try new foods.
- *Teachers:* Teachers lament the "poor eating practices" of their students and express some general interest in helping them eat better. Some teachers are very concerned about their own eating and are good role models for students.

Food and physical activity environment

General

Reviews, survey information, interviews of teachers and principal

- *More meals eaten away from home.* From 1977 to 1996, consumption of home meals dropped 14%, snacks away from home doubled, and eating at fast food restaurants on any given day increased 5 times (Beale, 2000).
- *Food advertising.* The average child sees 10,000 food ads per year. The food industry spends $10 billion each year to influence the eating behavior of children: $10 to $50 million for candy bars, $115.5 million for soft drinks, and in excess of $1 billion for McDonald's. In contrast, the National Cancer Institute's yearly budget for the 5 A Day campaign is $1 million (Nestle & Jacobson, 2000).
- *Portion size, price, and packaging.* Portion sizes have increased and the price per serving has decreased, and packaging is now an instrument of marketing (Young & Nestle 2003; Nielson & Popkin, 2003).
- *Changing modes of transport.* There is less walking, a lack of suburban sidewalks, and greater use of cars (U.S. Department of Transportation, 1997).

Specific

- The school provides breakfasts and lunches as part of the USDA national school meals program. It also provides à la carte meal items. The school has vending machines and a school store.
- Fruits and vegetables served in the school meals programs are not always very appealing.
- There are numerous fast food outlets and delis around the school.
- Physical education (PE) is required of students in middle school grades, but only once a week.
- The school is large and on several floors, so that students can get considerable exercise walking up and down the stairs.
- Students all live nearby and walk to school. There is a small park within five blocks of the school, with two basketball courts.

Resources: The youth are from low-resource families in a low-income urban neighborhood. *Existing school data*

Policies related to food in the target setting that might impede or facilitate healthful behaviors *Interviews, observations*

- Impact of vending machines and stores in schools. À la carte items in the cafeteria (Harnack et al., 2000) and items sold in school stores are often low in nutrient density, and the drinks are high in calories and added sugars (Wildey et al., 2000).
- The school has vending machines with mostly sweetened beverages, and school stores with mostly low-nutrient, high-energy-density, processed and packaged foods.
- The school does not have any policies related to the food environment, such as policies for foods in vending machines and school stores or for foods used for fundraising, as rewards by teachers, and at special events.

Informational environment: There are no attractive posters promoting fruits and vegetables in cafeteria. *Observations*

Step 2c: Identify individual and community assets

ASSESSMENT INFORMATION (*Record findings for relevant variables below, using separate sheets.*) **INFORMATION SOURCE**

School principal and teachers are very interested in an overweight prevention nutrition education program and will support it. Parents are also very supportive. *Observations, interviews*

Other

REFERENCES

Beale, C.L. 2000. A century of population growth and change. *Food Review* 23:16–22.

Centers for Disease Control and Prevention. 2000. *School Health Index for physical activity and healthy eating: A self-assessment and planning guide.* Atlanta, GA: Author. http://www.cdc.gov/nccdphp/dash.

Contento, I.R., J.S. Randell, and C.E. Basch. 2002. Review and analysis of evaluation measures used in nutrition education intervention research. *Journal of Nutrition Education and Behavior* 34:2–25.

Harnak L., J. Stang, and M. Story. 1999. Soft drink consumption among U.S. children and adolescents: Nutritional consequences. *Journal of the American Diet Association* 1999;99:436—441.

Liou, D., and I.R. Contento. 2001. Usefulness of psychosocial variables in explaining fat-related dietary behavior in Chinese Americans: Association with degree of acculturation. *Journal of Nutrition Education and Behavior* 33:322–331.

Michigan Department of Community Health. 2005. *The Healthy School Action Tool.* Lansing, MI: Cardiovascular Health, Nutrition and Physical Activity Section, Michigan Department of Community Health. http://www.mihealthtools.org/schools/.

Nestle M., and M.F. Jacobson. 2000. Halting the obesity epidemic: A public health policy approach. *Public Health Report* 2000;115:12–24.

Nielsen, S.J., and B.M. Popkin. 2003. Patterns and trends in food portion sizes, 1977–1998. *Journal of the American Medical Association* 289(4):450–453.

U.S. Department of Agriculture. 2000. *Changing the scene: Improving the school nutrition environment.* Alexandria, VA: U.S. Department of Agriculture, Food and Nutrition Service. http://www.fns.usda.gov/tn/Healthy/index.

U.S. Department of Transportation. 1997. *Nationwide personal transportation survey.* Lantham, MD: Federal Highway Administration, Research and Technical Support Center.

Wildey, M.B., S. Pampalone, M. Pelletier, M. Zive, J. Elder, and J. Sallis. 2000. Fat and sugar levels are high in snacks purchased from student stores in middle schools. *Journal of the American Dietetic Association.* 100:319–322.

Yaroch, A.L., K. Resnicow, and L.K. Khan. 2000. Validity and reliability of qualitative dietary fat index questionnaires: A review. *Journal of the American Dietetic Association* 100(2):240–244.

Young, L.R., and M. Nestle. 2003. Expanding portion sizes in the US marketplace: Implications for nutrition counseling. *Journal of the American Dietetic Association* 103(2):231–234.

CHAPTER 9

Step 3: Select Theory, Educational Philosophy, and Program Components

....

OVERVIEW   This chapter explores the importance of clearly stating the theoretical framework that will guide the development of program components as well as the assumptions or educational philosophy underlying the intervention.

OBJECTIVES   At the end of the chapter, you will be able to

- Select an appropriate theory or relevant model to design a given set of sessions or intervention
- Appreciate how nutrition educators' own philosophy about educational approach influences the nature of the nutrition education intervention
- Identify your own beliefs and philosophy about how nutrition and food content should be addressed
- Determine components and channels for your program

....

Introduction

Having a thorough understanding of our intended audiences, the issues that face them, and their environmental context is an important first step in designing nutrition education. We are now ready to design the "outputs" component of our logic model for nutrition education design. However, before rushing to do what we all like to do best—preparing presentations or designing exciting activities for a group—based on that understanding, we still have some preliminary planning to do. We will need to think through carefully how best to address the problems, issues, or interests identified, given the behaviors or practices that contribute to them and the influences on these practices.

In this preliminary planning step, you will

- Select the theory or create the conceptual model that will guide your program
- Articulate your philosophy about nutrition education
- Clarify your perspectives on nutrition content and issues
- Determine how many and which components your program will have

These factors are shown in Step 3 of our design model and are explored in detail in this chapter. The steps are listed in order. However, it should be noted that the components of our model are intimately related to each other, so you will probably go back and forth among them. Hence the arrows linking the components are bidirectional. After you have completed this preliminary planning step, you will be able to write educational objectives directed at the relevant determinants that can mediate change that you have identified and design appropriate theory-based educational strategies.

Selecting Theory and Creating an Appropriate Conceptual Model

We have said repeatedly that theory based on research, whether qualitative or quantitative, provides our best current understanding of why and how people take food- and nutrition-related action. It provides a useful mental map for what to address and how to do so. Selection of appropriate theory for the educational program is thus crucial. It will be helpful to first ask yourself the following questions, based on the information from Steps 1 and 2.

INPUTS: COLLECTING ASSESSMENT DATA		DESIGNING THE OUTPUTS			DESIGNING OUTCOMES EVALUATION
STEP 1 ←→ **Analyze needs and behaviors: Specify the behavior or action focus of the program** • Assess needs and identify audience: select need(s) or issue(s) to address • Identify behaviors of concern that contribute to need(s) or issue(s) • Select core behaviors or practices to address	**STEP 2** ←→ **Identify relevant potential mediators of program behaviors** • Identify potential personal psychosocial mediators • Identify potential environmental mediators	**STEP 3** ←→ **Select theory, philosophy, and components** • Select theory and/or create appropriate model • Articulate educational philosophy • Clarify perspectives on content • Determine program components	**STEP 4** ←→ **State educational objectives for potential mediators** • Select relevant mediators to address • State educational objectives for each selected mediator: —Personal psychosocial mediators —Environmental mediators	**STEP 5** ←→ **Design theory-based educational strategies and activities to address potential mediators** • Design strategies and activities for each selected mediator: —Personal psychosocial mediators —Environmental mediators	**STEP 6** **Design evaluation** • Design evaluation of program's impact on behaviors and mediators • Design process evaluation

● Given the duration, intensity, and scope of the intervention that is feasible based on practical constraints and resource considerations, will your program consist of only in-person sessions or will it be possible for your program to work in partnership with others to promote support for action by addressing the food and policy environments of the intended audience in addition to addressing person-related mediators of action? That is, will the program be able to address both personal and environmental mediators of behavior?

● What will be the overall educational goals of the nutrition education program? Your needs and issues assessment process yielded information on the behavioral focus of the program, the state of motivational readiness of the intended audience, and key relevant potential mediators of action or behavior change. Based on what you found out, will the program aim to increase awareness, promote active deliberation, and enhance motivation to take action? Or will it focus on building skills and the ability to take action? Will it aim to do both?

Once you have clarified these matters for yourself, you can then consider which theory is appropriate to use to design the intervention. A specific theory can be used, such as social cognitive theory, theory of planned behavior or the stages of change model. Or the theory can be based on qualitative interpretative research conducted with your own audience in Step 1. Box 9-1 summarizes key features of some of the most-used theories. We saw in earlier sections of this book that research evidence suggests that many theories converge in terms of key constructs: many terms are used for the same constructs that describe the mediators of behavior.

Your nutrition education sessions or program will use evidence and theory to address a specific issue or problem. Thus you must clearly lay out the theory or conceptual model for the intervention or program before you begin. This model will guide your nutrition education design. Consider the following in choosing your theory:

● *The nature of the audience.* For example, the health belief model, particularly the perceived risk variable, would not be useful for sessions or programs with children because they are not very concerned about their vulnerability to a health condition or disease. On the other hand, the perception of risk may be very valuable for adults, particularly older adults. The constructs of perceived benefits and perceived barriers to taking action in this model have been found to be useful in interventions with all ages.

● *The strength of the evidence for the theory constructs (mediators of behavior) used with the intended audience for the behaviors that you have selected as the focus of the program.* This is extremely important. Information on the nature of the evidence for various theories was explored in some detail in the first part of this book. But you should seek specific evidence from behavioral nutrition, nutrition education, or health education research for the behavior and audience you have selected, such as evidence from theory-based programs for increasing fruit and vegetable consumption among pregnant women, or eating more calcium-rich foods among adolescents.

You will then create an intervention model based on the theory you have chosen, incorporating evidence from ongo-

⬤ **BOX 9-1   Summary of Some Key Theories for Use in Nutrition Education**

Why Theories?
Theories help us do the following:
- Understand our audiences
- Design nutrition education interventions
- Understand how intervention works to promote change in diet and physical activity behaviors

Mediators
Mediators are influences on the behaviors of interest and come from theoretical or conceptual models of behavior. They mediate the behavioral outcomes in an intervention.

Key Theories
The theories summarized in the accompanying table are analyzed in terms of four issues:
- Motivation to change (why to change behavior or take action)
- Resources to change (how to change behavior or take action)
- Processes of change (what happens within the individual during the change process)
- Procedures or strategies of change (how to design an intervention)

	HEALTH BELIEF MODEL	**THEORY OF PLANNED BEHAVIOR**
Motivation	Level of perceived threat (severity + susceptibility) or the risk of a specific condition (readiness to act); perceived benefits and barriers (*outcome expectations*)	Positive and negative values of the outcomes of the behavior (*outcome expectations*) and the desire (or lack of desire) to comply with the expectations of important people in the person's life. Other motivators: personal norms, identities.
Resources	*Self-efficacy* influences the degree to which individuals engage in, persist at, and maintain behavior.	Perceived behavioral control (similar *to self-efficacy*).
Processes	Individuals obtain certain cues that stimulate or exacerbate their perceived threat of the disease (severity and/or susceptibility). Cue is either powerful enough or many small ones add up until a threshold is reached, at which time the person decides to take action. Which action is taken is based on perceived benefits and barriers (*outcome expectations*) and *self-efficacy* for the behaviors—the individual decides among alternative behaviors that could reduce threat.	When positive values of the outcomes of the behavior exceed the negative ones, leading to positive attitudes; social norms support behavior; and the individual has a perceived ability to carry out the behavior, the person forms an intention to take action. In the expanded version of the theory, the individual now makes implementation intentions and designs plans to carry out the behavior.
Procedures or strategies	Risk assessments and campaigns accompanied by information on strategies to reduce risk (*response efficacy*) and overcome barriers. Cues to action may work effectively in interventions, but there is little research on this	Not specifically addressed in theory, but some use of attitude-change strategies, focusing on outcome expectations and effect. In expanded version of the theory, use of goal setting and implementation plans to initiate behaviors

	SOCIAL COGNITIVE THEORY	**TRANSTHEORETICAL MODEL AND STAGES OF CHANGE**
Motivation	Achieve positive outcomes and avoid negative outcomes (*outcome expectations*).	Attain desired ends and avoid undesired ends: pros and cons of change (*outcome expectations*).
Resources	Skills and *self-efficacy* (skills are difficult to measure/study; thus, there is more focus on self-efficacy).	*Self-efficacy* and *pros and cons* in first three stages, self-efficacy in action stage. Resources for maintenance are not clearly specified.

(continued)

Box 9-1 (continued)

Processes	Attractiveness of the new behavior exceeds the negatives of that behavior, and a threshold is reached that leads the person to be motivated to try the new behavior. Whether the individual tries is determined by *self-efficacy*. Success increases self-efficacy, which increases the chances the behavior will be done again. *Self-control skills* can help people continue to do more difficult behaviors or be able to do behaviors in difficult situations.	Processes of change: the cognitive /experiential processes of consciousness-raising, dramatic relief, environmental and self-evaluation, and self-liberation more important in earlier stages; the behavioral processes of helping relationships, counterconditioning, stimulus control, and rewards more important in later stages; and social liberation important throughout.
Procedures or strategies	Goal setting and self-monitoring (*self-regulation and self-control processes*).	Activities that operationalize processes of change.

Source: Baranowski, T., K.W. Cullen, T. Nicklas, D. Thompson, and J. Baranowski. 2003. Are current health behavioral change models helpful in guiding prevention of weight gain efforts? *Obesity Research* 11(Suppl.):23S–43S.

ing research suggesting which specific theory constructs are most likely to serve as mediators of the behavior in an educational program for your particular audience. In creating your intervention model, you will specify the exact outcome expectancies, values, attitudes, affect, and self-efficacy issues (or other constructs you intend to address) and the exact supportive environmental changes you will seek to bring about. Because developing educational strategies directed at each of the mediators requires much time, energy, and other resources on your part, as well as time commitment and effort on the part of the intended audience, you will want to choose carefully the theory you use and those theory constructs that are most likely to serve as the mediators in your program. The integrative model of the determinants of behavior change discussed in Chapter 4, which combines chief features of the theory of planned behavior and social cognitive theory, is an example of an intervention model that combines compatible theories (see Figure 4-4).

Theory Use by Phases of Nutrition Education

This section discusses how theory may be useful in the different phases and components of the nutrition education intervention. The phases of nutrition education and key theories are described in Chapters 4 and 5 and summarized in Figure 9-1.

Pre-action, Motivational Phase of Nutrition Education

The educational goal in the motivational phase is to increase awareness, promote active contemplation, enhance motivation, assist the audience in understanding and resolving any ambivalence, activate decision making, and facilitate the formation of intentions to take action. Beliefs and attitudes, including feelings and emotions, are at the heart of the motivation to act, as we saw earlier in the book. This is a deliberative phase for individuals. The emphasis here is on *why to* take action and usually includes scientific evidence for why it is important to take action.

The theories and constructs outlined below are useful whether the nutrition education is one or several sessions long, a social marketing campaign, or an extensive program. In some cases, the entire program will be devoted to the educational goal of increasing awareness and enhancing deliberation and motivation for those in pre-action with respect to the selected behaviors. This design may be particularly relevant for an issue that is not familiar to audiences, such as safe food handling behaviors or folate and pregnancy. In other cases, the program may be more comprehensive, designed first to promote contemplation and increase interest and then to provide the intended audience with the abilities and opportunities to take action. In these cases, the theories and constructs that focus on motivation to act are useful in designing the motivational phase of the final intervention model

For interventions that focus on reaching those who are uncommitted, the following theories provide the most guidance on designing messages and activities that increase interest and enhance motivation. The outcome desired is the formation of an intention to act, based on active contemplation and a deliberative decision-making process. Individuals can, of course, choose not to act, and their decision needs to be respected. They will take action when they choose to do so and are ready.

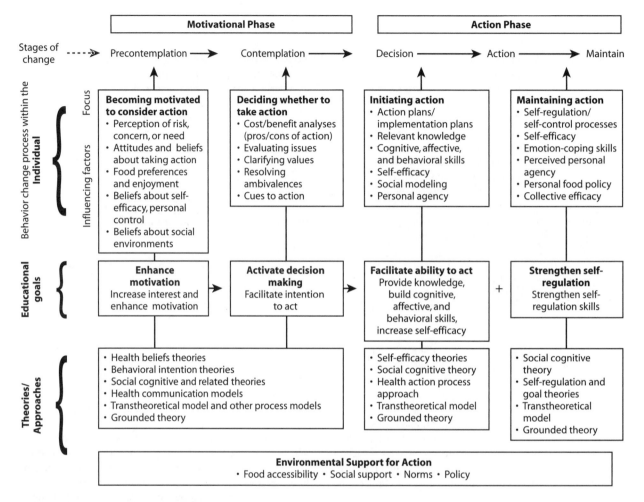

FIGURE 9-1 Conceptual framework for nutrition education.

- Psychosocial theories that focus on personal decision-making and motivational factors: attitude-change theories; the theory of planned behavior and its extensions that include considerations of affect or feelings, values, self-identities, and personal norms (including moral and ethical norms); the health belief model; risk perception theories; and the outcome expectancy and self-efficacy constructs of social cognitive theory
- Models of food choice addressing sensory-affective food factors and physiological factors, with their emphasis on food preferences and enjoyment, exposure to food and familiarity effects, emotions and mood, and physiological impacts of food on the body
- Models from grounded theory and interpretative research with this intended audience or applicable to this audience, with an emphasis on personal and cultural meanings and values and self-identities

Constructs in common that have been shown in many studies to be important motivators of food- and nutrition-related behavior and mediators of dietary change are the following:

- Outcome expectations (including perceived benefits and barriers or pros and cons of change)
- Attitudes or affect (feelings)
- Perception of risk/threat of current behavior (in some theories)
- Food preferences and enjoyment based on sensory-affective factors
- Self-efficacy or perceived control in performing the targeted behaviors
- Perceived social and personal norms and roles

Action Phase of Nutrition Education

Translating intentions into action is difficult for all of us, and assisting individuals to do so is a major task of nutrition education. Here the emphasis is on facilitating individuals' ability to take food-related actions or change their dietary behaviors. Individuals with strong intentions will form implementation intentions or begin making simple plans of action. Those with weak intentions may need some reminders and cues to action. Food- and nutrition-specific knowledge and skills are important, including food choice and food preparation skills. Critical evaluation skills may be important, where appropriate. The emphasis is on information and skills for *how to* take action.

In addition, skills in self-regulation, self-influence, exercising choice, and control of behaviors (including goal-setting and self-monitoring skills) are important in order for individuals to be able to act on their chosen motivations and intentions and to express agency. The following theories provide the most guidance in action-planning and self-regulation skills:

- Goal theories, which describe how people set goal intentions, make plans for attaining the goals, and maintain goal commitments (Gollwitzer, 1999; Bagozzi & Edwards, 1999)
- Social cognitive theory, with its emphasis on self-efficacy and self-regulation (Bandura, 1996)
- Self-efficacy and self-regulation theories (including the health action process approach) (Gollwitzer, 1999; Schwarzer, 1992; Sheeran, 2002; Sniehotta, Scholz, and Schwarzer, 2005). The transtheoretical model's emphasis on processes for relapse prevention (Prochaska & Velicer, 1997)

Constructs in common that have been shown in many studies to be important for facilitating the ability to act are as follows:

- Goal setting
- Self-efficacy
- Self-regulation skills, including goal setting and self-monitoring
- Food- and nutrition-specific knowledge and skills to enact goals, including food preparation or cooking skills, and critical evaluation skills where relevant

Both Motivational-Phase and Action-Phase Nutrition Education

In most instances, nutrition education will seek to include both motivational- and action-phase activities—both why-to and how-to education. This can occur at varying levels of depth and breadth. That is, one can begin with motivational activities and conclude with how-to activities in one session. Each of these components would, of course, be brief in this

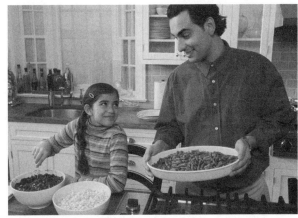

Preparing and cooking food with others reinforces nutritional goals.

instance. Or the activities can be spread over several sessions and even between components, so that health communications through the mass media, emphasizing motivational messages, can be accompanied by group sessions that focus on how-to skills.

- The extended theory of planned behavior is useful here, with its strong emphasis on motivation, accompanied by setting behavioral intentions or goals and developing implementation plans.
- The transtheoretical model, which describes processes of change for all stages and suggests that procedures or strategies for change can be based on these processes.
- Social cognitive theory. Often nutrition education interventions use social cognitive theory without the environmental component. This is not a true use of the theory but is a widespread practice. The health action process approach can also be used without the environmental component.

Promoting Relevant Environmental Supports for Taking Action on the Target Behaviors

Environments that provide opportunities to take action are important for the maintenance of action and dietary change. The following frameworks can provide guidance: social support and social network theories, coalition building, collective efficacy and empowerment frameworks, and policy building. For facilitating changes in the physical environment (food environment), coalition building and partnerships are crucial.

Constructs in common shown to be important for reducing impediments or barriers and increasing facilitators of behavior change are as follows:

- Enhancing social support for the action, including family support

- Influencing social norms to be more supportive
- Building coalitions to increase the availability and accessibility of foods and services to support the target behaviors and to promote relevant institutional policies and practices

Educational Interventions Directed at Both Phases of Nutrition Education and Accompanied by Relevant Environmental Supports

For nutrition education programs that are able to conduct activities that address both phases of nutrition education and create environmental opportunities to take action with respect to the targeted behavior(s), the following theories will be most useful: social cognitive theory, the health action process approach (Schwarzer, 1992; Sniehotta, Scholz, and Schwarzer, 2005) and the integrative model of the determinants of behavior change of the Institute of Medicine (2000), shown in Figure 4-4 (Chapter 4) and of others (Kok et al., 1996; Fishbein, 2000). The health action process approach is shown in Figure 9-2; it builds on the other theories and adds a time dimension. Other theories, such as extensions of the theory of planned behavior to include an action phase as described earlier, self-regulation theories, goal theories, and the transtheoretical (stages of change) model, can also be used if they are accompanied by coalition-building and collective-efficacy approaches for bringing about changes in the food and policy environments. The specific intervention model you will create will depend on current evidence from behavioral nutrition and nutrition education research and best practices.

Focusing on the individuals in context versus addressing multiple levels of the environment. We saw in Chapters 1 and 2 that our eating patterns are influenced by a myriad of factors. Ideally, we should thus address all those multiple lay-

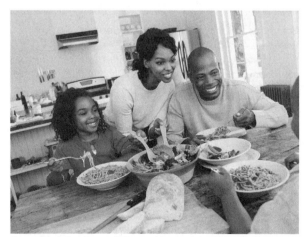

Our eating behaviors are influenced by a variety of factors.

ers of influences. However, many programs, particularly the small-scale programs conducted by most nutrition education practitioners, cannot address all these levels by themselves. Although nutrition education focuses primarily on activities conducted in person with groups and on indirect education through various kinds of media and social marketing, it also seeks to promote supportive environments by (1) educating individuals and organizations who are providers of food and nutrition services or who have policy-making power and authority over some aspect of the physical or social environment, and (2) working in collaboration with them to increase the opportunities for the intended audience to take action. These service providers and policy makers may include school food service personnel, food vendors in other settings, food-assistance programs, grocery stories and eating places, public health agencies, community leaders, and policy makers. If they become convinced of the importance of nutrition education, they can become intermediaries or partners in the nutrition education process.

To educate these policy makers, we can use the same theories and models described previously for our primary audience (i.e., models for enhancing motivation and facilitating the ability to take action), but now directed at a different audience. To build partnerships with these providers and policy makers, we will need to use models for coalition building and collective efficacy. These professionals and organizations may have a primary focus on addressing a variety of spheres of influence. For example, public health nutritionists focus on public health policy, systems, and services. Farmers provide food and focus on food system issues. School superintendents make decisions about the school environment. School food service professionals make decisions about which foods will be served. Effective nutrition education thus includes collaboration with a wide variety of individuals and organizations with differing interests and skills. You will need to decide on the kinds of collaboration you will be able to engage in given the scope of your program and the resources available to you.

Articulating a Philosophy of Nutrition Education for the Program

Regardless of the theory you have selected, your choice of *approach* to designing nutrition education sessions or programs and how you translate behavioral theory into educational practice will be very much influenced by your perspective or philosophy of nutrition education, so this philosophy should be clarified before you begin. As nutrition educators with considerable background in the natural sciences, we don't think of ourselves as using philosophy in our work, but we all do.

This book defines nutrition education as a set of educational strategies, accompanied by environmental supports, designed to facilitate the voluntary adoption of food- and

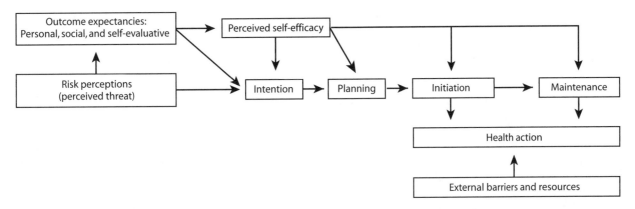

FIGURE 9-2 The health action process approach. *Source:* Used with permission of the author, R. Schwarzer, Freie Universität, Berlin, Germany.

nutrition-related behaviors that are conducive to long-term health and well-being. How we understand this process of facilitation, however, will be influenced by our philosophy, here referring to our system of values. We saw in Chapter 1 that for many reasons it is almost impossible for nutrition education to be value-free even if it wants to be. Hence the view of nutritionist Jean Mayer (1986) seems appropriate: that nutrition education has the value-laden goal of improving the health and well-being of individuals and communities. Indeed, nutrition education, along with health education, allied health professions, social work, and similar professions, is often described as a "helping" profession. There is, of course, a dilemma for us here, because there is a tension between the act of helping on our part and human agency or self-determination on the part of participants. For those of us in the nutrition profession, then, our philosophy about "helping" is particularly important.

This book has taken the position that nutrition education is about *facilitating* the voluntary adoption of behaviors conducive to health and well-being. This means that although food behaviors are voluntarily chosen, we have a role in enhancing awareness, promoting active contemplation, and assisting individuals to understand their own motivations and values and resolve their ambivalences so that they can decide whether or not to act. We also have a role in facilitating the ability to take action and enlarging individuals' environmental opportunities for action. You or your nutrition education team will need to carefully consider your *own* attitudes or convictions regarding this issue. We all bring with us to any educational activity many assumptions that we are not always aware of or do not articulate to ourselves or to others. Among these is what it means to us to be of help or, as some would prefer to say it, to be of assistance. Many of us say we want to make a difference in the world. What does that mean? Perhaps you believe your role is simply to provide information and skills, with the decision about taking action

entirely the personal responsibility of individuals. Or maybe you believe that the role of nutrition education is to encourage people to eat more healthfully.

One way to approach these issues, proposed by Brickman and colleagues (1982), is to think about who is responsible for the problem (that is, who is to blame for the current condition, such as a person's type 2 diabetes or obesity) and who is responsible for the solution in a given situation (that is, who is to control future events) and therefore what "helping" or "educating" means. Based on these attributions of responsibility, Brickman and associates proposed four models (Table 9-1):

- *Medical model:* Individuals are not responsible for problems or solutions. This philosophical perspective is called the medical model because in this instance neither the individual's health condition, such as type 2 diabetes or obesity, nor its solution is seen as the individual's responsibility. Individuals are *in need of treatment* by professionals, using medication or drugs,

TABLE 9-1 Models of Helping and Coping

Self Responsible for the Problem	Self Responsible for the Solution	
	High	**Low**
High	Moral model (Need motivation)	Enlightenment model (Need discipline)
Low	Compensatory model (Need power)	Medical model (Need treatment)

Source: Based on Brickman, P., V.C. Rabinowitz, J. Karuza, D. Coates, E. Cohn, and L. Kidder. 1982. Models of helping and coping. *American Psychologist* 37:368–384.

perhaps. Many professionals and group participants like the medical approach because it seems to promise a quick solution and permits people to accept assistance without being blamed for their condition. It may be a suitable model for certain situations or conditions, especially emergencies related to a medical condition such as diabetes. Achterberg and Trenkner (1990) note, however, that the medical model is a special case of the more general approach of paternalism. In this approach, the nutritionists are the experts, the dominant figures, who have the information—and hence power—and tend to take control of decisions, leaving little room for the autonomy of the audience members. Education using this model can be coercive because participants may not be told about acceptable alternatives and given a choice about which actions, if any, they wish to take. Even if benign, this approach can create dependency on the part of participants.

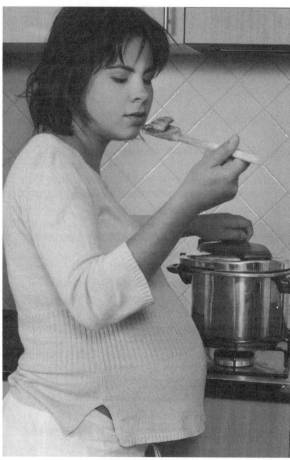

A pregnant woman's health goals may include preparing meals with the proper nutrients for two people.

- *Moral model:* Individuals are responsible for both problems and solutions. This philosophical perspective is at the other end of the spectrum from the medical model. Here the individuals are considered to have full personal responsibility for having created their problems and also for solving them. They have personal agency or control. They are primarily *in need of motivation.* This is a widely accepted perspective. In a free society with freedom of choice, and in a food system that offers 50,000 food items in the typical supermarket, individuals have control over their own food intake. Hence their health conditions are the result of their own choices and actions. The role of nutrition educators in this model is to increase interest and enhance motivation. However, this approach can result in "person blame," in which people are blamed for their conditions, such as heart disease. It becomes easy to ignore the fact that genetic factors affect health, as do powerful environmental forces and social conditions that shape and reinforce behavior, and resource considerations that limit choices for some.

- *Enlightenment model:* Individuals are responsible for problems but are not responsible for solutions. In this philosophical perspective, individuals recognize and accept that their lifestyles and health behaviors have led to problematic consequences (weight gain, hypertension, or type 2 diabetes) but feel that they cannot do much about it. They need to be enlightened about the true nature of their problem(s) and are primarily *in need of enlightenment and discipline,* which can often be supplied by some outside force. Thus, those in Overeaters Anonymous believe that they are responsible for their overeating or weight problems but need an outside authority or group to help them gain control over their behavior and their lives.

- *Compensatory model:* Individuals are not responsible for problems but are responsible for solutions. Here, individuals are not blamed for their current condition or problems but are held responsible for solving these problems. They have to compensate or cope with the particular problems they have. In this philosophical perspective, individuals are seen as suffering problems that are not of their own making, but which instead result from the failure of their social environment to provide them with the goods and services to which they are entitled, such as accessibility to nutritious, wholesome food or to education. Individuals are thus primarily *in need of power.* The role of the nutrition educator is to mobilize resources for them and/or to assist them to acquire the skills of collective efficacy or empowerment to deal effectively with the environment. When we refer to populations as "resource poor," we are acknowledging that the food or nutrition issues they may have are a result of environmental forces rather than their own actions.

Of these perspectives, Brickman and coworkers prefer the compensatory model because it is the only one that resolves the dilemma: it justifies the act of helping or assisting (because individuals are not responsible for their problems) but still leaves the individuals with active control over their lives (because they are responsible for using this help to find a solution if they wish). They also point out that it is important that the health professional (nutrition educator) and the intended audience have the same expectations and subscribe to the same philosophical perspective in terms of the particular intervention. At the least, they should be aware of each others' philosophical perspectives and resolve any differences in expectation.

Another way to look at the issue is to consider the relative responsibilities of the nutrition educator and the participants (Achterberg and Trenkner, 1990). This model is shown in Table 9-2. It is based on a model originally proposed to describe the relationships between clients and health providers, such as a physician (Roter, 1987). In this decision-making model, authoritative guidance is equivalent to the medical model in Table 9-1, and independent decision making is equivalent to the moral model. When no one takes responsibility for a health issue, no decision is made. However, this model proposes that there can be an active partnership between the educator and group members in which both are involved in joint decision making to arrive at mutually agreed-upon goals (Achterberg & Trenkner, 1990; Parham, 1990).

Others go further in emphasizing the fact that humans have agency or free will. People act, not just react. This free will, or the capacity to choose, gives human beings their unique place in the world and their human dignity. "The ability to choose provides human beings with the distinctive capacity for moral reasoning; that is, choosing on the basis of what we think is right, what we think we *ought* to do, and hence, our sense of moral responsibility, people decide what they want to do, and more significantly, at a higher, second-order level of thinking, whether they want to act on any given felt desire" (Buchanan, 2004, p. 150). In this approach, nutrition educators engage in a dialogue with individuals about ways of living that they find most worthwhile, exploring questions such as "Will losing weight help me to achieve the goals that I have set for myself? Is being physically fit the most important purpose in life?" Buchanan proposes that the nutrition educator and participants should be "fully engaged in mutual dialogue, deliberation, and debate with the aim of finding ways that we can work together to make this a better world" (Buchanan, 2004, p. 152). This model of nutrition education is similar to the moral model in that it emphasizes personal responsibility of the participant. However, a role *is* proposed for the nutrition educator, and it is similar to the joint decision-making, active participation role in the decision-making model in Table 9-2.

Self-determination theory suggests a similar approach (Deci & Ryan, 2000). This theory proposes that achievement of goal-directed behavior, and indeed of psychological development and well-being, is very much dependent on people's inherent need for autonomy, competence, and relatedness. Nutrition education that provides support for individuals' experience of autonomy, positive feedback in situations where individuals feel they are responsible for their competent actions, and a secure base of relatedness between educator and participants can lead to intrinsic motivation and integrated self-regulation or self-determination.

Health professionals have proposed, as we have here, that joint decision-making and mutual participation in the process of change proceeds best through a two-phase sequence in which motivation is first facilitated and supported by the nutrition educator or nutrition education program. This is a time to build trust, whereby feelings and expectations are expressed, and motivations are developed. In the second phase, skills are provided at a time when they are helpful, so that individuals can choose actions for change, internalize them, and then maintain the actions by themselves (Achterberg and Trenkner, 1990; Kolbe et al., 1981). Although the model of joint decision making and active participation was developed to describe one-on-one interactions, it can be applied to groups. In this case, joint decision making comes from (1) a thorough understanding of the group as the program is being designed, involving the group in the assessment process; and (2) designing session activities that are interactive, so that the audience's prior knowledge, feelings, and expectations can be incorporated and on-site corrections can be made to the lesson plan, if necessary, to suit the situation on the ground.

We have proposed two phases for nutrition education in this text, whereby in the early phase the emphasis is on

TABLE 9-2 Decision-Making Roles of Nutrition Educator and Group Participants

Nutrition Educator Responsibility	Participant Responsibility	
	Yes	**No**
Yes	Active participation	Authoritative guidance
No	Independent decision making	No decision making occurs

Sources: Modified from Achterberg, C., and L. Lytle Trenkner. 1990. Developing a working philosophy of nutrition education. *Journal of Nutrition Education* 22:189–193; and Roter, D. 1987. An exploration of health education's responsibility for a partnership model of client-provider relations. *Patient Education and Counseling* 9:25–31.

encouraging active deliberation and motivation, and in the later phase the emphasis is on empowerment through acquisition of relevant food and nutrition knowledge and skills and behavioral self-regulation skills, accompanied, where appropriate, by collective efficacy and advocacy skills to take action on the environment. Nutrition education provides the structure and educational resources to assist individuals as they seek to be motivated, willing, and able to take action, but individuals choose the goals that are important for them at any given time and by which alternatives to achieve that goal. That is, the nutrition educator has a role, and the individual has a role.

Achterberg and Trenkner (1990) provide some further thoughtful perspectives about nutrition education that are useful to consider at this time. One is that "life is open-ended," meaning that change is always possible. Thus, we should not give up on any group or individual. Maybe not now, but perhaps sometime later, the nutrition education messages and activities we have provided will become meaningful and acted upon. This also means that we can encourage the intended audience members to view change as always possible, if and when they choose to change. Maybe not now, but sometime in the future they may be in a better place to take action.

Another insight is that "humans are free agents." This makes behaviors hard to predict, because they have many rational and irrational determinants. Individuals should have "the freedom to choose their own motivations, beliefs and objectives in living; and the freedom . . . to select among alternatives that can, or might, bring about those objectives" (Achterberg & Trenkner, 1990). "Life is difficult" for both our intended audience and for us. We have to accept that our intended audience members have many issues and concerns in life, and nutrition may not be a high priority at the time of our nutrition education activity. We also have to accept that nutrition education is difficult and that we experience many professional dilemmas for which there are no easy solutions.

Nutrition Education in Action 9-1 and 9-2 contain example statements of the philosophies and perspectives of some programs. The philosophy and perspectives of the case study are shown at the end of the chapter.

Clarifying the Program's Perspective on Nutrition Content

All of us have a point of view about the content of nutrition education. This book has taken the stance that the content of nutrition education is broad, focusing on behaviors that are conducive to the health and well-being of individuals, their communities, and their food systems. This scope is similar to that stated by the Society for Nutrition Education in its mission and vision statements: "healthy, sustainable food choices" and "healthy people in healthy communities."

You, or the nutrition education planning group, will also need to clarify your own or the organization's stand on substantive issues related to the scope and content of the educational intervention that you are designing, both in broad terms and in specific ones. Now is the time to consider how the intervention will treat the issues in your program, such as the following:

- *Food production issues.* Will you consider how food is grown, processed, and transported in your recommendations regarding foods to eat? When you encourage a group to increase their fruit and vegetable intake, will you suggest any particular source? For example, will you recommend fruits and vegetables from all sources—fresh, frozen, canned, local, flown in from another country? If you will be working with a school or workplace to increase the number and variety of fruits and vegetables offered, will you be concerned about the source of these, such as whether they are from local farmers or whether they are organic? This will influence your messages as well as any environmental component that you may design, such as a farm-to-school approach.
- *All-foods fit.* Will you take the stance that there are no "good foods" or "bad foods," that is, that all foods fit into a healthful diet? Or will you take the stance that while all foods fit, some foods are more nutritious than others and use a "sometimes foods" and "anytime foods" approach, or some other approach?
- *Whole foods versus fortified and processed foods.* What will be your stance on using fortified foods (e.g., highly processed cereal fortified with vitamins) to obtain nutrients or on eating whole foods (e.g., whole-grain cereals)?
- *Weight.* Will you encourage health at every size or will you encourage weight control or weight loss along with healthy eating?
- *Breastfeeding.* Will you favor breastfeeding or bottle-feeding, or will you promote both as equally acceptable nutritional alternatives? This will influence your design of educational content.
- *Supplements.* Will you recommend supplements or not?
- *Sweetened beverages.* What will the intervention recommend on this issue, particularly if it is a school-based intervention that involves school meals or school food policy?
- *Genetically engineered foods.* What is your stance on genetically engineered foods? What will you say in your educational sessions? Will you be concerned about this issue when you choose foods for your environmental component, if you will have one?

NUTRITION EDUCATION IN ACTION 9-1

The Wellness IN the Rockies (WIN the Rockies) Project

Project Description and Philosophy

Project: WIN the Rockies is a research, education, and outreach project that seeks to address obesity innovatively and effectively.

Philosophy: People have responsibilities for their own health, but communities need to create environments that foster good health and provide healthy options.

Mission: To assist communities in educating people to

- Value health
- Respect body-size differences
- Enjoy the benefits of self-acceptance
- Enjoy healthful and pleasurable eating

Components for Adults, Children, and Patients

Adults

- *A New You: Health for Every Body.* Ten one-hour sessions for small groups that can be mixed, combined, or taught independently.
- *Cook Once: Eat for Two Weeks.* A family mealtime program that can be used in a class setting or as a do-it-yourself program. It involves recipes and food purchasing directions.
- *WIN Steps.* A community walking program.

Children

- *WIN Kids Lessons.* Thirteen lessons for youth that address food and eating, physical activity, and respect for body-size differences.
- *WIN Kids Fun Days.* A collection of 40 activities for youth.
- *WIN the Rockies Jeopardy.* A question and answer game for youth.

Patients

- *Goal-setting forms.* Health improvement goals for adult patients in consultation with their health care providers.

Source: University of Idaho, Montana State University, and University of Wyoming. 2005. A community-based research, intervention, and outreach project to improve health in Idaho, Montana, and Wyoming. www.uwyo.edu/wintherockies. Accessed 7/28/05.

Clarifying the Program's Perspective on Use of Educational Materials from a Variety of Sources

Nutrition education interventions are often not well funded and therefore cannot afford to develop and print their own high-quality educational materials. Instead, they use educational materials from a variety of sources. These are often of high quality and visually appealing. These sources may be from nonprofit voluntary organizations such as heart associations or cancer societies, or from the food industry or other businesses. You and your team should carefully discuss the pros and cons of using materials from other sources and decide your policy regarding the use of such materials. You might want to consider the following guidelines for good

practice that were established by the International Organization of Consumers Unions (1990):

- *Accuracy.* Information must be consistent with established fact or best evidence. It should be appropriately referenced so that it can be easily verified.
- *Objectivity.* All major or relevant points of view are fairly presented. If the issue is controversial, arguments in favor must be balanced by arguments against. The sponsor bias should be clearly stated, and reference to opposing views should be made.
- *Completeness.* The materials contain all relevant information and do not deceive or mislead by omission or commission.

NUTRITION EDUCATION IN ACTION 9-2

Team Nutrition Objectives, Philosophy, and Components

Overview
The U.S. Department of Agriculture's Team Nutrition is an integrated plan for promoting health in America's schools. The goal of Team Nutrition is to improve children's lifelong eating and physical activity habits through nutrition education based on the principles of the Dietary Guidelines for Americans and MyPyramid. promotes comprehensive, behavior-based nutrition education to enable children to make healthy eating and physical activity choices. Social cognitive theory is the foundation of efforts to help children understand how eating and physical activity affect the way they grow, learn, play, and feel today as well as the relationship of their choices to lifelong health. These efforts are designed to increase their understanding that healthy eating and physical activity are fun and that skills developed today will assist them in enjoying healthy eating and physical activity in later years.

Because studies show that eating habits established early in life tend to persist into adulthood, Team Nutrition focuses primarily, though not exclusively, on children in preschool, elementary, and middle school grades. All Team Nutrition messages are based on the *Dietary Guidelines for Americans* and MyPyramid.

Strategies
Team Nutrition has three strategies to change behavior:
1. Provide training and technical assistance to child nutrition food service professionals to enable them to prepare and serve nutritious meals that appeal to students and meet nutritional standards
2. Promote nutrition education in schools through multiple communication channels to build skills and motivation for children to make healthy food and physical activity choices as part of a healthy lifestyle. Flexible curriculum modules address the behaviors listed below.
3. Build school and community support for creating healthy school environments that are conducive to healthy eating and physical activity.

Behaviors
All program materials encourage students to make food and physical activity choices for a healthy lifestyle. They focus on five behavior outcomes:
- Eat a variety of foods.
- Eat more fruits, vegetables, and whole grains.
- Eat lower-fat foods more often.
- Get your calcium-rich foods
- Be physically active.

Team Nutrition Values
1. We believe that children should be empowered to make food and physical activity choices that reflect the *Dietary Guidelines for Americans*.
2. We believe that good nutrition and physical activity are essential to children's health and educational success.
3. We believe that school meals that meet the *Dietary Guidelines for Americans* should taste good and appeal to children.
4. We believe our programs must build upon the best science, education, communication, and technical resources available.
5. We believe that school, parent, and community teamwork is essential to encouraging children to make food and physical activity choices for a healthy lifestyle.
6. We believe that messages to children should be age appropriate and delivered in language they speak, through media they use, in ways that are entertaining and actively involve them in learning.
7. We believe in focusing on positive messages regarding food and physical activity choices children can make.
8. We believe it is critical to stimulate and support education and action at the national, state, and local levels to help children develop healthy eating and physical activity behaviors.

(continues)

Nutrition Education in Action 9-2 (continued)

Communication Channels

Six communication channels are utilized:

- Food service initiatives
- Classroom activities
- School-wide events
- Home activities
- Community programs and events
- Media events and coverage

These channels offer a comprehensive network for delivering consistent nutrition messages to children and their caretakers that will educate them about the importance of healthy eating and reinforce the messages through a variety of sources.

Source: U.S. Department of Agriculture, Food and Nutrition Service. 2005. *Changing the scene: Improving the school nutrition environment.* Alexandria, VA: Author. The numerous activities that are part of the program are available on the Web at http://www.fns.usda.gov/tn/. Accessed 7/25/05.

- *Nondiscriminatory.* The text and illustrations are free of any reference or characteristics that could be considered derogatory or that stereotype a particular group.
- *Noncommercial.* Sponsored material that is specifically designated as being for educational use should be clearly presented as such. Promotional materials should not be presented as "educational." There should be no implied or explicit sales message or exhortation to buy a product or service. Corporate identification should be used to identify the sponsor of the material and provide contacts for further information, but text and illustrations should be free of the sponsor's brand names, trademarks, and so forth.

Articulating Your Needs and Approach as a Nutrition Educator

Team members each need to clarify the following:

- Personal philosophy on nutrition education, if not answered previously.
- Skill level: experience in teaching, conducting workshops, designing health fairs, developing materials, and so forth; professional experience, such as in Cooperative Extension Service; level of understanding of nutrition and food and food systems issues (one or several courses in nutrition, graduate work).
- Preferred style of providing sessions for groups, such as lectures, discussion, hands-on activities, group work, field projects, food demonstrations, or cooking with groups.
- Personal priorities and motivations for being a nutrition educator. Why do you want to educate people about nutrition? What made you want to enter the field?

If you will be designing and/or delivering the nutrition education as a team, you may want to discuss these issues openly so that you can integrate team members' individual preferences and skills into the plan and create activities that use your complementary skills.

Selecting the Program Components or Channels

Depending on the scope of the intervention and the resources available, the program may consist of only a few sessions or of many components that involve many channels, such as group sessions, health fairs, lunch room signage, a Web component, or a media campaign.

Let us assume that you have chosen social cognitive theory as your theoretical framework. Thus you want the program to address the personal and environmental mediators of the behaviors targeted in your program. Because this theory is an extremely complex and complete model if used in its entirety,

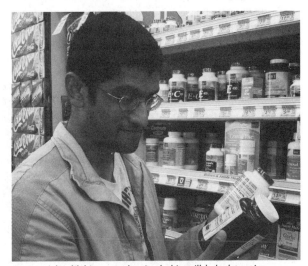

A person's health history and eating habits will help determine whether or not you recommend use of supplements.

▶ BOX 9-2 Elements of Effectiveness for Nutrition Education

General

- Nutrition education is more likely to be effective when it focuses on specific food choice behaviors or diet-related practices.
- Nutrition education interventions are more likely to be effective when they employ educational strategies that are directly relevant to the behavioral focus and are derived from appropriate theory and prior research evidence.

Communications and Educational Strategies for Enhancing Awareness and Motivation

- Addressing the motivators that have personal meaning for the particular population group is of primary importance.
- Taking into account the group's stage of motivational readiness to take action and adopt dietary change may improve effectiveness.
- Use of personalized self-assessment of nutritional status or food-related behaviors and feedback in comparison with recommendations can enhance motivation.
- Direct experience with food can enhance enjoyment of healthy food, motivation, and self-efficacy.
- Active participation is important.
- The effectiveness of communications through nonpersonal media such as letters, newsletters, and Web-based approaches can be enhanced by individually tailoring the messages.
- Mass media health campaigns can increase awareness of issues, affect beliefs and attitudes, and increase knowledge of targeted behaviors.
- A systematic audience-centered planning framework, such as social marketing, is a useful tool for targeting strategies to specific audiences.
- A variety of nontraditional channels show promise.

Strategies for Facilitating the Ability to Take Action and Maintain Behavioral Change

- Use of a systematic goal-setting and self-regulation process that fosters people's agency is most likely to be effective in facilitating individuals' ability to take action and maintain change. In this process, individuals are provided opportunities to conduct accurate self-assessments and compare them with recommendations; learn of effective behaviors for healthful and enjoyable eating; choose among alternatives to set their own goals; learn the cognitive, affective, and behavioral skills needed to achieve their goals; monitor their progress toward goal attainment; and experience a sense of agency or self-influence and control.
- Adequate attention to the complexity of food-specific issues is important.
- Use of small groups is likely to improve the effectiveness of nutrition education interventions.
- Social support such as family and peer involvement is important in all population groups and should be incorporated.
- Cultural appropriateness or sensitivity, along with behavioral theory, can enhance effectiveness.
- Long-term maintenance of food choices and behavior change is enhanced with (1) the use of a general framework, rather than a prescriptive diet, so as to enhance individuals' sense of control over their own diets; (2) continued experience of the new way of eating to increase familiarity and enjoyment; and (3) opportunity to develop personal food policies.

Environmental Interventions

- Educating and collaborating with policy makers, service providers, organizations, and agencies are important for promoting healthful food environments in schools, workplaces, and communities.
- Facilitating communities' collective efficacy or agency to create environments that foster good health and provide healthy options is likely to enhance individuals' ability to take action.
- Delivering nutrition education through multiple venues and directed at multiple levels of influence enhances dietary change.

Nutrition Educator Factors

- The credibility and trustworthiness of the nutrition educator enhance audiences' willingness to respond and accept the message. Open-mindedness and fairness engender a safe learning environment.
- Being organized is key to being effective. This allows for wise use of time and increased participant interest and engagement as well as enhanced credibility for the nutrition educator.
- The educator's ability to adapt to the situation on the ground is important for implementation of the intervention.
- Sensitivity to the audience is crucial to the effectiveness of nutrition education. This includes being appropriate in terms of developmental level and age-related concerns as well as sensitivity in terms of the culture and resources of the audience.

Sources: Contento, I.R., G.I. Balch, S.K. Maloney, et al. 1995. The effectiveness of nutrition education and implications for nutrition education policy, programs and research. *Journal of Nutrition Education* 127:279–418; Ammerman, A.S., C.H. Lindquist, K.N. Lohr, and J. Hersey. 2002. The efficacy of behavioral interventions to modify dietary fat and fruit and vegetable intake: A review of the evidence. *Preventive Medicine* 35(1):25–41; and Pomerleau, J., K. Lock, C. Knai, and M. McKee. 2005. Interventions designed to increase adults' fruit and vegetable intake can be effective: A systematic review of the literature. *Journal of Nutrition* 135:2486–2495.

you have decided that the intervention model will focus on only the following key personal potential mediating variables: physical outcome expectations (benefits, including taste), social outcome expectations (social norms), and self-evaluative expectations, along with self-efficacy as a motivational variable, and goal-setting and behavioral capabilities (food- and nutrition-related knowledge and skills) as variables that facilitate action and only modest environmental change.

You are now ready to brainstorm and then select how many and which program components you will design to address these mediators. As noted previously, your choice will depend to some extent on the scope of the intervention and the resources available. Box 9-2 summarizes the key elements that contribute to the effectiveness of nutrition education interventions, as determined by reviews of studies. You should consider these as you choose your channels and components.

Thus, for a workplace intervention, will you plan group sessions only, or will you use other channels as well, such as health fairs, lunch room food item signage, and a media campaign? Will you be able to facilitate changes in what is available in the cafeteria and/or vending machines? Will you be able to include a physical activity component? Will you be able to offer a family component?

For a school-based program, will you design a student classroom curriculum only? Or will you include food-tasting activities in the cafeteria, posters, and health fairs as well? For changes in the environmental determinants, will you be able to work with the school food service director to make changes in school meals? Will you be able to initiate or support a food or health policy council? Will you involve the parents? If so, how—through newsletters or activities to be taken home and activities to be done by students and family together? Will you organize family nights? For a food stamp–eligible population, will you design group nutrition education sessions for participants only? Will you include a mass media campaign? Will you be able to collaborate with others to make vouchers available for participants at farmers' markets?

In our continuing case study of increasing fruit and vegetable intake among middle school students, the components might include a classroom curriculum, a parent component, changes in school food policies and environment, and a school meals component.

The answers to these questions and the determination of how extensive your nutrition education intervention should be or how many components it should have depend on answers to questions such as the following.

1. What types of components or what channels are usually used in programs with this audience for the goal behaviors of your program that you identified in Step 1?

   Review the literature on evaluated, or even nonevaluated, programs. Look into programs described on the

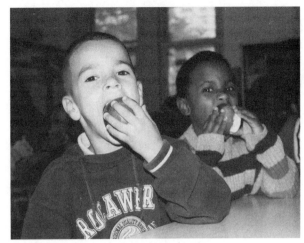

Every individual has a part in nutrition education.

Web. For programs with children and youth, the primary components are usually those directed toward school curricula, the school environment, the school food service, after-school programs, family, peers, and relevant community institutions such as the Girl and Boy Scouts to which youth may belong. With adults, the primary sites for nutrition education have been workplaces, community agencies, cooperative extension program sites, outpatient clinics, and churches. In these sites, program components are usually directed at the primary audience (e.g., employees; attendees of an organization's activities, such as a congregation) and their families.

2. What does the evidence suggest are the most effective components to use for your audience and behavior?

   The first section of this book has provided some evidence. You can now seek out more specific information for your intended audience (e.g., African American adolescent youth) and behavior (e.g., eating calcium-rich foods) from a review of research studies or existing effective programs. What intervention duration is needed to achieve action or change, based on the evidence?

3. What resources will you have? What is the time frame available?

   Personnel and skills: How many nutrition education personnel will be available for this program? What skills do you collectively possess? For development of the program, you will need skills in creating exciting activities for the audience, artistic skills to develop attractive materials, and desktop publishing abilities. To the extent possible, use resources that are already available. However, you still need to adapt materials for your own sessions and program. For delivery of the program, you will need skills in working with groups or in providing professional development regarding your project for others who will work with you, such as teachers or community leaders. If you plan on evaluating the program, you will also need skills in evaluation. This text seeks to help you acquire or hone these skills.

Time: You will need to allow time to develop the program, no matter how short or long it is: time for conducting the issue identification or needs analysis process, writing lessons, developing handouts, creating needed artwork, pilot testing (if your program is more than a one-time event), and developing evaluation instruments. In terms of implementation, you will also need to be clear about how much time will be available to you in the setting in which you intend to conduct the program. In schools, it is difficult to get more than six or seven 45-minute periods of class time. In community settings, attendance at more than three to six sessions is difficult to achieve. The time frame will determine how many goals and objectives you can write and how many activities you can conduct.

Money: You will need money for the handouts, student or participant activity sheets, and other materials that you develop. In schools, you usually also need money for binders for students and manuals and stipends for teachers. In nutrition education, money for food is always an important consideration. It is effective to bring samples of what you are talking about or food items to taste, or items to cook, if food preparation is being considered. This usually means that you will also need to supply plates and utensils for the group. If you use mass mailing, there are costs for mailing and postage and other media costs.

4. What collaborations will you include?

Many nutrition education programs need to involve collaborations with other people and organizations in order to accomplish nutrition education goals. You will need to seek these out: school district superintendents or principals, school food service directors, public health agencies, parent–teacher organizations, workplaces, community leaders and organizations, churches and other religious institutions, or existing task forces or coalitions.

5. What products will you need to produce?

Whether for one session or for a more extensive program, you will need to develop the materials you will use in the program. Even for one session with adults, you will need to develop a lesson plan plus all the materials you will use, such as overhead or PowerPoint slides, worksheets, and handouts. To the extent possible, use existing materials. For school-based programs, you will need a manual that includes the classroom component activities or curriculum; student activity worksheets and homework; and perhaps computer-based activities or videotapes, recipes for classroom food activities, or rewards. You may also need a teacher professional development manual. For environmental support activities, you may need to help school food service staff develop recipes. You may also need to develop school food service training manuals and cafeteria posters.

For workplace or community-based programs, you will need a manual that includes the lesson plans of group session activities, brochures, handouts, worksheets, and other materials. These materials all need to be designed to look catchy, inviting, professional, coherent, and appropriate to the audience as well as true to the goals and objectives of the program. The previous considerations of personnel, time, and money will help you decide how many of these materials you will be able to produce and who will produce them. Examples of program components and products are shown in Table 9-3.

Conclusions

Based on these considerations, you will need to decide which components to incorporate into your program. You may plan group sessions with the audience only, or secondary audience activities as well. For example, in a school-based setting,

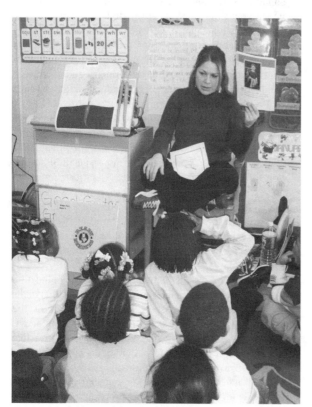

Connecting children with how food is grown is important in some nutrition education programs: Reading a letter from Farmer Betty.

TABLE 9-3 Potential Program Components and Products: Examples

Program Components	Potential Program Products
School-based program	Classroom curriculum or manual of lessons/activities for the 12 sessions
Classroom component: 12- session program	Student activity sheets and homework
	Audiotapes and videotapes
	Computer and website activities
	Incentives and rewards
	Snack preparation and taste-testing recipes
Teacher professional development sessions: 2	Teacher professional development manual
Family involvement component:	
• Educational sessions: 2	Family educational session manual (2 sessions)
• Other activities	Family educational session materials
	Family activities done by family and youth at home (5)
	Newsletters and other mailed information (2)
	Recipes and tip sheets for family activities (10)
	Family fun nights (2) protocols
School environment (through collaborations)	
• School food service changes	School food service professional development manuals; menu modification manual
• School food policies	School food environment assessment tools
	School food and health policy councils' recruitment and activity protocols
	School food and health policy manuals
• School informational environment	Classroom and cafeteria posters
Workplace programs	
Worksite educational component	
• Kickoff event	Protocol for kickoff activities
• Educational sessions: 6	Manual of lessons/activities for the 6 sessions
	Activity sheets, handouts
• Activities	Health fair protocol
	Food demonstration protocol
	Cholesterol screening equipment and education protocol
	Nutrition quizzes
• Information distribution	Brochures and self-assessment with feedback materials
Worksite environment component (through collaborations)	Worksite food environment assessment tools
	Employee councils' recruitment and activity protocols
• Worksite food service offerings	Recommended menu offerings/modification manual
• Catering policies	Catering policy document
• Information environment	Nutrition information in cafeterias (signage) and vending machines
Family component	Family newsletters, activity sheets, recipes, tip sheets
Community programs	
Community educational component: 4 sessions	Manual of lessons/activities for the 4 sessions
	Activity sheets, handouts
	Snack preparation and taste-testing recipes
	Cooking classes: Protocols for teaching skills, recipes
	Incentives and rewards
Social marketing component	Social marketing materials
Farmers' market component: 2 tours	Manual for farmers' markets tours
	Recipes and handouts

you may choose to plan activities for the children only or for teachers and parents as well. With adults in the workplace, you may choose for the intervention to be directed at employees only, or you may plan to involve managers and the families of employees. The intervention activities may involve direct education with group sessions only; an extended program; use of audiovisual or print media, including Web-based activities; health fairs; billboards; and other community activities. You may decide to capitalize on the opportunities to collaborate with others to increase the opportunities to engage in the particular food choices or behaviors targeted by the intervention through policy changes or changes in the food environment.

Some examples of the philosophy, vision, and components of programs were shown earlier. Box 9-3 adds an example of the types of components recommended for school-based program to promote healthful eating habits.

Your Turn

Using Worksheet 9-1, review the issue or need that is of concern, your intended audience, and the behaviors that are the focus of your sessions or program. You and/or your planning group should now select the theory you will use to design the nutrition education intervention and create the specific intervention model. Now is also the time to clarify the philosophical perspective of the program in terms of educational approach and food and nutrition content. You should also determine the number of components and which channels or venues you will use. *At this point, you do not need to plan the details of activities for these various venues and channels.* That will come in the next few chapters. Here you need only decide which components and channels you will incorporate so that you can write goals and objectives and design appropriate activities for each of these components.

> ### BOX 9-3　Guidelines for School Health Programs to Promote Healthful Eating

Based on the available scientific literature, national nutrition policy documents, and current practice, the Centers for Disease Control and Prevention provided the following broad recommendations for ensuring a quality nutrition program within a comprehensive school health program.

- *Policy:* Adopt a coordinated school nutrition policy that promotes healthy eating through classroom lessons and a supportive school environment.
- *Curriculum for nutrition education:* Implement nutrition education from preschool through secondary school as part of a sequential, comprehensive school health education curriculum designed to help students adopt healthy eating behaviors.
- *Instruction for students:* Provide nutrition education through developmentally appropriate, culturally relevant, fun, participatory activities that involve social learning strategies.
- *Integration of school food service and nutrition education:* Coordinate school food service with nutrition education and other components of the comprehensive school health program to reinforce messages on healthy eating.
- *Professional development for staff:* Provide staff involved in nutrition education with adequate pre-service and in-service professional development that focuses on teaching strategies for behavioral change.
- *Family and community involvement:* Involve family members and the community in supporting and reinforcing nutrition education.
- *Program evaluation:* Regularly evaluate the effectiveness of the school health program in promoting healthy eating and change the program as appropriate to increase its effectiveness.

Source: Centers for Disease Control and Prevention. 1996. Guidelines for school health programs to promote lifelong healthy eating. *Morbidity and Mortality Weekly Report* 45(RR-9):1–41.

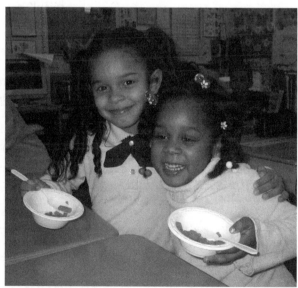

School food service can provide an opportunity for children to taste and enjoy new vegetables.

You are now ready to embark on a most interesting, and challenging, process: writing the educational goals and objectives that will address the mediators of the targeted behavior that you identified in Step 2, using the theory or conceptual map you have selected in Step 3 to guide your intervention. This task is described in the next chapter.

Case Study

The case study for our ongoing hypothetical program to promote more healthful eating by adolescents appears here. Five behaviors were identified as being of nutritional concern, but we have the space to explore only one of them—eating more fruits and vegetables. The case study presents the theory, educational philosophy, and components for Taking Control: Eating Well and Being Fit. Use it as an example to help you think through your philosophy, select your theoretical framework to design your own nutrition education sessions or program, and select the components you will incorporate.

Questions and Activities

1. Describe at least three criteria that nutrition educators should use to select which theory to use for a given nutrition education program or session.
2. From what you have learned, what are the arguments for and against combining constructs from different theories into an intervention model for a nutrition education program?
3. List, and briefly describe, three theory constructs in common to several theories that are useful in interventions that focus on increasing awareness and enhancing motivation. How might these constructs be used in developing your intervention model?
4. List, and briefly describe, three constructs in common to theories that are useful in interventions that focus on facilitating the ability to take action. How might these constructs be used in developing your intervention model?
5. Compare, contrast, and critique the medical, moral, enlightenment, compensatory, and joint decision-making models for helping and coping, indicating when and how each of them might be used in nutrition education or even if they should be used.
6. What factors should you consider as you are selecting components for your program?

WORKSHEET 9-1   **Select Theory, Philosophy, and Components**

Create a document in which you state the following for your program:

Issue and audience: _____

_____

_____

Target behaviors, practices, or actions that are the focus of the program: _____

_____

_____

Philosophy of educational approach: _____

_____

_____

Perspective on nutrition content and issues relevant to the behaviors recommended by the program: _____

_____

_____

Components: _____

_____

_____

Theoretical model for program _____

_____

_____

CASE STUDY 9-1   Step 3: Theory, Educational Philosophy, and Components

Through our analysis using the worksheets in Step 1, we identified the following.

Issue and Audience
A major national and local issue of concern is the high prevalence of overweight among youth. The mission of our agency is to work with low-income youth and their families. The primary audience we have selected is middle school youth in a school setting. The focus of the program is thus as follows: overweight prevention among middle school youth.

Target Behaviors or Practices of the Program
From Step 1, the behavioral goals of the program identified for youth are to
- Increase intake of fruits and vegetables (youth to aim for 2.5 cups or more a day)
- Decrease amount of sweetened beverages consumed each day (aim for no more than 8 ounces a day)
- Decrease number of packaged high-fat, high-sugar snacks so that they contribute no more than 150 calories a day (targets for drinks and snacks are based on the discretionary calories allowance for this age group)
- Increase physical activity to 10,000 steps a day and participate actively, when possible, in gym or other school-sponsored physical activities

Philosophy of Educational Approach
We will thus develop a program for middle school youth to address the issue of prevention of overweight. The issue of weight will not be addressed directly; instead, healthful eating and activity patterns will be emphasized.

This program believes that youth have responsibilities for their health and the power to make healthful food and activity choices, but that they need the necessary understanding, motivation, and tools to take charge in today's difficult environment. The program also believes that it is the responsibility of the school and home to provide an environment that is supportive and makes healthful options available.

The aim of this program is to assist youth increase awareness of their own behaviors and of environmental forces influencing their choices, and to enhance their ability to make healthful food choices and to overcome environmental barriers. Activities will provide them with tools to take charge of their own eating and activity patterns through goal-setting and self-regulation processes. Hence, the philosophy is that regardless of how the teens acquired their eating patterns, they need motivation to act and a sense of agency. It also recognizes that individuals need appropriate skills and environmental support, thus suggesting a compensatory model.

The aim will be carried out through a program directed at personal mediators that includes two phases: a phase that encourages analysis of self and environment, understanding, deliberation, and motivation and a phase that focuses on skills to take action. The program will also include an environmental component to provide support and increase options for the behaviors identified.

Perspective on Nutrition Content and Issues
It is also the position of this program to encourage youth to eat foods that are minimally processed, naturally nutrient dense, and fresh and local to the extent feasible given resource and availability constraints.

Components
The program will consist of three components:
- A classroom curriculum component
- A parent component
- Changes in the school environment to increase options for healthful eating.

Title of project: Taking Control: Eating Well and Being Fit

Theoretical Model for Program
From evidence in the literature and the assessments in Steps 1 and 2, we created the model shown here. It is based on the integrated model of behavior change (Institute of Medicine, 2000).

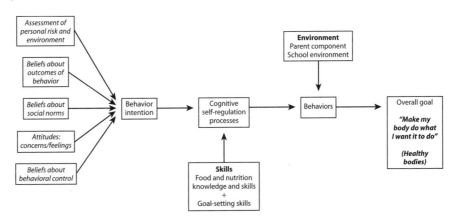

REFERENCES

Achterberg, C., and L.L. Trenkner. 1990. Developing a working philosophy of nutrition education. *Journal of Nutrition Education* 22:189–193.

Bagozzi, R.P., and E.A. Edwards. 1999. Goal striving and the implementation of goal intentions in the regulation of body weight. *Psychology and Health* 13:593–621.

Bandura, A. 1997. Self-efficacy: The exercise of control. New York: WH Freeman.

Brickman, P., V.C. Rabinowitz, J. Karuza, D. Coates, E. Cohn, and L. Kidder. 1982. Models of helping and coping. *American Psychologist* 37:368–385.

Buchanan, D. 2004. Two models for defining the relationship between theory and practice in nutrition education: Is the scientific method meeting our needs? *Journal of Nutrition Education and Behavior* 36:146–154.

Deci, E.l., and R.M. Ryan. The "what" and "why" of goal pursuits: Human needs and the self-determination of behavior *Psychological Inquiry* 2000;11(4):227–268.

Fishbein, M. 2000. The role of theory in HIV prevention. *AIDS Care* 12(3):273–278.

Gollwitzer, P.M. 1999. Implementation intentions—strong effects of simple plans. *American Psychologist* 54:493–503.

Institute of Medicine. 2002. *Speaking of health: Assessing health communication strategies for diverse populations.* Washington, DC: National Academy Press.

International Organization of Consumers Unions. 1990. Code of good practice. In *IOCU code of good practice and guidelines for business sponsored educational materials used in schools.* Policy statement. London: International Organization of Consumers Unions.

Kok, G., H. Schaalma, H. De Vries, G. Parcel, and T. Paulussen. 1996. Social psychology and health. *European Review of Social Psychology* 7:241–282.

Kolbe, L.J., D.C. Iverson, W.K. Marshal, G. Hochbaum, and G. Christensen. 1981. Propositions for an alternate and complementary health education paradigm. *Health Education* 12(3):24–30.

Mayer, J. 1986. Social responsibilities of nutritionists. *Journal of Nutrition* 116:714–717.

Parham, E. 1990. Applying a philosophy of nutrition education to weight control. *Journal of Nutrition Education* 22:194–197.

Prochaska, J.O., and W.F. Velicer. 1997. The transtheoretical model of health behavior change. *American Journal of Health Promotion* 12:38–48.

Roter, D. 1987. An exploration of health education's responsibility for a partnership model of client-provider relations. *Patient Education and Counseling* 9:25–31.

Schwarzer R. 1992. Self-efficacy in the adoption and maintenance of health behaviors: theoretical approaches and a new model. In *Self-efficacy: Thought control of action*, edited by Schwarzer R. London: Hemisphere Publishing Corporation.

Sniehotta F.F., U.R. Scholz, and R. Schwarzer. 2005. Bridging the intention-behavior gap: Planning, self-efficacy, and action control in the adoption and maintenance of physical exercise. *Psychology and Health* 20: 143–160.

Step 4: State Educational Goals and Objectives to Address Potential Mediators of Program Behaviors and Actions

OVERVIEW This chapter describes key issues in translating behavioral theory into educational objectives and environmental support objectives and describes how to do so.

OBJECTIVES At the end of the chapter, you will be able to

- Appreciate the importance of writing educational goals and objectives for nutrition education sessions and programs
- Write general educational objectives to achieve the behavioral goals of the session or program
- Write specific educational objectives to guide specific learning experiences or activities within each session or component directed at the potential personal mediators of behavior identified in Step 2
- Write educational objectives to guide activities directed at those decision makers and policy makers who can promote environmental supports of the program's targeted behaviors

SCENARIO

A middle school has invited a nutrition educator to speak at a school assembly of several health classes (about 100 students) about "the importance of good nutrition." She designed a 45-minute presentation using computer slides. Starting with a description of what teens typically eat, she discussed the components of a healthy diet, covering the major recommendations of the government's guidelines, and then talked about the importance of eating more fruits and vegetables and how to add them to the diet; of eating fewer high-energy-dense, high-fat, high-sugar foods; the importance of regular meals during the day and of selecting healthy snacks and portion sizes; and the importance of being physically active and how to be more active. She began to notice the teens were getting restless. When she ended, one teen came up, very worried, and said, "This isn't going to be on the final exam, is it? That was a lot of information and I couldn't write it all down." Another said, "I got rather confused and couldn't follow everything you said, so I'm not sure what I should be eating." Later she told a colleague about her experience. Her colleague asked her, "What was the overall educational objective of your talk? What did you hope to accomplish?" She was rather surprised. "I didn't have a specific objective," she said. "This was the only time they were going to hear about nutrition in their health class this year, so I just wanted to make sure they got lots of information so that they could make wise choices."

COMMENT

What is going on here? The nutrition educator had not clearly thought through the goal for the session, or the specific educational objectives. She had rambled on, providing a good deal of interesting information but no identifiable message. So it is not surprising that the teens would leave with no clear understanding of what to do to eat well. A clear behavioral goal and several specific educational objectives would have helped to focus the presentation and enhanced the ability of the youth to make healthy choices. Sometimes less is more—when it is well focused.

INPUTS: COLLECTING ASSESSMENT DATA		DESIGNING THE OUTPUTS			DESIGNING OUTCOMES EVALUATION
STEP 1 ←→ **Analyze needs and behaviors: Specify the behavior or action focus of the program** • Assess needs and identify audience: select need(s) or issue(s) to address • Identify behaviors of concern that contribute to need(s) or issue(s) • Select core behaviors or practices to address	**STEP 2** ←→ **Identify relevant potential mediators of program behaviors** • Identify potential personal psychosocial mediators • Identify potential environmental mediators	**STEP 3** ←→ **Select theory, philosophy, and components** • Select theory and/or create appropriate model • Articulate educational philosophy • Clarify perspectives on content • Determine program components	**STEP 4** ←→ **State educational objectives for potential mediators** • Select relevant mediators to address • State educational objectives for each selected mediator: —Personal psychosocial mediators —Environmental mediators	**STEP 5** ←→ **Design theory-based educational strategies and activities to address potential mediators** • Design strategies and activities for each selected mediator: —Personal psychosocial mediators —Environmental mediators	**STEP 6** **Design evaluation** • Design evaluation of program's impact on behaviors and mediators • Design process evaluation

Introduction

This step is *the* most crucial step in the design of theory-based nutrition education: the process of translating behavioral theory and research findings into educational activities. This is the step that is most difficult for those trained in foods and nutrition. We have learned a good deal of nutrition information and are eager to transmit that information to a variety of audiences. Even though we have read about the theories and evidence, such as those described in the first part of the book, and we have gone through Steps 1 and 2, we are likely to ignore them at this stage in our eagerness to proceed. However, by stating our goals and objectives we are giving shape to our sessions or programs and making them more effective.

In Step 1 of the procedural model for designing theory-based nutrition education, we identified the behavioral focus of the program and specified one or more core or target behaviors or practices that the program would address. In Step 2, we identified relevant determinants of these behaviors that influence the current behavior of our intended audience and those that are potential mediators for achieving the program's target behaviors. In this step we write *educational goals and objectives* directed at these mediators of behavior in order to achieve the program's targeted behavioral goals. You will go back and forth between this step and the next, because in the next step you will select educational strategies and design practical learning experiences that also address these mediators of behavior change.

Why Write Goals and Objectives?

Most of us *like* to develop educational activities for audiences and can be very creative. For example, having identified that

teenagers are not eating enough calcium-rich foods, we may immediately think of many activities that we could do to get teenagers interested in eating more of these foods. However, in the rush to develop activities, we often do not make clear the *purpose* of each activity. We may then end up with learning experiences that are active and fun but may not be specifically directed at achieving the behavioral goals of the program. These activities can be said to be *hands-on* but not necessarily *minds-on* activities.

Writing goals and objectives is *not* a favorite activity of nutrition educators—it seems to be an artificial formality. Yet, as nutrition educators, we usually have a purpose in mind for each activity; in essence, we have implicit goals or objectives. Making these explicit allows us to see whether they serve the purpose of the nutrition education program, and whether they are based on theory constructs and research evidence from both quantitative and qualitative sources. *Every* educational activity that you design should first have an explicit educational objective.

What Are Goals and Objectives?

Many different terms are used with similar meanings: *goals, objectives, performance objectives, performance indicators, behavioral objectives, educational standards, nutrition competencies,* and so forth. We should not be rigid about which terms to use. In this text, we use the terms *goals* and *objectives* with the following meanings:

- *Goals give focus to the intervention.* They describe the purpose, expectations, or desired ends of nutrition education stated in general terms. Such focusing is necessary whether for a program of several months' duration involving many components or for one or two sessions.

- *Objectives provide a road map on how to proceed.* They describe how to address the goals that have been identified. Objectives are stated in terms of specific actions to be taken to achieve the goals.

Educational Goals and Objectives

These describe the *educational* goals and objectives of the intervention for group participants, stated in general terms (program educational goals) or in specific learner terms (educational objectives or learner objectives) to help shape the design of educational activities and learning experiences to reach the identified behavioral goals. These are similar to instructional goals and objectives in the field of education. To confuse matters, however, instructional objectives are often called behavioral objectives in the field of education. In this text, *behaviors always* refers to food- and nutrition-related actions and practices, *not* to behaviors that demonstrate that cognitive learning has taken place. For example, "Participants will be able to verbally describe the food groups of MyPyramid and how many servings we should eat from each" is not considered a "behavioral objective" here even though it would be considered so by educators. We consider it a *cognitive objective*. To confuse matters even further, the health promotion and nutrition education fields talk about "goal setting" as a strategy for assisting individuals to make changes in their own personal behavior. We described that process in detail in Chapter 5. In this situation, group participants are asked to state personal behavioral "goals" that they will try to achieve ("I will eat two additional fruits and vegetable servings each day this week"). We use the term *goal setting* with this standard behavioral theory meaning in the context of behavior change skills and strategies.

Learner-Centered Education and Goals and Objectives

Learner-centered education is education in which the learner is central. It takes into account and values participants' or learners' prior knowledge, experience, and assets, includes activities that are engaging, and accepts the notion that learners are primary influencers of how the group will go. Thus it is sometimes thought that designing educational plans (lesson plans) based on stating clear goals and objectives is not necessary. But that is not the case. A good needs analysis will help you understand the group, and you need to conduct the sessions in a way that is flexible to allow you to follow group interests to some degree. However, you still need goals and objectives and lesson plans to provide a map for how to proceed. Without a clear plan, discussions can ramble, and no clear message come through. Participants often leave such sessions frustrated. Indeed, designing learning-centered education or facilitated dialogue takes more work and planning as you design learning tasks for the group.

Determine Educational Goals to Achieve the Actions or Behaviors Targeted by the Program

To achieve the behavioral goals of the program through educational means, you need to think through carefully your educational goals. These will guide your educational activities within and among program components. Throughout the text we have noted that research evidence has suggested that behavior change generally occurs through two main phases: a motivational, pre-action, deliberative phase and an action or implementation phase. We also stated that nutrition education can thus be seen as having two major educational goals: to increase awareness and enhance motivation to act (for those in the motivational, deliberative phase) and to facilitate the ability to take action (for those in the action phase). For the intervention you are planning, you or your nutrition education team should think through whether you will address one or other of the goals or both, based on your problem analysis results from Step 1. Carefully review each of the program components and decide the educational goal for each of the components. For example, what is the educational goal of the health fair component you are planning for a college campus or a workplace? To enhance awareness and increase motivation for taking action? To draw attention to other components that will provide skills, such as a cooking class?

In our case study of middle school teens, for example, there are several *behavioral goals*, such as the following:

- Youth will increase their intake of fruits and vegetables.
- Youth will increase their walking to 10,000 steps a day and participate actively, when possible, in gym or other school-sponsored physical activities.

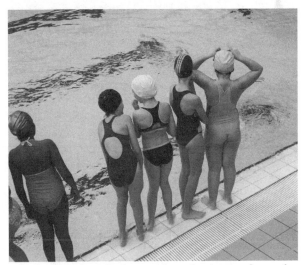

School-sponsored exercise classes such as swimming are a fun way for students to meet their physical activity requirements.

The *educational goals* could be that the program will do the following:

- Increase awareness in youth of the importance of fruits and vegetables in the diet and enhance motivation to eat them through a school curriculum and school-wide activities
- Facilitate the ability to act by providing opportunities to gain relevant food and nutrition knowledge and practice food-related skills and self-regulation skills through a school curriculum
- Educate decision makers and work with them to increase opportunities for youth to engage in healthful eating at school and home through an educational component with parents and policy initiatives in the school

Your perspective, or philosophy, on nutrition education that you identified in Step 3 will influence how you state your educational objectives. As you prepare to write your educational goals and objectives, think through who you consider to be responsible for the food issues or nutritional problems you have identified for this particular intended audience and who is responsible for the solution. Do you believe that the group needs activities to facilitate motivation, empowerment, discipline, or treatment, or some combination of these?

Your perspective, or philosophy, on food and nutrition content that you identified in Step 3 will also influence how you state your educational and environmental support objectives. Because educational objectives guide the content and strategies of the sessions, you will need to think through some issues: Is the objective of your intervention to increase fruit and vegetable intake regardless of source? Or will your objectives take into account the source of fruits and vegetables, such as local in season? Will all forms of fruits and vegetables—frozen, fresh, or canned—be presented as acceptable? In terms of environmental support objectives, will you plan to use whole or locally grown fruits and vegetables for foods served in the cafeteria, such as through a farm-to-school approach or farm-to-cafeteria approach? Or again, will all sources be equally acceptable?

Write Educational Objectives to Address Mediators of Targeted Behavior

Program components that are directed at personal psychosocial mediators of the target behaviors will focus on personal motivational factors and decision-making processes for those in the pre-action phase of dietary change, and on cognitive self-regulation skills for those in the action and maintenance phases of dietary change. Personal mediators are those that rest within the individual and have the potential of being influenced by educational or learning experiences. You will recall that personal determinants of behavior are represented as constructs in theories and may serve as mediating variables in a nutrition education program. These potential mediators include perceived risk, attitudes, affect/feelings, perceived benefits and barriers, outcome expectations, values, perceived responsibility, self-identify, self-efficacy, social norms, and goal-setting skills.

Select Relevant Mediators to Address for Identified Audience

You have already selected the theory to guide your sessions. The list of personal mediators of the selected behaviors obtained from the Step 2 assessment, expressed in terms of theory constructs, may be quite long at this point. Select those that can be realistically addressed in the sessions or program to enhance motivation or increase behavioral skills, or both, given the time and resources you have available. The list should be reduced to a manageable number based on the strength of the evidence of an association between the given mediator and the targeted behavior change itself and how sensitive the mediator is to change by an educational intervention. (In a research intervention, these might be the secondary outcomes.) You should think through carefully what you can actually accomplish in the time you have. We all have the tendency to try to cover too much.

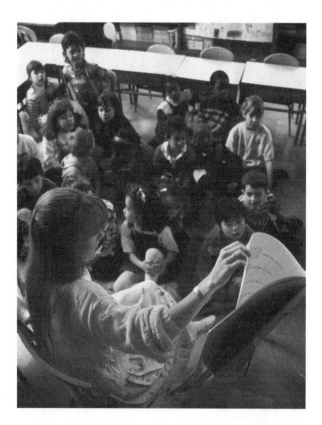

Developmentally appropriate educational objectives are important for nutrition education with children.

Write Educational Objectives for Each Potential Personal Mediator

For each personal mediator of behavior change, write one or more educational objectives to guide the design of educational activities to address that mediator. These objectives provide ways to convert mediators to a form that is useful for guiding the design of learning activities.

The objectives are expressed in terms of the learner or participant and are thus often called *learning objectives*. This term is often used interchangeably with *educational objectives* because learning is what the participant does, and educating is what we do to encourage learning. Both terms refer to the same activity with the same desired outcomes. Both terms are used in this text, but *educational objectives* will be favored to remind us of what we must do as nutrition educators to encourage learning. They should *not* be a statement of what the *nutrition educator* will do, such as "demonstrate a food preparation technique" or "show a film," or even what the intended audience member will do, such as "discuss" or "make a salad." Instead, objectives answer the following question: What will the nutrition education *participant* need to know, feel, or be able do differently in terms of the specific mediators of behavior in order to achieve the behavioral goals?

Learning objectives are often called *behavioral objectives* in the field of education. This term comes from the behaviorist school of psychology, which insists that we can only know if true learning has occurred if it results in observable "behaviors." Here, 2 + 2 = 4 is considered a behavior. Such "behavioral objectives" are widely used by school educators. Nutrition educators need to keep in mind the differences in terminology when working with teachers. In this textbook, however, as noted before, *behavior* always refers to observable actions in relation to food or nutrition and not to cognitive or affective learning outcomes.

When writing objectives, you should first write some *general* educational or learning objectives to guide the development of educational strategies that will lead to achievement of the behavioral goals over the course of several sessions or across several components. Review your findings from Step 2 and identify the three to six major mediators that you think you have time to cover and that will contribute to increasing the group's ability to enact the goal behaviors. Write general educational objectives directed at these mediators.

You then write *specific* learning objectives that will guide the development of specific educational activities to achieve the general educational objectives. These specific learning objectives guide the design of *each* of the specific educational activities or learning experiences within individual sessions or program components as identified by the general educational objectives. There will be many of these, depending on the length of each session or the extensiveness of the program component. Specific learning objectives state exactly

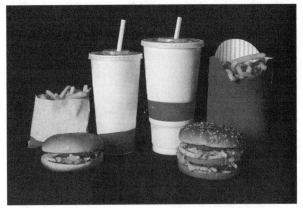

The increase in portion sizes from the 1970s to the present day is substantial.

what the learner will be able to do; are measurable; and are related to achievement in terms of a particular personal mediator of action or behavior change, such as self-efficacy, perceived benefits, perceived behavior control, goal setting, and so forth. Specific educational objectives have the following form: "At the end of the session/program, participant will be able to . . ." followed by a verb such as *describe, state, identify, translate, judge,* and so forth.

In practice, you will probably go back and forth between general and specific objectives, and even between objectives and educational activities. As you come up with exciting and relevant activities, you should think carefully about their purpose (specific objectives) in achieving the behavioral goals of the program and how they relate to the general educational objectives. If they do not serve any of the identified larger purposes, you should drop the activities, no matter how exciting. However, at this point you may want to rethink your general objectives. Perhaps they need to be changed to accommodate the specific objectives and activities because you consider them important to achieving the behavioral goal.

The sequence goes something like this for a given session. Think about the question "What is one key message that will assist the group to understand, feel, or do something differently as a result of this session?" That can become the title of your session. For example, if you have found from Step 1 that portion sizes of high-fat and/or high-sugar foods are a problem among youth, the title of a session might be "Portion sizes matter." Then review your findings from Step 2 and identify the two or three key mediators that you think you have time to cover using interactive methods and that will contribute to increasing the group's ability to enact the goal behaviors. You might want the group members to

- Increase their awareness of the large portion sizes of today's sodas and fast foods and how they have increased over time (consciousness-raising; perceived risk)

- Understand the impacts of those increased portion sizes on body functioning and weight (outcome expectations)
- Increase their awareness of what they are eating (self-assessment), so that they can choose portions more wisely (behavioral capability)

These become the general educational objectives.

See the case study at the end of this chapter for an example of how to write general and specific educational objectives directed at mediators of behavior expressed as theory constructs.

We have identified the potential mediators of the targeted behaviors listed in the left column. The general educational objectives for these mediators are shown in the right column.

Potential Mediators	General Educational Objectives
Motivation-Related Potential Mediators	
Perceived threat	Evaluate their own intake of fruits and vegetables (F&V) compared to recommendations
Outcome expectations: taste, convenience, other benefits	Demonstrate understanding and appreciation of the importance of eating a variety of F&V
Action-Related Potential Mediators	
Self-efficacy	Demonstrate increased self-efficacy in eating a variety of F&V each day
Behavioral capability	Demonstrate increased knowledge and skills in incorporating F&V into their daily food patterns
Goal setting	Prepare action plans using goal-setting and decision-making skills to increase their consumption of F&V

The specific educational objectives are related to the assessments of potential mediators in Step 2 as shown here.

Potential Personal Mediators of Behavior	Findings from Step 2: Needs Assessment/ Relevant Literature	Specific Learning Objectives for Personal Mediators

Write Educational Objectives in Three Domains

Educators categorize "learning" tasks, and hence educational objectives, as falling into three domains: the cognitive, affective, and psychomotor (Bloom, 1956). *Cognitive domain* objectives aim to promote abilities in thought, understanding, and cognitive skills; *affective domain* objectives aim to promote changes in attitude, feeling, or emotion; and *psychomotor domain* objectives aim to promote improvement in physical or manipulative skills. The effectiveness of nutrition education is improved if activities are designed to engage participants in these three domains of head, heart, and hand. Thus, nutrition educators must check that their objectives address all three domains of learning. Within each domain, learning tasks are considered to range in a graded sequence from simple to complex. Nutrition educators should ensure that their objectives are set at the appropriate level of complexity for any given task and, as important, that any given session or program includes objectives for more complex understandings and attitudes, as well as the simple ones.

Figures 10-1 and 10-2 later in this chapter provide detailed outlines of the learning tasks in the cognitive and affective domains and a list of verbs that you can use as you write educational objectives in each of these domains.

Cognitive (Knowing or Thinking) Domain

As human beings we are thinking beings. Just about everything we do involves our thinking about it and interpreting it in some way. Thus, all of nutrition education involves providing knowledge in some form. However, information can serve many purposes. For example, information can make us aware of issues, ideas, and conditions about ourselves or people in general that we never knew before. We might refer to this as *awareness*. Information about the latest scientific findings regarding the relationships between diet and health might make us thoughtful about the importance of eating well. If we then record our food intake for three days and compare it with the recommendations, we may realize that our personal diets are not so healthful, and we may truly become concerned about our own eating patterns. These different pieces of information may be called *why-to information*, because they help us to consider why to take action. This information, based on nutrition science and dietary guidance, has motivational power because it provides us with information about the perceived risk of a condition, and perceived benefits or taking action and can be called *motivational knowledge*, as we saw in the first part of this book. Many of the constructs or variables of social psychological theories that are representations of the personal motivating mediators of behavior, such as values, attitudes, social norms, or self-efficacy, are called *social cognitions*. Such information about our social world, though not based on nutrition science findings, is information nevertheless and belong in this category of motivational knowledge.

Knowledge can also serve an *instrumental* or *how-to function*. Information such as how much of which foods we can eat to foster health, the food pyramid, label reading, standard serving sizes, food composition, and so forth is important for guiding individuals on how to make healthful choices. The relative importance of the two kinds of knowledge often depends on the issue being addressed. For issues that are relatively new to the group, such as food safety, food bio-terrorism, or eating locally, why-to knowledge may be more important, whereas for issues that are quite familiar, such as eating fruits and vegetables, how-to knowledge may be more important. As you can see, all educational objectives have some cognitive dimension.

Both social cognitions (or why-to information) and behavioral capabilities and self-regulation skills (or how-to information) can range widely in terms of degree of complexity. Educational objectives can range from simple recall of facts to highly original and creative ways of combining and synthesizing new ideas. A taxonomy or classification system of cognitive domain objectives that is commonly used in education was developed by Bloom and colleagues (1956). It describes six levels of under-standings that an educational experience or strategy can aim for developing in learners, beginning with *knowledge* and then moving through *comprehension* to the ability to *apply* information to new decision-making situations

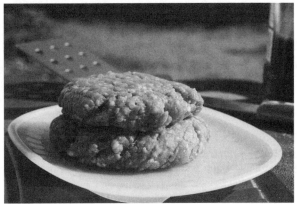

Learning to properly prepare and cook raw meat is a central part of how-to knowledge of food safety.

and the ability to *analyze or synthesize* information, and finally ending with *evaluation,* or wisdom regarding taking action on food and nutrition matters. Figure 10-1 illustrates these levels.

Levels of complexity of learning tasks

Useful verbs

Knowledge	Comprehension	Application	Analysis	Synthesis	Evaluation
(Recalling information as it is learned)	(Reporting information in a way other than how it was learned to show understanding)	(Applying learned information to a new context)	(Taking learned information apart)	(Putting together parts and elements into a unified organization or whole)	(Judging the value of something using appropriate criteria)
define	translate	interpret	distinguish	compose	judge
repeat	restate	apply	analyze	plan	appraise
record	describe	use	differentiate	propose	evaluate
list	recognize	demonstrate	appraise	design	rate
recall	explain	dramatize	calculate	formulate	compare
name	discuss	practice	experiment	arrange	value
state	express	illustrate	test	assemble	revise
underline	identify	modify	compare	collect	score
label	locate	operate	contrast	construct	select
tell	report	predict	criticize	create	choose
	review	schedule	diagram	set up	assess
		shop	inspect	organize	estimate
		sketch	debate	manage	measure
			inventory	prepare	conclude
			question	relate	justify
			relate		criticize
			solve		
			examine		
			categorize		

FIGURE 10-1 Cognitive domain: Levels of thinking.

Source: Adapted from Bloom, B.S. et al. 1956. *Taxonomy of educational objectives. Handbook I: The cognitive domain.* New York: David McKay.

Depending on the findings of the needs analysis in Step 2 with respect to the difficulty of the behavior change and the motivations and skills of the target group, educational strategies in the cognitive domain may be designed to bring about measurable changes in understanding at different levels of difficulty or complexity.

1. *Knowledge: Recalling information very much as it was learned.* At the lowest level of learning, this involves recall and memory. When you set objectives at this level, it means that you will design learning activities that will result in group participants being able to remember or recall specific pieces of information, terminology, and facts such as which foods are in which food groups or which foods are sources of which nutrients. For example, your aim is that the learning activities you design will result in participants' being able to state the names of the food groups in MyPyramid and how many servings a typical adult needs from each group. For the reader, it means the ability to define the various constructs in theories described in the first part of this book.

2. *Comprehension: Ability to grasp the meaning of material.* This level represents the beginnings of understanding.

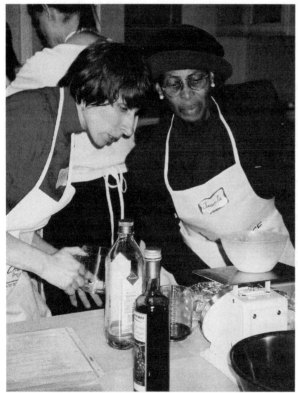

Cookbooks, friends, family, and community centers can all be used as sources for finding and learning new recipes.

It means that individuals are able to make sense of the information and to paraphrase it in their own words. The individuals may even be able to extrapolate the information to new but related ideas and implications, making simple inferences. For example, when you set educational objectives at this level, you are aiming for group participants to be able to understand general disease risk information and apply it to themselves, or to understand the benefits of eating fruits and vegetables.

3. *Application: Use of information in new and concrete situations.* At this level of learning, individuals are able to carry over information, principles, concepts, or theories learned in one context to a completely new one. When you set objectives for the session at this level, you are aiming for group participants, after learning how to set goals to increase their consumption of fruits and vegetables, to be able to apply goal-setting principles to a new behavior, such as eating more foods high in calcium. For the reader, an objective set at this level is for you to be able to apply what is learned in this book to the design of new educational activities and programs.

4. *Analysis: Taking information apart so that its organizational structure can be understood.* This level involves breaking information into its components to identify the elements, the interactions between them, and the organizing principles or structures. It also involves distinguishing fact from opinion, and relevant from extraneous issues or events. For example, educational objectives set at this level may aim for group participants to be able to compare and contrast the impacts of low-fat and low-carbohydrate diets on weight and health, or to debate the benefits and barriers of breastfeeding versus bottle-feeding.

5. *Synthesis: Putting information together in a unique or novel way.* At this level, individuals are able to reassemble information and experiences into a unified framework in order to create new meaning or to think about the situation in a new way. For the intended audience, it involves the ability to use what they are learning and experiencing in the program in a new way to affect their food practices and eating experience. For the reader, it means being able to integrate ideas from the different parts of this book to create new ways of thinking about nutrition education curricula and programs.

6. *Evaluation: Judging the value of something for a particular purpose.* Here individuals are able to make judgments about the worth of information and experiences based on well-accepted external criteria (such as relevance to stated purposes) or on internal criteria (organization and meaning). These criteria may be given to, or created by, individuals themselves. Objectives at this level include elements of all the previous levels, as well as conscious value judgments based on the criteria. For the intended

nutrition education audience, for example, it may mean the ability to evaluate the merits of different ways to assist children to learn good eating habits, or the ability to reach sound judgment regarding food and nutrition matters based on evidence. For the reader, it means the ability to evaluate the merit of different theories and educational strategies based on evidence.

Affective (Feelings) Domain

We are not only thinking beings but also feeling beings. The affective domain is associated with feelings, attitudes, values, appreciation, and interests. Educational strategies in the affective domain may be designed to result in different levels of the participants' affective engagement with the material or activity and commitment to taking action regarding food and nutrition, beginning with awareness or willingness to *receive or attend to* a message at the lowest level and moving through *responding* to it, *valuing* the message to the point of commitment to it, *organizing* their life around the message (e.g., developing a personal food policy to eat only organic vegetables), and finally to *characterization* of themselves by their commitment to the value system (e.g., becoming known to be health-conscious people). Figure 10-2 illustrates these levels.

For nutrition education to be effective, the intended audience must not only understand the message or information but also value it and believe it to be relevant and important to them. The affective domain objectives focus on a process of affective engagement and internalization, categorizing into levels the inner growth that occurs as individuals become aware of, and later adopt, the attitudes and principles that assist in forming value judgments that guide their actions. Krathwohl, Bloom, and Masia (1964) identified five levels, which are described in the following list. As you design your sessions, you will need to decide the level of affective engagement you wish for your audience. For example, do you want the group to just *receive* your message or do you want the group to be actively engaged and to *value* it? Do you want them to value the message enough to *make a commitment*? A general strategy is for the session (or several sessions) to provide opportunities for the group to move from lesser degrees of affective engagement and commitment to greater degrees of commitment.. Therefore the objectives will be set at ever higher levels in the classification scheme described in the following list.

1. *Receiving: Paying attention.* At this level, the participants are willing to listen to the nutrition educator or other form of communication and become aware of the ideas communicated. From a purely passive role, they may advance to willingness to attend to the communication despite distractions or competing stimuli. When you set objectives at this level, it means that you expect partici-

pants to be willing to listen to a message, such as the importance of eating fruits and vegetables, but that is about all.

2. *Responding: Active participation.* This level involves willingness to participate in something, although not necessarily with enthusiasm at first. From obedient participation (perhaps a health professional has insisted that participants attend these nutrition education sessions), individuals may advance to voluntary response and, indeed, to a pleasurable feeling or satisfaction in participation. If you set educational objectives at this level, it means that you expect that from being onlookers during group nutrition education activities, individuals will move toward participating in these activities and find that they enjoy them. Or objectives may be set even higher, expecting individuals to move from complying with the expectations of the educator, to start developing their own positions and taking responsibility for themselves. Objectives at this level take the form of aiming for changes in attitudes, motivations, and self-efficacy.

3. *Valuing: Consistent behavior reflecting positive regard for something.* At this level, the issue or behavior is considered to have worth. This sense of worth ranges from acceptance of the value to a deep-enough commitment to the value that it is reflected in observable behavior. Behavior reflects a belief or an attitude. Thus, this level is characterized by motivated behavior in which individuals' commitments guide their behaviors. This is the level that is most appropriate for nutrition education. When you set objectives at this level, it means that you aim for the learning activities that you design to increase participants' value for the targeted behavioral goal or issue so much that they are willing to take action. At the lower end, this may mean tentative behavior in keeping with advice from others, with readiness to reevaluate. At the upper end, individuals develop conviction about the behavior or issue, resulting in commitment. They have less need to be motivated by the need to comply with others and have begun to internalize their own viewpoints and values as a basis of action. For example, stating your educational objective at this level means that you intend for individuals to move from ambivalence, to deciding to eat more fruits and vegetables each day, and then to actually doing so.

4. *Organization: Behaving according to a set of principles.* Here individuals have established a conscious basis for making choices. They understand that there are other values beside their own. Objectives at the organization level are concerned with assisting individuals to bring together different values, resolve conflicts among them, and begin to build an internally consistent value system—a set of criteria—for guiding behavior. Individuals are aware of the basis of their own attitudes and values and are able to defend them. They begin to develop their own personal food policies. For example,

Levels of commitment and integration

1. Receiving (Paying attention)	2. Responding (Active participation)	3. Valuing (Behavior based on positive regard for something)	4. Organization (Behaving according to a set of principles)	5. Internalizing values (Behaving according to consistent world-view)
Stages 1.1 Awareness 1.2 Willingness to receive 1.3 Controlled or selected attention	**Stages** 2.1 Acquiescence in responding 2.2 Willingness to respond 2.3 Satisfaction in response	**Stages** 3.1 Acceptance of a value 3.2 Preference for a value 3.3 Commitment to a value	**Stages** 4.1 Conceptualization of a value 4.2 Organizing values into a system	**Stages** 5.1 Has a generalized value system controlling behavior 5.2 Characterized by a value system
Explanation for each stage 1. Aware with no position taken 2. Willingness to receive or attend to information 3. Will not avoid stimulus	**Explanation for each stage** 1. Complying with expectations of educator 2. Stating or defending own position 3. Beginning of own emotional response with satisfaction Opinions/position formation	**Explanation for each stage** 1. Tentative acceptance with readiness to reevaluate 2. Conviction 3. Commitment or loyalty to a position, group, or cause No longer motivated primarily by value to comply with others; beginning to internalize own viewpoint	**Explanation for each stage** 1. Conceptualizing one's important values and understanding they may be different from those of others 2. Building an internally consistent value system for guiding behavior by resolving conflicts and creating a unique value system Developing one's own values or policies to guide action Able to defend own position	**Explanation for each stage** 1. Integration of value into one's consistent, total world-view that guides behavior 2. Person's behavior is consistent, predictable, and characterized by the values Person has developed a consistent and recognizable way of life guided by a set of values

←-------- *Adjustment or Behavior* ------------------------→
←------ *Values and Attitudes* ------→
←-------- *Appreciation* ------→

| **Key verbs** asks, chooses, describes, follows, gives, holds, identifies, locates, names, points to, selects, replies, uses | **Key verbs** answers, assists, aids, helps, complies, conforms, greets, discusses, labels, tells, reads, performs, reports, practices, writes, recites, selects | **Key verbs** completes, demonstrates, explains, initiates, joins, justifies, proposes, reports, selects, shares, studies, works | **Key verbs** adheres, alters, arranges, combines, compares, completes, defends, explains, generalizes, integrates, modifies, orders, organizes, relates, synthesizes | **Key verbs** acts, discriminates, displays, influences, listens, modifies, performs, practices, proposes, qualifies, questions, revises, serves, solves, verifies |

FIGURE 10-2 Affective domain: Levels of affective engagement.

Source: Adapted from Krathwohl, D.R., B.S. Bloom, and B.B. Masia. 1964. *Taxonomy of educational objectives: The classification of educational goals. Handbook II: Affective domain.* New York: David McKay; and Grunland, N.E. 1978. *Stating behavioral objectives for classroom instruction.* New York: Macmillan.

if you set educational objectives at this level, it means that you intend for your learning experiences or activities to lead individuals now to use health, or ecological concerns, social justice issues, or personal, social, or cultural values, as a *consistent* criterion for making choices about food- and nutrition-related issues.

5. *Characterization by a value or a value complex: Behaving according to a consistent worldview.* At this level, values are integrated into some kind of internally consistent worldview so that the person is recognized by these values. The individual has developed a characteristic lifestyle. If objectives are set at this level, it means that you expect that the educational activities or learning experiences you design will lead participants to a change in worldview and a lifestyle consistent with that worldview. For example, you expect that as a result of your educa-

tional activities, the individual will practice a new way of eating so consistently that he or she becomes known as a vegetarian or an ecologically conscious, or "green," consumer.

Note on "values" and "behaviors" in the context of educational objectives. As you can see, individuals achieving objectives set at the valuing level of the affective domain begin to demonstrate observable behaviors that reflect these values. Thus, educational objectives to achieve food- and nutrition-related behavioral goals will normally be set at the valuing level of the affective taxonomy. Long-term or more intense nutrition education may be able to assist individuals to understand and internalize their values to the extent of establishing a conscious basis for making choices, such as developing their own personal food policies. There is often miscommunication between nutritionists and educators regarding terminology, which we need to be aware of. When nutritionists talk about objectives to facilitate behavior change, educators talk about educational objectives in the affective domain at the valuing level or above. This chapter keeps these two sets of terminology separate. Thus, according to our scheme, program behavioral goals are achieved through educational objectives set at the valuing level or above.

Psychomotor Domain

The emphasis in the psychomotor domain is on the development of psychomotor skills, even though some degree of understanding and varying degrees of emotion may also be involved. This domain involves a graded sequence from simple to complex. At the lowest level, participants *observe* a more experienced person perform the activity (e.g., preparing a recipe), then are able to *imitate* it, and then *practice* it so that conscious effort is no longer necessary and it has become somewhat habitual in nature; finally, the individuals may be able to *adapt* the activity.

1. *Observing.* When objectives are set at this level, individuals observe a more experienced person performing the skill. Sometimes, the reading of directions substitutes for this experience. However, usually reading is supplemented with direct observation, such as watching someone preparing a salad or recipe.
2. *Imitating.* When objectives are set at this level, you provide opportunities for individuals to follow directions and sequences under close supervision. It may require conscious effort on the part of individuals to carry out the actions in sequence.
3. *Practicing.* When objectives are set at this level, you provide opportunities for the entire sequence to be performed repeatedly, so that conscious effort is no longer required. The actions become more or less habitual, and we can say that the individuals have acquired the skill.

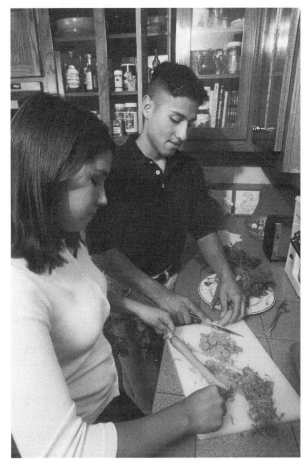

Healthy cooking habits can be formed at any age.

Perhaps the individuals have learned to prepare recipes with vegetables in them, or to modify recipes to make them lower in fat.
4. *Adapting.* Objectives at this level involve the ability to adapt or modify the actions to improve the outcome even further. This may mean the ability to adapt learned recipes to individual or family tastes.

Overall

Educational objectives need to specify which kinds of strategies should be designed: ones in the cognitive domain only? The affective domain only? Or both? Will you have the opportunity to assist individuals to develop psychomotor skills as well? In reality, most activities in the food and nutrition area will involve both the cognitive (knowing) and affective (feeling) domains. It may be possible to address the psychomotor domain by including food preparation. In the cognitive/knowing domain, educational strategies should attempt to assist the intended audience to do more difficult learning tasks, such as application or evaluation, and not just the easier tasks, such as recalling information. In the affective/feeling domain, it is preferable to design activities that actively engage participants and assist them to actively contemplate and value the message to the point of being willing to try the recommendations. Too often, objectives are set to achieve the lower levels of audience engagement, such as just listening and receiving the message (through lectures, for example). Box 10-1 contains examples of learning objectives directed at mediators of behavior within the three domains.

Note on writing detailed specific objectives. In the educational world, writing specific "behavioral" objectives is based on the premise that learning is the *observable* response to a specific stimulus. That is, the achievement of each objective needs to be demonstrated by a specific observable action (Bloom, 1956; Krathwohl, Bloom, & Masia, 1964; Grunland, 1978). The following elements are usually included:

1. The behavior expected of the learner
2. The conditions under which the behavior is to be demonstrated

Thus, specific objectives will usually take the following form:

Given_____(here name the condition or stimulus), the learner (participant) will _____ (here name the desired response).

For example, "Given information on the government's food pyramid for healthy eating, the participant will be able to place foods into the correct food groups."

Often a third element is added: the degree of mastery required. In this case the objective might be "Given information on the government's food pyramid for healthy eating, the participant will be able to place 12 foods into the correct food groups with 80% accuracy."

You may follow this format if you wish. However, our advice is that for nutrition education purposes, it is not necessary to follow this format slavishly. In addition, you may not need to write out the specific learning domains and levels for each educational objective. However, it is *very* important to be aware of, and to target, the different domains and levels in each session or throughout the program to ensure that nutrition education activities are directed at a range of levels of difficulty and that head, heart, and hand are all engaged.

Write Educational and Support Objectives to Address Potential Environmental Mediators of the Targeted Behaviors

Environmental mediators are those influences on the selected behaviors that reside outside the individual that may mediate change. From the environmental factors that may mediate the goal behaviors identified in Step 1, select those that you will be able to realistically target in the intervention to increase environmental support, given the available time and resources. In most instances, achievement of environmental support objectives involves educating and working in partnership with food or service providers, policy makers, or individuals and organizations that have decision-making authority over the environmental factors that you have identified as potentially relevant mediators of change. These might include school food service directors, school principals and superintendents, grocery store managers, parent–teacher organizations, farmers, food assistance programs, or community leaders and organizations.

First write *general* environmental support goals for changes in the environment to increase the opportunities of the intended audience to engage in the program goal behavior or behaviors. For our case study, this might include the following:

- The school food service will provide more fruits and vegetables in the school meals and other food venues.
- School policies will ensure many opportunities for students to taste fruits and vegetables.
- Parents will make fruits and vegetables more accessible to their children, and encourage their children to eat them.

Your perspectives on food and nutrition content issues will influence your selection of specific actions regarding the environment. For example, will you encourage the food provider to offer fresh fruits and vegetables (rather than canned) when possible? Will you encourage the use of local sources to the extent possible, such as through a farm-to-school program?

Write Educational and Support Objectives for Each Interpersonal-Level Environmental Mediator

Social support can be an important environmental mediator of individuals' eating patterns. This is especially true for our case study, in which children's willingness and ability to take recommended action is very much influenced by parental or family actions. Hence a parent/family component can be planned to assist them to be more supportive of their children's attempts to eat healthfully.

Parents or family are external to the students. At the same time, they represent a new audience for whom general and specific educational objectives will need to be written, in a process similar to that for the students described earlier. See the case study for details of behavioral goals, general educational objectives, and specific educational objectives for the parent/family component.

> **BOX 10-1 Examples of Learning Objectives Directed at Mediators of Behavior Within the Three Domains**

In each example, the objective is preceded by the following phrase: "At the end of the program (or session), the participants will be able to . . ."

Motivational Mediators

1. **Concern for the problem or issue.** Demonstrate appreciation of their own susceptibility to heart disease (by naming people in their family who have died of heart disease and discussing how that made them feel).
   Affective domain: Responding level.

2. **Perceived risks.** Demonstrate the understanding that a diet high in fat increases their risk of heart disease (by correctly answering a questionnaire at the end of the program or session).
   Cognitive domain: Comprehension level. *Affective domain:* Responding level.

3. **Outcome expectations/perceived benefits.** Demonstrate the understanding that a diet high in fruits and vegetables reduces their risk of heart disease and cancer (by correctly answering a questionnaire at the end of the program or session).
   Cognitive domain: Comprehension level. *Affective domain:* Responding level.

4. **Values.** Appreciate the importance of overcoming psychological barriers to eating a lower-fat diet (by orally describing one barrier and listing one action the learner will take in the next week to overcome that barrier).
   Cognitive domain: Comprehension level. *Affective domain:* Valuing level.

5. **Self-efficacy.** Demonstrate belief in their ability to prepare foods lower in fat (by proposing to bring in a lower-fat recipe to share with the group next session).
   Cognitive domain: Comprehension level. *Affective domain:* Valuing level.

6. **Social influence.** Appreciate the role of peers in influencing food choices (by noting one instance in which the participant did not eat what peers ate and describing how that made the participant feel).
   Cognitive domain: Comprehension level. *Affective domain:* Valuing level.

Action Mediators: Facilitating the Ability to Take Action

1. **Knowledge.** Understand the dietary advice for reducing risk of cancer (by listing three of the relevant dietary guidelines without looking at materials).
   Cognitive domain: Comprehension level.

2. **Skills.**
   a. **Cognitive.** Demonstrate ability to apply the recommendations from MyPyramid (by comparing own 24-hour dietary intake to recommendations and describing implications for self).
      Cognitive domain: Evaluation level.
   b. **Affective.** Demonstrate resistance to peer pressure to eat high-fat foods (by eating a salad at lunch and not the high-fat choice of peers, and appropriately explaining/defending own choice).
      Cognitive domain: Evaluation level. *Affective domain:* Organization level.
   c. **Behavioral capability.** Demonstrate ability to stir-fry vegetables (by imitating demonstration in class by preparing identical dish at home).
      Cognitive domain: Comprehension level. *Psychomotor domain:* Imitation level.
   d. **Self-regulation skills.** Engage in systematic planning to change their own diet (by identifying a behavior that they wish to change, developing an action plan to make the change, self-monitoring the change, and sharing with the group their progress in attaining the goal).
      Cognitive domain: Evaluation level. *Affective domain:* Valuing level.
      Demonstrate satisfaction in achieving a personal dietary change goal (by rewarding self with seeing a movie).
      Affective domain: Valuing level.

3. **Social support.** Demonstrate ability to share feelings about chosen diet to friends and family and to seek support from them (by asking family to support their own macrobiotic eating pattern).
   Cognitive domain: Comprehension level. *Affective domain:* Valuing level.

Write Educational and Support Objectives for Each Potential Organizational- or Community-Level Environmental Mediator

In order to promote environments that facilitate the enactment of the actions, behaviors, or practices targeted by the program, we need to increase the awareness of key decision makers and policy makers regarding the importance of the health, food, or nutrition issue that the program is seeking to address and the behaviors that will contribute to health. Thus we need to write educational and support objectives for this new audience.

Using our case study as an example, this may mean seeking changes in the school environment to make it more supportive of the behaviors targeted by the program. See the case study for details of the objectives for the school environment component.

Your Turn

Use the Step 4 worksheets to write your own educational goals and objectives for a hypothetical or real intervention. These educational objectives and environmental support objectives will guide the development of nutrition education strategies and environmental support activities to be delivered through a variety of channels. Step 5, discussed in Chapters 11 and 12, describes how to design appropriate activities.

Case Study

This chapter presents a case study of nutrition education designed to encourage adolescents to eat more fruits and vegetables. The case study lays out the following features.

For the classroom component:

- The program's behavioral goals for the adolescents
- The educational goals of the program
- The general educational objectives to address potential personal psychosocial mediators of the behaviors, based on the theory model created for the program.
- The specific educational (learning) objectives for the potential mediators. For each of these specific educational objectives we add information on the domain in which the educational activities should occur, and the anticipated level of cognitive difficulty or affective engagement for the group for each activity within each domain.

For the parent component:

- Behavioral goal for parents
- General educational objectives
- Specific educational objectives

For the school component:

- Educational objectives for decision-makers
- Objectives for the food environment
- Objectives for food policy
- Objectives for the school social support and information environment

---

Questions and Activities

1. Describe briefly three reasons why it is important to write educational goals and objectives for nutrition education, no matter how brief.
2. What are learning objectives? Describe carefully the relationship between learning objectives for a program or session and the potential mediators of behavior or practices (which are identified in Step 2 of the design process).
3. Distinguish between an educational goal, general educational/learning objective, and specific educational/learning objective.
4. Objectives are often described as being written in the *cognitive, affective,* or *psychomotor* domains of learning. What do we mean by these terms? How do they guide learning?
5. For practice, select three potential mediators of the behavior of increasing the intake of calcium-rich foods among teenage girls and state *general* educational/learning objectives directed at each. Write one for each domain of learning.
6. For practice, write *specific* educational/learning objectives for the following potential mediators of the behavior of increasing the intake of calcium-rich foods among teenage girls. For each objective, indicate the learning domain and level.
   - Outcome expectations/perceived benefits
   - Perceived self-efficacy
   - Personal action goal

STEP 4 WORKSHEETS   **State Educational Goals and Objectives to Address Mediators of Behavior**

In this step we state educational goals and objectives directed at the potential mediators of the target behaviors. Begin by reviewing all the worksheets that you completed in Steps 1, 2, and 3.

WORKSHEET 10-1   **Translating Behavioral Theory into Educational Goals and Objectives**

In this worksheet you will translate the information you collected in Steps 1 and 2 plus your thinking and planning in Step 3 into educational goals and objectives to guide your intervention. As a result of the needs analysis process in Steps 1 and 2, you should proceed as follows.

1. **Restate the program's target behaviors or behavioral goals from Step 1.**
   [*For example: Middle school students will increase their intake of fruits and vegetables, will drink fewer sweetened drinks, and will increase their walking.*]

   _____

   _____

   _____

2. **Determine the educational goals of the program to achieve these behavioral goals.**

   • _____

   • _____

3a. **State (briefly) the theory model developed in Step 3 that you will use to guide the development of the nutrition education program.** [*For example: Social cognitive theory*]

   _____

   _____

b. **From the theory model developed in Step 3, state the potential personal psychosocial mediators (theory constructs or variables) of the target behavior that you will address in the intervention.** [*For example: Self-assessment of risk, outcome expectations, social norms, preferences, etc.*]

   • _____

   • _____

   • _____

   • _____

4. **Write *general* educational objectives to address the potential personal psychosocial mediators you have selected.**

   - _____
   - _____
   - _____
   - _____

5. **Write *specific* educational (learning) objectives for each of the potential personal mediators or theory constructs listed above.** Mediators in Table A have been placed in motivating and behavioral change categories to remind you to consider both categories of constructs. However, you can use other categories as appropriate, based on the intervention model you have created.

TABLE A Specific Educational Objectives for Personal Mediators of Selected Behavior

Potential Personal Mediators of Behavior	Findings from Step 2: Needs Analysis and Relevant Literature	Specific Educational Objectives for Personal Mediators
Motivating mediators [*Examples*] Perceived risk Perceived benefits Outcome expectations Self-efficacy	[*For each mediator, list the following.*] *Current motivation:* *Potential motivators:*	*At the end of the session/program, participants will be able to:* • • • •
Behavior change mediators [*Examples*] Behavioral capabilities	[*For each mediator, list the following.*] *Current food and nutrition knowledge and skills for the behavior:* *Potential facilitators of change:*	*At the end of the session/program, participants will be able to:* • • • •
Self-regulation skills	*Current goal-setting skills:* *Potential facilitators:*	

6. **Review specific educational objectives for their appropriate domains and levels.** Now review your objectives, and designate their domain (cognitive, affective, or psychomotor) by writing C, A, or P next to each. Then designate their level within the domains. For the cognitive domain, "knowledge," "application," and "higher-order" designations may be sufficient. This will help ensure that the educational objectives are appropriately targeted. Do you have objectives that address the affective domain of feelings as well as the cognitive domain of understanding? Are psychomotor domain objectives included, if relevant? Are the objectives stated so as to guide the development of activities that will lead to a range of learning, from the simple to the complex? Will they address affect/feelings and values at the appropriate level? See case study for examples.

7a. **Write general educational and support objectives for the potential environmental mediators that influence achievement of behavioral goals.**

- _____

- _____

- _____

b. **Write specific educational objectives and environmental support objectives for each component of the program.**
   Complete a worksheet like the one shown in Table B for each environmental component that you wish to address: interpersonal, organizational/community, or policy and systems.

TABLE B Specific Educational Objectives for Environmental Mediators

Potential Environmental Mediators	Findings from Step 2: Needs Analysis and Relevant Literature	Specific Environmental Educational Support Objectives
	Current situation:	•
		•
		•
	Potential supportive actions:	•

CASE STUDY 10-1   Step 4: State Educational Goals and Objectives to Address Mediators of Behavior

In this step we state educational goals and objectives directed at the potential mediators of the target behaviors: eating well and being fit.

1. **Restate the program's target behaviors or behavioral goals from Step 1.**

   From Step 1, the behavioral goals of the program are for youth to
   - Increase intake of fruits and vegetables (youth to aim for 2.5 cups or more a day)
   - Decrease amount of sweetened beverages consumed each day (aim for no more than 8 ounces a day)
   - Decrease number of packaged high-fat, high-sugar snacks so that they contribute no more than 150 calories a day (targets for drinks and snacks are based on the discretionary calories allowance for this age group)
   - Increase physical activity to 10,000 steps a day and participate actively, when possible, in gym or other school-sponsored physical activities

2. **Determine the educational goals of the program to achieve these behavioral goals.**

   The program will seek to
   - Increase awareness in youth of the importance of fruits and vegetables in the diet and enhance motivation to eat them through a school curriculum and school-wide activities
   - Facilitate the ability to act by providing opportunities to gain relevant food and nutrition knowledge and practice food-related skills and self-regulation skills through a school curriculum
   - Educate decision makers and work with them to increase opportunities for youth to engage in healthful eating at school and home through an educational component with parents and policy initiatives in the school.

3a. **State (briefly) the theory model developed in Step 3 that you will use to guide the development of the nutrition education program.**

   The theory to be used is an integrated general model of the determinants of behaviors change of the Institute of Medicine as shown in Case Study 9-1.

   b. **From the theory model developed in Step 3, state the potential personal psychosocial mediators (theory constructs or variables) of the target behavior that you will address in the intervention.**

   Motivation-related mediators:
   - Perceived threat
   - Outcome expectations: taste, convenience, other benefits
   - Perceived barriers
   - Social outcome expectations (social norms)

   Action-related mediators:
   - Self-efficacy
   - Behavioral capability (food- and nutrition-related knowledge and skills)
   - Personal action goals/implementation intentions
   - Self-regulation (SR) skills

4. **Write *general* educational objectives to address the potential personal mediators you have selected.**

   For the purposes of illustrating the writing of educational objectives for this case example, we will focus on only one of the behaviors—eating more fruits and vegetables—although all are equally important to assist youth to eat healthfully and maintain a healthy weight.

   The general educational objectives to achieve the behavioral goal of increasing fruit and vegetable intake might be as shown in Table A.

TABLE A

Mediators	General Educational Objectives *Adolescents will be able to:*
Outcome expectations Scientific knowledge of benefits	Demonstrate understanding and appreciation of the importance of eating a variety of fruits and vegetables (F&V)
Personal risk assessment	Evaluate their own intake of F&V compared with recommendations
Barriers	Identify barriers to intake of F&V and propose ways to overcome them
Preference/sensory-affective response to eating F&V Positive attitudes to eating F&V	Express enjoyment of and positive attitudes toward eating a variety of F&V
Behavioral intention	State intention to increase own F&V intake
Self-efficacy	Demonstrate increased self-efficacy in eating a variety of F&V each day

Behavioral capability	Demonstrate increased knowledge and skills in incorporating F&V into their daily food patterns
Self-regulation/goal-setting skills	Prepare action plans using goal-setting and decision-making skills to increase their consumption of F&V

5. **Write *specific* educational (learning) objectives for each of the personal potential mediators.**
   Table B is an example of specific educational objectives for the student group sessions component of our ongoing example, focusing only on the fruit and vegetable intervention with adolescents.

TABLE B

Personal Mediators of Behavior	Findings from Step 2: Needs Analysis and Relevant Literature	Specific Educational Objectives for Personal Mediators
Motivation-related mediators		*At the end of the session/program, participants will be able to:*
Perceived threat	*Current motivation:* No sense of urgency about eating F&V *Potential motivators:* Personalized risk	Describe health risks of eating too few F&V. Evaluate personal risk of not eating enough F&V.
Outcome expectations Benefits	*Current:* Understand benefits of F&V in general but don't see immediate benefits *Potential motivators:* If taste good, etc.; immediate benefits for health (skin, eyes)	Appreciate that F&V taste good and are enjoyable to eat. State benefits: energy, convenient, build strong bones and muscles for athletic performance.
Barriers: Taste, convenience	*Current:* Expensive, taste bad, inconvenient, go bad quickly	Identify barriers to eating F&V. Propose ways to overcome barriers.
Social outcome expectations (social norms)	*Current motivation:* Friends do not eat vegetables; unaware of media influence *Potential motivators:* Make veggies cool; make participants aware of lack of media attention to F&V	Describe the role of the peers in influencing food choices. Appreciate that vegetables are cool to eat.
Action-related mediators		*At the end of the session/program, participants will be able to:*
Self-efficacy	*Current motivation:* Not familiar with different F&V; not confident; unwilling to venture *Potential motivators:* Exposure to new foods	State the key features and health benefits of a variety of new F&V (a "rainbow of colors"). State satisfaction in trying new F&V.
Behavioral capability (food- and nutrition-related knowledge and skills)	*Current motivation:* Need skills to choose and prepare F&V snacks *Potential motivators:* Making learning skills fun and convenient	Describe how these F&V can be used in meals and as snacks. Compare the nutrient content of F&V snacks with processed and packaged energy-dense snacks. Prepare simple recipes using F&V.
Personal action goals/ implementation intentions Self-regulation (SR) skills	*Current motivation:* Impulse eating of high-fat, high-sugar snacks and beverages; weak intentions to eat F&V; low SR skills *Potential motivators:* Learn goal-setting and self-monitoring skills	State personal goals to eat more F&V; develop clear implementation plan for goals. Appreciate the importance of recognizing hunger and satiety cues during a busy day. Develop plan, incorporating F&V, to satisfy hunger when it occurs and to follow plan during a busy day; monitor progress toward that goal; reward self when goal is achieved.

6. **Review specific learning objectives for their appropriate domains and levels.**

    Now we examine the learning objectives that we have written, to ensure that they are written in all domains of learning and are set at the appropriate level of complexity for the issues and learning tasks. Table C shows the results.

TABLE C

Phase of Nutrition Education	Personal Mediator of Behavior	Specific Learning Objectives for Each Mediator	Learning Domain with Level
Pre-action *Educational goal:* Increase awareness and enhance motivation	Perceived threat	*At the end of the session/program, learner will be able to:* Describe the health risk of eating too few F&V.	Affective domain: *Responding level* Cognitive domain: *Comprehension level*

	Outcome expectations
	  Taste
	  Convenience
	  Health benefits
		Appreciate that fruits and vegetables taste good
		State benefits: energy, convenient, build strong bones and muscles for athletic performance.
			Affective domain: *Valuing level*
			Cognitive domain: *Comprehension level*

	Social outcome expectations (social norms)	Appreciate that vegetables are cool to eat.	Affective domain: *Valuing level*
Action *Educational goal:* Facilitate the ability to take action	Behavioral capabilities (food- and nutrition-related knowledge and skills)	State the key features and health benefits of a variety of new F&V (a "rainbow of colors"). State satisfaction in trying new F&V. Describe how these F&V can be used in meals and as snacks. Compare the nutrient content of F&V snacks with processed and packaged energy-dense snacks. Prepare simple recipes using F&V.	Cognitive domain: *Comprehension level* Affective domain: *Responding level* Cognitive domain: *application level* Cognitive domain: *Analysis level* Psychomotor domain: *Imitation level*
	Personal action goals/implementation intentions	State personal goals to eat more F&V; develop clear implementation plan for goals.	Cognitive domain: *Application level* Affective domain: *Valuing level*
	Self-regulation skills	Appreciate the importance of recognizing hunger and satiety cues during a busy day. Develop plan, incorporating F&V, to satisfy hunger when it occurs and to follow plan during a busy day; monitor progress toward that goal; reward self when goal is achieved.	Cognitive domain: *Application level* Affective domain: *Synthesis level*

Parent Component
Behavioral Goal for Parents
- Parents will make a variety of fruits and vegetables available and accessible to their children.

General Educational Objectives of the Parent Component
- Parents will demonstrate understanding and valuing of the importance for their children of eating a variety of fruits and vegetables.
- Parents will be able to provide social support to each other.
- Parents will develop skills in preparing and making fruits and vegetables accessible for their children.
- Parents will demonstrate commitment to providing fruits and vegetables for their children.

TABLE D Specific Educational Objectives

Personal Mediators of Behavior	Findings from Step 2: Needs Analysis and Relevant Literature	Specific Educational Objectives for Personal Mediators
Motivation-related mediators		*At the end of the session/program, parents will be able to:*
Outcome expectations Taste Convenience Benefits	*Current motivations:* Not high priority in food choice for children; not familiar with different F&V	State benefits: energy, important for healthy growth, build strong bones and muscles for athletic performance.
	Children not familiar with different F&V, do not like the taste of vegetables; unwilling to venture	State the importance of eating a "rainbow of colors." Value importance of providing many opportunities for children to become familiar with different F&V.
Action-related mediators		*At the end of the session/program, parents will be able to:*
Barriers	*Current motivations:* F&V expensive, inconvenient to prepare for children, go bad quickly	Describe ways to select F&V to lower cost. Describe how F&V can be used in meals and as snacks.
Self-efficacy	*Current motivations:* Lack confidence in preparing F&V; lack confidence in effective parental skills for increasing F&V intake of children.	Possess skills in quick and easy preparation methods and recipes using F&V.
Social norms/social support	*Current motivation:* Friends do not eat or serve vegetables; no media support *Potential motivators:* Supportive friends; awareness of lack of media attention to F&V	Appreciate that other parents and media personalities share their challenges and successes.
Behavioral capability (food- and nutrition-related knowledge and skills)	*Current motivations:* Need skills in ways to cut expenses of buying F&V, skills in storing, and recipes using quick and easy preparation methods.	Demonstrate skills to make F&V readily accessible and available to their children.
Behavioral intention	*Current status:* Parents are interested but do not seem to be able to act on their motivations. *Potential motivators:* Issuing a call to action.	State a commitment, in writing, to make F&V readily accessible and available to their children.

School Environment Component

TABLE E Environmental Objectives

Potential Environmental Mediators	Findings from Step 2: Needs Analysis and Relevant Literature	Educational and Environmental Support Objectives
Decision makers' awareness and motivation	*Current:* School administrators have many priorities, and healthful food environment is not of high importance. School food service must be financially self-supporting—fruits and vegetables (F&V) are expensive. *Potential motivation to be supportive:* Data on financial viability of healthful eating policies; legislation on policies.	*Educational objectives* *School administrators:* Increase importance of benefits of healthful school environment for health, learning, and financial situation of school. *School food service:* Increase awareness of options for increasing F&V intakes by students.
Food environment	*Current:* Students are unfamiliar with F&V and do not like taste. *Potential supports:* Opportunity to taste; tasty F&V items available in school meals.	• School will provide many opportunities for students to taste F&V. • School food service personnel will increase F&V in meals, obtained from local farmers in a farm-to-school program.
Food policy	*Current:* Students are unfamiliar with F&V. *Potential supports:* Tasty F&V items available in school meals, vending machines, and school stores at reasonable price.	*Policy and systems objectives* Through collaboration with stakeholders: • Establish school food policy council to develop guidelines for foods available in school. School council to be made up of administrators, food service staff, teachers, and students. • School food service personnel will provide healthful low-fat, high-vegetable meals. • Develop guidelines for items in vending machines and school stores. • Vending machines will carry healthful fruits and vegetable items. • Vendors will supply healthful F&V items in vending machines • School stores will carry healthful F&V items.
School social support	*Current:* No support for healthful F&V by school staff and among other teens. *Potential:* Peer models involved in healthy food-related activities; celebrity role models.	Educational objectives • Increase importance of healthful eating among teachers personally; increase importance of their being examples to students. • Increase social modeling by valued celebrities.
Information environment	*Current:* No role models of teens eating healthful F&V; few ads. *Potential:* Provide posters, newsletters.	Educational objectives • Develop posters of teens eating healthful F&V for cafeteria; newsletter to family.

REFERENCES

Bloom, B.S., M.D. Engelhart, E.J. Furst, W.H. Hill, and D.R. Krathwohl. 1956. *Taxonomy of educational objectives. Handbook I: The cognitive domain.* New York: David McKay.

Grunland, N.E. 1978. *Stating behavioral objectives for classroom instruction.* New York: Macmillan.

Krathwohl, D.R., B.S. Bloom, and B.B. Masia. 1964. *Taxonomy of educational objectives: The classification of educational goals. Handbook II: Affective domain.* New York: David McKay.

Step 5a: Design Theory-Derived Educational Strategies to Address Potential Mediators of the Motivation for Action

OVERVIEW   The focus of this chapter is designing strategies for why to take action, in particular, selecting theory-based educational strategies and designing practical educational activities to address potential mediators of program-targeted behaviors in order to increase awareness, promote contemplation, and enhance motivation. The information in Chapters 3 and 4 will help you with this step in the design process.

OBJECTIVES   At the end of the chapter, you will be able to

- Describe the kinds of theory-based strategies to address potential mediators of target behaviors that focus on increasing awareness, promoting contemplation, and enhancing motivation
- Design specific educational activities or learning experience*s* to make practical the theory-based educational strategies designed to address potential mediators of target behaviors
- Recognize the importance of using a systematic instructional design process for designing and sequencing educational strategies
- Sequence the educational objectives and strategies to create an educational plan or lesson plan

SCENARIO

A nutrition educator new to a community agency has learned from talking with others that the women who use the nutrition services of her agency tend to eat fast food items that are high in saturated fat and calories. They do not eat many vegetables and do not like them, but they do like to eat some familiar fruits. The nutrition educator decides that when she next makes a presentation, she will focus on helping the women value the importance of adding more vegetables to their diet.

Some days later these women attend a session she teaches. She lectures on the government's food pyramid, the different food groups, and the number of servings from each group that they should have. She then focuses on the vegetables group, the nutrients in some popular ones, and the number of servings they should eat. When she later sees them at a local coffee shop, she observes the women ordering their usual items that are high in saturated fat and calories. None of them ordered any vegetables.

COMMENT

What is going on here? The nutrition educator selected a valid affective objective—to help participants value eating fruits and vegetables; in essence, she aimed to encourage positive attitudes. However, the educational format she used—a lecture—was highly didactic and cognitive, and inappropriate to the objective. It is a common practice for nutrition educators to focus solely on traditional cognitive activities when in fact they are trying to accomplish affective and behavioral change objectives. When directed to affective and behavioral objectives, the instructional strategies and content should emphasize motivational factors such as beliefs, attitudes, feelings, personal and cultural values, peer pressure, and community norms.

Introduction

With your educational goals and objectives directed at the potential mediators of the actions or behaviors targeted by the program now set, you are ready to create some educational activities to address them. As you can see from the procedural model for designing theory-based nutrition education, in Step 5 you select theory-based educational strategies and design educational activities or leaning experiences to address the mediators of behavior that you selected in Step 4.

Theory-based educational strategies are ways to operationalize constructs of psychosocial theory describing mediators of behavior change for educational and instructional purposes. *Educational activities* or *learning experiences* are the numerous ways in which strategies are carried out in practice. Thus, the theory construct of perceived threat for osteoporosis may be a potential motivational mediator of eating more calcium-rich foods to reduce the threat. The educational strategy chosen may be confrontation of the audience with the risks. The educational activities or learning experiences might involve showing trigger films, pictures, charts, and striking national or local statistics, telling personal stories, or having the audience identify those in their families who have osteoporosis and describe their experiences.

The logic framework introduced in Chapter 3 provides a framework for planning. Our *inputs* are the resources we invest as well as the needs analysis process we conduct. Our *outputs* are our intervention activities through a variety of venues and the theory-based strategies that we use within these activities and venues to accomplish our goals. These include strategies to address potential motivational mediators and action mediators. Depending on the duration and intensity of the intervention, you may be able to incorporate environmental support activities as well.

Gaining Audience Interest and Engagement

Influential educators such as Dewey (1929) and Tyler (1949) make a clear distinction between content presentations and actual learning experiences. A learning experience is the interaction between learners and external conditions through which learning takes place. Learning takes place through the active behavior of learners. Education is what we do; learning is what the program participants experi-

INPUTS: COLLECTING ASSESSMENT DATA		DESIGNING THE OUTPUTS			DESIGNING OUTCOMES EVALUATION
STEP 1 ←→ **Analyze needs and behaviors: Specify the behavior or action focus of the program** • Assess needs and identify audience: select need(s) or issue(s) to address • Identify behaviors of concern that contribute to need(s) or issue(s) • Select core behaviors or practices to address	**STEP 2** ←→ **Identify relevant potential mediators of program behaviors** • Identify potential personal psychosocial mediators • Identify potential environmental mediators	**STEP 3** ←→ **Select theory, philosophy, and components** • Select theory and/or create appropriate model • Articulate educational philosophy • Clarify perspectives on content • Determine program components	**STEP 4** ←→ **State educational objectives for potential mediators** • Select relevant mediators to address • State educational objectives for each selected mediator: —Personal psychosocial mediators —Environmental mediators	**STEP 5** ←→ **Design theory-based educational strategies and activities to address potential mediators** • Design strategies and activities for each selected mediator: —Personal psychosocial mediators —Environmental mediators	**STEP 6** **Design evaluation** • Design evaluation of program's impact on behaviors and mediators • Design process evaluation

ence and accomplish. (Although we usually learn a great deal as well!) Mere educator intentions, however, will not result in learning. Mere presentation of information by us may not result in learning. The dynamic engagement of the participants with the content is essential. This is the basis of all good education and is emphasized in learning-centered education.

By *learning* we do *not* mean simply learning of facts and figures, or cognitive information and skills such as the number of calories in a teaspoon of sugar or how to read a food label. We mean an interaction between learners (program participants) and the activities we have designed that results in active contemplation about issues, changes in how participants view the world, an examination of their values, and changes in their expectations, attitudes, and feelings about food and nutrition, and, indeed, in their actions. Learning takes place through many venues—formal, nonformal, and informal—and we are all learners throughout life. This is where the true challenge of nutrition education design rests. It calls on us not only to have a firm grasp of food and nutrition content, but also to design creative, productive, and meaningful experiences to address mediators of behavior in order to bring about specified goals and objectives. This involves creative risk taking on the one hand and careful organization on the other hand. We design the educational strategies that provide learning experiences for participants. Hence the two terms are often used interchangeably. This book uses the term *theory-based strategies* to describe ways to address potential mediators of behavior change; the term *educational activities* or *learning experiences* is used for the numerous ways in which strategies are carried out in practice.

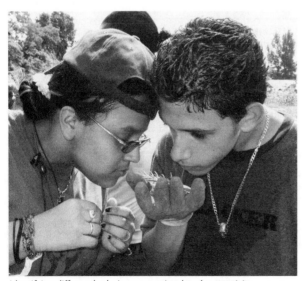

Identifying different herbs is an engaging, hands-on activity.

Getting Started

Many nutrition educators find this step to be the most creative and enjoyable part of nutrition education planning: designing messages and activities that are theory based and engaging, fun, and relevant to the intended audience. This is the time to brainstorm numerous ideas for translating objectives into activities! These activities need to be based on a thorough understanding of the audience. If you are designing these sessions with a colleague or a group, it is usually helpful if one of you brings in ideas for some tentative activities for the session(s) and the others provide feedback and brainstorm. You may designate one person to do the actual writing of the lesson plans/educational plans, or you may all take turns writing the lessons. A *lesson plan* (or *educational plan*) is a plan for the educational activities that you will conduct with any group, in nonformal as well as formal settings. Lesson plans, in modified form, also guide educational content and activities conducted through other channels (e.g., newsletters, posters). They are similar to the notion of "messages" in social marketing approaches.

Before you begin, however, you will find it useful to consult the following specific information sources to help you in the process:

- *Research literature* from information in Part I of this text, particularly Chapters 3 and 4, and current nutrition education studies or best practices on effective strategies to enhance motivation for health- and food-related behaviors for your intended audience and for the behavioral goals selected for your program.
- *Programs, activities, and materials produced by other interventions* that might serve as useful models if they incorporate theory as recommended here. Suitable evaluated programs or materials may already be available for use. There is no point reinventing the wheel. Many materials developed with government funding can be found on the Internet, so go online to learn more about the program or materials. Review the program materials and talk to the individuals and organizations that developed the lessons if you have questions. However, it is extremely important that the educational strategies and learning experiences be based on clearly identified theory and evidence (or that you can identify the theory variables being addressed even if the program developers did not make the theory clear). Ask yourself these questions:
  - Does the program or activity address your program's specified behavioral goals and educational objectives?
  - Did the program using these materials have positive outcomes? Which key strategies did it use? Is there evidence as to which strategies were most effective in addressing the mediators of behavior?

- *Needs analysis information* that you gathered in Step 1 about characteristics of the intended group that affect learning: for example, data showing the importance of peers for teenagers, or life stage considerations for women with children. A review of the kinds of magazines, books, and other media that the intended audience uses most often, or trusts the most, will be helpful.
- Audience background considerations from Step 1 are crucial at this point:
  - Cultural background considerations in terms of learning activity preferences
  - Educational level: Years of schooling completed
  - Academic skills, literacy level
  - Physical and cognitive developmental level (children)
  - Special needs: If the group is an adult group, will children be present? Can child care be provided during the sessions or will you need to design activities for both mothers and their young children? Does the group have special learning disabilities or physical handicaps?
  - Emotional needs: What is going on emotionally in the lives of the audience? How will this influence their ability to hear the nutrition education message?
  - Social needs: Do they know each other? Does getting together satisfy a social need as well as an educational one?
- *Audience-preferred learning styles or instructional formats* from Step 1, such as lectures, films, discussion, hands-on activities, group work, or field experiences such as supermarket tours.

Creating Opportunities for Active Participation and Learning

As you design activities, keep in mind that generally we remember

- 10% of what we read
- 20% of what we hear
- 30% of what we see
- 50% of what we hear and see
- 70% of what we say and write
- 90% of what we both say and do

A major way to encourage active participation is the use of *hands-on activities*. Hands-on activities enhance motivation by giving participants a sense of involvement with the learning at hand. For example, label reading can be taught in a hands-on way in which participants handle real food packages, containers, and cans (empty) to determine healthful choices. Such an activity is much more motivating than simply lecturing to participants about "how to read a food label." When conducting demonstrations, it is effective to have audi-

> ### BOX 11-1 Special Challenge of Nutrition Education with Low-Resources Audiences in Low-Income Neighborhoods
>
> Adopting healthful eating patterns is difficult for most people. It is especially difficult for low-resources individuals for a variety of reasons. Some of the reasons identified in studies include the following:
>
> - Financial limitations due to low resources
> - Lack of time, since many work long hours
> - Lack of availability of quality healthful foods at affordable prices in neighborhood
> - Family customs and habits
>
> Low-income consumers want to ensure that no one in the family goes hungry. They will thus strive to get enough food energy for all at low cost. An economic analysis of diets has found an inverse relationship between the energy density of foods, defined as available energy per unit weight (kilocalories per gram), and energy cost (dollars per kilocalorie). This means that diets based on refined grains, added sugars, and added fats cost less than the diets recommended by nutrition educators that are based on lean meats, fish, fresh vegetables, and fruit. On a *calorie per dollar* basis, bread, cookies, and even chocolate are cheaper than fruits and vegetables. One study found that adding fat and sweets to the diet *lowered* adjusted diet costs, whereas adding fruits and vegetables *increased* adjusted diet costs.
>
> Nutrition education must keep these economic considerations in mind when working with low-resources audiences. Institutional- and policy-level activities are also essential to complement group-level activities.
>
> *Sources:* Palmieri, D., G.W. Auld, T. Taylor, P. Kendall, and J. Anderson. 1998. Multiple perspectives on nutrition education needs of low-income Hispanics. *Journal of Community Health* 23(4):301–316; and Drewnowski, A. 2004. Obesity and the food environment: Dietary energy density and diet costs. *American Journal of Preventive Medicine* 27(3, Suppl. 1):154–162.

ence members come up to perform some aspects of the demonstration activities (e.g., spooning out the amount of fat in various fast foods) or to participate in a drama presented to the others. This not only provides active participation for some members, but also encourages peer social norms.

Another example of active participation is *role playing*, in which the person enacts the role of someone else by improvising rather than reading a script. Role playing attitudes counter to our own can be a powerful technique in facilitating deliberation and change in our views of ourselves, of other people, and of an advocated viewpoint or behavior.

You can also engage learners in *discussion* among themselves in dyads, triads, or small groups about such topics as why it is so hard to get our children to eat vegetables, why we have a hard time carrying out our intentions to eat more healthfully, what are some ideas for healthful meals in minutes, or how to make food choices in a manner that promotes local farms. Such an approach encourages cooperative learning. Research on cooperative learning indicates that when people participate in small group activities, they are more likely to deliberate on the issues, examine their own attitudes, and desire to learn more (Johnson & Johnson, 1987).

Facilitated discussion is a commonly used approach to group sessions that fosters active participation. Facilitated discussion is based on dialogue and exchange between the nutrition educator as facilitator of the group and group participants. It avoids lecturing, instead focusing on open-ended questions, active listening, and respect for the ideas of everyone in the group to promote active participation and weave a meaningful learning experience for all. It can include the kinds of cooperative learning discussed earlier. Facilitated discussion is described in greater detail in Chapter 15.

Constructing an Instructional Framework to Deliver Educational Strategies

The major task in translating theory into practice is to design, sequence, and deliver theory-based educational strategies in such a way as to achieve the behavioral goals and educational objectives we have selected.

Chapter 1 defined nutrition education as a combination of educational strategies, accompanied by environmental supports and policy, designed to facilitate the voluntary adoption and maintenance of behaviors conducive to health. This means that nutrition education consists of a set of learning activities that are systematically designed and organized with a purpose in mind. Designing nutrition education thus presents the challenge of selecting and organizing a logical and productive sequence for the educational strategies or learning experiences. The plan for the educational strategies is referred to as a lesson plan, activity plan, educational plan, curriculum, or program. Instruction is the means or method for making the plan operational. The curriculum or program is the *what*, and instruction is the *how*. In our case, the *what* are the *mediators* of behavior change—the theory constructs—that the program addresses, and the *how* are the educational *strategies* we use to operationalize mediators and the *activities* that translate the strategies into *learning experiences*.

Creating an instructional framework to deliver the educational strategies thus requires two activities: (1) selecting the strategies that are based on theory constructs and operationalizing them, and (2) organizing and sequencing the strategies appropriately. We will provide a brief overview of these two activities and then devote the remainder of the chapter to describing how to conduct them.

Designing Educational Strategies to Address Potential Mediators of Behavior Change

Educational strategies are ways to operationalize theory constructs so that educational means can be used to address potential mediators of behavior change. These strategies can be used in delivering nutrition education through a variety of channels and are based on the evidence reviewed earlier in this book and on ongoing research (Contento et al., 1995; Lytle & Achterberg, 1995; Ammerman et al., 2002; Pomerleau et al., 2005). Figure 11-1 depicts the conceptual framework for nutrition education used throughout Part I of this book, this time showing how educational strategies and activities derived from theory can specifically address the educational goals and potential mediators of behavior change. Note that this model reflects the increasing evidence that the process of taking action or making change involves two phases: a motivational phase and an action phase (Armitage & Conner, 2000; Schwarzer, 1992). The potential mediators of change may be different for these two phases. Strategies derived from theory constructs for these mediators are thus likely to be different in each phase. The strategies from theory that are useful in the motivational phase are described in this chapter; those more useful in the action phase are described in the next chapter.

You may select from among these educational strategies those that are based on those mediators of change that are based on the theory you have selected or the conceptual model you have created for the intervention, serve your educational goals, and that reflect your nutrition education philosophy. That is, some strategies are relevant if you plan to use the health belief model, others if you plan to use the theory of planned behavior, and probably all of them if you are using the integrative model or health action process approach model that is the basis of the nutrition education conceptual framework of this book. There are many overlaps among theories, so many of these strategies will serve several theories.

This chapter describes strategies to operationalize social psychological theory constructs that represent potential personal mediators of the target behaviors. These strategies focus on increasing awareness of issues and risks, promoting active contemplation, enhancing motivation, and facilitating behavioral intentions. Chapter 12 describes strategies that operationalize social psychological theory constructs that represent potential personal mediators of change that assist individuals to develop action plans, build food- and nutrition-related skills, and strengthen their self-regulation

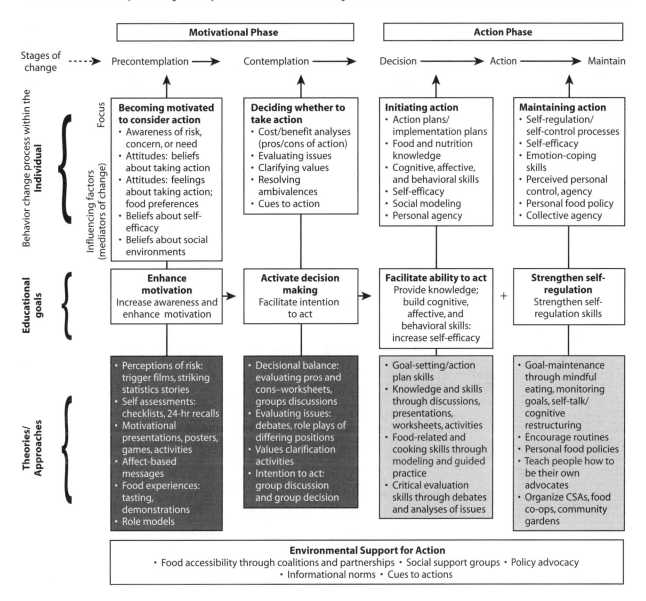

FIGURE 11-1 Conceptual framework for nutrition education: designing educational strategies to address educational goals and mediators of behavior.

skills. Although the educational strategies are separated into two chapters, you will most likely need to go back and forth between these two chapters as you design your strategies.

We recognize, of course, that people are integrated wholes—that thinking, feeling, and action are not linearly organized but closely interconnected. For example, learning new skills, such as cooking, may help people act on their motivations; at the same time, the new skills may increase self-efficacy, which is likely to enhance motivation. Furthermore, the immediate social environment, such as family and friends, may provide social support for change but may also

prove to be a barrier to change. In addition, individuals who are already in attendance at groups you have planned are probably the more interested and concerned ones. However, it is often the case that individuals attend sessions because others have suggested or required that they attend, or because they think they are ready to make changes but are not. Hence, assisting them to review and reflect on their motivations is still useful and important.

Table 11-1 summarizes these educational strategies, along with the kinds of practical educational activities or learning experiences you can create to operationalize these strategies.

TABLE 11-1 Linking Theory, Strategies, and Educational Activities

Potential Mediator of Behavior Change (Theory Construct)	Theory-Based Strategies for Potential Mediators of Behavior Change	Practical Educational Activities, Learning Experiences, Content, or Messages
Perceived risk	Confrontation with risks • Increase salience of issues or concern about problems. • Convey threat or use fear communications (TTM: Consciousness-raising and dramatic relief)	Trigger films, pictures, charts, striking national or local statistics, personal stories, role plays, demonstration Clear image of threat (e.g., film clips on effect of high-saturated-fat diet in clogging arteries) Demonstration using plastic tube clogged with fat and colored water to show blockage
Awareness	Self-assessment • Provide personalized self-assessments to counter optimistic bias (TTM: Self-reevaluation)	Self-assessment checklists; food or activity records or recalls
Outcome expectations	Information about outcome expectations (why-to information) • Persuasive communications about positive outcomes • Information on response efficacy or effectiveness of taking action	Presentations, visuals, demonstrations of scientific evidence regarding dietary practices and health or disease risk; nutrient–health relationships (antioxidants for eye health; nutrients and bone health) Motivational activities
Perceived benefits	Information about perceived benefits of taking action or motivators with personal meaning for the intended audience (why-to information)	Messages or educational activities that provide arguments for the desired action or practice to emphasize "what's in it for me?" Personal health benefits Other personal, family, or community benefits
Attitudes/affect	Reflection on affect/feelings	Attitude statements and discussion; learner-centered activities; emotion-based messaging
Self-efficacy and perceived barriers	Decrease perception of barriers or negative outcomes	Brainstorming; discussion of barriers and ways to overcome them
Food preferences	Direct experience with healthful food	Food tastings, demonstrations, cooking
Social norms	Awareness of social norms and social expectations	View print & TV ads; discuss impact of others
Habit	Bring to consciousness automatic behaviors, habits, or routines	Checklists of current practices; self-observation tool
Behavioral intention	Decisional balance: Analysis of pros and cons of action, and choice among actions Values clarification • Resolving resistance and ambivalences Anticipated regret Group decision and public commitment (TTM: Self-liberation)	Worksheets or discussions to analyze pros and cons of action; choices Values clarification worksheets for individuals, or group activities Imagery activities Group discussion followed by group decision on goals for action, and public commitment
Goal setting	Goal setting and implementation or action plans	Teach goal-setting skills, provide contracts/pledges or action plan forms

Potential Mediator of Behavior Change (Theory Construct)	Theory-Based Strategies for Potential Mediators of Behavior Change	Practical Educational Activities, Learning Experiences, Content, or Messages
Behavioral capability (how-to information)	Food- and nutrition-related knowledge and cognitive and behavioral skills to engage in actions (tailor to prior knowledge, beliefs, attitudes, and values) Teaching of how-to information Building food and nutrition skills Active methods Discussion and facilitated discussion Guided practice	Discussions, presentations, or learning experiences to teach needed food- and nutrition-related knowledge and skills to engage in behavior; food preparation skills
Self-efficacy	• Social modeling of behavior • Guided practice to encourage mastery of behavioral skills • Exhortations or persuasion so as to overcome doubt	Make the desired actions easy to understand and do: • Clear instructions • Demonstration of the behavior by respected social model • Direct experience (e.g., food preparation or cooking) with guidance and feedback • Give feedback on performance, emphasizing achievements and difficulties already overcome
Reinforcements	Provide reinforcements and rewards	Verbal praise, tee-shirts, drawing for prizes, or awards
Self-regulation	Strengthen self-regulation skills (self-influence or self-control) • Self-monitoring skills for progress toward goal • Goal maintenance • Coping self-efficacy • Managing cues from environment	Identify and prioritize competing goals Provide self-monitoring forms and tips Protecting action goals from distractions: Mindful eating Conscious attention (self-talk) and planning ahead Developing strategies for coping with difficulties
	Developing personal policies, routines, and habits (TTM: counter-conditioning, rewards management, stimulus control)	Tip sheets on personal policies for purchasing foods, meal patterns (e.g., always eat breakfast; bring lunch to work), eating out
Social support	Social support (TTM: Helping relationships)	Create supportive group environment; encourage buddy system
Cues to action	Provide cues to action	Billboards, grocery bags, media messages, news articles, refrigerator magnets and key chains with messages

TTM = Transtheoretical model.

Organizing and Sequencing Educational Strategies: Instructional Design

The instructional design principles of Gagne (1965, 1985) and a step model of health communications (McGuire, 1984) can help us think about the sequencing of strategies. Gagne's theory of instruction has been widely used to design instruction using a variety of media (e.g., oral, written, computer based, Web based) for a variety of audiences (e.g., children, adults). Instruction can be seen as the deliberate arrangement of events in the individual's environment to make learning happen and also to make it effective (Gagne, 1994). A theory of instruction is thus about how to select and arrange *events of instruction* to provide support for the internal processes of learning. Later in this chapter we describe how to sequence educational strategies according to Gagne's instructional design principles. The end result will be one or a series of educational plans or lesson plans. We provide one such educational plan for our case study in this chapter, and another educational plan in Chapter 12.

Selecting Educational Strategies That Operationalize Theory Constructs That Are Potential Personal Mediators of Action or Change

Enhancing motivation focuses on "what's in it for me?" It requires us to select educational strategies that operationalize theory constructs that are potential *motivational mediators* of action or behavior change derived from theory and nutrition education research evidence, such as beliefs and attitudes. These strategies will assist individuals to become aware of critical food-related issues; better understand their own needs, wants, feelings, motivations, and factors that seem to control their behaviors; actively contemplate the issues; resolve ambivalences; and then choose to take action—or not to do so—given their life circumstances. At the end of this process, if they intend to make a change, we can use strategies that operationalize *action mediators* derived from theory, such as implementation intentions or action plans, to carry out the change by addressing mediators of behavior change, the subject of the next chapter. It is important to remember that individuals make changes in their behavior only when they see the need to change, when the contemplated change touches other deeper values they have, and when they want to change. In addition, biological predispositions and powerful environmental forces make it difficult to change, so that the role of education needs to be placed in context.

How we address potential mediators (theory constructs) to increase deliberation and enhance motivation in practice will depend to a certain extent on the theory we have chosen, the channels we use, and the audiences with whom we work. In instances when we are able to work with small groups, we may be able to engage in more direct dialogue and debate about the issues, risks, and problems. In other circumstances, other activities, such as health communications through a variety of channels, will be useful to get attention, to raise issues, and to promote active contemplation. Media campaigns and other channels of health communications that use social marketing principles can be especially useful here.

Awareness is often considered the first step of the dietary change process. So how do we increase awareness in individuals who are not aware of an issue or of the impacts of their behavior on health or other outcomes? Both instructional theory and communications theory point to the importance of gaining people's attention from the outset. This can be done by presenting messages on the positive or negative consequences of the behavior or practice in a way that is striking, memorable, and respectful of the audience, inspiring individuals to care. Messages can address the potential behavioral mediator of *perception of risk*, or they can focus on the positive—the potential behavioral mediator of *perceived benefits of action*.

Table 11-1 shows how strategies are derived from theory-based mediators of change and how they shape the educa-

tional experiences or learning experiences used in nutrition education. From among the strategies, choose those that are appropriate for your targeted behavior and intended audience. Not all strategies will be appropriate for all situations. Your assessment in Step 2 will guide your choices. In addition, do not attempt too much in your sessions. People can usually process only small amounts of information at a time, so provide only what is relevant and needed to achieve the objectives. The rule of thumb is, plan to cover half as much in twice the time as you think it will take!

Educational Strategies Based on the Theory Construct of Risk Perceptions

Several theories propose that a sense of concern about an issue or a perception of personal risk is important for individuals to be in a state of readiness to act. Although such perceived risk or concern is not the most immediate or direct mediator of behavior, it is often a necessary and important first step. People are often either unaware of an issue or have an optimistic bias. People thus need enough knowledge of potential problems to warrant action, but not so much as to elicit denial or paralyze them. It is often useful to start with learning experiences or messages to provide more accurate understanding of an issue or perceptions of risk. The strategies discussed here are similar to those designed to address the consciousness-raising and dramatic relief/emotional arousal processes of change in the transtheoretical model (Table 11-2).

Provide Personalized Self-Assessments to Provide Realistic Appraisal and Correct Optimistic Bias

Self-assessment of food-related behaviors that is personalized and compared with recommendations can be an effective motivational activity as a starting point for nutrition education. People love to find out about themselves! Accurate self-assessment is key: people are often not aware of their own dietary intake status and do not perceive a need to change. Knowing about their actual behaviors can help them become more interested in deliberation of issues, and more motivated. Such personalized feedback may also counteract the tendency to be optimistically biased and encourage individuals to consider changes in their dietary behaviors based on their true risk. As noted earlier in this book, research with the precaution adoption process model suggests that when individuals first become aware of a concern or risk, they tend to disregard it as irrelevant or unimportant, then they believe that it may be significant for others but not for themselves, and then finally they believe that it is relevant to themselves personally. Only then will they take action.

Individuals can complete checklists that provide information specific to the intervention's behavioral goals, such as how many fruits and vegetables they are actually consuming, the number of sweetened beverages or milk products con-

TABLE 11-2 Transtheoretical Model: Processes Associated with Stages of Change and Implications for Intervention Strategies

Processes of Change	Stages When More Often Used	Brief Description of Change Process Within the Individual	Intervention Strategies
Consciousness-raising	PC to C	Increasing one's awareness about causes and consequences, seeking new information about healthy behavior	Increase awareness of individuals' eating patterns (e.g., F&V intake) through self-assessment and feedback, confrontations, media campaigns
Dramatic relief/emotional arousal	PC to C	Emotional experience of threat followed by relief if action is taken	Personalizing risk, personal testimonies, role playing, trigger films, media campaigns to address feelings
Environmental reevaluation	PC to C	Assessing how one's behaviors affect others and the physical environment	Empathy training, documentaries
Self-reevaluation	C to Prep to A	Appraisal of one's image of oneself	Assisting individuals to clarify their values; imagining themselves as active and healthy; believing that behavior change is part of their identity
Self-liberation	C to Prep to A	Believing in ability to change; consciously making a firm commitment to act	Commitment-enhancing techniques such as contracting and public group decisions
Helping relationships	A to M	Enlisting social support for the healthy behavior change	Build rapport; create a supportive environment through groups, buddy systems, and calls
Counterconditioning	A to M	Substituting alternative thoughts and behaviors for less healthful eating behaviors	Teach new ways of thinking (self-talk) about behavior; new food- and nutrition-related skills
Reinforcement and rewards management	M	Increasing rewards for healthful eating and decreasing rewards for unhealthful eating practices	Overt rewards such as tee-shirts; incentives; verbal reinforcement; teaching individuals to reward themselves
Stimulus or environmental control	M	Removing cues to less healthful eating and adding cues for more healthful eating	Provide instruction on how to restructure environment; refrigerator magnets with reminders; tip sheets
Social liberation	All	Selecting and advocating for environments that support healthful food practices	Provide environmental supports such as more F&V in schools or worksites; advocacy; policy

PC = precontemplation; C = contemplation; Prep = preparation; A = action; M = maintenance; F&V = fruits and vegetables.

sumed in a day, or how many times they eat breakfast in a week. Another example of self-assessment in group settings might be asking the group to complete a 24-hour food intake recall, and then have members individually compare their intakes with the food pyramid recommendations. Or you can analyze the intakes of the group and use those average data as the starting point for nutrition education. For example, you can collect such data during your needs analysis process in Step 1, calculate the averages, and display them in a handout or slide when you meet with the group. This is particularly useful if the group is a low-literacy audience. Studies show, however, that in group settings, such assessments are more effective when people analyze their own data than when data are analyzed for them. Thus, self-analysis is preferable when time permits and the level of education enables people to do so.

In the Powerful Girls Have Powerful Bones campaign created by the Centers for Disease Control and Prevention (www.cdc.gov/PowerfulBones/), girls can complete a

"Bone Health Habit Quiz" online to find out how they are doing in terms of diet and physical activity related to bone health, or a "Powerful Girl Quiz" to find out how much they know about bone health. The website is colorful and motivating, and the quizzes are engaging. The participant gets a score and recommendations for what to do. Nutrition Education in Action 11-1 reproduces the Powerful Girl quiz.

Checklists can also be devised to see how "green" individuals' food shopping practices are (based, perhaps, on where the food comes from or its degree of packaging). Or a checklist, with a scoring system, can be devised for positive behaviors that contribute to nutritional well-being. Group members can also complete short instruments that provide them with information on their own stage of readiness to make changes in their diet. In the area of physical activity, pedometers can be very motivating. Health risk appraisals are examples of self-assessments. As noted before, personal feedback must be accompanied by information on effective actions that individuals can take to deal with the threat or by information on potentially better alternative behaviors.

Self-assessments can be modified to involve assessment of relevant community or organizational behaviors and practices. Members of an organization or community can do an assessment about food-related practices and resources to provide themselves with a true picture of the extent of risk or the severity of an issue. For example, children can first do a 24-hour food recall on themselves in terms of the packaging they disposed of at each eating occasion. Then they can do a study in their schools to investigate how much packaging their school throws out after each lunch, from which they can calculate the amount disposed of by all schools in their city or in the United States.

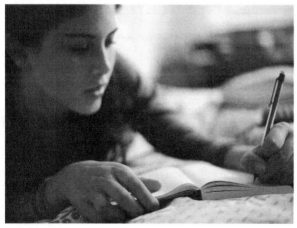

Self-assessment is a powerful tool.

Increase Awareness of Risks and Concerns: Why-To Knowledge

As we saw in Chapter 4, an appeal to fear about the threat of a condition is effective only if it is accompanied by information on effective actions that people can take to reduce the threat, and these actions appear easy to accomplish. Research evidence suggests that a sense of threat may be important, particularly on some issues such as food safety behaviors, but it is an empirical question whether fear will be useful for your particular audience and, if so, what the optimal level of threat might be. You must determine this information from your activities in Step 1. It has been suggested that fear may be useful for taking precautions against future problems but is counterproductive in dealing with existing problems.

When using the risk perception approach, the first part of the message is designed to create a motivation to avoid risk or danger. In group settings, trigger films, pictures, charts, striking national or local statistics, personal stories, and other consciousness-raising strategies can be used to bring to life and make relevant issues of concern based on scientific evidence, such as the increase in obesity rates, breastfeeding rates, increasing portion sizes, bone loss, and metabolic syndrome in adolescents. Such activities can also be used to bring other issues to awareness, such as the rate of loss of farm land, how much of school lunch is thrown away daily, or the amount of disposable service materials (paper plates, sporks, etc.) thrown away each day from the school (students could also do a study to find out). Visuals are especially powerful, such as pictures or actual food products (packages only) to show the portion sizes of various food products and beverages served in movie theaters, fast food outlets, and elsewhere. Media campaigns are especially useful here.

The second part of the message should be designed to show that people can take specific actions that will reduce the threat or danger and should provide exact instructions for when, how, and where to take action.

An example of an activity on cancer risk perception in a group setting to illustrate the notion of risk is to have individuals count off using 1 through 4. All those who are 1s are asked to gather in a group, and all the others in a second group. Those in the first group are told they have a high risk of getting cancer, and the others do not. But then, those in the first group who eat four cups or more of fruits and vegetables a day are asked to move to the second group, illustrating that they can reduce their risk by their food choices. Likewise, those in the second group who eat fewer fruits and vegetables are asked to move into the first group, illustrating that they can increase their risk by their dietary behaviors. This activity needs to be followed by specific instructions about what group participants can do to increase their fruit and vegetable consumption and about how to engage in other preventive actions, such as increasing physical activity and getting regular checkups with physicians.

NUTRITION EDUCATION IN ACTION 11-1

The Powerful Girl Quiz: A Motivational Self-Assessment

Are You as Bone-Health Savvy as You Think? Yeah, you're smart about school, guys, and the real scoop on all the hot bands. But do you know enough about powerful bones? Take this quiz to see how much you really know. If you score high enough, you just might win a cyber trophy.

1. You're babysitting your little sister and you have to make a healthy dinner with vegetables. What should a bone-smart babysitter pick?
   a. French fries — Potatoes are a vegetable, right?
   b. Broccoli — With low-fat cheese for even more calcium.
   c. Skip the vegetable, Mom will never know.
   d. Lima beans — Your sister can't stand them.
2. Mom and Dad are away! You could drink soda all day, but for strong bones you . . .
   a. Slurp up the soda anyway.
   b. Drink fruit punch.
   c. Go for fat-free or low-fat milk and orange juice with added calcium.
   d. Drink diet soda.
3. Its been storming for days and you're tired of being shut in. What is the best way to get some weight-bearing physical activity?
   a. Forget it and catch up on TV reruns.
   b. Find a comfy chair and chat on the phone.
   c. Do some stretches while watching movies. At least it's some activity.
   d. Clear some space and jump rope.
4. You're eating out with friends after a basketball game. Everyone orders chicken tenders and soda, but for healthy bones you order. . .
   a. Chicken tenders and soda too — why be difficult?
   b. Chicken tenders and low-fat milk — a yummy way to get calcium.
   c. Nothing — there's no healthy fast food.
5. Your best pal won't drink milk or eat yogurt or cheese, either. But calcium is important for strong bones. What can you do?
   a. It's really none of your business.
   b. There aren't any other foods with calcium.
   c. Tell her about other foods with calcium like broccoli and orange juice with added calcium.
   d. Who needs calcium? Isn't weight-bearing physical activity enough?
6. It's Saturday and you're playing basketball with friends when it starts to rain! What should a powerful girl do?
   a. Tell your friends they might as well go home.
   b. Get out your board games.
   c. Pick a few CDs and make up dance routines.

Answers are then given on the website, and individuals taking the quiz can add up their points to see how they stack up.

Source: Centers for Disease Control and Prevention. 2006. Powerful bones. Powerful girls. http://www.cdc.gov/PowerfulBones/quizzes/index.html.

Educational Strategies Derived from the Theory Construct of Outcome Expectations or Perceived Benefits

Increase Perception of Positive Outcomes or Perceived Benefits of Taking Action: Why-To Knowledge

A major task in promoting contemplation and enhancing motivation is to design activities that focus on beliefs about the potential desirable outcomes or benefits of the given behaviors. Such beliefs are powerful motivators of behavior through their impact on attitudes, intentions, and the formation of goals. In many situations, a focus on benefits is the best way to gain the attention of the intended audience.

Information about desirable outcomes is usually stated in the form of reasons for the action. These reasons are of two kinds: benefits based on scientific or other kinds of evidence for the effectiveness of taking action, which we have referred to as *why-to knowledge*, and benefits that are of personal importance to individuals. Here is the time to present the scientific studies and data that make a case for a role of diet in health, weight control, disease prevention, or bone health or for the importance of breastfeeding for infant health. For those nutrition educators interested in food sustainability issues, this is the time to talk about the benefits of eating locally and so forth. Here is also the time to explore benefits of a personal nature.

As an attention-getter at the beginning of a session or series of sessions, or as part of a media campaign, the benefits of action should be presented in a way that is brief, catchy, and memorable. When benefits are explored in greater detail later in the instructional sequence, more food and nutrition data can be presented and explored. Perceived benefits can be presented through striking statistics, such as on the benefits of breastfeeding in reducing infections in infants when working with pregnant women. The anticipated benefits or positive outcomes of recommended skills and behaviors can also be communicated by use of such methods as films, posters, games, role plays, or excerpts from magazines popular with the intended audience. The beneficial effects of various food- and nutrition-related behaviors, such as eating more vegetables, can be presented in terms of health benefits or of benefits for the sustainability of the food system. Use of vivid and personal material is more likely to be effective.

For most audiences, the emphasis should be on short-term benefits, such as feeling better, having more energy, looking more attractive, providing satisfaction in doing something good for oneself or for the community, or improving the availability of local foods. Such an approach is more likely to be effective than emphasizing the long-term benefits such as reduced disease risk, a longer life, or leaving enough fossil fuel for people in the 22nd century. In one study, an attempt to increase consumption of the school lunch was accomplished by communicating the message that eating school

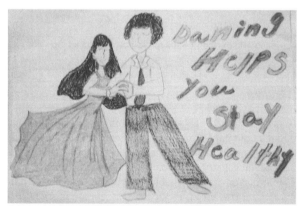

Drawing personal beliefs is a vivid example of personal motivators. (Courtesy of Linking Food and the Environment, Teachers College Columbia University.)

lunch was "cool" and by linking it with something perceived as positive—sports: a Training Table program highlighted how nutritious foods boost athletic performance. Activities must be fun, engaging, and involve active participation to the extent possible.

We must bear in mind, of course, that we all have many conflicting beliefs about the consequences of the same behavior: rich desserts may be fattening, but they taste good; breastfeeding may be good for the infant, but is embarrassing to do when outside the home. In addition, the relative importance of different benefits, or reasons for action, may differ depending on the behavior and the group or audience. For example, for the behavior of eating fruits and vegetables, being cool may be important for teenagers, and creating clear skin may be important for young women; improving the health of the baby may be important for pregnant women, whereas reducing cancer risk may be important for men. Immediate benefits usually carry more weight than benefits in the future, particularly for teenagers. Thus, the messages about benefits or positive anticipated outcomes of action must be based on those that are personally meaningful to the specific group.

A focus on positive outcomes for taking action is especially useful for mass media campaigns. Here the elaboration likelihood method (ELM) of communication can be especially useful (Petty & Cacioppo, 1986). As we discussed in Chapter 4, this method proposes that individuals differ in their ability and motivation to process educational messages thoughtfully. Hence, our messages need to take into account the recipients' ability to process the messages and encourage their motivation to do so. Simply providing more arguments may not increase effectiveness; it is the quality of the arguments that is important. To increase participants' *ability* to process messages, make your messages straightforward and clear, repeat or reinforce them, and present them with a minimum of distractions. To address the issue of *motivation* to process messages, make messages unexpected or novel, memorable, culturally appropriate, and most important, *personally relevant*, stressing positive outcomes important to the intended audience. Messages can involve humor, warmth, or other attributes that are appropriate for a given audience. The messages can be expressed in terms of what participants will gain from taking action as well as what they will lose by *not* taking action. These principles apply whether the messages are delivered through mass media, brochures, newsletters, or in a group setting.

The 5 A Day campaign message was stated as "Eat 5 a Day for Better Health," the latter words (*for better health*) being the argument for, or the benefit of, eating five fruits and vegetables. This message was chosen based on results from focus groups, which found that the benefits of feeling better, health, and weight control were most salient to consumers. Interestingly, the potential benefit of "cutting my risk of getting cancer in half" was not considered credible, and that of "feeling less stress and a little more in control of my life" from eating fruits and vegetables was met with skepticism. Thus, your educational activity must be specific to the benefits that you have identified as relevant to the intended audience. The message was later "freshened" to "Five a day the color way: eat your colors every day to stay healthy and fit."

The VERB campaign, created by the Centers for Disease Control and Prevention (CDC) for children aged 9 to13, is designed to increase physical activity through targeted advertising, promotions, and events for tweens. The CDC has developed a variety of VERB materials to help organizations that work with children connect VERB to their programs, classes, and activities. It is an excellent example of a campaign that is based on making the outcomes meaningful for teens, based on research regarding potential motivators (see Nutrition Education in Action 11-2). So although the rationale for the program is that there are health risks to inactivity and health benefits to being active, those are not the motivators (or expected outcomes) used with participating youth.

Individuals' actions and choices are always embedded in larger values. The perceptions of benefits discussed previously can be considered instrumental values—that is, values to bring about specific outcomes. The larger values are end-state or terminal values, such as self-respect, a sense of accomplishment, equality, pleasure, true friendship, or wisdom. These are discussed later in the chapter in the section "Assist Groups to Clarify Their Values."

Decrease Perception of Negative Outcomes or Barriers to Taking Action

Nutrition education seeks not only to increase the perceptions of benefits but also to decrease the perceptions of barriers to taking action. For some behaviors, reducing the negative outcomes of action is more important than increasing the positive effects or benefits of action. In the language of social marketing exchange theory, nutrition education helps the audience see that the costs they incur in taking action are outweighed by the benefits they will receive. You should have identified the barriers or perceived costs specific to your intended audience for the program's target behaviors or practices in Step 2. Here we describe potential activities and learning experiences to operationalize these strategies.

We can assist the group to share and understand the difficulties and identify their (or their family members') barriers to healthful eating practices. This can be done by having the group identify barriers and list them on newsprint, and then asking the group to brainstorm ways of overcoming these barriers. You can facilitate and add your own suggestions. This is a useful strategy for all age groups. This is the time to address and, if appropriate, change individuals' misconceptions about their ability to act. For example, for the barrier

of the cost of fruits and vegetables, suggestions can be made about buying in season. For the barrier that fruits and vegetables easily go bad, suggestions can be made about how to store them to reduce spoilage, or to buy other forms, such as frozen or canned. For embarrassment about breastfeeding in public places, suggestions can be made as to how to do this unobtrusively. Misconceptions can also be factual in nature, such as the belief that eating calcium-rich foods can increase "hardening of the arteries."

Educational Strategies Derived from the Theory Construct of Self-Efficacy

Enhance Self-Efficacy: Make the Desired Actions Easy to Understand and Do

Self-efficacy is important for both motivation and taking action. In the motivational phase of nutrition education, perceived barriers are closely related to, and often mirror, self-efficacy and perceived behavioral control. That is, as barriers are overcome, self-efficacy increases, and as self efficacy increases, perceived barriers decrease. In this phase of nutrition education, therefore, increasing self-efficacy is about reducing the perceived difficulty of taking action. Using examples of valued social models enacting the behavior, such as sports figures or successful breastfeeding moms, is an effective strategy.

Here the focus is on making the behavior that is the target of the intervention easy to understand and carry out. In a group setting, you can elicit from the group tips and write them up on newsprint. Individuals who have been successful in engaging in the targeted behavior can share their experiences. In using social models, the audience must see that the outcomes of the behavior are clearly beneficial to the model.

In one example with inner-city teens, nutrition educators led the group through calculations that showed that packaged snacks from vending machines and their local stores actually cost more than making their own simple snacks or even fruit that could easily be carried around. They then had the teens assemble simple snacks from basic ingredients that they liked, such as raisins and nuts. The nutrition educators also calculated the time it took to make or assemble the snacks, showing how time did not have to be a barrier.

Educational strategies to increase self-efficacy can also involve mass media messages. An interesting mass media campaign to increase fruit and vegetable intake involved billboards in the community, along with flyers, that had on them a drawing of a specific fruit or vegetable accompanied by a relevant message, all with a similar format. For example, a drawing of a banana was accompanied by the message "Peel. Eat. How easy is that?" (Iowa Department of Public Health, 2005).

NUTRITION EDUCATION IN ACTION 11-2

VERB: A Physical Activity Campaign for Tweens

The VERB campaign, created by the Centers for Disease Control and Prevention (CDC, 2006), works to increase physical activity through targeted advertising, promotions, and events for tweens. The CDC has also developed a variety of VERB materials to help organizations that work with children connect VERB to their programs, classes, and activities.

The VERB vision: All youth leading healthy lifestyles.

The VERB mission: To increase and maintain physical activity among tweens (youth ages 9–13).

Campaign audiences: The main audience for the campaign is tweens. Other important audiences are parents and adult influencers, including teachers, youth leaders, physical education and health professionals, pediatricians, health care providers, and coaches.

Teens can go on the website (www.verbnow.com) for ideas for physical activity and participate in all kinds of online activities with other teens. Parents are also urged to participate: (www.verbparents.com, English; www.NAFS.org, Spanish).

Rationale for Campaign

The underlying rationale for the campaign has to do with risks to children of inactivity and the benefits of being physically active, such as strengthening muscles, bones, and joints; controlling weight; and improving overall health. Physical activity also helps to develop skills that can benefit children for life, including goal setting and achievement, getting along with others, leadership, and teamwork. Other research shows that physical activity can help increase concentration, reduce anxiety and stress, and increase self-esteem—all of which may have a positive effect on students' scholastic achievement. These important benefits of being physically activity are *not,* of course, particularly meaningful to the tween audience.

What Moves Tweens

Meaningful motivators for this age group are based on VERB research findings: Children this age respond to the spirit of adventure, discovery, and finding their own thing. So adults can help tweens discover new activities that they enjoy.

- Give away small prizes such as stickers, pins, or water bottles to reward tweens for being active. Prizes serve as great incentives for kids.
- Design activities with input from the kids. They will be more inclined to participate because they want to, not because they have to, do something.
- Some tweens prefer activities with a competitive edge, whereas others simply like playing a game with friends. Find out their preferences. All tweens will experience the rewards of being active if it is enjoyable for them.
- Tweens, especially girls, like social interaction with friends. It makes playing actively more fun and offers opportunities for peer recognition and praise.
- Praise kids just for trying something new and getting active. Your encouragement means a lot to them.

Campaign Outcomes

After one year, the VERB campaign had

- Narrowed the gap in physical activity between girls and boys
- Resulted in lower-income tweens becoming more physically active, despite greater barriers to being active
- Reached extraordinarily high awareness levels among tweens (74% nationally and 84% in high-dose communities) and very high understanding (90% nationally) of the campaign's core messages to be physically active and have fun

More specifically, evaluation measures demonstrated significant increases in physical activity as a direct result of VERB in the following key groups (Huhman et al., 2005):

Children 9–10 Years Old (8.6 million national population)

- 34% increase in free-time physical activity sessions nationally
- 32% decline in the number of sedentary 9- to 10-year-olds in high-dose communities

Girls (10 million national population)

- 27% increase in free-time physical activity sessions nationally
- 37% decline among least active in high-dose communities

(continued)

Nutrition Education in Action 11-2 (continued)

Tweens from Lower- (<$25,000; 4.5 million national population) to Lower-Middle-Income ($25,000–50,000; 6 million national population) Households
- 25% increase in free-time physical activity sessions nationally among lower-middle-income households
- 31% decline among least active from lower-income households in high-dose markets
- 38% decline among least active from lower-middle-income households in high-dose communities

These analyses included children from all racial/ethnic groups. Older tweens, boys, and tweens from middle- to higher-income households also showed some increases in physical activity, but those increases were not statistically significant.

References

Centers for Disease Control and Prevention. 2006. Youth media campaign: VERB. http://www.cdc.gov/youthcampaign/; and Huhman, M., L.D. Potter, F.L. Wong, et al. 2005. Effects of a mass media campaign to increase physical activity among children: Year 1 results of the VERB campaign. *Pediatrics* 116:e277–e284.

Educational Strategies Derived from the Theory Construct of Attitudes and Feelings Related to Taking Action

Increase Reflection on Attitudes and Feelings About Program Goal Behaviors or Practices

Beliefs about the outcomes of behavior constitute the cognitive component of attitudes and are a major motivator of behavioral intention, as we have seen. However, the affective component of attitudes, reflecting feelings, is also a powerful motivator. Nutrition education can assist individuals to understand their own feelings and emotions about food- and nutrition-related behaviors so that they can make changes where necessary to serve their own interests in improving health. Positive attitudes and feelings often come about from positive experiences from educational activities such as tasting and preparing food. However, they can also arise from having group members explore their feelings, not just their thoughts, about the behaviors central to your program. This can be done through a process of attitudes clarification.

Present some attitude statements and ask the group to discuss them or to explore them individually. You can also use the strategy of forming an attitude line. For example, you can verbalize an attitude statement such as the ones listed below and have participants line up from "Strongly Agree" to "Strongly Disagree." Alternatively, the four corners of the room can be used as "attitude corners": Strongly Agree, Agree, Disagree, and Strongly Disagree. Whatever the format, individuals should be encouraged to discuss their response with their peers. Examples of attitude statements are as follows:

Exclusively breastfeeding is best for my baby.

Healthful foods take too long to prepare.

People should have more willpower when they make food choices.

Eating food from local farms is very important for the health of the planet.

Attitudes and feelings about food also result from the sensory-affective responses generated from our experience with food. We should thus provide opportunities for pleasurable experiences with healthful food, as described later in the chapter.

Build on Personal Meanings

Lead a facilitated dialogue or a set of learner-centered activities to explore the personal and functional meanings that individuals give to food and eating. For example, it has been found that adolescents often use eating certain foods, such as junk foods, as a way to express their independence and personal will, challenge parental authority, and test boundaries. Many women see food as an enemy. Build on the personal meanings that you identified in Step 1.

Provide Direct Experience with Food to Enhance Enjoyment of Healthful Foods

Study after study shows that taste is a powerful determinant of food choice. Taste is in some ways an anticipated outcome of eating a food, but it also has an important physiological component. To emphasize the tastiness of healthful foods, nutrition educators should design activities that include tasting foods prepared in a healthful and delicious way.

Although active participation in general (such as group activities, checklists, or self-appraisals) is important in enhancing motivation and self-efficacy, hands-on food-related activities are important enough to be considered a special category (Liquori et al., 1998; Ammerman, 2002). Cooking or food preparation can provide vivid and motivating experiences when participants are physically involved in the activities (that is, not just watching a food demonstration). An example is the Cookshop Program, in which students were actively involved in cooking in classrooms (and eating what they cooked) (Liquori et al., 1998; Levy & Auld, 2004). Classes in which students cooked were compared with classes that involved active hands-on activities but did not include preparing food. Although both groups increased in knowledge, only the group that cooked changed its behavior to eat more of the whole grains and vegetables that were offered in the school lunch.

Educational Strategies Derived from the Theory Construct of Social Norms and Social Expectations

Increase Awareness of Social Norms and Social Expectations

Social norms and social expectations are also important mediators of behavior, as we have seen. You can design activities in which groups or intended audience members can be made aware of the influence of social norms on their behaviors. For example, mothers in the Women, Infants and Children (WIC) program can be provided with activities that analyze TV and print ads about women as mothers feeding their children and can be asked to share their feelings about the ads. Schoolchildren can be asked to conduct a survey of Saturday morning food ads, analyze them, and design an ad campaign they think would be effective in increasing the consumption of fruits and vegetables.

Group members can analyze the many other social sources of influences on food choice, such as when eating at work, in the cafeteria, and at home, or eating out with friends. You can also assist the groups to identify what important others think they should be doing, such as their spouses', partners', or mothers' approval or disapproval of breastfeeding (injunctive norms). Materials, films, and statistics can be used to indicate how individuals similar to the target group are engaging in the healthful behaviors, such as other WIC women breastfeeding, other teenagers drinking water instead of sweetened beverages, and so forth (descriptive norms). You can use peer educators to deliver the nutrition education, as has been done in programs with adolescents and with older adults, or you can use sports figures for adolescents, either in person or through other channels such as videos or brochures. You can discuss your own experiences or that of other credible social models. When designing mass media communications, whether visual or print, you can use messages from important people with whom audience members identify. Posters can be designed that show attractive people like themselves (e.g., other schoolchildren or other WIC mothers) enjoying eating the particular foods being emphasized in the intervention.

Skills for resisting social pressure are also important. Suggestions can be made about how to handle various social situations in which choosing the recommended foods or enacting the goal behaviors of the program will be difficult (such as office parties, social gatherings). In addition, the effects of the participants' behavior on others can be brought to awareness—such as the behaviors of parents in terms of impacts on their children's eating patterns, that of older siblings on younger siblings, and even that of teenagers on their friends. This is the environmental reevaluation strategy from the transtheoretical model (TTM).

Educational Strategies Derived from the Theory Construct of Beliefs About the Self

Clarify Self-Representation and Self-Evaluative Beliefs

Self-representations such as self-identity or social identity can be explored. Develop activities for individuals to explore such issues as "I think of myself as a health-conscious consumer," "I think of myself as someone who is concerned about environmental issues," "as a good mother," and so forth. You can also use the strategy of self-reevaluation from TTM to help individuals assess their images of themselves and rethink these images in positive terms.

Develop discussion questions or activities to explore individuals' perceptions about their responsibilities and moral obligations, both personal and social (e.g., as a mother, a spouse, or a citizen), in relation to the focus issue of your nutrition education session or program. Help individuals explore ideal-self versus actual-self discrepancies by devising messages or activities to help individuals become aware of their ideals, where they come from, and how realistic or healthful they are. Individuals can then make decisions about how to handle this awareness. In similar fashion, ought-to-be self versus actual-self discrepancies can be explored through activities that bring to awareness sources of the "oughts," such as being a good mother or being thin, and how to handle them. Active methods of self-exploration and understanding, debates of pros and cons, and discussions are likely to be the most effective strategies, although films and written materials can also be helpful if used appropriately.

Educational Strategies Derived from the Theory Construct of Habits and Routines

Bring to Consciousness Automatic Behaviors, Habits, or Routines

Many of our behaviors appear to occur without much thought. As we have seen, this results from the frequent pairing of foods and situations in which they are consumed. Nutrition education activities can bring to awareness such attitude–situation cues so that individuals can choose to change behaviors if they wish. For example, you can devise activities to assist individuals to identify cues that seem to trigger behavior directly (such as the smell of baked products or the sight of ice cream) or to identify the chain of events leading to eating a second helping so that individuals will be conscious of what they are doing.

Habit or routines are also important motivators of behavior. Nutrition education activities can be designed to bring the less positive routines (e.g., eating high-calorie snacks) to consciousness so that they can be considered and replaced by more positive routines or habits. Because these more positive behaviors may require more effort (e.g., cutting up fruits and vegetables), tip sheets, checklists, or activities can be designed to assist individuals to develop the new routines.

Provide Cues to Action

In many instances, individuals are motivated to some degree but need reminders to take action. Refrigerator magnets, bookmarks, grocery bags, and pencils with messages on them can provide cues to action. Mass media messages can also be very useful. Billboard messages can serve this role. You can also use more intensive methods, such as telephone calls, email messages, or mailed reminders.

A nutrition intervention at a college campus based on social cognitive theory illustrates how a variety of the strategies described here were used to increase students' awareness, attitudes, outcome expectations, and behavior-related how-to knowledge in order to increase the behaviors of increased fruit and vegetable intake and decreased fat intake. The program, called Right Bite, is discussed in Nutrition Education in Action 11-3. Note the many theory variables that were addressed and the activities used to address them.

Designing Education Strategies to Address Behavioral Intentions

Focus on Resolving Ambivalences and Making a Commitment

After the nutrition education activities have provided individuals with the opportunity to become more aware of their personal wants, feelings, and behaviors, to understand their own motivations and the factors that seem to control their behaviors, and to deliberate on the issues, we should now provide them with the opportunity to resolve any ambivalences that they have and to make a decision to take action, or not to do so, given their life circumstances. As we have noted before, individuals' attitudes and their beliefs about the outcomes of a behavior are numerous and may often conflict and compete. Ambivalence reflects the coexistence within individuals of both positive and negative beliefs about outcomes for the same behavior (e.g., eating chocolate is both delicious and fattening), as well as numerous conflicting feelings or attitudes. Individuals can pursue many alternative wishes or actions, and they will have to select among them. This is especially true for food choices and dietary behaviors.

We describe several strategies that you may find useful to activate decision making, assist individuals to resolve ambiv-

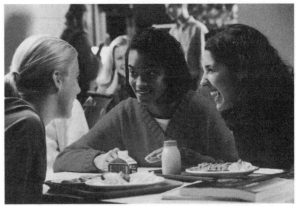

The influence of peers affects eating patterns of adolescents.

alences, and facilitate the formation of a behavioral intention or a goal intention. These strategies involve both cognitive and affective domains. In general they involve individuals' evaluations of the feasibility and desirability of the action or practice. Several of these strategies are similar to the transtheoretical model's strategies for self-reevaluation and self-liberation.

Provide Opportunity to Analyze the Pros and Cons of Action and of Choices Among Actions: Decisional Balance

Nutrition educators can provide opportunities for individuals to analyze all the benefits or pros of taking action and the cons or costs of taking action through worksheets or discussions. Individuals should also examine the reverse—that is, what they will lose by *not* taking action. This can be done using a pros and cons grid:

	Pros	Cons
If I don't take given action		
If I do take given action		

Participants can then make a decision as to whether to take action.

Individuals do not make decisions about taking action in a vacuum. Any given action is an alternative among several potential actions: for example, eating fruit for dessert or eating cheesecake, breastfeeding or bottle-feeding, and going running or watching television. Worksheets thus should help individuals evaluate and make choices among alternative behaviors competing for their time and attention.

Assist Groups to Clarify Their Values

Values are an important basis for action. As we have seen, individuals are motivated to take action if the action will lead to outcomes or goals they value. These are instrumen-

NUTRITION EDUCATION IN ACTION **11-3**

The Right Bite: A Nutrition Education Program for College Students Using Social Cognitive Theory

Right Bite Components	Description	Individual Responsible for Implementation	Social Cognitive Theory Constructs
Small group presentations	Nutrition education to small student groups. About 10 different presentations were prepared.	Peer educators	Outcome expectations
Personal follow-up (diet analysis)	One-on-one nutrition assessment and evaluation.	Peer educators	Outcome expectations; behavioral knowledge
Poster campaign	Campus role models such as the president of the college and well-known faculty members were featured in posters throughout campus.	Students in nutrition department	Outcome expectations; reinforcement; situation
Dorm contests	Healthy eating scavenger hunt.	Peer educators	Reinforcement; situation
Information tables at high-traffic areas	Nutrition information presented informally. Tables were supervised by peer educators.	Peer educators	Reinforcement
Brochure racks in dorms	Selected nutrition and exercise information was offered at dorms. Peer educators were responsible for replenishing supplies.	Peer educators	Behavioral knowledge; reinforcement
"Dear Foody" column in the campus newsletter	Brief newspaper column giving quick nutrition tips. Addressed topics of interest or concern to students.	Graduate assistant	Outcome expectations; impediments
Point-of-purchase information in campus cafeteria and vending machines	Specific nutrition analysis information about food choices.	Graduate assistant and cafeteria employees	Reinforcement
Website	Presented general program and nutrition information.	Graduate assistant	Reinforcement; impediments
Cafeteria tours	Offered specific tips on developing a healthy eating style.	Peer educators	Outcome expectations; Impediments
Right Bite video	Student role models illustrated benefits of healthy eating style. Addressed most barriers identified through students focus groups during the first year of implementation.	Students in the university communication department	Impediments

Source: Evans, M.E., and M. K. Sawyer-Morse. 2002. The Right Bite Program: A theory-based nutrition intervention at a minority college campus. *Journal of the American Dietetic Association* 102(Suppl):589–593.

tal values, such as taste, losing weight, looking attractive, or being liked by friends. You can assist the group to explore these values and to evaluate the importance of these values to them. However, we also make choices based on larger, end-state values, such as self-respect, sense of accomplishment, equality, social recognition, pleasure, true friendship, an exciting life, a world of beauty, inner harmony, freedom, happiness, mature love, wisdom, a worthwhile life, and so forth (Rokeach, 1973; Buchanan, 2000). For some individuals, these values are much more important than short-term, instrumental values. Again, individuals need to clarify for themselves how their current behaviors relate to these larger values and what changing these behaviors would mean to them in terms of these values.

Several activities can be used to assist people to clarify their values. You can present some value statements and ask participants to discuss or explore them in dyads and triads. One powerful activity that will help participants understand and process their feelings is to assemble pictures from magazines, photographs taken in the community, or drawings showing people engaging in different food- or health-related activities such as shopping for food, going to a farmers' market, preparing food, breastfeeding, eating at fast food restaurants, weighing themselves, or running. Show these pictures to participants and have them either write down or verbally report the feelings evoked by each picture. The answers can be coded, tallied, and reported back to the group as a whole to discuss. Participants may be surprised at their own feelings in response to the pictures, as well as those of others. The next phase is to explore why particular emotions or feelings came up and to develop some understanding of these feelings, especially the problematic ones. The group can then come up with some ways to explain the problems depicted or implied by the pictures and to solve them. The Freiere *conscientizacion* process involves this process (Freiere, 1970, 1973).

Affect/Feelings: Reflection on Potential Anticipated Regret

Anticipated regret or worry about the consequences of acting or failing to act has been shown to be a motivator of preventive health behavior. Individuals can be stimulated to visualize or imagine how they will feel about themselves after they have made the decision to act or not to act. Will they regret their choice?

Resolving Resistance and Ambivalence

To be effective, nutrition education strategies and messages need to enhance positive thoughts, feelings, and actions in recipients. Inevitably, however, group participants or message recipients may resist what is being said. Resistance to change can be useful because it contributes to human consistency and prevents people from constantly swinging from one opinion or behavior to another. Manoff (1985) points

out that potential cognitive and emotional "resistance points" of the audience, or their barriers to taking action, must be known, understood, and decisively resolved in the communication process if awareness of the recommended action is to be translated into action. That is, the effectiveness of nutrition education is improved if the potential internal dialogues of the audience disagreeing with the message are acknowledged, empathy with them is expressed, counterarguments are provided where appropriate or reassurance is given that the doubts do not interfere with taking action, and a way is provided for people to be able to comfortably give up the resistance. This does not imply manipulation of the audience. On the contrary, it means understanding the social, cultural, religious beliefs and practices, economic conditions, and political realities of the audience and making the nutrition message relevant and actionable.

We need to assist individuals to resolve their ambivalences and objections, but not in a defensive way. The task is to present the other side in a neutral, professional tone. Here we take three examples of internal dialogues or objections of program participants and provide a sample dialogue that aims to dispel these doubts.

Internal dialogue of group participant or message recipient: "My grandfather ate a high-fat diet and smoked all his life and didn't get heart disease, so why should I worry?"

Nutrition educator. A counterargument approach might go something like this: "Some of you may have had a grandfather or grandmother who ate unhealthy diets and smoked and yet lived to a ripe old age. However, that grandparent was lucky. You may or may not be so lucky. If that grandparent had 50 friends and half of them practiced poor health habits (as your grandparent did) and the other half ate healthful foods, exercised, and did not smoke, on the average the latter group would live longer, healthier lives. Taking care of yourself lowers your risk of developing chronic diseases such as cancer, heart disease, and stroke."

Internal dialogue: "My mother is always bugging me about doing the right thing to control my diabetes. I hate being told what to do—I'm just not going to do it!"

Nutrition educator. Teenagers are often angry at their parents, and counterargument would not be listened to. Using an acknowledging approach, the communication with newly diagnosed teenage diabetics might go like this: "I am sure that for many of you, your mothers tend to nag you about taking care of your diabetes. But controlling your diabetes is not your mother's job—it's yours. Consider following your doctor's instructions, but not for your mother's sake. Do it for yourself. You are worth it. Your mother means well; you need only to reassure her that you've got it under control, and that her way of showing concern is not helpful."

Internal dialogue: "What you say I should do is so difficult I'm feeling powerless."

Nutrition educator. What persons like this need is encouragement. Try a reassuring communication: "What I've recommended to you need not be accomplished in one day. Even the highest slopes can only be climbed one step at a time. Making changes to eat more ecologically is no different. You can't change the ways things are all at once. Think about one small step you are ready to change—today. For example, you may decide that you will bring your own bag to the grocery store to carry back your groceries rather than have the store put groceries in plastic bags. When you feel good about your progress, you can move on to the next action."

Other internal dialogues of program participants might include the following:

- "What you are saying is so complicated you are making me feel incompetent!"
- "You can talk all you want about eating more fruits and vegetables, but stores in my neighborhood don't carry many of them, and they're expensive."

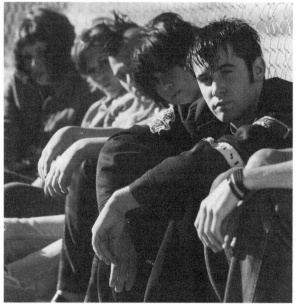

Sometimes teenage rebellion can be a factor in dietary decision making.

- "Often I don't do all I'm supposed to do for my hypertension, and nothing bad happens, so I'm not going to take all this too seriously."
- "My mother never breastfed me and I turned out all right. Also, none of my friends are breastfeeding, so why should I breastfeed my infant?"

Formation of behavioral intentions is best facilitated if you know the specific potential internal dialogues, ambivalences, and objections most commonly occurring in a given group, talk about them and resolve them in a presentation, or provide opportunities for the group members to discuss them openly and resolve them in the group discussion.

Group Decision Making and Public Commitment

Individuals are more likely to follow through with a specific action or behavior pattern if their attitudes and commitments are made public than if they are kept private, particularly if their peers hold them accountable for fulfilling their commitments. To the extent that individuals, acting in the absence of coercion, make a commitment in front of others to take action, they come to see themselves as believers in that kind of activity. In addition, taking a stand publicly makes the action less likely to be denied or forgotten and more resistant to challenge in subsequent situations when the behavior can be enacted (Halverson & Pallack, 1978).

As a result of his research on such issues as group dynamics and social influence, social psychologist Lewin concluded that commitment to an action was greater when social influence or the social support of the group was involved. During World War II, when food rationing and conservation were important concerns, Lewin conducted a series of experiments to change food habits (Lewin, 1943; Radke & Caso, 1948). He compared several methods with a "group decision" method in which group discussion was followed by the group setting definite goals for action. These goals could be set up by the group for the group as a whole or by each individual in the group setting. Either way, a public decision was made to try the targeted behavior, through a show of hands or verbal statements. No attempt was made to force a decision, nor were high-pressure sales techniques used.

In one study with housewives, the target behavior was using organ meats such as hearts, lungs, liver, and kidneys instead of the more common cuts of meat. In the control group (or lecture condition), a nutritionist discussed the advantages of using organ meats—low cost, nutritional value, and importance to the war effort. The information was provided in an enthusiastic but formal lecture format, with no group interaction. Recipes for "delicious dishes" were handed out. In the group decision situation, the nutritionist very briefly discussed similar information as for the lecture situation. The group then exchanged views on potential barriers to using organ meats (e.g., their families might not like kidneys, kidneys smell bad during cooking). The nutritionist made suggestions from time to time for dealing with these barriers, but only after group members themselves had expressed their concerns and discussed with each other ways to overcome the barriers. Group members then publicly voted on their decision to serve organ meats during the following week. In follow-up interviews in the women's homes seven days later, it was found that only 10% of the women in the lecture condition reported serving one of the three targeted organ meats, whereas 52% of the women in the group decision method condition reported trying one of these meats.

In the second study, a request for change (via an announcement) was compared with group decision for increasing the intake of whole-wheat bread by male college students in dormitory settings. A third study compared individual instruction with group decision for getting mothers to give their babies the proper amount of cod liver oil and orange juice. These two comparisons also demonstrated that the group decision method was substantially more effective in changing behavior than the other methods.

The group decision method of Lewin was used with success more recently in the Family Heart Study (Carmody et al., 1986), which was designed to reduce the risk of cardiovascular disease. About 200 families met monthly in small groups of 8 to 12 families over a five-year period. At each meeting, the nutritionist was present and provided some educational activities. However, much of the time was devoted to group members sharing successes and problems and then making a group decision and public commitment for actions that families would take during the coming month.

These studies indicate that a process wherein groups of peers mutually share concerns, ask for public commitments from each other, and then hold each other accountable for fulfilling their commitments to the group can exert a powerful effect on individuals' self-image, commitment, and action taking. Nutrition educators can encourage such group decision and public commitment to assist individuals to bridge the intention–behavior gap.

Intention Formation
Educational strategies can assist individuals to evaluate the desirability and feasibility of taking a particular action or making a particular behavior change and then make a decision. If they decide to take action, their decision is then their behavioral intention or goal intention. It is best to assist individuals to clearly state their behavioral intention, preferably in writing (e.g., through a commitment form, contract, or pledge). Alternatively, they can make the commitment orally in the group. As discussed earlier, when group participants make public commitments, they hold each other accountable and also provide social support to each other to fulfill their commitments.

In the context of a nutrition education program, this intention is usually the program's behavioral goal. If the program's behavioral goal is quite specific, such as for program participants to eat four or more cups of fruits and vegetables daily, the behavioral intention is stated as "I intend to eat four or more cups of fruits and vegetables daily." If the program's goal is quite broad, such as healthy eating, then individuals will choose actions they want to take to achieve the goal and express their personal, individualized goal. How to assist individuals to translate these intentions into action is the subject of the next chapter.

Using Instructional Design Theory to Organize and Sequence Educational Strategies: The Educational or Lesson Plan

As we noted earlier, instruction can be seen as the deliberate arrangement of events in the individual's environment to make learning happen and to make it effective (Gagne, 1994). A theory of instruction is thus about how to select and arrange *events of instruction* to provide support for the internal processes of learning.

Gagne's theory of instruction (1965, 1994) has been widely used to design instruction using a variety of media (e.g., oral, written, computer based, Web based) for a variety of audiences (e.g., children, adults). Gagne's instructional design principles and a step model of health communications (McGuire, 1984) can help us think about the sequencing of educational strategies directed at the mediators of behavior change.

In Gagne's scheme, instruction involves nine steps, beginning with the event of gaining attention, then moving on to informing learners of the objective of the session, building on prior learning, presenting new information, providing "learning guidance," eliciting the performance, providing feedback, assessing performance, and enhancing retention and transfer. For our purposes, the term *instruction* is used in its broadest sense, involving not only instruction in formal settings but also educational messages and activities through a variety of channels in various settings, including informal settings and mass media. *Learning* is also used in its broadest sense, including not only verbal information but also changes in skills, attitudes, and behaviors. Thus, an *instructional design* is one in which the events of instruction are arranged in a sequence that mirrors and provides instruction for each of the sequences in the internal mental processes involved in dietary change, such as we have described in this text.

Kinzie (2005) has modified Gagne's process into a five-step process for use in health education design, as shown in Table 11-3. The step model of health communications (McGuire, 1984) similarly focuses on the design of activities that facilitate people's internal movement in response to a message from paying attention to the message to understanding the message, to attitude change and skills acquisition, to making a decision, to adopting the behavior, to reinforcement, and finally to consolidating the new behavior within their lifestyle.

Both of these models suggest that at any given session, or for a media campaign, instructional events should proceed from focusing on gaining attention, through enhancing interest and motivation, to facilitating adoption and maintenance of a behavior. Table 11-3 shows how educational strategies can be used to address the theory-based mediators of health behavior change in each sequence of instructional events. Educational strategies derived from health behavior theory are listed in italics in the table.

The sequencing suggested by instructional theory and the health communications framework provides practical guidance on how to arrange educational strategies within a session or over several sessions into an instructional sequence, leading to a *plan for instruction* or *lesson plan.*

- Motivational or promotional activities are usually conducted first, whether within a series of sessions or in a multicomponent nutrition education intervention. The

nutrition science information you present in this phase is of a *why-to* nature. However, motivational activities are still needed throughout the intervention to promote active deliberation and to reinforce motivation.

- Strategies to facilitate the ability to take action usually follow motivational activities. The food and nutrition information you present in this phase is of a *how-to* nature.

Table 11-4 provides a brief summary of how the theory-based educational strategies we have described in this chapter can be arranged into a sequence of instructional events to generate a lesson plan.

If you are conducting only one session, it is unlikely that you will be able to cover all five events of instruction and all the strategies. However, it is helpful to follow the general sequence in each session. You can select one or two strategies within each event of instruction to focus on. If you have the opportunity to conduct several sessions, you can start with the motivational-phase activities and continue with action-phase activities in the second and later sessions. Even

TABLE 11-3   Use of Educational Strategies to Address the Theory-Based Mediators of Health Behavior Change in a Sequence of Instructional Events

Gagne's Sequence of Events of Instruction as Modified by Kinzie for Health Behaviors *(Educational strategies)*	McGuire's Step Model of Health Communications
Gain attention *Threat: Fear and health losses* *Benefits: Health benefits*	Exposure/attention to the message Interest or personal relevance of the message
Present stimulus/new material, building on prior learning *Tailor messages to audience's prior knowledge and values* *Demonstrate effectiveness of the desired behavior (response efficacy)* *Make desired action easy to understand and do (self-efficacy)*	Understanding the message Personalizing the behavior to fit one's life (learning what message recommends) Accepting the message about change (attitude change) Remembering the message and continuing to agree with it
Provide guidance *Use credible social models*	Skills (learning how to do what message recommends)
	Storing and retrieving information to use when needed for action
Elicit performance *Provide authentic practice and feedback*	Decision (based on bringing the message to mind) Acting according to decision Receiving positive reinforcement for behavior
Enhance retention and transfer *Provide social supports* *Deliver behavioral cues*	Consolidating the behavior into one's life (maintaining it)

Sources: Kinzie, M.B. 2005. Instructional design strategies for health behavior change. *Patient Education and Counseling* 56:3–15; and McGuire, W.J. 1984. Public communication as a strategy for inducing health-promoting behavioral changes. *Preventive Medicine* 13:299–313.

in this instance it is helpful to start each session with an event to gain attention, and then provide short motivational activities to strengthen the group's attitudes, reinvigorate their motivation, and renew their commitment to act before moving into skill building in the food and nutrition area and in self-regulation.

If you are addressing more than one behavior, you will go through this instructional design sequence for each of the behaviors, such as eating fruits and vegetables and avoiding highly processed, high-energy-density snacks. Sometimes the strategies for achieving behavioral goals can be combined—for example, we can encourage fruits and vegetables as snacks to replace highly processed, high-energy-density snacks.

Sequencing by the Transtheoretical Model's Stages of Change

You can also sequence educational activities and learning by individuals' stage of readiness to make dietary changes. Table 11-2 describes the ten processes of change of the transtheoretical model. Educational activities that facilitate the

movement through the stages of motivational readiness form a sequence rather similar to the events of instruction and steps of health communication just described. Although all the processes of change are used in all stages, in general experiential processes are used more often during the early stages of motivational readiness, and behavioral processes are used more often during the later stages of change. In the early stages, the experiential processes of change emphasized are consciousness-raising, dramatic relief, environmental reevaluation, and self-reevaluation. In the later stages, the processes often used for behavior change are the relapse prevention strategies of counterconditioning, management of reinforcements, control of environmental stimuli, and social liberation (see Chapter 5 for details). Consequently, if you wish to design educational activities and learning experiences by stages of change, you can use intervention activities that are appropriate for each stage.

Your Turn

You can now apply the information in this chapter to the design of educational strategies to address the mediators that

TABLE 11-4 Sequencing Nutrition Education Strategies to Address Theory Constructs

Phase of Nutrition Education	Sequence of Events of Instruction	Theory-Based Nutrition Education Strategies
Motivational phase: Enhancing motivation, active contemplation, and decision making (why to take action)	Gain attention	*Threat:* Increase awareness of concerns and risks; self-assessment *Benefit:* Increase perceived benefits of taking action: scientific information on why to take action; personal benefits
	Present stimulus or new material, building on prior learning	*Outcome expectations or perceived benefits:* Demonstrate effectiveness of the desired behavior through scientific research data *Barriers/self-efficacy:* Make desired action easy to understand and do Increase reflection on affect/feelings about taking action Address social norms and social expectations Bring to consciousness automatic behaviors, habits, or routines
	Provide guidance	Provide direct experience with food Pros and cons of action: Assist with resolving resistance and ambivalences Clarify values Group decision and public commitment
Action phase: Facilitating the ability to take action (how to take action)	Elicit performance and feedback	Set goals Provide food- and nutrition-related knowledge and cognitive skills to engage in actions *Self-efficacy:* Make the desired actions easy to understand and do Provide social models
	Enhance retention and transfer	Provide reinforcements and rewards Strengthen self-regulation skills Assist individuals to develop personal policies, routines, and habits Provide cues to action

you identified and the educational objectives that you have stated. These strategies should then be sequenced into an instructional plan for how to proceed, showing the events of instruction. The resulting plan goes by many names, such as the *lesson plan* or *education plan* for a single session, a *curriculum* for several sequenced sessions, a *media message plan*, or the *intervention guide* for an intervention with many components. Designing activities is a very fluid process in which you go back and forth between designing activities and sequencing them appropriately. After pilot testing, you may want to change or rearrange activities.

How you will arrange your sequence of educational strategies will depend on many factors that are specific to the needs of your audience and the theory guiding your intervention. In general, though, you want to begin each session or series of sessions with activities to gain the attention of the group, move to activities to enhance motivation and promote contemplation, and then focus on activities to facilitate decision making and the formation of intentions to take action. The same systematic process is needed for the design of all nutrition education messages and activities, such as brochures, newsletters, posters, media messages, or campaigns. Strategies for assisting individuals to translate intentions into action are described in Chapter 12.

It is useful to first develop a lesson plan outline using a table format as shown in the case study. The table format enables you to see whether you have addressed all the educational objectives that you set and whether the activities are appropriate in terms of domain of learning and level of complexity. You may be able to conduct the actual sessions using this table format, or you may need to convert the table into a narrative lesson plan or some other format that you will actually use when you are with a group. A sample lesson plan using both the table and narrative formats is provided in the case study. A worksheet is also provided at the end of this chapter for you to use to develop your educational plan for a real or hypothetical educational session.

If your program is more than a one-time event, all the learning experiences designed should be extensively pilot tested with the intended audience. If food is used, test the recipes and preparation procedures for taste acceptance and feasibility. Using focus groups, direct observation, and interviews, assess whether activities are acceptable and effective with the intended audience.

Case Study

We will now apply the information in this chapter specifically to our ongoing case study to illustrate the processes of selecting appropriate theory-derived educational strategies to address potential motivational mediators and of designing practical educational activities and learning experiences that are specific, fun, and enjoyable for group participants and that will allow them to achieve the educational objectives we wrote in Step 4.

As you recall, we have been focusing on the sessions that address our first behavioral goal: to increase intake of more fruits and vegetables. These sessions have been titled "The Whys and Whats of Colorful Eating." We use the logic model conceptual framework to design the inputs, outputs, and outcomes for our sessions (Figure 11-2).

Our *inputs* include the funding organization's contributions, the nutrition educator, classroom teachers, materials, classroom space, and partners.

Our *outputs* include our intervention activities and our intervention strategies. Among the intervention activities are the classes that we will conduct, the parent or family component, and the school component, including working with policy makers. In terms of designing the intervention itself, we will design strategies directed at (1) potential motivational-phase mediators for this teenage group to eat more fruits and vegetables, such as perceived risks of not eating enough and perceived benefits of eating fruits and vegetables, as well as preferences for fruits and vegetables and social norms; (2) potential action-phase mediators, such as developing action plans and practicing food- and nutrition-related skills and self-regulation skills; and (3) potential environmental support activities directed at the family and school environment.

This chapter focuses on designing strategies to address the motivational-phase mediators. The case study presents the lesson plan or educational plan outline for the first of two hypothetical sessions—this one directed at motivational-phase strategies. Thus, the box in Figure 11-2 showing strategies directed at potential motivational-phase mediators is highlighted. The case study session directed at action-phase strategies is presented in Chapter 12.

The case study presents an example of the table format of a lesson plan. We build on the table that we created in Step 4 showing the educational objectives for each mediator of behavior or theory construct. In the second column of the table, we list the events of instruction to help us sequence our activities during the session appropriately. In the third column, we list each of the potential mediators of behavior change—which are also the theory constructs—from Step 4 that the lesson will address. In this column we also list the theory-based strategies that are derived from the potential mediators. For each mediator, we then list the specific educational objectives that we stated in Step 4. In the final column, we indicate all the practical educational activities, learning experiences, or messages that we plan to use to carry out the educational strategies.

For use in the actual educational session, the table format is converted into a narrative format. The narrative for the session is also shown in the case study.

The education plans or lesson plans as presented here may seem quite specific, detailed, and almost rigid. It is important to have such a plan, but it is understood that you will apply the lesson plans more fluidly. Even using learner-centered education and facilitated dialogue approaches does not remove the necessity to develop strong, theory-based lesson plans. You may find yourself needing to adapt the lessons to the situation on the ground. You will interact with the group and adjust the content and activities as needed. How you will do this in practice in a group setting is described in Part III of this book, which is about methods of implementing and delivering nutrition education (see Chapter 15).

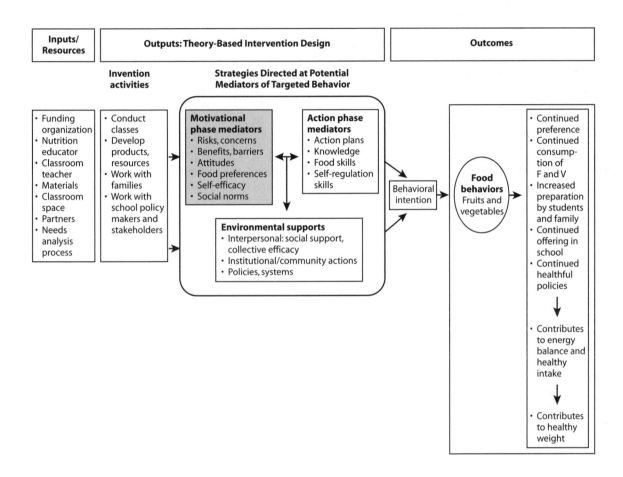

FIGURE 11-2 Logic model conceptual framework for case study: The Whys and Whats of Colorful Eating.

Questions and Activities

1. In the context of this book, what do we mean by *educational strategies*? Define and describe. How are they related to educational activities or learning experiences?

2. Describe carefully the relationship between educational strategies, potential mediators, theory constructs, and diet-related action or behavior change.

3. Compare what we mean by *instruction, instructional framework,* and *instructional design*. How are these terms related to educational strategies?

4. State the five events of instruction and a give a one- to two-sentence description of each.

5. Give one specific example of an educational activity or learning experience that can be used to teach or implement each of the following theory-based educational strategies:
   a. Perceived risk
   b. Outcome expectations/perceived benefits
   c. Attitudes
   d. Habit
   e. Behavioral intention
   f. Cues to action

6. For practice, state one educational strategy for each of the potential motivational mediators of the behavior of increasing intake of calcium-rich foods among teenage girls shown in the accompanying table. For each strategy, describe at least one educational activity or learning experience.

Potential Motivational Mediator	Educational Strategy	Educational Activity or Learning Experience
Outcome expectations/perceived benefits		
Perceived risk		
Affect/feelings		
Behavioral intention		

STEP 5A WORKSHEETS Design Theory-Derived Educational Strategies to Address Potential Motivational Mediators

WORKSHEET 11-1   **Lesson Plan Worksheet**

Title of session: _____

Behavioral goal: _____

Educational goal: _____

General educational objectives: Participants will be able to

- _____

- _____

- _____

- _____

Phase of Nutrition Education and Educational Goal	Sequenced Events of Instruction	Potential Mediator of Behavior Change *(Theory-based strategies*)*	Specific Educational Objectives for Mediator	Review Learning Domain and Level**	Practical Educational Activities, Learning Experiences, Messages, or Content
Pre-action phase *Educational goal:* Enhance awareness, contemplation, and motivation (focus on why-to information)	Gain attention		*At the end of the session or program, learner will be able to:*		
	Present new material (building on prior knowledge)				
	Provide guidance				
	Elicit performance and feedback				
	Enhance retention and transfer				

*Theory-based strategies addressing mediators of behavior change are shown in italics in the third column.
**Review learning objectives for domain and level within domain to ensure that they are set at appropriate levels.

CASE STUDY 11-1   Step 5a: Sample Lesson Plan Outline for a Motivational, Pre-action Phase Lesson

Title of session: The Whys of Colorful Eating

Behavioral goal: Adolescents will increase their intake of a variety of fruits and vegetables (F&V).
Educational goal: Enhance awareness, contemplation, and motivation
General educational objectives: Adolescents will be able to

- Demonstrate understanding and appreciation of the importance of eating a variety of fruits and vegetables
- Evaluate their own intake of fruits and vegetables compared with recommendations
- Identify barriers to intake of fruits and vegetables and propose ways to overcome them
- Express enjoyment of, and positive attitudes toward, eating a variety of fruits and vegetables
- State intention to increase own fruit and vegetable intake

Phase of Nutrition Education and Educational Goal	Sequenced Events of Instruction	Mediator of Behavior Change (*Theory-based strategies**)	Specific Educational Objectives for Mediator	Review Learning Domain with Level**	Practical Educational Activities, Learning Experiences, Messages, or Content
Pre-action, motivational phase *Educational goal:* Enhance awareness, contemplation, and motivation (focus on why-to information)	Gain attention		At the end of the session or program, learner will be able to:		Gain attention by bringing in a variety of F&V of different colors, shapes, and sizes: ask group to guess names and talk about them. Today will focus on the *whys* of eating a rainbow of colors, and next time will focus on the *whats*.
	Present new material (building on prior knowledge)	Outcome expectations *Health benefits/ pros of behavior*	State benefits of eating F&V: energy; hair and skin; build strong bones and muscles for athletic performance	Cognitive domain: *comprehension* Affective domain: *valuing*	Use a worksheet activity, or have group volunteer benefits of eating F&V; list on newsprint. Build on prior knowledge and experience (grounding or anchoring).
			State the key reasons for eating a variety of F&V ("a rainbow of colors")	Cognitive domain: *comprehension level* Affective domain: *Valuing level*	Emphasize the need for variety of intake (a colorful plate). List the five colors: blue/purple, green, white, yellow/orange, and red. Provide scientific evidence that eating F&V makes for strong bodies; clear up misconceptions.

Phase of Nutrition Education and Educational Goal	Sequenced Events of Instruction	Mediator of Behavior Change (*Theory-based strategies**)	Specific Educational Objectives for Mediator	Review Learning Domain with Level**	Practical Educational Activities, Learning Experiences, Messages, or Content
		Personal risk *Self-assessment; personalizing risk*	Describe risks to health from eating too few F&V Evaluate personal risk of not eating enough F&V	Cognitive domain: *comprehension level* Affective domain: *Valuing level*	Checklist, or 24-hour recall, of own intake of F&V and compare with recommendation for number and colors: Is there a rainbow on your plate?
	Provide guidance	Barriers/self-efficacy *Overcoming barriers*	Identify barriers to eating F&V Propose ways to overcome barriers to eating F&V Describe ways in which F&V can be easy to eat	Cognitive domain: *comprehension level* Affective domain: *valuing level*	Group brainstorms barriers to eating F&V; list on newsprint. Group brainstorms ways to overcome barriers. Group discusses ways to make behavior easy to do.
		Social norms *Exposing peer pressure; modeling*	Describe the role of peers in influencing food choices Appreciate that vegetables are cool to eat	Affective domain: *valuing level* Affective domain: *valuing level*	Students express what peers say when they eat F&V. Provide relevant models (media models, stories) eating F&V, showing it is cool.
		Food preferences *Direct experience with food*	Appreciate that fruits and vegetables taste good	Affective domain: *valuing level*	Provide a fruit salad or vegetables and dips for tasting.
	Elicit performance and feedback	Behavioral intention *Values clarification Decisional balance*	Evaluate the pros and cons of eating a variety of colors State an intention to add one fruit or vegetable a day to diet	Cognitive domain: *evaluation level* Affective domain: *valuing level*	Group activity: Present value statements and discuss in group. Worksheet for each person to record pros and cons of adding F&V to diet. Make decision about actions to take— individually or share with group.

* Theory-based strategies addressing mediators of behavior change are shown in italics in the third column.

** Review learning domain and level of objectives of within domain, if possible, to ensure appropriate mix of objectives.

"The Whys and Whats of Colorful Eating"

The Whys of Colorful Eating: Motivational Phase Lesson, Narrative format

Overview of Content
(50 to 60 minutes)

1. Introduction, overview, gain attention
2. Brainstorm and record on newsprint the benefits of eating F&V
3. Emphasize importance of different colors
4. Fill out 24-hour recall checklist to assess colorfulness of F&V intake
5. Brainstorm and use newsprint to record barriers to eating F&V
6. For each barrier, brainstorm and record on newsprint ways to overcome barriers and discuss ways to make it easier to eat all the colors of the rainbow
7. Discuss influence of peers and provide alternate models
8. Appreciate the rainbow of fruits and vegetables by tasting F&V
9. Group values discussion
10. Pros and cons worksheet of adding F&V to your diet
11. Goal-setting and wrap up

Materials

- 5–10 different F&V, such as eggplant, blueberries, zucchini, kale, green grapes, jicama, potato, carrots, kumquat, tangerine, tomato, strawberry
- Copies of the 24-hour recall checklist and pros/cons and goal-setting worksheets
- Fruit salad or vegetables and dip
- Newsprint
- Markers
- Pencils or pens

Lesson plan

1. **Introduction.** Overview, gain attention (3 minutes)
   Demonstrate the wide variety of colors that are found in F&V. Hold up F&V. Ask the following series of questions to facilitate conversation: What is the name of this food? Have you seen this food before? Have you eaten this food before? Are there other foods that are similar in color? Are there other foods that are similar in shape? Encourage participation from the whole group. Discuss *why* it is important to eat a rainbow of colors. (Address any behavior problems immediately and talk about the importance of creating a positive, supportive environment.)

2. **Benefits of F&V.** Brainstorm and record on newsprint (6 minutes) *(Perceived benefits)*
   "Now that we are familiar with how a variety of different F&V look, we are going to continue to explore what we already know about F&V. Let's make a list of some of the benefits of eating a wide range of F&V."
       Discussion will follow; ensure that the following benefits of eating F&V are covered: Provides essential vitamins, minerals, fiber, and other nutrients; can increase energy; helps make hair and skin healthy; builds strong bones and muscles for athletic performance; decreases risk for certain diseases.

3. **Benefits of F&V**. Emphasis on importance of different colors (3 minutes) *(Perceived benefits)*
   List the following colors on newsprint: blue/purple, green, white, yellow/orange, red. Emphasize a need for a variety of different color F&V. Different colors reflect the presence of different phytonutrients. Explain that by eating all different colors, they are eating a wide range of different nutrients. Tell students that instead of needing to remember that orange color vegetables are filled with carotenoids and dark blue/purple fruits, like blueberries, are filled with resveratrol, they should remember to eat the rainbow and they will eat all the different nutrients they need! Ask the group if there are any questions in order to clear up misconceptions.

4. **Self-assessment of intake**. 24-hour recall checklist to assess colorfulness of F&V intake (9 minutes) *(Self-assessment of risk)*
   Distribute checklist and ask participants to think about what F&V they ate yesterday (or during the past week). Each participant should write down the F&V they ate from each color group. Discussion starters: Is there a rainbow on your plate? What colors are you missing?

5. **Barriers to eating F&V**. Brainstorm and record on newsprint (5 minutes) *(Perceived barriers)*
   Make a list of the reasons why it is sometimes hard to eat all the colors of the rainbow. Ask students what prevents them from eating all the different colors.
       Ensure that the following topics are mentioned: lack of time, not available, my parents don't buy/cook them, dislike taste.

6. **Overcoming barriers.** Brainstorm and record on newsprint ways to overcome each barrier and discuss ways to make it easier to eat all the colors of the rainbow (6 minutes) *(Self-efficacy)*
       Based on the list of barriers, ask for suggestions on ways to overcome each barrier. For example: lack of time: pre-cut vegetables; whole fruit for a snack; dislike taste: provide culturally appropriate suggestions on how to prepare.
       Ask for other suggestions about how to eat a variety of foods. If there is a color that most participants seem to be lacking, this is the time to focus on that particular color.

7. **Social influences.** Discuss influence of peers and provide alternate models (5 minutes) *(Social norms)*
       What might your friends say when you choose to eat F&V or bring them as a snack? Allow for adequate discussion time.
       If the participants suggest that it might be seen as "uncool," provide alternate stories or media models that show F&V consumption as "cool." Make sure that the models are appropriate for the specific age, gender, and culture of the group.

8. **Tasting F&V**. Appreciate the rainbow of fruits and vegetables by tasting F&V (10–20 minutes)
       Provide a rainbow fruit salad or a rainbow vegetable plate with dips for the participants to enjoy. Depending on time and facilities, allow participants to prepare the snack.

9. **Group values discussion** (5 minutes) *(Values clarification)*
       Now that you have discussed the importance of eating a rainbow of F&V, and ate a great snack with a rainbow of colors in it, ask the participants for their thoughts now about F&V. Facilitate discussion by presenting value statements using a scale of 1–10, such as, How important is it to you to eat a rainbow of different F&V? How likely do you think it is that you will eat a rainbow of different F&V during the next week?

10. **Pros and cons** of adding F&V to your diet (5 minutes) *(Decisional balance)*
       Hand out pros and cons worksheet. Ask the participants to write at least three personal pros and three cons about eating a rainbow of different colored F&V.

11. **Goal-setting and wrap up** (8 minutes) *(Goal-setting)*
       Review the reasons why and ways to increase the colorfulness and number of F&V in diet. Encourage participants to make a clear statement about what actions they will take in the next week. For some it might be adding one F&V a day to their diet, for others it might be adding a different color F&V. Take a few minutes to fill out the worksheet.
       Ask participants, Will some of you now share the goals you set for yourself? After a participant reads his or her goal, ask if others have a similar goal. Encourage the members of the group to support each other in reaching their goals.

Thank the group and include any reminders about future meetings or events.

REFERENCES

Ammerman, A.S., C.H. Lindquist, K.N. Lohr, and J. Hersey. 2002. The efficacy of behavioral interventions to modify dietary fat and fruit and vegetable intake: A review of the evidence. *Preventive Medicine* 35(1):25–41.

Armitage, C.J., and M. Conner. 2000. Social cognition models and health behavior: A structured review. *Psychology and Health* 15:173–189.

Buchanan, D.R. 2000. *An ethic for health promotion: Rethinking the sources of human well-being.* New York: Oxford University Press.

Carmody, T.P., J. Istvan, J.D. Matarazzo, S.L. Connor, and W.E. Connor. 1986. Applications of social learning theory in the promotion of heart-healthy diets: The Family Heart Study dietary intervention model. *Health Education Research* 1(1):13–27.

Contento, I., G.I. Balch, S.K. Maloney, et al. 1995. The effectiveness of nutrition education and implications for nutrition education policy, programs, and research: A review of research. *Journal of Nutrition Education* 27(6):277–422.

Dewey, J. 1929. *The sources of a science of education.* New York: Liveright.

Freiere, P. 1970. *Pedagogy of the oppressed.* New York: Continuum.

———. 1973. *Education for critical consciousness.* New York: Continuum.

Gagne, R. 1965. *The conditions of learning.* New York: Holt, Rinehart, & Winston.

———. 1985. *The conditions of learning and theory of instruction.* 4th ed. New York: Holt, Rinehart, & Winston.

Halverson, R., and M. Pallack. 1978. Commitment, ego-involvement and resistance to attack. *Journal of Experimental Social Psychology* 14: 1012.

Iowa Department of Public Health. 2005. Pick a better snack. http://www.idph.state.ia.us/pickabettersnack/.

Johnson, D.W., and R.T. Johnson. 1987. Using cooperative learning strategies to teach nutrition. *Journal of the American Dietetic Association* 87(9 Suppl.):S55–S61.

Kinzie, M.B. 2005. Instructional design strategies for health behavior change. *Patient Education and Counseling* 56:3–15.

Levy, J., and G. Auld. 2004. Cooking classes outperform cooking demonstrations for college sophomores. *Journal of Nutrition Education and Behavior* 36:197–203.

Lewin, K. 1943. Forces behind food habits and methods of change. In *The problem of changing food habits. Bulletin of the National Research Council.* Washington, DC: National Research Council and National Academy of Sciences.

Liquori, T., P.D. Koch, I.R. Contento, and J. Castle. 1998. The Cookshop Program: Outcome evaluation of a nutrition education program linking lunchroom food experiences with classroom cooking experiences. *Journal of Nutrition Education* 30(5):302.

Lytle, L., and C. Achterberg. 1995. Changing the diet of America's children: What works and why? *Journal of Nutrition Education* 27(5):250–260.

Manoff, R.K. 1985. *Social marketing: New imperatives for public health.* New York: Praeger.

McGuire, W.J. 1984. Public communication as a strategy for inducing health-promoting behavioral changes. *Preventive Medicine* 13:299–313.

Petty, R.E., and J.T. Cacioppo. 1986. *Communication and persuasion: Central and peripheral routes to attitude change.* New York: Springer-Verlag.

Pomerleau, J., K. Lock, C. Knai, and M. McKee. 2005. Interventions designed to increase adults fruit and vegetable intake in adults can be effective: A systematic review of the literature. *Journal of Nutrition* 135:2486–2495.

Radke, M., and E. Caso. 1948. Lecture and discussion-decision as methods of influencing food habits. *Journal of the American Dietetic Association* 24:23–41.

Rokeach, M. 1973. *The nature of human values.* New York: Free Press.

Schwarzer, R. 1992. Self-efficacy in the adoption of maintenance of health behaviors: Theoretical approaches and a new model. In *Self-efficacy: Thought control of action,* edited by R. Schwarzer. Washington: Hemisphere.

Tyler, R.W. 1949. *Basic principles of curriculum and instruction.* Chicago: University of Chicago Press.

CHAPTER

12

Step 5b: Design Theory-Derived Educational Strategies to Address Potential Mediators of the Ability to Take Action

OVERVIEW The focus of this chapter is on designing strategies for how to take action; in particular on selecting educational strategies and designing practical educational activities or learning experiences to address potential mediators of behavioral change in order to facilitate the ability to take action. The information in Chapter 5 will help you with this step in the design process.

OBJECTIVES At the end of the chapter, you will be able to

- Describe the kinds of theory-based strategies to address potential mediators that are particularly important in facilitating the ability to take action
- Design specific educational activities or learning experiences to make practical the theory-based educational strategies designed to address potential mediators of target behaviors
- Sequence the educational objectives and strategies to create a lesson plan or educational plan.

SCENARIO

A nutrition educator has been asked to make a presentation to a group of community women who are interested in being able to provide their families with better diets. They are very busy and use many processed foods to save time. The nutrition educator decides that he will teach them about label reading. He therefore enlarges a food label and puts it on poster board and an easel. He spends the next 20 minutes going over each of the items in the label and explaining what it means. He also goes over the ingredient list. He notices that the group is getting restless.

COMMENT

What is going on here? His general educational objective is appropriate. He is providing the group with important skills they need. However, to develop skills, the audience should have the opportunity to practice the skills in an active manner. Thus, he could have increased his effectiveness by bringing in packages of different foods and using one or two of these as demonstrations. Then he could have given them the packages (always empty) to practice reading package labels. Doing the activity in pairs can increase the comfort level of participants and increase learning by discussing labels while reading them.

Introduction

Eating is very personal—and we like our eating patterns. Making changes in them is usually undertaken with some ambivalence: we want to eat for health, but we also gain psychological satisfaction, a sense of belonging to our culture, and enjoyment from our food. And eating is not optional, unlike some other health-related behaviors such as smoking. Therefore our choices usually require trade-offs and difficult decisions. Not surprisingly, translating intentions into action is often fraught with difficulties. Even when we are motivated to make changes, we are not always able to act on our interests and motivation because of the press of other concerns and barriers. This intention–action gap is a common phenomenon to which we can all attest. How, then, can we improve individuals' abilities to act on their motivations? What educational strategies can we design that would facilitate the translation of intentions into action?

The evidence suggests that there are two major approaches: we can assist individuals to strengthen their *self-regulation skills*, particularly the skill of setting goals, and we can foster supportive *environments* that make the action easier to do. This chapter focuses on the first approach. The next chapter focuses on the second. The environment presents many challenges to eating healthfully and being active, so individuals need knowledge and skills to navigate the environment successfully. At the same time, health promotion efforts should seek to make the environment easier to navigate.

Self-regulation models propose that progress toward engaging in an action or practice will not occur simply because individuals judge that the behavior or practice is highly desirable and feasible. Motivation alone is not sufficient to initiate health-promoting personal change. Bridging the intention–behavior gap requires, in addition, that individuals form specific action goals and specific action plans to achieve these action goals. For actions that are complex, as they are for dietary change, maintenance of the behaviors over the long term requires continuing to pursue these action goals, even in the face of difficulties, and employing additional self-regulation processes that focus on the ability of individuals to make choices and to direct and control their own behavior.

Research evidence is providing information on the efficacy of a number of strategies that can help individuals transform motivation into action and the maintenance of behavior. In general, the process requires the food- and nutrition-related knowledge and skills necessary for taking action, and enhanced self-regulation skills to use those knowledge and skills in the service of taking action.

In Chapter 11, we described how to design theory-based strategies to influence mediators of behavior change that would increase awareness of concerns and risks, promote active contemplation and enhance motivation, and facilitate behavioral intentions. In this chapter we describe how to design theory-based strategies, educational messages, and learning activities to achieve those objectives developed in Step 3 that influence mediators of behavior change that focus on increasing individuals' ability to take action. Consequently, this chapter describes theory-based strategies to assist individuals to

- Develop implementation intentions or action plans (initiate action)
- Build food- and nutrition-related skills
- Strengthen self-regulation skills

INPUTS: COLLECTING ASSESSMENT DATA		DESIGNING THE OUTPUTS			DESIGNING OUTCOMES EVALUATION
STEP 1 ⟷	**STEP 2** ⟷	**STEP 3** ⟷	**STEP 4** ⟷	**STEP 5** ⟷	**STEP 6**
Analyze needs and behaviors: Specify the behavior or action focus of the program	**Identify relevant potential mediators of program behaviors**	**Select theory, philosophy, and components**	**State educational objectives for potential mediators**	**Design theory-based educational strategies and activities to address potential mediators**	**Design evaluation**
• Assess needs and identify audience: select need(s) or issue(s) to address	• Identify potential personal psychosocial mediators	• Select theory and/or create appropriate model	• Select relevant mediators to address	• Design strategies and activities for each selected mediator:	• Design evaluation of program's impact on behaviors and mediators
• Identify behaviors of concern that contribute to need(s) or issue(s)	• Identify potential environmental mediators	• Articulate educational philosophy	• State educational objectives for each selected mediator:	—Personal psychosocial mediators	• Design process evaluation
• Select core behaviors or practices to address		• Clarify perspectives on content	—Personal psychosocial mediators	—Environmental mediators	
		• Determine program components	—Environmental mediators		

In designing your sessions or program, you will most likely go back and forth among these various strategies and between strategies in this and Chapter 11.

Selecting Theory-Derived Strategies to Facilitate the Ability to Take Action

Your selection of educational strategies will depend on the theory or model for the intervention that you created in Step 3 and your educational philosophy. Increasing evidence suggests, however, that for this phase, self-regulation models, social cognitive theory, some processes of the transtheoretical model, and grounded theory from extensive interviews are the most helpful (Pelican et al., 2005; Bisogni et al., 2005). As we saw in Chapter 5, studies suggest that the key tasks of nutrition education in this phase are to assist individuals to initiate action, acquire the needed food- and nutrition-related knowledge and skills, and maintain action through the strengthening of self-regulation. The educational strategies for these tasks are described in this section.

Remember, *educational strategies* are ways to operationalize each of the personal mediators of behavior change for educational and instructional purposes, and hence the mediators and strategies are often called by the same name. Table 12-1 shows the connections between theory constructs, potential mediators of change, and educational strategies and learning experiences, as we discussed in the last chapter.

It is important to design educational activities that are engaging and fun, involve the affective as well as the cognitive domain, and include the psychomotor domain where appropriate. As we noted in Chapter 11, people generally remember 10% of what they read, 20% of what they hear, 30% of what they see, 50% of what they hear and see, 70% of what they say and write, and 90% of what they say as they do a thing (Wiman & Mierhenry, 1969).

Action Planning: Development of Implementation Intentions or Action Plans

How can we assist individuals to move from motivation to action, from intention to reality? Theory and evidence suggest that the following theory-based educational strategies are useful.

Clarify Behavioral Goals (Goal Intentions)

We need to start with assisting individuals to state their behavioral goals or goal intentions clearly. These are called *proximal goals* in social cognitive theory. Stating a clear goal intention is usually understood by individuals as committing themselves to an action, resulting in a sense of control, of determination, and of obligation to realize the action or behavior. In a behavior-focused nutrition education intervention, *personal* behavioral goals will reflect the *program's* behavioral focus. If the program's behavioral goal is that program participants will eat five fruits and vegetables daily, the individual's personal behavioral goal is stated as "I will eat five fruits and vegetables daily." However, the program behavioral goal may be quite general ("participants will eat a healthy diet" or "eat fewer high-fat foods, more fruits and vegetables, and be physically active"), and hence there may be several behavioral goals (Step 3). In this case, the participants may choose among them those actions that they want to commit to taking—maybe they will commit to eating lower-fat foods or eating more fruits and vegetables but not both.

Action Plans

Translating behavioral intentions and goals into action is greatly facilitated by the formation of implementation intentions (Armitage, 2004). These are also called *action goals*. Some audiences prefer the term *action plans* because the word *goals* seems too lofty. The term *contracting* is sometimes also used because it involves a contract between the person and himself or herself. These implementation intentions or action goals are volitional (conscious-choice) strategies that are designed to ensure that the behavioral goal or goal intentions are translated into action. Thus, whereas behavioral goals take the form of "I will eat more fruits and vegetables daily," action goals or implementation intentions take the following form: "In the next week, I will add orange juice at breakfast, eat a fruit for a snack mid-afternoon, and add one vegetable to my dinner in the evening."

Implementation intentions are effective because they link the specific actions to a given situation, so that when the situation arises, such as breakfast time, individuals do not have to think and make a new decision each time (Gollwitzer, 1999). Such planning ahead means the behavior will require less mental effort each time. This is especially important because healthful food- and nutrition-related behaviors are often perceived as difficult or even unpleasant to implement, even if they are desirable and feasible (e.g., switching from a high-fat to a low-fat diet, switching from eating mostly takeout to cooking one's own food, starting to exercise daily, or buying local foods). You should provide action goal or action plan worksheets for individuals to complete. Have someone else in the group sign as a witness to the action plan, and where appropriate and comfortable for the group to do so, have the group participants discuss with each other their action plans. Such verbalization can enhance a sense of commitment.

Skill Building in Food- and Nutrition-Related Knowledge and Skills

We have said before that how-to knowledge is not enough for individuals to take health-related actions or to make changes in their diets—motivation is necessary. However, how-to or instrumental knowledge *is* necessary for individuals to act on their motivations and achieve their behavioral goals and action plans. Thus, individuals need both motivation and

TABLE 12-1 Linking Theory, Strategies, and Educational Activities

Potential Mediator of Behavior Change (Theory Construct)	Theory-Based Strategies for Potential Mediators of Behavior Change	Practical Educational Activities, Learning Experiences, Content, or Messages
Perceived risk	Confrontation with risks • Increase salience of issues or concern about problems • Convey threat or use fear communications (TTM: Consciousness-raising and dramatic relief)	Trigger films, pictures, charts, striking national or local statistics, personal stories, role plays, demonstration Clear image of threat (e.g., film clips on effect of high-saturated-fat diet in clogging arteries) Demonstration using plastic tube clogged with fat and colored water to show blockage
Awareness	Self-assessment • Provide personalized self-assessments to counter optimistic bias (TTM: Self-reevaluation)	Self-assessment checklists; food or activity records or recalls
Outcome expectations	Information about outcome expectations (why-to information), specific and personal • Persuasive communications about positive outcomes • Information on response efficacy or effectiveness of taking action	Presentations, visuals, demonstrations of scientific evidence on dietary practices and health or disease risk; nutrient–health relationships (antioxidants for eye health; nutrients and bone health); motivational activities
Perceived benefits	Information about perceived benefits of taking action or motivators with personal meaning for the intended audience (why-to information)	Messages or educational activities that provide arguments for the desired action or practice to emphasize "what's in it for me?" Personal health benefits; other personal, family, or community benefits
Attitudes/affect	Reflection on affect/feelings	Attitude statements and discussion; learner-centered activities; emotion-based messaging
Self-efficacy and perceived barriers	Decrease perception of barriers or negative outcomes	Brainstorming; discussion of barriers and ways to overcome them
Food preferences	Direct experience with healthful food	Food tastings, demonstrations, cooking
Social norms	Awareness of social norms and social expectations	View print and TV ads; discussion of impact of others
Habit	Bring to consciousness automatic behaviors, habits, or routines	Checklists of current practices; self-observation tool
Behavioral intention	*Decisional balance:* Analysis of pros and cons of action, and choice among actions *Values clarification:* Resolving resistance and ambivalences Anticipated regret Group decision and public commitment (TTM: Self-liberation)	Worksheets or discussions to analyze pros and cons of action, and choices Values clarification worksheets for individuals, or group activities Imagery activities Group discussion followed by group decision on goals for action, and public commitment
Goal setting	Goal setting and implementation or action plans	Teach goal-setting skills, provide contracts/pledges or action plan forms

Potential Mediator of Behavior Change (Theory Construct)	Theory-Based Strategies for Potential Mediators of Behavior Change	Practical Educational Activities, Learning Experiences, Content, or Messages
Behavioral capability (how-to information)	Food- and nutrition-related knowledge and cognitive and behavioral skills to engage in actions: tailor to prior knowledge, beliefs, attitudes, and values Teaching of how-to information Food and nutrition skills building Active methods Discussion and facilitated discussion Guided practice	Discussions, presentations, or learning experiences to teach needed food- and nutrition-related knowledge and skills to engage in behavior; food preparation skills
Self-efficacy	Social modeling of behavior Guided practice to encourage mastery of behavioral skills Exhortations or persuasion so as to overcome doubt	Make the desired actions easy to understand and do: • Clear instructions • Demonstration of the behavior by respected social model • Direct experience (e.g., food preparation or cooking) with guidance and feedback • Give feedback on performance, emphasizing achievements and difficulties already overcome
Reinforcements	Provide reinforcements and rewards	Verbal praise, tee shirts, drawing for prizes, or awards
Self-regulation	Strengthen self-regulation skills (self-influence or self-control) • Self-monitoring skills for progress toward goal • Goal maintenance • Coping self-efficacy • Managing cues from environment Developing personal policies, routines, and habits (TTM: Counter-conditioning, rewards management, stimulus control)	Identify and prioritize competing goals; provide self-monitoring forms and tips; protect action goals from distractions: mindful eating; conscious attention (self-talk) and planning ahead; develop strategies for coping with difficulties Tip sheets on personal policies for purchasing foods, meal patterns (e.g., always eat breakfast, bring lunch to work), eating out
Social support	Social support (TTM: Helping relationships)	Create supportive group environment; encourage buddy system
Cues to action	Provide cues to action	Billboards, grocery bags, media messages, news articles, refrigerator magnets and key chains with messages

TTM = transtheoretical model.

ability to act, both why-to information and specific how-to knowledge and skills, in order to carry out the actions.

Knowledge and Cognitive Skills

After individuals intend to take action, they may still need specific knowledge and skills in order to carry out the actions. For example, individuals may not know how to select foods for optimal health from the 50,000-item supermarket; evaluate the nutrition information that bombards them from maga-

zines, newspapers, television news, advertising, and friends; or interpret medical information provided by their physicians. Food and nutrition education activities must therefore be directed at increasing basic knowledge and complex cognitive skills that will enhance people's power to take thoughtful action.

It is also important to find out what your audience already knows, so that you can build on their current knowledge. This will help you avoid providing information they already know, which can come across as condescending, or information that is too complex. In a group setting, encourage the audience to share information with each other.

Now is the time to provide how-to information (factual knowledge) about foods, nutrients, dietary guidelines, and label reading and ways to apply the information in the audience's daily eating plans (procedural knowledge). In the case of our fruits and vegetables example, individuals now need information such as how many cups a day they should eat, the importance of eating a variety of colors, and tips on when and how to add them to one's diet. As nutrition educators, we are very good at these kinds of activities! Review existing programs or curricula for ideas; use available materials if they are suitable for your nutrition education intervention, or design your own activities. Here is the opportunity to use your creativity and imagination.

In discussing educational goals and objectives in Step 4, we reminded you to write objectives that addressed several levels of thinking in the cognitive taxonomy, ranging from knowledge (recall of information) through comprehension, application, analysis, and synthesis to evaluation. Table 12-2 summarizes these levels of knowledge skills. Do not focus only on basic factual knowledge. All age groups are capable of all levels of learning; it is only the sophistication of the language and concepts that may differ. For example, do not assume that for young children or low-literacy audiences, educational activities should be set at low levels of cognitive learning such as recall of information or comprehension. Even second graders can evaluate. It is good practice to include information on the cognitive level of each activity in your lesson plan to ensure that activities are well distributed across levels.

Provide factual knowledge and comprehension. As we have seen, knowledge has been defined for the purposes of developing educational programs as "the recall of specifics and universals, the recall of methods and processes, or the recall of a pattern, structure, or setting" (Bloom, Krathwahl, & Masia, 1964, p. 201). In the area of food and nutrition, knowledge might include the ability to recall such facts as the recommended guidelines for healthful diets appropriate for an individual's age, sex, and stage of life; which foods to select in order to meet the guidelines; serving sizes and how many servings one should eat of each food group in the food pyramid; and the ecological impact of different food processing techniques and packaging materials. Comprehension might involve understanding why fruits and vegetables are important in the diet or how to read a label.

Such information can be provided through lectures, handouts, slides, discussions, and demonstrations. Just as nutrition messages are more likely to be motivating if they are vivid and personal, so also how-to nutrition information, especially for the general public, is more likely to be remembered if it is vivid end understandable in everyday terms.

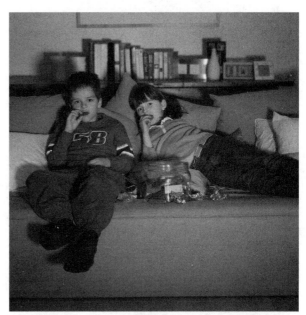

Consider all of the messages that children receive about food, and where they get those messages.

Graphs can be made using "foods" visually as units instead of abstract numbers (e.g., a stack of five teaspoons on top of each other instead of a plain bar graph to display the number of teaspoons of fat in foods). Show photographs or models of foods to help the audience estimate portion sizes, or bring in boxes or containers of foods to show nutrient composition. (Tip: Containers should be empty, so that audience members don't ask to take the foods home! This has the added advantage that you can use the containers again.) Demonstrations can be very effective, such as spooning out onto a plate the number of teaspoons of fat in a hamburger or burning a cracker to show that it has "calories" in it. (Tip: Use a cracker that has a lot of fat and a loose weave for oxygen to get in.) Other methods involve newsletters, flyers, and Web-based programs depending on the behavior or practice and the channel chosen (e.g., mass media or in-person). Correcting misconceptions at this time is very important if they constitute barriers to program participants' ability to take action.

Stimulate higher-order thinking. Food and nutrition issues are often complex. To take action and maintain behavior change requires not only knowledge of facts but also development of conceptual frameworks on which to hang isolated messages, called *knowledge structures* or *schemas*. Skills in analysis, synthesis, and evaluation are important here. Building such skills is more difficult than providing factual information. Analysis may involve comparing the sugar content of different beverages or the fat content of different fast

TABLE 12-2 Knowledge: Levels of Thinking

Levels of Thinking	Description
Knowledge	Recalling information as it is learned
Comprehension	Reporting information in a way other than how it was learned to show understanding
Application	Applying learned information to a new context
Analysis	Taking learned information apart into components so that its organizational structure may be understood
Synthesis	Putting together parts and elements into a unified organization or whole, with emphasis on creating new meaning or structure
Evaluation	Making judgments about the value of something using appropriate criteria

Source: Adapted from Bloom, B.S. 1956. *Taxonomy of educational objectives. Handbook I: Cognitive domain.* New York: David McKay.

foods. Synthesis may be planning a day's menu to incorporate nine servings of fruits and vegetables (or just a plan as to when individuals will incorporate nine fruits and vegetables in a day). Evaluation may involve rating several different food sources of calcium to select the best source based on some criterion such as price or impact on the body, or evaluating the amount of energy used to produce different types of food packaging. Active methods are usually more effective with most audiences: worksheets and hands-on, minds-on activities are appropriate to help people see connections between concepts and develop their conceptual frameworks for the given issue.

Skills in Critical Evaluation and Problem Solving

Depending on the behavior or practice and the channel chosen (e.g., mass media or in-person), nutrition education may include activities directed at enhancement of critical reasoning skills to evaluate complex and controversial issues or to understand food and nutrition policies. Food choice criteria have become more complex, involving not only health concerns but also, for many people, concerns about the ecological consequences of consumption (conventional? organic? local?), moral/ethical concerns (to eat meat or not), social justice concerns (who produced the food? under what working conditions?), and food safety concerns. Thus, critical thinking skills are needed so that people can make informed trade-offs between criteria in making food choices.

Individuals also need such skills so that they can examine the arguments on both sides of an issue—for example, whether to reduce dietary fat or carbohydrate to lose weight, eat organic versus "regular" fruits and vegetables, or breast-feed or bottle-feed their infant. They need critical evaluation skills to analyze and resolve contradictions and develop personal policies that will guide their food-related activities on an ongoing basis. A cognitive understanding of the food system and its impacts provides a context for action. Food- and nutrition-related behaviors are also embedded in larger social, economic, and political contexts that need to be understood for the continued maintenance of change.

Trigger films or audiotapes can be used, followed by discussion, to enhance critical thinking skills so as to be able to evaluate controversial issues or develop complex understandings. The arguments for and against certain practices can be volunteered by the group and recorded on newsprint in a brainstorming format and then discussed and perhaps voted upon. Carefully designed activities such as written or oral critiques or debates can also be used to encourage analysis of issues. Here participants should focus on the claims of the position, the evidence for and against the position and the strength of such evidence, and conclusions based on this evaluation of the evidence. When selecting opposing groups for a debate, to the extent possible assign group members to argue for the position that is contrary to their own personal position: this will greatly facilitate discussion and debate based on evidence rather than personal conviction. Use of these activities will depend on the learning style preferences of the audience as well as their comfort level with them. However, debates are interesting for all and should be considered. Low literacy does not preclude oral debates.

Affective Skills

Unlike some health-related behaviors such as smoking, food consumption is not optional. Food is needed for survival, and any changes in diets are undertaken with some ambivalence. Survival and quality of life require that appetite and enthusiasm about eating be maintained. Yet people recognize that they may need to change some of their food practices for health reasons even if these current practices are psychologically or culturally beneficial. Or they may want to take action on food system issues to support broader goals and values (such as supporting local agriculture), even though doing so is personally inconvenient and more expensive.

In discussing educational goals and objectives in Step 4, we reminded you to write objectives that addressed several levels of engagement in the affective taxonomy, ranging from receiving (awareness and willingness to receive your message) through responding, valuing, organizing, and internalizing values. Table 12-3 summarizes these levels of affective engagement.

TABLE 12-3 Levels of Affective Engagement

Levels of Commitment and Integration	Description
Receiving: Paying attention	1. Awareness with no position taken 2. Willingness to receive or attend to information 3. Will not avoid stimulus
Responding: Active participation	1. Complying with expectations of educator 2. Stating or defending own position 3. Beginning of own emotional response with satisfaction
Valuing: Behavior based on positive regard for something	1. Tentative acceptance with readiness to reevaluate 2. Conviction 3. Commitment to the behavior or action; beginning to internalize own viewpoint
Organization: Behaving according to a set of principles	1. Conceptualizing one's important values and understanding that they may be different from those of others 2. Building an internally consistent value system for guiding behavior by resolving conflicts and creating a unique value system
Internalizing values: Behaving according to a consistent worldview	1. Integration of value into one's consistent, total worldview that guides behavior 2. Person's behavior is consistent, predictable, and characterized by the values

Source: Adapted from D.R. Krathwahl, Bloom, B.S., and B.B. Masia. 1964. *Taxonomy of educational objectives. Handbook II: Affective domain.* New York: Longman.

Your activities should seek an appropriate level of affective engagement by your audience. Maybe you wish only for groups or audiences to become aware of an issue (mass media campaigns may seek this level). Or you may seek for your audience to actively respond during your sessions or program, participating instead of just observing, and beginning to respond with satisfaction to the educational activities and to form their own opinions. Most educational programs aim for the valuing level of engagement. Here individuals make a commitment to the action recommended by the program, perhaps at first tentatively, but later with conviction. At that level of commitment, individuals are ready and willing to take action, moving from intention to action. Review your activities to see if they encourage engagement and commitment. Depending on the issue and the audience, you may be able to design activities that assist individuals to build an internally consistent value system for guiding behavior by resolving conflicts and developing their own policies to guide action. See Chapter 10 for more details on the affective taxonomy.

Skills in the cognitive and affective domains accompany, and are usually integrated with, skills in the behavioral domain. For example, to be able to carry out a behavior, individuals need to be able to accurately observe and interpret a situation, to understand their own feelings in the situation, to change self-talk or how they think about the situation

from ways that are less accurate or productive to ones that are more productive (a process that is often called *cognitive restructuring*), to evaluate their own abilities to perform the behavior, to express themselves in ways appropriate to situations and persons, to express personal objectives, and to negotiate demands in an assertive and appropriate way.

Facilitated discussion or dialogue in small groups is one way nutrition educators can deal with feelings and emotional issues. In facilitated discussion, group members share feelings and experiences. The process is described more fully in Chapter 15. Participants can also be divided into groups of three or four in which they can talk over questions such as the following: What is the hardest thing about trying to change the way we eat? What are some successful ways we have changed other habits that could be applied to this particular dietary behavior?

Skills Mastery or Guided Practice (Behavioral Rehearsal)
Self-efficacy is an important mediator of behavior change in the action phase of nutrition education. Self-efficacy may increase with increased level of skills, but self-efficacy is not the same thing as skills. Self-efficacy involves both skills and the confidence that individuals can consistently use them even in the face of impediments or barriers. Social cognitive theory argues that a person's feeling of self-efficacy or competence in being able to carry out a behavior is crucial in

whether that person will perform the target behavior (Bandura, 1986). Furthermore, an increased perception of control or feeling of success comes from becoming more skillful in performing the desired behavior. Skill acquisition is thus an essential step leading from intention to behavior.

Skills include behavioral skills such as food shopping, household food management skills, and time management skills. Shopping skills such as using a shopping list, stocking up on bargains, and using coupons have been shown to be related to nutrient intake in low-income households and are thus important. Physical skills include such skills as preparing foods, cooking, breastfeeding, growing a vegetable garden, and participating in sports.

A review of the many methods for facilitating mastery of skills yields the following three specific instructional methods (Thoresen, 1984) that can be applied to the acquisition of food preparation, cooking, breastfeeding, safe food handling, and other food- and nutrition-related skills.

- *Clear instructions to individuals on how to perform the desired behavior.* Nutrition educators can enhance individuals' sense of confidence in their own abilities to carry out the goal behaviors or think analytically about issues when they provide individuals with clear and realistic instruction on how to perform the behavior or evaluate evidence critically. Examples include teaching participants how to make tasty low-fat meals, add fruits and vegetables to the diet, store fruits and vegetables correctly so that they do not spoil quickly, plant a vegetable garden, breast-feed, or handle foods safely in the home kitchen. Such teaching can be done by direct verbal instruction, using audiovisual media, role playing, or written instructions.

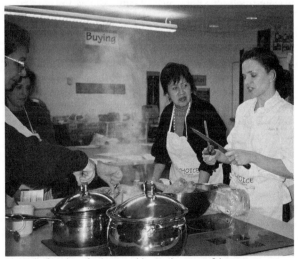

The skill of cooking fresh vegetables can boost confidence.

- *Social modeling, in which the skills are demonstrated.* Food demonstrations are a notable example. Such demonstrations can be live, on videotape, through visual mass media such as television, or in printed materials. Note the popularity of food shows and cooking demonstrations on television. Modeling is a powerful factor in motivating behaviors as well as an important instructional tool. We have to realize that as nutrition educators we are always modeling behavior, whether formally or informally, and whether we are aware of it or not. An unfortunate example of modeling is a situation in which nurses in Papua New Guinea were verbally encouraging breastfeeding among poor mothers but were bottle-feeding their own infants (Zeitlin & Formacion, 1981). The good health of the nurses' infants was interpreted by the poor mothers as evidence of the benefits of bottle-feeding, and thus they emulated the nurses' practice rather than what they said.

- *Guided practice with feedback.* This method is highly effective in both teaching skills and increasing self-efficacy. Cooking has been shown to improve cooking-related knowledge, attitudes, and behaviors more than food demonstrations (Levy & Auld, 2004). Here you create opportunities for individuals to practice the behavior (e.g., cooking a particular food) and provide them with specific feedback immediately after they have performed the desired behavior. Encouragement is useful because it can overcome participants' self-doubts. Early in the skills acquisition process, individuals should be encouraged to try out skills without evaluation by you or by themselves so that they can focus their attention on the skills to be acquired. This, of course, requires food preparation or cooking facilities to be available. However, many nutrition educators have developed ways to make cooking demonstrations, and even cooking by participants, possible by bringing with them all the needed food and equipment, including portable butane stoves or electric hot plates. Supermarket tours can enhance skills in shopping practices that are nutritionally healthy and ecologically sound.

Taken together, these three procedures result in a strategy referred to as *guided practice, behavioral rehearsal,* or *skills mastery.* You provide a demonstration of the desired behavior or skills, create opportunities for participants to practice what they observed with guidance on the performance of the task, make suggestions for improvement where necessary, and encourage them in their actions.

Complexity of Dietary Behavior Changes

Making dietary changes requires attention to a specific recurring array of behaviors and many specific actions that constitute the behavior, such as food shopping, eating out, or food preparation practices. It is the cumulative effects of these behaviors that have an impact on health. The environment in which dietary choices have to be made is quite challenging. One study found, for example, that in order to eat more fruits and vegetables, individuals said that they had to make more visits to stores, eating at friends' houses became more difficult, and buying takeout meals became more problematic (Anderson et al., 1998).

Making changes in food intake involves different behavioral categories, such as the following:

- Decreasing or avoiding certain foods, food constituents, or beverages
- Adding foods to the diet
- Modifying foods

More specifically, for fat intake, Kristal, Shattuck, and Henry (1990) identified the following dimensions of dietary behavior as relevant based on anthropological theory and their own research:

- Excluding high-fat ingredients and preparation techniques
- Modifying high-fat foods
- Substituting specially manufactured low-fat food for their higher-fat counterparts
- Replacing high-fat foods with low-fat alternatives

For vegetable intake, on the other hand, the relevant behavioral dimension is *adding* vegetables to the diet—specifically, adding vegetables to mixed dishes, including vegetables at lunch and dinner, eating raw vegetables, and eating salads (Satia et al., 2002).

The psychological, educational, and practical tasks may be very different for these two behaviors. Learning to avoid fat (or salt) means being able to recognize which types of foods it may be found in, learning to read food labels, and acquiring new food preparation techniques. Psychologically, it may mean giving up certain foods. Fruits and vegetables are easier to recognize, so this requires less education. In addition, psychologically, eating fruits and vegetables is about adding foods to one's diet and not having to give up certain favorite foods. Sometimes these behaviors are complementary, so they can be addressed together—for example, eating fruit rather than a high-fat snack between meals.

These behaviors are of course very culture bound and hence must be investigated for each intended audience. In addition, dietary behaviors are complex and the psychological motivations and skills needed are different depending on the food; these factors need to be considered when planning nutrition education.

Strengthening Self-Regulation Processes

Self-directed change comes about when individuals are not only motivated but can exercise self-regulation. Self-regula-

tion involves processes of self-influence and self-directedness through which individuals develop the ability to influence and control their own actions or behaviors though their own efforts: this is often referred to as *self-control*. Hence, the action phase of health behavior change is also referred to as the *volitional, conscious-choice,* or *action-control phase*. Several models describe the process (Bandura, 1997; Gollwitzer, 1999; Schwarzer & Renner, 2000). Self-regulation is not achieved through willpower but through the development of self-regulation skills. Such skills are needed for both action initiation and action maintenance. Nutrition education interventions must therefore create opportunities for individuals to develop these skills and, through these, develop a sense of agency.

Two examples in which the development of a sense of agency was the central focus of the intervention are provided in this chapter's features. Nutrition Education in Action 12-1 describes the Squire's Quest program, and Nutrition Education in Action 12-2 describes the Choice, Control, and Change program.

Chief among the strategies to achieve self-regulation skills is the process known to professionals as goal setting, which was discussed in Chapter 5 (Locke & Latham, 1990; Shilts, Horowitz, & Townsend, 2004; Cullen, Baranowski, & Smith, 2001). Although the term *goal setting* seems to be only about setting goals, as used by professionals it refers to a systematic behavioral change *process* that involves many of the educational or behavioral change strategies described earlier. The steps in the process are described slightly differently by different researchers and professionals, but they contain the same essential features.

Note: The strategies described here use the language of nutrition education professionals. You would not necessarily use the same terms with the public. Examples are given of terms to use with the intended audience for each strategy.

Goal Setting

Goal setting works to motivate, bridge the intention–action gap, and maintain action in nutrition education program participants for a variety of reasons. It engenders a sense of commitment to the goal. By planning ahead, participants do not have to make a new decision every time a food choice situation arises, thus leading to less mental burden and to development of a routine. The statement of a goal sensitizes individuals so that they are more conscious or mindful as they make food choices. It gives them a sense of control over their own behavior. It builds their perceptions of self-efficacy and mastery. It creates self-satisfaction and a sense of fulfillment from having achieved their goals, and contributes to the cultivation of intrinsic interest through active involvement in the process.

Goal setting is an example of exercising control over one's own behavior, or exercising agency, and is similar to the pro-

NUTRITION EDUCATION IN ACTION 12-1

Squire's Quest! A Multimedia Game

Increased consumption of fruits and vegetables by children have immediate benefits in terms of healthier growth and development and may reduce the risk of chronic disease later in life. Nutrition education can thus play an important role by addressing the mediators of eating more fruits and vegetables. Research evidence suggests that the most important mediators for children are increased availability and accessibility, preference, and skills in making fruit and vegetable recipes when they are responsible for making their own snacks. Squire's Quest was designed to increase consumption of fruits and vegetables in fourth grade children by addressing these mediators.

Program

Squire's Quest was designed as a 10-session, computer-based, interactive multimedia game, with each session lasting about 25 minutes. The game was based on the following background story: the kingdom of 5A Lot was being invaded by the Slimes (snakes) and the Mogs (moles), who were desirous of destroying the kingdom by destroying its fruits and vegetable crops. The king (Cornwell) and the queen (Nutritia) were leading their knights to defeat the invaders. The knights had such names as Sir Sarah See-a-Solution and Sir Alex Try-to-be-Right. The program invited children to commit to being a squire in the first session, and to seek to become knights in order to help the king and queen.

The squire had to face many challenges in this quest. These involved acquiring skills and setting goals related to eating more fruits, juice, and vegetables. The squire prepared FJV (fruit, juice, and vegetable) recipes in a virtual kitchen and had the help of a wizard through the challenges. Many of the sessions were delivered by the castle robot. The children participated in decision-making activities, choosing between their favorite FJV and a more common snack. The decision criteria provided were based on the most important outcome expectancies reported by the child at baseline. Before the end of each session, the squire set goals to make a recipe during that session, eat a FJV serving as a meal or snack, or ask for FJV to be available at home. Through this game, children learned about serving sizes and finding and buying FJV, and acquired practice in decision-making, goal-setting and problem-solving skills as well as practical skills such as preparing recipes in the virtual kitchen. Computers were provided to the schools and the intervention was conducted in five weeks.

Evaluation

The program was evaluated with 1,578 fourth grade students in 26 schools. The schools were matched in pairs and within matched pairs, schools were randomly assigned to intervention or control conditions. The behavioral outcome was assessed immediately after the program based on four days of dietary intake data obtained through a multiple pass, 24-hour dietary intake interview with the children. Results showed that children participating Squire's Quest increased their FJV intake by 1.0 servings more than the children not receiving the program. This suggests that psychoeducational multimedia games can serve an effective venue through which to provide nutrition education to children.

Source: Baranowski, T., J. Baranowski, K.W. Cullen, T. Marsh, N. Islam, I. Zakeri, L. Honess-Morreale, and C. DeMoor. 2003. Squire's Quest! Dietary outcome evaluation of a multimedia game. *American Journal of Preventive Medicine* 245:52–61.

cess of self-liberation in the transtheoretical model. Several reviews have shown that the goal-setting process can be very useful in the dietary arena (Cullen, Baranowski, & Smith, 2001; Shilts, Horowitz, & Townsend, 2004). A goal-setting worksheet that you can use with your audience is provided at the end of the chapter (Worksheet 12-1).

The word *goal* is used widely by the public and by professionals with many different meanings. Goals can refer to a variety of levels of states to be achieved. There are *end goals*, which express long-range, deeply valued end states that serve an orienting function to life, such as being healthy, being self-fulfilled, enjoying a high quality of life, contribut-

ing to the community, or living a life worth living. Behaviors to achieve these end goals may include eating healthfully or being physically active, among others. *Intermediate goals*, or *instrumental goals*, are behaviors or practices that people can engage in to achieve these end goals, such as eating a healthful diet or walking to get exercise (to support an end goal of a healthy life). Finally, there are *specific action goals* for specific actions we can take to achieve these intermediate goals, such as "I will drink orange juice each morning for breakfast." Many different terms are used by different models or theories to refer to these differing levels of goals. In the goal-setting process, we generally focus on the intermedi-

NUTRITION EDUCATION IN ACTION 12-2

Choice, Control, and Change

The Choice, Control, and Change (C3) program is an inquiry-based science education and health program for overweight prevention among middle school students. Given an environment that encourages overeating and sedentary behavior, the goal of C3 is for youth to become competent eaters who have a sense of agency and are able to navigate this environment. Students collect scientific evidence to enable them to understand why and how healthful eating and ample physical activity are important. It is thus both a science education curriculum as well as a behavior-focused, theory-based nutrition education intervention. It addresses both why to and how to eat healthfully. The why-to information explores the interplay of biology, personal behavior, and the food system and meets various national standards for science education. The how-to information focuses on teaching cognitive self-regulation skills and enhancing agency.

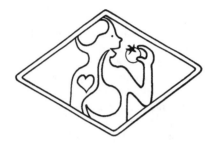

The program consists of 24 sessions of hands-on, exciting science activities:

- *The balancing act:* Students learn about energy balance in the human body and collect food intake (energy input) and activity (energy output) data on themselves.
- *Food, exercise, and health*: Students explore how food and activity choices relate to health and explore the reasons why obesity, diabetes, and heart disease are increasing in our society.
- *Our food environment:* Students explore influences on their food choices such as their food environment, portion sizes, and the ads they watch.
- *Moving toward health:* Students analyze their own food and activity data and discuss, debate, and defend any changes they would like to make to their own eating and activity.
- *Overcoming barriers:* Students collect data on ways that our society presents challenges to maintaining healthful habits.
- *Guided goal setting:* Students select actions that they will take to make their body perform for them and practice self-regulation skills to become competent eaters and movers. They select one food-related behavior from among several, such as drinking fewer sweetened beverages, eating fewer packaged snacks, or eating more fruits and vegetables. In the physical activity area, the goal for youth is to walk more, and students are given pedometers.

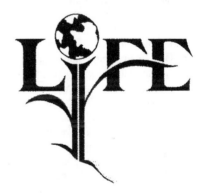

Courtesy of Choice, Control and Change curriculum, Linking Food and the Environment Program, Teachers College Columbia University www.tc.edu/centers/life.

- *Confirming competence:* Students integrate their understanding of the science connecting food and activity to health and confirm their personal health commitments.

Students in the program significantly reduced the reported frequency (days per week) and amount (packages per day) of candy, sweetened beverages, and packaged salty and sweet snacks, as well as the portion size of sweet snacks. They also reported walking more.

Source: Choice, Control, and Change is a curriculum module of the Linking Food and the Environment (LiFE) program from Teachers College Columbia University. Available at www.tc.edu/centers/life. The logos are used with permission.

ate or instrumental behavioral goals (or goal intentions) and on action goals to achieve them. These action goals are the same as implementation intentions. There are different ways to describe the goal-setting process (Cullen, Baranowski, & Smith, 2001; Shilts, Horowitz, & Townsend, 2004). One way is suggested in the following.

1. Choose the behavioral goal (or goal intention). The process of choosing behavioral goals can arise from external or internal sources. In self-directed change, it is usually some emotional experience or some consciousness-raising understanding that initiates the decision to take action. In the context of a nutrition education intervention, the behavioral goals come from the needs analysis that you conducted in Step 1 of the nutrition education design model. The effectiveness of assigned, self-selected, or collaboratively (group) set goals has been compared. Evidence seems to suggest that effectiveness does not differ by type, but that the suitability of different types may depend on several factors such as the age of participants, their readiness to change, and the type of behavior being targeted (Bandura, 1986; Shilts, Horowitz, & Townsend, 2004). Group goal setting does not automatically ensure that all individuals are equally involved or have bought into the goals. It appears that once people believe in a goal's importance and get immersed in the process, the goal itself becomes more important than how it was set.

For a behavior-focused intervention, a *guided* goal-setting process may be particularly appropriate, with the behavioral goals being assigned but specific action goals being chosen by the program participants. That is, the behavioral goals for individuals are the same as the behavioral goals specified by the intervention or program, such as eating a healthier diet, improving bone health through eating more calcium-rich foods and being more physically active, eating more fruits and vegetables, and so forth. If the program's behavioral goal is quite broad, such as "participants will eat a healthier diet," then the individual will have some choices to make. The individual's behavioral goals are stated as follows: I will (or I intend to)

- Increase my intake of fruits and vegetables (or, more specifically, I will eat more than 2.5 cups of fruits and vegetables daily)
- Decrease my intake of high-fat, high-sugar foods
- Increase my intake of calcium-rich foods
- Increase my purchases from local farmers

Depending on the duration and intensity that is possible for your program, you will usually want the participants to select only one or two goals to work on.

2. Select or develop a self-assessment tool for participants. Self assessment involves identification of specific actions that participants are currently engaging in that relate to the behavioral goals of the intervention program, such as eating a healthier diet, improving bone health through eating

more calcium-rich foods and being more physically active, eating foods produced locally, and so forth.

For example, if the intervention or program's behavioral goal is to reduce fat in the diet, then participants need to identify the foods in their diet that contribute to their fat intake. Is it the amount of meat they are eating, or the number of rich desserts? If the goal of the intervention is to increase fruit and vegetable consumption among audience members, how many servings are they now eating in a day? If the program's behavioral goal is to encourage eating locally produced foods, then how often do the participants visit farmers' markets or look for foods in the supermarket that are labeled as being local? This may further the recognition of the need for change. Participants can also identify the determinants of their behavior so as to gain the information needed for setting realistic goals. The self-assessment usually involves some kind of recording method, such as food records of one to three days, 24-hour dietary recalls, or checklists of the targeted foods or practices. Figure 12-1 shows an example of a self-assessment tool for recording food intakes; it is for the EatFit program described in Chapter 5.

3. Develop a system for scoring the self-assessment tool and generating appropriate goals. This system could be as simple as adding up the scores for different behaviors assessed in the self-assessment tool. An example is shown in Worksheet 12-1 at the end of the chapter.

4. Provide instruction for setting effective action goals or action plans. Action goals should be clear and quantifiable, close in time, and attainable (Bandura, 1986; Locke & Latham, 1990; Shilts, Horowitz, & Townsend, 2004).

- *Clear and quantifiable (specificity).* The action goal should be specific. General action goals have been shown to be ineffective for achieving changes in behavior. Specific goals provide clear targets for action, indicating the type and amount of effort needed to achieve the goal. An example might be "I will drink orange juice for breakfast and add a vegetable to lunch" (to increase intake of fruits and vegetables from one to two cups daily).

- *Close in time (proximity).* Action goals to be accomplished in the immediate future are more likely to be effective than those set for a longer time frame, since in the latter case, it is easy to postpone action. For example, "I will eat 2.5 cups of fruits and vegetables *today* by having orange juice at breakfast, eating a fruit for a mid-morning snack, adding a salad to lunch, and eating two vegetables for dinner" is likely to be more effective than stating "I will eat more fruits and vegetables this month."

- *Reachable (difficulty).* The action goals should be difficult yet reachable. Those that are challenging but clearly attainable through extra effort are more likely

My Eating Record

1) Write down the foods you eat and drink as you go through the day.
2) Begin your record in the morning with the first thing you eat or drink and finish at bedtime with the last thing that you eat or drink.
3) Include those foods and drink consumed during breakfast, lunch, and dinner and do not forget to write down your snacks and munchies. A piece of gum, and drink from the water fountain, a taste of cookie dough all count, so write them down.
4) Make sure to check out the hunger rating scale at the bottom of your food record: write down how hungry you were *before* you began to eat.

Help! How much did I eat?

1 cup = a handful
1 ounce of cheese = 4 dice
1 tsp = the tip of your thumb
1 tablespoon = the size of your thumb
1/2 cup = the size of an ice cream scoop
3 ounces of meat = a deck of cards
1 medium-size fruit = 1 tennis ball
12 fluid ounces = 1 can of soda

Once you're done, log onto www.eatfit.net to see how your eating rates

Name: _____

1 Day Eating Record

FIGURE 12-1 Example assessment tool from the EatFit program: Eating record. *Source:* Shilts, M.K., M. Horowitz, and M. Townsend. 2004. An Innovative innovative approach to goal setting for adolescents: Guided goal setting. Journal of Nutrition Education and Behavior 36:155–156. Courtesy of M.K. Shilts, M. Horowitz, and M.S. Townsend, University of California, Davis.

Food/Beverage	Type/Description	Preparation	Amount Eaten	Where Did You Eat/Drink It?	Hunger Rating
Bread	*Whole wheat*	*Toasted*	*1 slice*	*Kitchen*	*7*

Hunger Rating Scale

1 —— 2 —— 3 —— 4 —— 5 —— 6 —— 7 —— 8 —— 9 —— 10

starving   pretty   a little   not   pretty   stuffed
              hungry   hungry   hungry   full

to be motivating and satisfying. Difficult goals require more effort to achieve than easy ones. It is the discrepancy between where we are and where we want to be that is motivating. Motivation can be sustained by setting progressively more difficult action goals, assuming that they are seen as reasonable and within reach. Very difficult or complex changes should be broken down into smaller units, and goals set for each of the units. The maxim is that the goal should be small enough to achieve but large enough to matter. For example, rather than set one action goal "to eat less fat and sugar and to eat more fruits and vegetables," individuals should set separate action goals and make them specific, such as "to add one dark green vegetable to my diet each day this week" or "to eat ice cream only twice this week."

It is best to recommend that program participants set relatively small and easily accomplished goals at first, moving on to more difficult actions when these are successfully accomplished. Also, it is wise to ask participants not to completely eliminate any favorite foods in the beginning—no matter how fatty or high in sugar or ecologically unwise they may be. This line of reasoning is based on research that success raises judgments of self-efficacy or competence, whereas repeated failure lowers them. Anticipation of self-satisfaction in achieving the goals and the experience of success can increase the sense of personal control and sustain commitment to the decision. As the saying goes, "Nothing breeds success like success." Setting a goal to eat 1 cup each of fruits and vegetables each day for someone who normally eats one-half cup can constitute a difficult but attainable goal, whereas eating more than 2.5 cups probably does not. The individual could work up to more than 2.5 cups over time.

Regarding the question of whether to strive for small changes or large ones, some studies show that those who made action goals for the most drastic reductions in fat intake met with the greatest success (Barnard, Akhtar, & Nicholson, 1995; Brunner et al., 1997). Some researchers conclude that advising individuals to make small goals may discourage them from making sufficient changes to experience the benefits of the change. In these studies, however, the individuals for whom this is true are those who are highly motivated, feel at high risk of disease, or want to prevent a reoccurrence of a disease. They may find it easier to clear out their food cabinets of current items and start anew (e.g., replacing all highly processed items with whole-grain products). Most individuals, however, find that small changes are more effective. (You might want to check with your audience as to whether small changes or big ones would be easier for them.)

5. Create a contract, pledge, or challenge sheet. Commitment to an action goal is the personal resolve to pursue the goal and is affected by several factors: the goal must be valued and seen as attainable. Thus, action goals that support

values that are personal and long term are more likely to sustain commitment. (Perhaps the goal is not really about health per se, but about some personal standard that is important, such as taking care of oneself.) Small commitments that will eventually lead to larger ones can be sought first. Setting an action goal increases effort, as we have noted previously, as well as concentration and persistence. Personal commitment is strengthened by pledges that bind the individual to future action. The motivational effect of binding ourselves to future action is largely due to not wanting to renege on an agreement we have made. This is especially true if the goal is highly valued.

It is helpful to provide some kind of agreement form or worksheet on which group participants can state their commitment or pledge (Figure 12-2). The actual form is often called a *contract* because it involves a contract between the person and himself or herself. The word *contract* may not work with your audience. You should pilot test your form with the target group to find a term that is most appropriate for them. For example, it can be called an *action plan*. Each participant should sign one. Given that public commitment enhances the likelihood of following through on a pledge, it is best to have another member of the group, a friend, or family member also sign as a witness. Table 12-4 contains some tips to go with the contract form, which can be made into a handout for the group. Some nutrition educators who work in classroom settings with younger children, who might lose contract forms, have students voluntarily sign a class book instead. The children then check off when they have attained the goal. This is often called a challenge sheet.

6. Build skills. In many instances, program participants will need to hone their existing skills or learn new ones in order to carry out the behaviors to which they have committed themselves. Becoming more skillful in performing the desired behavior also results in an increased perception of control or feeling of success. The program needs to design strategies and activities to assist individuals to do so. These should include enhancing behavioral capabilities or specific food- and nutrition-related knowledge, cognitive skills, and behavioral skills, including food preparation. Possible activities to build skills were described in an earlier section of this chapter.

7. Develop a tracking and feedback system (self-monitoring and self-evaluation). The next step is for individuals and groups to track their progress to see how well they are doing compared with their action goals. Self-observation and self-evaluation are considered extremely important in the self-regulatory process. Such feedback can be provided through a tracking system that you develop for use by individuals. This may be quite easy for behaviors that are clearly visible or identifiable, such as eating fruits and vegetables. However, other behaviors may not be so easy, such as reducing fat in foods. In the latter case, you could come up with some clear definitions of higher-fat and lower-fat foods to make tracking possible. You can review the completed tracking forms and give individual feedback as well. Or the participants could give oral reports in group settings, if the action goals have been made public. In this case, individuals will get feedback from the group also. Both individual and group feedback can be used, depending on the conditions under which the action goals were set. The focus should be on positive accomplishments rather than failures.

Figure 12-3 shows the tracking system used in the EatFit program for middle school students. The system consists of a graph in the form of a thermometer (one thermometer for tracking a student's eating goal and another for his or her fitness goal). Students shade in the thermometer starting at the bottom (cold) and move toward the hot end of the thermometer as they judge that they are reaching their goal.

8. Create rewards and encouragement. Achievement of the action goals can be rewarded by program staff, by collective action on the part of the participants, or by the individuals themselves, depending on the situation. Nutrition educators can provide reinforcement in many ways: verbal encouragement, smiles, and an approving, nonjudgmental tone of voice in all interactions with the group; or material rewards such as key chains, magnets, tee-shirts, or sweat shirts to those who participate or complete the program. For example, tee-shirts appear to be quite motivating to runners. A founder of the New York City Road Runners Club used to say, "Never underestimate the power of a tee-shirt!" Indeed, some runners are known to select races on the basis of the tee-shirts being given out. You can also give out raffle tickets to be drawn for prizes upon completion of the contract. The hidden messages in these reinforcements should be consistent and support the spoken, overt message. For example, rewarding children for being physically active with high-fat, high-sugar food products would not be supportive of the message. Present participants with certificates of achievement when they achieve their goals.

Individuals can also reinforce themselves in tangible ways, such as buying a new piece of clothing or a new piece of exercise equipment, or through their affective reactions, such as praising themselves when they meet their goals and problem solving when they fall short. Physiological and external reinforcements also influence goal achievement. Thus, knowledge that one's serum cholesterol level has declined can enhance an individual's commitment to eating a low-fat diet. Similarly, it can be very reinforcing when individuals notice that they no longer have to exert themselves as much during exercising because of their increased fitness. Other reinforcements might include comments from others that they look healthier or that they are performing their jobs better (because of their increased fitness).

9. Problem solving. When participants do not attain their action goals, assist them to engage in problem solving and

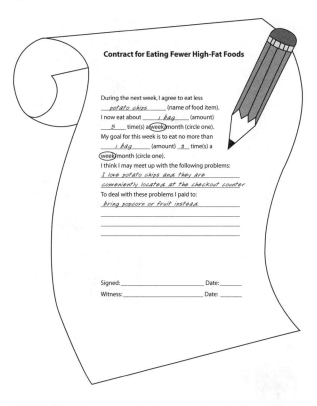

FIGURE 12-2 Sample completed contract for eating fewer high-fat foods.

TABLE 12-4 What Works and Doesn't Work in Making Changes

What Works	What Doesn't Work
Setting realistic goals and breaking your goal into small steps you can achieve	Setting unrealistic goals
Allowing for your food dislikes	Trying to include foods you don't like
Making small changes	Making drastic changes
Choosing foods you can get easily	Choosing foods you have to search for
Getting support from your family and friends	Trying to make changes all by yourself
Being flexible: compromising in some situations	**Being rigid:** trying to live up to your changes with absolutely no exceptions

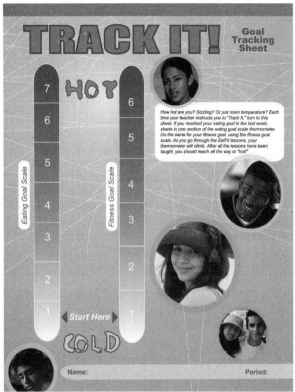

FIGURE 12-3 The EatFit program's goal tracking sheet. Source: Shilts, M.K., M. Horowitz, and M. Townsend. 2004. An Innovative innovative approach to goal setting for adolescents: Guided goal setting. *Journal of Nutrition Education and Behavior* 36:155–156. Courtesy of M.K. Shilts, M. Horowitz, and M.S. Townsend, University of California, Davis.

decision making to find more effective ways to attain the goals they set or to set new ones that are more attainable.

Goal Maintenance (Relapse Prevention)

In the area of food and dietary behavior, goal maintenance is a more appropriate concept than relapse prevention. As noted before, eating is not optional and is not a single behavior, such as smoking, that one can change and then relapse. Instead, eating requires daily food choices and constant trade-offs among numerous alternative actions. Healthy food practices need to be maintained for the long term—indeed, permanently. Studies have found that no magic food changes are involved in making dietary changes. In interventions designed to lower fat intake, for example, people made changes in all four high-fat food groups: the greatest changes were in the fats/oils, red meat, and dairy food groups, and the least in the grains group (Burrows et al., 1993). In interventions directed at fruits and vegetables, people made changes through conventional eating habit changes such as adding

fruit juice as a snack or including a vegetable at lunch (Cox et al., 1998). Adding foods to the diet, such as fruits and vegetables, appears easier to do and maintain than removing a food or a food constituent such as fat.

An effective approach is to use a general dietary framework, not a prescriptive diet. This gives individuals control over their diets. You can provide them with more than one way to change their diets and give alternative menu suggestions to enhance their ability to make their own trade-offs. Another effective approach is to devise and provide to program participants some sort of self-monitoring system that is feasible and easy to use. For foods that are easily identifiable, such as fruits and vegetables, such a system is relatively simple—counting items and estimating the amounts in foods. In the dietary fat arena, visible fats are easily identified (such as butter and oils), and changes can be monitored. However, many nutrients are not visible, such as fat, salt, or fiber. Here some kind of point system needs to be devised for self-monitoring purposes, and label reading skills become important.

In general, whereas the initial motivation for change is driven by *anticipated* positive consequences of making the change, maintenance of change is motivated by *actual* positive experiences from the change, such as finding that eating healthful food is satisfying and pleasurable. Consequently, a number of other self-regulatory processes besides goal setting are important for maintaining a food-related behavior once action is taken.

Prioritizing competing goals. Managing conflicting goals and competing priorities is at the heart of self-regulation for maintaining the behavior chosen. A major ongoing challenge in maintaining healthful practices is setting priorities between conflicting goals or desires, such as between the goal to eat more healthfully and a personal agenda that may involve work-related aspirations that do not leave much mental and physical time for planning and eating healthfully. At this time, the chosen behavioral goal, such as to eat healthful lunches at work, needs to be evaluated in relation to competing goals, such as the desire to be a productive worker and hence not to be gone too long from one's desk, and needs to be protected from these competing goals if the chosen goal is determined to be more important. We should remember that implementing a new, more healthful behavior, such as adding fruit to the diet, does not automatically reduce less healthful habits such as eating high-fat, high-sugar snacks. Encourage participants to review each goal they are trying to achieve (e.g., eating fruits and vegetables, breastfeeding) in terms of its positive value to them, how important or desirable it is to them, how it relates to their larger life goals, how they will feel about achieving or not achieving the goal, and how much they have already invested, and then to reaffirm their commitment to their chosen goal. Your role is that of a collaborator and coach.

Protecting action goals from distractions (mindful eating). Goal maintenance relies on conscious control and attention. It is important to assist participants to protect their goals from being interrupted and given up prematurely due to competing distractions. For example, a table that is full of tasty, high-fat foods presents a distraction to someone who has chosen the goal of eating lower-fat foods. Ask individuals to identify potential distracting situations and to make plans ahead of time to ignore these anticipated distractions. This can be done by participants' verbally describing or imagining the situation and rehearsing exactly what they will do and the positive outcomes they can expect from staying with their goals. You can also remind individuals just to be mindful about what they eat: think before they eat.

Attributions and counterconditioning (self-talk). When individuals attempt to make changes in their eating patterns, they will likely experience both successes and failures. Their attributions of why they were successful or not will influence their sense of self-efficacy and future behavior. If they think their success (for example, in cooking) was due to a stable cause, such as their ability, they will have a higher expectation of success the next time compared with individuals who attribute their success to something unstable, such as luck. After failure, these effects are reversed. These attributions are sometimes called *self-talk*. You can assist individuals to develop more accurate attributions and new ways of thinking or self-talk. For example, encourage individuals to tell themselves they are not clumsy, but skillful, and to recognize that the great dish they have prepared is due to the skills they have acquired, not luck, and to tell themselves they can do it again. This process is called *counterconditioning* in the transtheoretical model.

Focusing on higher-order behavioral goals in the achievement of action goals. Higher-order behavioral goals can provide stability and facilitate choices among specific action goals in difficult situations. Encourage participants to focus on the major goal when they are in difficult situations. For example, individuals may find themselves unable to eat the vegetables at lunch they had planned because of a birthday party for a coworker. They can fulfill their personal social goal at lunch and "reschedule" an extra vegetable serving at dinner to achieve their major health goal of eating more fruits and vegetables.

Linking action goals to self-identity. If the chosen goals can be seen as part of the identify of intervention participants, they are less likely to be devalued or postponed when competing goals emerge (such as deadlines at work). For example, if individuals come to think of themselves as health-conscious or ecologically responsible eaters, they will be more likely to stay with their action goals to eat more fruits and vegetables.

Coping Self-Efficacy
Goal maintenance also relies on emotion-coping strategies, such as the ability to ignore feelings of worry or of disap-

pointment in not meeting the goals we set. These strategies are important because many desirable food- and nutrition-related practices require effort—for example, seeking out farmers' markets in order to eat locally, or learning to cook so as to gain control over what we eat. Optimistic beliefs about our ability to deal with barriers, though a major hindrance in getting us motivated, may be helpful here because a new behavior may turn out to be much more difficult to adhere to than we had anticipated. These beliefs are sometimes referred to as *coping self-efficacy*. Examples are "I can stick with a healthful diet even if I have to try several times until it works" or "I can stick with a healthful diet even if I need a long time to develop the necessary routines" (Schwarzer & Renner, 2000). Or again, "I can stick with a healthful diet even when others in the family do not wish to do so." Thus, the nutrition educator should help program participants become aware that they have coping resources. Here again, having people practice positive, action-oriented self-talk (or cognitive restructuring) can be useful, reminding themselves that they are capable of taking action.

Cue Management (Stimulus Control)
Cue management or stimulus control is the process in which individuals remove cues to less healthful eating and add cues for more healthful eating. Provide instruction to program participants on how to restructure their personal environments. For example, they can reduce the number of less healthful foods in the household and keep them out of sight, or make them less accessible and convenient. Such foods can be purchased and eaten occasionally or as treats. On the other hand, fruit can be washed, ready to eat, and left on the counter or in the refrigerator. Likewise, vegetables can be washed, cut

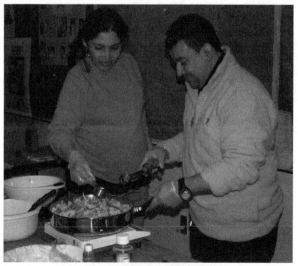

Learning to cook and eat healthy at the WIC clinic.

up and ready to eat, and conveniently placed in the refrigerator. If a goal is to reduce the number of plastic bags used for groceries, then canvas bags can be placed on the front door knob or in the car, ready for use in the grocery store.

Developing Routines and Habits

A major aim during the maintenance phase of dietary change is for the new behaviors to become automatic or habitual (Bargh & Barndollar, 1996). When we repeatedly perform a behavior in a specific context (such as drinking orange juice at breakfast), the motivation (to eat more fruit) and its implementation instructions (drink orange juice at breakfast) become so integrated that as soon as we experience the situation (breakfast) the specific action is triggered in memory without the need for conscious decision making. Thus, repeated context-specific action will lead to increasingly effortless enactment of the behavior.

Setting goals helps to initiate new habits. At first, achieving the goals will require conscious control, but repetition of the action will lead to more unconscious control over behavior. Help program participants to develop routines. Assure them that even difficult behaviors will become easier when they become more routine (such as making a lunch to bring to school or to work each day).

Familiarity or Repeated Experience with Healthful Food

An important aim of nutrition education is for individuals to enjoy eating healthful foods. As we saw earlier in the book, there is considerable evidence that repeated experience with a food can increase liking and preference for it. Studies have found that those who decide to eat less salt eventually come to like foods with less salt. In the case of fat intake, when individuals use fat substitutes to reduce the fat content of their diet, they still like the taste of fat, but when they switch to naturally low-fat foods, they decrease their liking for the fatty taste (Mattes, 1993; Grieve & Vander Weg, 2003). One study of long-term maintenance of a low-fat diet found that using fat substitutes was easily adopted but did not contribute much to dietary fat reduction, whereas avoiding fat as a flavoring (such as sauces on vegetables or butter on bread) and eating less meat were difficult to adopt but contributed the most to reducing the overall fat content of the diet (Bowen et al., 1993). It should be noted that the former represents a substitution of one product for a similar one and is not a behavioral change, whereas the latter actions represent a change in behavior. Many of the study participants felt deprived, but those who successfully maintained the diet regimen found they no longer liked the taste of fat (Urban et al., 1992). It is clear that *we eat what we like, but we also come to like what we eat.* Hence, remind program participants to stay with their chosen dietary change long enough for them to come to like the new foods and, indeed, to find them pleasurable to eat.

Personal Food Policies

The ultimate goal in nutrition education is for individuals themselves to be able eventually to take control of their food choices and practices by using self-regulatory processes such as those described in this chapter. These processes will help them develop the skills necessary for influencing not only their own personal behavior but also the environments in which their food choices are made. Individuals can be encouraged to develop personal food policies to guide their dietary choices and food-related actions. They can decide, for example, that they will always eat breakfast, always have a vegetable at lunch, eat desserts only once a week, buy organic or local foods whenever there is a choice, shop at farmers' markets in season, (only once a week or whatever frequency) eat at a fast food chain restaurant, and so forth. These food policies will help guide decisions on an ongoing basis.

Management of Social Context

Most eating occurs in a social context, even if many meals are eaten alone. For example, food purchasing requires consideration of household needs. Thus, the mother of the household may decide to drink nonfat milk, but the rest of the family insists on whole milk. Should she then buy both kinds? Does she have space to store both kinds? If she decides to eat more plant-based, whole-grain meals, whereas the other family members want to eat hamburgers and french fries, will she make two meals? Or will she cook for herself and let the others fend for themselves? She will have to make trade-offs and negotiations between her desire for health for herself and her desire to maintain good family relationships. And of course mothers of young children also need encouragement and skills in feeding their children. Facilitated group discussions can be invaluable here as individuals meet with others like themselves to share ideas and challenges and how to overcome them. The nutrition educator can provide valuable assistance in the process. An example of such an intervention is discussed in Nutrition Education in Action 12-3.

Figure 12-4 summarizes the educational strategies and activities that are useful in action-phase sessions or program components.

Your Turn

We will now apply the information in this chapter to the process of selecting appropriate educational strategies and designing learning experiences to achieve each of the behavioral goals or goal intentions identified by the participant or the program. As we saw in the last chapter, these strategies should be sequenced as events of instruction to provide a plan for how to proceed. We refer to the resulting plan as the *lesson plan* or *educational plan,* even though it will be used for in-person group activities with all ages and in all settings, particularly nonformal ones. By now you will probably realize that designing learning experiences or activities is a

NUTRITION EDUCATION IN ACTION 12-3

Sisters in Health: An Experiential Program Emphasizing Social Interaction to Increase Fruit and Vegetable Intake Among Low-Income Adults

Sisters in Health was a community-based program to increase fruit and vegetable intake among low-income women that was designed to be implemented in small groups in real-life community settings, to be flexible, and to be easy to implement by community nutrition educators. It was based on facilitated group discussion and experiential learning, in which group members were interactively involved in discussing their knowledge, experiences, problems, and solutions with other group members.

Program

The program consisted of six 90-minute weekly meetings for groups of approximately 10 women, facilitated by community nutrition paraprofessionals trained through the Cooperative Extension Service. The program was based on extensive formative research or needs assessment.

Each session included the following:

- A welcome or warm-up activity, such as how the family liked the new dish tried at home
- A food preparation and tasting experience, such as creating and tasting a salad bar
- A group learning activity, such as adding or subtracting ingredients from a salad to boost nutrient density
- A take-home challenge, such as making at least one "enhanced salad" at home
- Feedback on the meeting and for planning the next one
- Low-cost incentives, such as cooking utensils and notebooks for recipes

All groups received the sessions "Getting Started," which focused on participants' familiarity with and preferences regarding fruits and vegetables, and "All About Me," which focused on recommendations and portion sizes. Four other sessions were chosen by the group (from eight), on topics such as "Scoring with Salads," "Kids and Vegetables," "Easier than Pie: Fruit Anytime," and "Beat the Clock with Meals in Minutes." Such an approach combined flexibility and the needs and interests of the group with the need for preprepared education plans for effective education.

Evaluation

The program's impact was evaluated in a nonrandom sample of 269 low-income adults in 32 intervention and 10 control groups using a quasi-experimental, pre- and postprogram evaluation design in which a control group received a budgeting or parenting program of the same duration and intensity. Intervention groups reported an increase in fruit and vegetable consumption, measured by a brief screener, of 1.6 times a day (compared with 0.8 in the control groups). Knowledge of the number of servings people should eat and self-efficacy did not increase (they may have already been high), but attitudes, knowledge of preparation methods, and satisfaction with how vegetables turned out did increase significantly. Group support, active learning experiences, food tastings, and food skill development were thus effective in increasing fruit and vegetable intake in these low-income adults.

Source: Devine, C.M., T.J. Farrell, and R. Hartman. 2005. Sisters in Health: Experiential program emphasizing social interaction increases fruit and vegetable intake among low-income adults. *Journal of Nutrition Education and Behavior* 37:265–270.

---

very fluid process, so that you will be going back and forth between designing activities, sequencing them, and writing educational objectives. In addition, after pilot testing, you may want to change or rearrange activities.

It is useful to first develop a lesson plan outline using a table format as shown in the previous chapter. The table format enables you to see whether you have addressed all the potential mediators of behavior change and educational objectives that you set and whether the activities are appropriate in terms of domains of learning and level

of complexity. Worksheet 12-1 at the end of the chapter can be used to develop your own real or hypothetical session.

You may be able to conduct the actual sessions using this table format, but you will probably need to convert it into a narrative lesson plan for use when you are with a group. You may also design other formats as appropriate for your situation. Regardless of teaching format, starting with a table format is crucial for gaining an overview of your strategies and checking whether you have incorporated the strategies

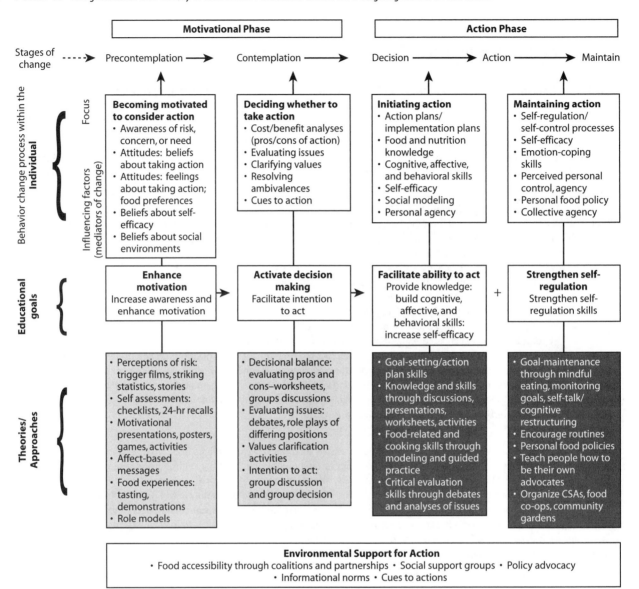

FIGURE 12-4 Conceptual framework for nutrition education: action-phase educational strategies and activities.

that have been shown to be effective. Such a format is shown for our ongoing case study.

Do not try to cover too much in one session. It is our tendency to want to share with our audiences all that we know and are enthusiastic about. But individuals cannot process too much information at one time (Achterberg, 1998). Focus on one overarching theme in each session related to the behavioral goals, two to four supporting concepts (general educational objectives), and a limited number of specific theory-based strategies (specific educational objectives). The

rule of thumb is to cover half as much in twice the time you think is needed.

If the lessons are not just a one-time event of one or several sessions, all the activities as designed should be extensively pilot tested with the intended audience. If food is used, test recipes and preparation procedures for taste acceptance and feasibility. Using focus groups, direct observation, and interviews, assess whether activities are acceptable and effective with the intended audience.

Case Study

We will now apply the information in this chapter specifically to our ongoing case study to illustrate the process of selecting appropriate educational strategies for each of the mediators we selected to address and of designing fun, enjoyable educational activities and needed content for group participants to achieve the educational objectives.

We have been focusing on the sessions that address the behavioral goal of increasing intake of fruits and vegetables. These sessions have been titled "The Whys and Whats of Colorful Eating." The logic model for our case study that we presented in the last chapter is shown here again as Figure 12-5, now with the box showing strategies directed at potential action-phase mediators highlighted. The case study educational plan directed at such action-phase strategies is presented at the end of this chapter, using the outline table format.

We build on the table that we created in Step 3 showing the educational objectives (and learning domain and level) for each mediator of behavior change or theory con-

struct. In the second column of the table, we list the events of instruction to help us *sequence* our activities during the session appropriately. In the third column we list each of the *potential mediators* of behavior change—which are also the theory constructs that the lesson will address. In this column we also list the theory-based *strategies* that will be used to address the potential mediators. For each mediator, we then list the *specific educational objectives* that we stated in Step 3. In the final column, we indicate all the *practical educational activities, learning experiences, or messages* that we plan to use to carry out the educational strategies.

The narrative form of the lesson is also shown for the case study. This is probably what you will take with you to implement the lesson or session. Some nutrition educators like to put the information on index cards and use those in the session.

The lesson plans as presented may seem quite specific and detailed. However, it is very important to have such plans. As noted before, using learner-centered education and facilitated

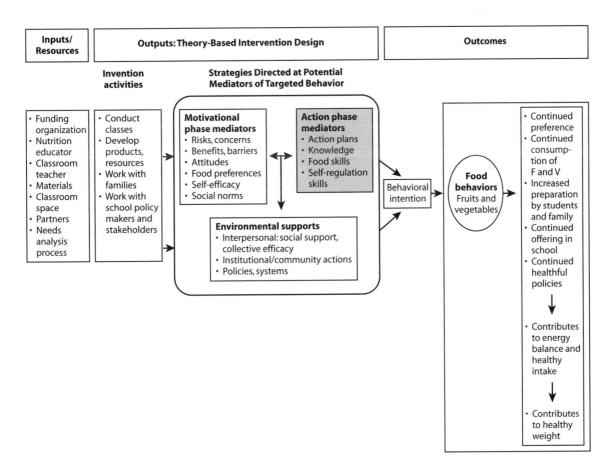

FIGURE 12-5 Logic model conceptual framework for case study: The Whys and Whats of Colorful Eating.

dialogue approaches does not remove the necessity for careful planning. It is understood, however, that you may find yourself needing to adapt the education plans to the situation on the ground and to the backgrounds and interests of the *specific* group with whom you are working. Practical delivery methods are described in more detail in Part III of this book (see Chapter 15).

Questions and Activities

1. Why are goal setting and the development of action plans important for the effectiveness of nutrition education interventions? Discuss.
   a. What are three characteristics of effective action goals?
   b. Describe some practical ways that goal setting can taught.

2. Describe three kinds of specific educational activities or learning experiences that you could conduct to strengthen self-regulation skills.

3. For practice, state one educational *strategy* for each of the following potential mediators that facilitate the ability to increase the intake of calcium-rich foods among teenage girls. For each strategy, describe at least one *educational activity or learning experience*.

Potential Mediator of the Ability to Take Action	Educational Strategy	Educational Activities or Learning Experiences
Perceived self-efficacy		
Social support		
Cues to action		

STEP 5B WORKSHEETS Design Theory-Derived Educational Strategies to Address Potential Motivational Mediators of the Ability to Take Action

| WORKSHEET 12-1 | Goal-Setting Worksheet: A Call to Action |

Step 1: Get the facts.

To find out more about your eating and physical activity habits, complete the following questionnaire:

How many days last week did you . . . ?

Eating Habits	Number of Days
Eat five or more servings of fruits and vegetables each day	
Drink or eat calcium-rich foods such as yogurt, milk, or cheese	
(etc.)	
Total	
Physical Activity: Lifestyle	
Climbed stairs that were more than two flights	
Walked to a friend's house, store, or park, or walked around the mall	
Total	
Physical Activity: Aerobic	
Exercise for a total of 30 minutes or more (speed walk, jog, bicycle)	
Dance, do aerobics, or other fun movement for a total of 30 minutes for more	
Total	

Based on my scores for **Eating Habits** and **Physical Activity: Lifestyle** and **Physical Activity: Aerobic**, I recognize that my eating habits are not what I want them to be. In particular, I need to make the following change (e.g., eat more calcium-rich foods):

_____

Step 2: Choose a major goal.

In order to make the change above, my major goal is (e.g., I will eat three or more servings of calcium-rich foods each day):

_____

Step 3: Find out how you rate.

Track what you are doing. In order to make a realistic plan to reach your major goal, you need to know what you are doing now with respect to that goal. Keep track of the following for one day:

- How often you ate the food (e.g., calcium-rich foods)
- How much you ate
- What would be a healthy substitute

Step 4: Make a plan of action and try it out.

   a. Choose action goals to achieve the major goal and make a plan of action. Choose action goals that are based on your own current behaviors and habits that you identified above.
      - *Challenging but realistic.* Choose specific actions that you realize are difficult but that you can clearly reach.
      - *Very specific* (e.g., "I will drink orange juice for breakfast and add a vegetable to lunch").

- *Timely*. Preferably it should be actions that you will take today or this week. For example, "I will eat 2.5 cups of fruits and vegetables *today/this week* by having orange juice at breakfast, eating a fruit for a mid-morning snack, adding a salad to lunch, and eating two vegetables for dinner."

b. Make a contract or pledge. Have a friend or family member sign it.

Step 5: Check-in for change.

At the end of one week, review how you are doing.

During the last week (or other period), I (*place an X on the scale*)

10	9	8	7	6	5	4	3	2	1
Completely fulfilled my contract				Somewhat fulfilled my contract					Did not fulfill my contract

My major difficulties were:

1. _____

2. _____

3. _____

My major successes were:

1. _____

2. _____

3. _____

In the future, I can do the following things to overcome the difficulties I've had:

1. _____

2. _____

3. _____

Step 6: Recommit to your contract or make a new one for a more difficult behavior.

_____

_____

WORKSHEET 12-2   **Lesson Plan Worksheet**

Title of session: _____

Behavioral goal: _____

Educational goal: _____

General educational objectives: Participants will be able to

- _____

- _____

- _____

- _____

Phase of Nutrition Education and Educational Goal	Sequenced Events of Instruction	Potential Mediator of Behavior Change (*Theory-based strategies**)	Specific Educational Objectives for Each Mediator	Review Objectives for Learning Domain and Level**	Practical Educational Activities, Learning Experiences, Messages, or Content
Pre-action phase Educational goal: Enhance awareness, contemplation, and motivation (focus on why-to information)	Gain attention		*At the end of the session or program, learner will be able to:*		
	Present new material (building on prior knowledge)				
	Provide guidance				
Action phase Educational goal: Facilitate the ability to take action (focus on how-to information)	Elicit performance and feedback				
	Enhance retention and transfer				

* Theory-based strategies addressing mediators of behavior change are shown in italics in the third column.

** Review learning objectives for domain and level within domain to ensure that they are set appropriately.

CASE STUDY 12-1   **Step 5b: Sample Lesson Plan Outline for an Action-Phase Lesson**

Title of session: The Whats of Colorful Eating

Behavioral goal: Adolescents will increase their intake of a variety of fruits and vegetables.
Educational goal: Facilitate the ability to take action
General educational or learning objectives: Adolescents will be able to

- Demonstrate increased self-efficacy in eating a variety of fruits and vegetables (F&V) every day
- Demonstrate increased knowledge and skills in incorporating fruits and vegetables into their daily food patterns
- Prepare action plans using goal-setting and decision-making skills to increase their consumption of fruits and vegetables

Phase of Nutrition Education and Educational Goal	Sequenced Events of Instruction	Mediator of Behavior Change (*Theory-based strategies**)	Specific Educational Objectives for Mediator	Review Learning Domain with Level**	Specific Educational Strategies, Learning Experiences, Messages, or Content
Action phase Educational goal: Facilitate the ability to take action (focus on how-to information)	Gain attention				Ice-breaker: In dyads, individuals discuss one time they felt really good about their eating and another when they did not, and why.
	Present new material (building on prior knowledge)	Behavioral capabilities *How-to knowledge: Food- and nutrition-related knowledge and cognitive skills*	State the key reasons for eating a variety of F&V ("a rainbow of colors") Compare the nutrient content of F&V snacks with processed and packaged energy-dense snacks Estimate serving sizes of F&V	Cognitive domain: *comprehension* Cognitive: *evaluation level* Cognitive: *comprehension level*	Review reasons for eating a variety of F&V; key nutrients in them, health benefits, and need for variety of intake. Show commonly eaten packaged energy-dense snacks; worksheet for students to calculate and compare fat and vitamin C content with F&V. Show serving sizes; engaging group activity for estimating serving sizes (e.g., group contest for correct answers)

Phase of Nutrition Education and Educational Goal	Sequenced Events of Instruction	Mediator of Behavior Change (*Theory-based strategies**)	Specific Educational Objectives for Mediator	Review Learning Domain with Level**	Specific Educational Strategies, Learning Experiences, Messages, or Content
	Provide guidance	*How-to knowledge: Food skills*	Describe how these F&V can be used in meals and as snacks; prepare simple recipes using F&V	Cognitive: *application level*	Present tips on how to use F&V in meals and snacks.
				Psychomotor: *Imitation level*	Provide exciting cooking experience if possible; or teens in groups make different snacks from new fruits and/or vegetables: salads, salsa.
			State satisfaction in trying new F&V	Affective: *valuing level*	
					Teens eat foods/snacks they prepared.
		Goal setting *Personal action goals*	State clear personal action goals to eat more F&V	Cognitive domain: *application level* Affective domain: *valuing level*	Teach skills in goal setting and in developing action plans to achieve personal action goals; provide contract forms.
			Make action plan to eat all the colors during a given week	(Same)	Worksheet for action plan to eat all the colors during the following week.
	Elicit performance and feedback	Self-regulation skills *Goal-setting; self-monitoring*	Appreciate the importance of recognizing hunger and satiety cues during a busy day	Affective: *valuing level* Cognitive: *synthesis level*	Activity to teach students to identify hunger, mood, and cues for food intakes.
			Develop plan, incorporating F&V, to satisfy hunger when it occurs and to follow plan during a busy day	Affective: *organization level*	Provide action planning form for adolescents to plan F&V to eat during a busy day; make contract; develop way to monitor progress toward that goal; reward self when goal is achieved.
					If more than one session, provide opportunities for feedback, rewards, and new goals.

* *Theory-based strategies* addressing mediators of behavior change are shown in italics in the third column.

** Review learning domain and level of objectives of within domain, if possible, to ensure appropriate mix of objectives.

"The Whys and Whats of Colorful Eating"

The Whats of Colorful Eating: Action Phase Lesson, Narrative format

Overview of Content (50 to 65 minutes)

1. Introduction and icebreaker
2. Review reasons for eating a variety of fruits and vegetables (F&V)
3. Worksheet comparing fat and vitamin C between various foods
4. Group serving size activity
5. F&V snack and meal tips
6. Prepare and eat a snack
7. Goal-setting and action plans for eating a variety of different color F&V
8. Hunger and mood discussion
9. Goal-setting and action plans for eating F&V when hungry, and wrap-up

Materials

- Worksheet to record fat and vitamin C content in food items
- Energy-dense snack labels (e.g., candy bars, chips, cookies, and chocolates)
- Various F&V (e.g., lettuce, broccoli, different size apples, grapefruit, banana)
- Game prizes (e.g., stickers, temporary tattoos, pencils, small bounce balls)
- Bowls
- Blank paper and pencils
- F&V for snack
- Utensils necessary to prepare the snack (e.g., knives, cutting board)
- Action Plan worksheets

Lesson plan

1. **Introduction and icebreaker.** (8 minutes)

   Greet participants and introduce the lesson, the whats of colorful eating—*what* you can do to make sure you eat a rainbow of different colored F&V every day. Instruct participants to pair up with a partner they do not usually work with.

   The pairs will individually discuss a time they felt really good about their eating and another time when they did not, and why. Allow discussion for a few minutes and then ask pairs to switch speakers. Bring group back together. Ask if anyone wants to share his or her experience during the icebreaker. Remind the group that positive participation is encouraged.

2. **Review reasons for eating a variety of F&V.** (2 minutes) *(Perceived benefits)*

   Begin by reviewing the reasons to eat a colorful range of F&V. Ensure the following are mentioned: provides essential vitamins, minerals, fiber, and other nutrients; can increase energy; helps make hair and skin healthy; builds strong bones and muscles for athletic performance; and decreases risk for certain diseases.

3. **F&V can be wonderful snacks**. Worksheet comparing fat and Vitamin C content between common snack foods. (8 minutes) *(How-to knowledge)*

   Now that the reasons for eating F&V have been discussed, compare the fat and amount of Vitamin C found in some common snack foods with the fat and Vitamin C found in F&V. Provide nutrition labels of a few different energy-dense snack items, such as chips. Ask the participants to fill out the worksheets. Discussion: How did the energy-dense snacks compare with the F&V in terms of fat and Vitamin C? How surprised are you at the difference?

4. **Estimating serving sizes.** Group activity. (10 minutes) *(Food-related skills)*

   Explain that knowing why we should eat F&V is as important as understanding how much we are eating when we have a portion of F&V. Divide into teams and play a game to guess the serving size, with the winner winning a prize.

   Take prepared bowls filled with a variety of different foods that have been previously measured for their portion size. Show each group the first bowl, for example one filled with lettuce, and ask each group to write down how many servings are in the bowl. If the bowl was filled with two cups, each group that guesses two servings will get a point. Continue the game with different F&V and portion sizes. Discussion: What do you think about the size of a serving? How often do you think about the serving size when you eat a food? Do you usually eat larger or smaller portions than the recommended serving size?

5. **F&V snack and meal tips.** (3 minutes) *(Food-related skills)*

   Ask participants to share one of their favorite F&V snacks, or ways to eat F&V at a meal. Ensure tips such as leaving fruit on the kitchen table to grab as a snack or cutting up a lot of veggies to make an easy grab-and-go snack are mentioned. Suggest having a piece of fruit at breakfast, F&V for snack, a salad during lunch or dinner, and discuss ways to cook vegetables.

6. **Snack time!** Prepare and eat a snack. (10–30 minutes) *(Food-related skills)*

   Snack suggestions: veggies and dips, such as hummus, lemon yogurt, peanut butter, fruit salad, green salad with dressing.

   Make sure all the participants are involved in the preparation. Encourage everyone to taste the food. Let the group know that positive feelings about the food should be shared, but negative ones should not. Remember to practice good food safety and clean up when you are done.

7. **Time to take action**. Goal-setting and action plans for eating a variety of different color F&V. (5 minutes) *(Self-regulation skills)*

   Discuss the importance of practicing what has been learned every day. Encourage participants to set personal goals for eating more F&V by filling out the action plan worksheet. For example, set incremental goals of eating three different colors of F&V one week, four different colors the next week, and then all five the following week. Provide time for the students to fill in the worksheets. Ask if any of the students want to share what their goals are and how they hope to achieve them.

8. **Planning ahead.** (4 minutes) *(Self-monitoring skills)*

   A sample lecture is as follows: *The school day can be very busy, beginning from the moment you wake up. Many of you don't have time to eat breakfast before you leave the house, and then you rush from class to class. That means you can get quite hungry. Then you grab whatever is easiest to eat and whatever is at hand, so it is almost impossible to include F&V in your day. This happens to all of us. These ups and downs can affect our mood and our ability to learn. However, we can plan ahead, and carry some foods with us to eat when we get hungry and are not near food—such as bananas or apples.*

   Instruct students to review their action plans and make them more specific: They can now write action plans that focus on bringing F&V with them and eating them when they are hungry. Participants can list three occasions when they anticipate they will be hungry during the day and write down specific actions they will take to incorporate F&V during these times.

9. **Self-monitoring**.

   Discuss ways to monitor progress. Encourage the members of the group to support each other and remember to reward themselves when they meet their goals!

Thank the group and include any reminders about future meetings and events. If the group will continue to meet in the future, plan to follow up with the participants' successes and struggles working towards their goals.

REFERENCES

Achterberg, C. 1998. Factors that influence learner readiness. *Journal of the American Dietetic Association* 88:1426–1428.

Anderson, A.S., D.N. Cox, S. McKellar, J. Reynolds, M.E. Lean, and D.J. Mela. 1998. Take Five, a nutrition education intervention to increase fruit and vegetable intakes: Impact on attitudes towards dietary change. *British Journal of Nutrition* 80(2):133–140.

Armitage, C. 2004. Evidence that implementation intentions reduce dietary fat intake: A randomized trial. *Health Psychology* 23:319–323.

Bandura, A. 1986. *Foundations of thought and action: A social cognitive theory*. Englewood Cliffs, NJ: Prentice-Hall.

———. 1997. *Self-efficacy: The exercise of control*. New York: WH Freeman.

Bargh, J.A., and K. Barndollar. 1996. Automaticity in action: The unconscious as repository of chronic goals and motives. In *The psychology of action: Linking cognition and motivation to behavior*, edited by P.M. Gollwitzer and J.A. Bargh. New York: The Guildford Press.

Barnard, N.D., A. Akhtar, and A. Nicholson. 1995. Factors that facilitate compliance to a low fat intake. *Archives of Family Medicine* 4:153–158.

Bisogni, C.A., M. Jastran, L. Shen, and C.M. Devine. 2005. A biographical study of food choice capacity: Standards, circumstances, and food management skills. *Journal of Nutrition Education and Behavior* 37:284–291.

Bowen, D.J., H. Henry, E. Burrows, G. Anderson, and M.H. Henderson. 1993. Influences of eating patterns on change to a low-fat diet. *Journal of the American Dietetic Association* 93:1309–1311.

Brunner, E., I. White, M. Thorogood, A. Bristow, D. Curle, and M. Marmot. 1997. Can dietary interventions change diet and cardiovascular risk factors? A meta-analysis of randomized controlled trials. *American Journal of Public Health* 87:1415–1422.

Burrows, E.R., H.J. Henry, D.J. Bowen, and M.M. Henderson. 1993. Nutritional applications of a clinical low fat dietary intervention to public health change. *Journal of Nutrition Education* 25:167–175.

Cox, D.N., A.S. Anderson, J. Reynolds, S. McKellar, M.E.J. Lean, and D.J. Mela. 1998. Take Five, a nutrition education intervention to increase fruit and vegetable intakes: Impact on consumer choice and nutrient intakes. *British Journal of Nutrition* 80(2):123–131.

Cullen, K.W., T. Baranowski, and S.P. Smith. 2001. Using goal setting as a strategy for dietary behavior change. *Journal of the American Dietetic Association* 101:562–566.

Gollwitzer, P.M. 1999. Implementation intentions: Strong effects of simple plans. *American Psychologist* 54:493–503.

Grieve, F.G., and M.W. Vander Weg. 2003. Desire to eat high- and low-fat foods following a low-fat dietary intervention. *Journal of Nutrition Education and Behavior* 35:93–99.

Kristal, A.R., A.L. Shatttuck, and H.J. Henry. 1990. Patterns of dietary behavior associated with selecting diets low in fat: Reliability and validity of a behavioral approach to dietary assessment. *Journal of the American Dietetic Association* 90:214–220.

Levy, J., and G. Auld. 2004. Cooking classes outperform cooking demonstrations for college sophomores. *Journal of Nutrition Education and Behavior* 36:197–203.

Locke, E.A., and G.P. Latham. 1990. *A theory of goal setting and performance*. Englewood-Cliffs, NJ: Prentice-Hall.

Mattes, R.D. 1993. Fat preference and adherence to a reduced fat diet. *American Journal of Clinical Nutrition* 57:373–377.

Pelican, S., F. Vanden Heede, B. Holmes, et al. 2005. The power of others to shape our identity: Body image, physical abilities, and body weight. *Family and Consumer Sciences Research Journal* 34:57–80.

Satia, J.A., A.R. Kristal, R.E. Patterson, M.L. Neuhouser, and E. Trudeau. 2002. Psychological factors and dietary habits associated with vegetable consumption. *Nutrition* 18:247–254.

Schwarzer, R., and B. Renner. 2000. Social cognitive predictors of health behavior: Action self-efficacy and coping self-self-efficacy. *Health Psychology* 19:487–495.

Shilts, M.K., M. Horowitz, and M. Townsend. 2004. An innovative approach to goal setting for adolescents: Guided goal setting. *Journal of Nutrition Education and Behavior* 36:155–156.

Thoresen, C.E. 1984. Strategies for health enhancement overview. In *Behavioral health: A handbook of health enhancement and disease prevention*, edited by J.D. Matarazzo, S.M. Weiss, J.A. Herd, and N.E. Miller. New York: John Wiley & Sons.

Urban, N., E. White, G. Anderson, S. Curry, and A. Kristal. 1992. Correlates of maintenance of a low fat diet in the Women's Health Trial. *Preventive Medicine* 21:279–291.

Wiman, R.V., and W.C. Mierhenry. 1969. *Editors, educational media: Theory into practice*. Columbus, OH: Charles Merrill.

Zeitlin, M. and C.S. Formacion. 1981. *Nutrition in developing countries. Study II. Nutrition education*. Cambridge, MA: Oelgeschlager, Gunn, O'Hain.

Step 5c: Design Strategies to Address Potential Environmental Mediators of Action

OVERVIEW   The focus of this chapter is on designing strategies to address potential environmental supports for participants to take action on behaviors or practices targeted by the program. The information in Chapter 6 will be especially helpful to you with this step in the process.

OBJECTIVES   At the end of the chapter, you will be able to

- Describe general types of strategies that can be used to address potential environmental mediators of the actions, behaviors, or practices targeted by the intervention
- Recognize the importance of collaboration with decision makers and policy makers
- Select, from the potential environmental mediators of the goal behaviors identified in Step 1, those that are to be targeted in the intervention to increase environmental support
- Use theory, current nutrition education research, and existing evaluated programs to design specific strategies to address the relevant environmental support objectives written in Step 4

Introduction

We saw in the last chapter that a major way to assist individuals to bridge the intention–behavior gap is to encourage them to set goals, plan ahead, develop routines, and make personal policies regarding the action or behavior. This process increases commitment and reduces effort because individuals do not have to make decisions anew in every situation. A second way to assist individuals to bridge the intention–behavior gap is to promote environmental supports for the targeted behaviors and thus increase the *opportunities* and *support* for participants to take action, which is the subject of this chapter.

INPUTS: COLLECTING ASSESSMENT DATA		DESIGNING THE OUTPUTS			DESIGNING OUTCOMES EVALUATION
STEP 1 ←→ **Analyze needs and behaviors: Specify the behavior or action focus of the program** • Assess needs and identify audience: select need(s) or issue(s) to address • Identify behaviors of concern that contribute to need(s) or issue(s) • Select core behaviors or practices to address	**STEP 2** ←→ **Identify relevant potential mediators of program behaviors** • Identify potential personal psychosocial mediators • Identify potential environmental mediators	**STEP 3** ←→ **Select theory, philosophy, and components** • Select theory and/or create appropriate model • Articulate educational philosophy • Clarify perspectives on content • Determine program components	**STEP 4** ←→ **State educational objectives for potential mediators** • Select relevant mediators to address • State educational objectives for each selected mediator: —Personal psychosocial mediators —Environmental mediators	**STEP 5** ←→ **Design theory-based educational strategies and activities to address potential mediators** • Design strategies and activities for each selected mediator: —Personal psychosocial mediators —Environmental mediators	**STEP 6** **Design evaluation** • Design evaluation of program's impact on behaviors and mediators • Design process evaluation

In the socioecological approach (McLeroy et al., 1988; Green & Kreuter, 1999; Gregson et al., 2001), as we have seen, interventions are directed not only at personal psychosocial mediators of behavior change but also at factors in the interpersonal, organizational, community, and policy spheres of influence to make them more health enhancing.

Some researchers suggest that environments may influence us through conscious and unconscious processes (Kremers, de Bruijn, Visscher et al., 2006). Conscious processes result in impacts on behavior through psychosocial cognitions. For example, the lack of healthful foods in a neighborhood may reduce our sense of self-efficacy, and high prices for such foods may result in a negative attitude toward healthful foods. Changes in these cognitions can become mediators of change in intentions and behavior. Unconscious processes operate through a "mindless" or automatic route in which behaviors are automatically elicited by the environment through environment-behavior links. This route exists because our cognitive capacity is limited and automatic processes free our conscious capacity from having to consider, make choices, and deal with every aspect of our lives all the time. We automatically and unconsciously engage in actions in response to environmental cues. For example, as soon as breakfast time arrives, we may reach for the donut without much thought, or whenever there is an advertising break in a television program, we head for the refrigerator for a snack. Thus, even with motivation, knowledge, and skills, we often still face difficulties in taking action because of automatic responses to the environment and environmental obstacles. Consequently, the environment must be addressed if nutrition education is to be effective.

We can think of nutrition educators as using two primary practical approaches in creating environmental supports for the behaviors that are the focus of their programs: a direct role with the intended audience and an indirect, collaborative role in which they work with others to bring about changes in the environment to support actions by their intended audience. A direct role includes strategies that nutrition educators can use to create informational and social supports for their intended audience. These might include creating support groups for the program participants, working with peer educators, developing a family component to support school- or worksite-based programs, and creating informational environments that reinforce behavior and change social norms.

The indirect role is where nutrition educators work in collaboration with those who provide food and services (such as food assistance programs and public health departments) and those who have decision-making power and authority in other fields that affect the lives of our participants, such as policy makers at city and state levels. These individuals and groups can be considered to be gatekeepers. Our role here is to educate them about the importance of the issues that are the focus of our program, and to develop collaborations with

them in order to bring about changes in the relevant food environments. In many instances, such as with food service directors in schools and workplaces or leaders in the community, the "education" will be collegial and quite informal, through activities such as individual meetings, presentations to potential coalition members, or task force meetings. If these individuals or organizations are convinced of the importance of your program goals, you will then work in collaboration with them to provide professional development to their staffs and other activities as needed. In many instances, the educational route may be both direct and indirect: for example, you may want to develop an educational program for parents so that they can be supportive of their children, who are the primary audience of your intervention, and you may also work with them as partners on school health policy councils.

Figure 13-1 shows a possible community nutrition education logic model and summarizes the kinds of activities we can conduct at various levels of influence on target behaviors. This chapter focuses on activities at the interpersonal, organizational, and community levels as they are relevant to design of a specific program. In designing activities, you select from among the potential environmental educational and support objectives that you wrote in Step 4 for your program goal behaviors those that can be realistically targeted in the intervention, given your available time and resources. Environmental mediators are those influences on the program goal behaviors that reside outside the individual.

Promoting Environmental Supports for Program Behavioral Goals

Designing Theory-Based Strategies to Increase Interpersonal Social Support and Informational Support

Nutrition educators can promote supportive environments by addressing social support, a potential environmental mediator of behavior. Here we seek to strengthen existing social networks to make them more supportive of the food- and nutrition-related behavioral goals of your program, such as increasing breastfeeding rates and duration (e.g., by involving the family in the intervention); to develop new networks that are supportive of participants' desire to take action; and to provide informational support as reinforcements and cues to action. These activities can be considered to be interpersonal-level support strategies.

Making Existing Networks More Supportive of Program Participants Through Educational Activities

You can design activities to encourage members of participants' current social networks to be more supportive. These networks might include parent associations in schools, employee associations at workplaces, or groups that meet regularly in communities and organizations.

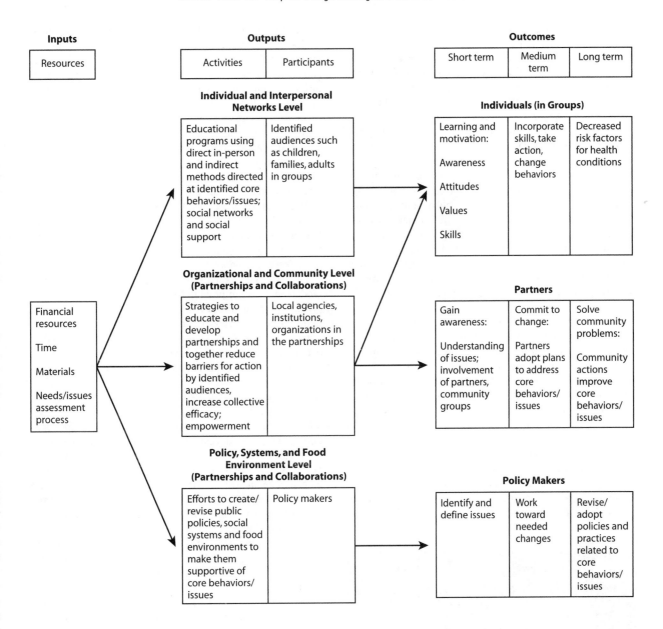

FIGURE 13-1 A nutrition education logic model addressing multiple levels of intervention. Source: Based on Community Nutrition Education (CNE) Logic Model, Version 2: Overview, January 2006. Helen Chipman, National Coordinator, Food Stamp Nutrition Education, CREES/USDA, and Land Grant University System Partnership. http://www.csrees.usda.gov/nea/food/fsne/logic.html. Used with permission.

Parental support. For programs directed at preschool or school-aged children in school settings, parents are external to the students and are hence part of students' external environment. In this case, parents represent a new "audience" for whom general and specific educational objectives will need to be written and educational activities designed in a process similar to that for the students, as described in the last two chapters.

The most general approach is to design sessions with parents so that they can support their children's attempts to eat healthfully. These sessions will be based on your assessments in Steps 1 and 2 (Chapters 7 and 8) and the goals and objectives that you stated in Step 4 (Chapter 10). Our ongoing case study has been with middle school youth, addressing the goal of increasing their intake of fruits and vegetables. A potential program for parents is shown in the case study section at the end of this chapter.

In most communities, parents are very busy, and getting parents to attend nutrition education sessions may not be feasible. You will need to use alternate channels and design alternate educational activities that will fit into their busy schedules. Carefully determine the educational objectives of these alternate channels. In general, they are similar to the ones listed earlier: to stimulate awareness and interest, provide food- and nutrition-related knowledge and skills, and elicit parental support for your program, for example, by increasing the accessibility of the foods targeted by your program.

For programs in elementary schools, it is most effective to develop activities that children can do at home that require parental participation. Families can accumulate points for these activities, for which they can receive incentives and reinforcements. For programs with teens, colorful brochures featuring the targeted foods can be distributed to parents with school mailings; special program newsletters with activities, recipes, discount coupons, and information on the benefits of the targeted behaviors can be sent; and calendars with monthly eating tips can be distributed. You can provide taste testings, media displays, and activities at parent–teacher organization meetings and hand out colorful brochures. Again, the educational objectives of these materials should be clear.

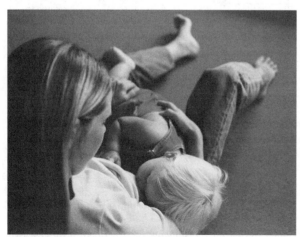
Breastfeeding mothers need peer and social support.

Family support for adults. In workplaces and outpatient clinics, it may be possible to provide educational activities for families to help them create a home environment that is supportive of participants' attempts to engage in needed or desired actions, such as eating more fruits and vegetables or diets that are lower in saturated fat. Activities that have been found to be effective are written learn-at-home programs distributed through participants at the workplace, family newsletters, and family activities related to program goals that can be incorporated into workplace family holiday parties or picnics. For each of these activities, goals and objectives need to be developed so that the purposes of the activity are clear.

Peer educators as social support. Peer educators have been used in a variety of settings, such as in schools, with low-income families through the Expanded Food and Nutrition Education Program (EFNEP), with older adults, and for breastfeeding promotion, as described in Chapter 6. The role of peer educators is not only to teach sessions and serve as models, but also to provide social support. You will need to provide professional development wherein you help them understand the purposes and content of the program. They are a new audience to educate, and hence you will need to determine a set of goals and objectives for their training and develop appropriate theory-based educational strategies.

Developing New Social Networks That Are Supportive of Change

Social support is incorporated into many health interventions through the development of new social groups, such as weight control groups at work, HIV support groups at a health center, cooking classes, or behavioral change sessions with participants in a program. Programs can also initiate new social networks in which individuals participating in the intervention can help each other (such as forming walking groups or buddy systems).

Support groups. Nutrition programs frequently create social support by providing regular structured occasions for participants to meet and support each other. Such structured social support was identified in a review of nutrition education as one of the key elements that contributed to effectiveness (Ammerman et al., 2002). Weight loss interventions routinely incorporate social support groups (e.g., Weight Watchers). Interventions in schools, workplaces, and communities have also incorporated social support groups. Increasing social support through social networks means increasing one or more of the following kinds of support:

- *Emotional support:* Expressions of empathy, caring, love, and trust
- *Informational support:* Advice and suggestions
- *Appraisal support:* Information that is useful for self-evaluation
- *Instrumental support:* Tangible support and resources

A social support group session must be carefully designed and facilitated: it is not just a matter of getting a group together and talking. Write educational objectives for the sessions and design activities for each objective. In other words, develop an educational plan. However, you will implement it through facilitated dialogue and mutual support. The structure or agenda usually involves the following: individuals share how they did during the previous week or time interval in terms of successes and challenges (focus on successes); group members assist each other from their own wealth of experience; the nutrition educator provides content where necessary and designs learning tasks to promote active engagement and maintain support; worksheets, handouts, food tasting, or cooking are provided when feasible; and time is set aside for the development of action plans or goal setting for the next session. Design a manual for the group leader with all this information if this is not you and also a manual for participants. For participants, hand out session packets each time as you go along.

During the session, your role is to be a facilitator to guide the discussion. The participants are experts on their lives, even though you may be an expert on food and nutrition information. (Even here, participants can be very knowledgeable.) They come with prior experience and expertise. Invite them to share with each other and create dialogue. Build on the strengths of the group members and not their deficits.

Mutual support. You can also foster social support by encouraging program participants to help each other through such strategies as forming buddy systems or walking clubs, creating an e-mail listserve to share ideas, experiences, and resources, or going out to eat together and practicing learned behavioral skills.

Creating Informational Supports for Program Behavioral Goals

To support the behavioral goals of the program, you can place information in public forums to serve as environmental supports by being cues to action. For example, you can institute point-of-choice labeling of targeted foods such as fruits and vegetables or lower-fat foods in grocery stores or workplaces, distribute key chains that have program messages on them, hang posters on walls, and place flyers or brochures on tables in settings where program participants eat, such as cafeterias.

Information in public spaces can help establish social and community norms that are supportive of the behavioral goals of the program. For example, posters about breastfeeding in pediatricians' offices, or posters on eating fruits and vegetables in restaurants, company cafeterias, health centers, and community centers, can encourage people to see these behaviors as the social norm. Billboards in the community can also help to establish norms and serve as cues to action. Promotions through other media, such as radio and maga-

zines, can also be supportive of the behavior change that is targeted by the intervention.

Designing Supportive Policy, Systems, and Food Environment Change Activities Through Collaborations and Partnerships

It is increasingly clear that many of the food- and nutrition-related issues of key concern cannot be addressed by nutrition educators working alone. We must work in collaboration with others to address issues such as overweight prevention, decreasing chronic disease risk, decreasing food insecurity, increasing intakes of fruits and vegetables, and increasing consumption of food from local farmers, because changes in behavior require organizational- and community-level support as well as interpersonal support and individual action. In the context of program design, we need to collaborate with providers of foods and services and others who have policy-making power and authority so as to increase the availability and accessibility of foods at the institutional/organizational and community levels that will support the program's behavioral goals. Thus, changes in foods offered at nutrition education intervention sites, such as schools, workplaces, community centers, soup kitchens, food banks, or supermarkets, require that we work with partners to modify policy, systems, and the food environment.

To bring about changes at such sites may require use of both motivational- and action-phase educational activities, this time directed at new audiences such as food service providers, administrators, or managers at an institution or policy makers in organizations and communities. Professional development workshops and incentives will be important here. Changes in the food offered may require changes in organizational policy and union rules so that food service staff can make the changes. This will require negotiations and advocacy. Making such food changes possible may also require changes in physical facilities at sites such as schools or other locations, so that foods can actually be cooked or prepared on site. These changes will require resources and collective action. Families and local organizations, such as parent–teachers associations, community groups, city councils, and health-related voluntary organizations (e.g., heart associations or cancer societies) may also become new audiences for your program in order to support the behavioral goals for your primary audience.

Collaboration, Partnership, and Collective Efficacy

Collaboration has been described as "a fluid process through which a group of diverse, autonomous actors (organizations or individuals) undertakes a joint initiative, addresses shared concerns, or otherwise achieves common goals. It is characterized by mutual benefit, interdependence, reciprocity, concerted action, and joint production" (Rosenthal, 1998). In degree of involvement, collaboration ranges from loose networks through cooperation and coordination of effort to full collaboration. Collaboration has long been practiced in the field of nutrition. For example, nutrition educators have long collaborated with school food service personnel and with food assistance programs such as the Food Stamps Program, the Women, Infants and Children (WIC) program, and congregate meals programs for older adults to provide nutrition education in these contexts. Nutrition educators can also collaborate with public health departments in health promotion programs, with farmers in farm-to-school programs, or with community groups in gardening projects in schools and communities.

Collaborations include a range of structural relationships, and different terms are often used to describe these (Rosenthal, 1998; Gregson et al., 2001). The exact names are not important because they are often used interchangeably. One arrangement is the *strategic partnership,* formed for a single purpose or for a multifaceted venture. Partnerships are formed for reasons of organizational self-interest and pragmatism and can be for the long or short term. Partners have distinct resources and expertise that, if pooled, can expand possibilities for everyone: the whole becomes greater than the sum of its parts. Partners share responsibility and ownership of the effort or product. Another arrangement might be *coalitions* or *consortia,* in which organizations, institutions, and sectors unite to develop a comprehensive approach. The focus is on social change, empowerment, and community building, and the activities include planning, community organizing, advocacy, and program development.

Service integration collaborations are another arrangement. In this case, the integration is created at the policy or administrative level so that systems of service can be integrated for a specific area or population. *Problem-solving collaborations* are sometimes created to solve a complex problem where differing parties have different views on an issue. An example is a task force formed to explore a problem issue and make recommendations (Rosenthal, 1998). Some collaborations are

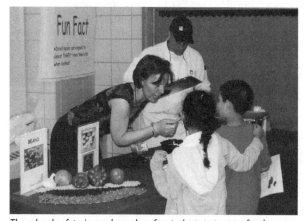

The school cafeteria can be a place for students to try new foods.

quite loose, others have legal arrangements with each other, and still others may have a common governing body.

We will use the general term *collaboration* or *partnership* to describe the variety of arrangements in which nutrition education is involved. The U.S. Department of Agriculture's Team Nutrition program (www.fns.usda.gov/tn/Healthy/index.htm) is an example of many groups in a given community working in collaboration to bring nutrition education and healthful foods to specific schools. The collaborative arrangements have varying degrees of formality. The many activities that are part of the program are described on the Web.

Collaborations can lead to a sense of collective efficacy. The group makes plans to address specific issues or achieve specific objectives (somewhat like goal setting for individuals). When the group is successful at bringing about change on one issue, the members feel self-efficacious and ready to take on other issues.

Although collaborations can mobilize material resources and peoples' knowledge, skills, and enthusiasms to achieve desired goals in a way that is not possible for small groups alone, there are costs as well. Collaborative efforts are complex, requiring time and effort. Successful collaboration requires the following: a shared and agreed-upon vision and mission, reached by consensus through open dialogue, negotiation, and problem solving; a unique purpose that is meaningful to members; clear tasks that are specific and empowering; a sense of productivity and efficiency; a skilled convener who can facilitate team building and conflict resolution; broad-based involvement in decision making; open, frequent communication; benefits that accrue to members for participation; relationships that are based on trust, openness, and respect; power sharing; and adequate resources (Rosenthal, 1998).

It is likely that your program will be enhanced by having a collaboration with some other group. Indeed, it may be that an environmental support component to your program is made possible only by such partnership. For example, the environmental change objectives of your nutrition education curriculum in a school might require that you work in partnership with school food service personnel, school administrators, school health councils, and perhaps also school–parent associations. Similarly, changes in foods in many other settings, such as workplaces, might require your first educating, and then entering into collaborations with, food vendors in those settings. In Chapter 10 you wrote several environmental support objectives for your program. Here we describe examples of how they can be translated into action.

Policy and Food Environment Activities in Schools

Students in schools where à la carte foods and snack and beverage vending machines are available eat fewer fruits and vegetables at lunch (Cullen et al., 2000, 2004) and fewer fruits and vegetables and more saturated fat during the entire day

(Kubik et al., 2003). Hence, changing the food environment means making changes in a variety of venues: school meals offerings, vending machines, à la carte offerings, food items in school stores, and foods used for fundraising programs and as rewards by teachers. These changes are all difficult to achieve, as we discussed in Chapter 6. You will need different partners to bring about changes in these different venues because different people have decision-making power and authority over each venue, such as principals, food service personnel, teachers unions, and parent associations.

Legislation now requires every local district that participates in the federal school meals program to develop and implement a wellness policy. Such a policy must

- Include nutrition guidelines for all foods available on the school campus during the school day
- Include goals for nutrition education, physical activity, and other school-based activities designed to promote student wellness
- Establish a plan for measuring the implementation of the policy
- Involve parents, students, and representatives of the school food authority, school board, administrators, and public in development of the policy

Although school *districts* have developed such policies, some plans are incomplete or may not been implemented fully in each *school*. Policies also need to be evaluated and updated from time to time. Nutrition educators can serve as a valuable resource.

Schools and school districts can also call on a variety of other resources to help them in the process. The Centers for Disease Control and Prevention's *Guidelines for School Health Programs to Promote Lifelong Healthy Eating* (CDC, 1996) has identified various strategies to improve the school food environment (in addition to guidelines for school curricula). The U.S. Department of Agriculture's Team Nutrition program has created *Changing the Scene: Improving the School Nutrition Environment* (USDA, 2000), which provides a comprehensive, step-by-step how-to guide. The National Association of State Boards of Education has also developed a policy document, *Fit, Healthy and Ready to Learn* (Bogden, 2000). Many food- and nutrition-related professional organizations also provide suggestions for developing such policies, such as the USDA (www.fns.usda.gov/tn/Healthy/wellness-policy_resources.html), the American Dietetic Association (www.eatright.org), and a coalition of food and nutrition organizations known as the National Alliance for Nutrition and Activity (www.schoolwellnesspolicies.org). The School Nutrition Association provides outgoing reports about local wellness policies (www.schoolnutrition.org).

Depending on the scope and duration of your school intervention and the resources you have, you may incorporate the following strategies in assisting schools in implementing, revising, or updating the wellness policy to support healthy eating.

Work with the school team and foster buy-in by others: School health councils or school nutrition advisory councils. Legislation for the wellness policy requires that many stakeholders be involved. The CDC recommends that school nutrition policy "incorporate input from all relevant constituents of the school community: students, teachers, coaches, staff, administrators, food service personnel, nurses, counselors, public health professionals, and parents" (CDC, 1996). This usually means working with an existing group that is often known by various names, such as a school nutrition advisory council, school health policy council, or coordinated school health team. The existence of school health councils increases the likelihood of having health policies in schools (Brener & Kann, 2004). However, such formal councils may not be present or functioning in all schools (Wechsler et al., 2001).

As a nutrition educator, you can contribute to the process by providing information to school administrators about the importance and benefits of conducting an assessment to describe the food environment of the school. Although school administrators are highly concerned about academic achievement issues, they are also interested in health. You may also work with teacher and parent associations to familiarize them with the purpose of such a council and member responsibilities. Potential student members can be solicited from the recommendations of the principal and teachers. Developing and maintaining such a council can be a challenge (Kubik, Lytle, & Story, 2001). The team should consist of those who are willing to make a commitment to participate actively and to stay involved.

Conduct a school food environment assessment. An accurate description of current food-related practices and policies provides a framework for discussion and decision making, permits the school that you are working in to devise an appropriate action plan to implement its wellness policy, and provides a means by which to monitor progress. Several widely used assessment tools are available to help with the process, such as the School Health Index (SHI) from the CDC (2004a, 2004b), the Changing the Scene assessment tools from the USDA's Team Nutrition program (USDA, 2000), and the Healthy Schools Action Tool (HSAT) from the Michigan Department of Community Health (2005), which is based on the CDC and the Team Nutrition instruments. (You can use one of these tools as part of your assessments in Step 1.) These instruments are quite general, seeking information on broad policies such as the degree of commitment to nutrition and physical activity, quality meals, and a pleasant eating experience. You may want to be more specific. If the school has not already fully implemented its current wellness policy, you might use the following questions from the TEENS intervention (Kubik, Lytle, & Story, 2001):

- Does the school have a written food policy? Is nutrition addressed in it?
- Does the school have an ongoing nutrition or health advisory council?
- Does the school have a soft drink policy?
- Do teachers/faculty use food as a reward or incentive?
- Does the school use food for fundraising?
- Does the school permit food promotion and advertising?
- If the school already has a good nutrition wellness policy, is it being implemented? How is the school monitoring implementation?

There are different ways to collect the necessary data. It is considered best that the school nutrition advisory council, school health policy council, or health action team conduct this assessment. You may help the group develop an assessment tool (or monitoring tool if a policy is already in place) and administer it. Or you may interview key informants, such as the school principal or assistant principal, using a list of questions such as the above. In addition to interviews, you will want to make direct observations of the foods and beverages available through various venues, such as school meals, vending machines, school stores, or competitive foods in the cafeteria (Kubik, Lytle, & Story, 2001). This means that you will need to devise some kind of coding scheme that is fairly simple and directed only at the behaviors of interest to your program. For example, the TEENS intervention, which focused on increasing intake of fruits and vegetables and decreasing fat consumption, came up with a list of food items to promote, foods to neither promote or limit, and foods to limit (Kubik, Lytle, & Story, 2001) and characterized foods in various venues according to this scheme.

Develop an action plan. Whether implementing a policy or revising it, the group's task is now to analyze the school's food and nutrition assessment data that have been collected, come up with a shared vision, identify areas needing improvement, and develop action plans. Such actions might include activities to ensure that more healthful foods are available or to increase the proportion of more healthful to less healthful foods, recommending pricing practices, developing policies regarding competitive foods and beverage contracts, or developing alternative ways for teachers to reward students in class (Kubik, Lytle, & Story 2001; Kramer-Atwood et al., 2002). Your role as the nutrition educator is to provide technical assistance in the form of relevant research data and to help the group think through issues and make choices. Here the philosophy of your nutrition education program, articulated in Step 3, will be important. For example, will the school implement nutrition standards for competitive foods and beverages so that less healthful items will not be available, or will alternative items be stocked, leaving the choice to students (Kubik, Lytle, & Story, 2005)?

Put the plan into action. The team may come up with very creative, manageable but meaningful activities that are supportive of your program's behavioral goals. For example, in the TEENS study, the nutrition advisory council set the policy that 50% of items offered in the school store should come from the "foods to promote" list; that instead of using high-fat, high-sugar foods as rewards for students, teachers would use "healthy food" coupons that students could redeem in the school cafeteria for baked chips, fruit, or low-fat desserts; and that they would produce and display posters advertising healthy choices (Kubik, Lytle, & Story, 2001). Your role is to provide technical assistance and advice.

It should be noted that implementing food policies is fraught with barriers. Often opponents object to the policies for a variety of reasons and put enormous pressures on schools not to change, particularly when revenues are at stake. For policies to be actually implemented requires political will on the part of school administrators and parental support. In addition, it has been found that even though extra funding can initially enable schools to provide quality lunches, success cannot be sustained without changes in students' preferences for unhealthful foods and parental and community involvement in fostering healthy eating behavior. Coordination and communication among food service staff, teachers, and health educators have been found to be essential, as well as school-wide nutrition education (Cho & Nadow, 2004), confirming that both individual-level and environmental-level strategies are needed so that individuals have both the willingness as well as opportunity to take action.

Changes in school meals. All schools are interested in offering quality meals that children will eat and a pleasant atmosphere in which to eat them. If you would like the school meals to be more supportive of your nutrition education program's behavioral goals, plan to meet with the school food service manager to discuss how you might collaborate. For example, if your program goal is to increase children's consumption of fruits and vegetables (or whole grains, or low-fat, high-calcium foods), you can discuss how the school meals program can be supportive, given the constraints of budget and staff. Clarify what your role will be. Perhaps the school food service staff are already providing the foods you are targeting but need help with promotion. Maybe they could use some technical assistance with menu modification or with staff development. View the process as a collaboration of persons who have different but complementary knowledge and skills that are needed to enhance healthful eating.

Team Nutrition provides an example of collaborations between schools, parents, nutrition educators, members of the community, policy makers, and other stakeholders in improving the eating patterns of youth in schools. Some examples of successes are discussed in Nutrition Education in Action 13-1.

Use of local foods in schools: Farm-to-school programs. Many schools are introducing salad bars using fresh produce

NUTRITION EDUCATION IN ACTION 13-1

Making It Happen: School Nutrition Success Stories

As we have seen before, the Team Nutrition program of the U.S. Department of Agriculture (USDA) is an example of nutrition education that is directed at both the individual and environmental levels. Team Nutrition focuses attention on the important role that nutritious school meals, nutrition education, and a health-promoting school environment all play in helping students learn to enjoy healthful eating and physical activity. In particular, it encourages collaboration among many partners, such as school food service personnel, teachers, school administrators, parents, and community organizations, to achieve these student outcomes. Such collaborations can help to establish wellness policies for schools.

Examples of what some school districts have done are described in a set of "success stories" collected by the Centers for Disease Control and Prevention (CDC) and Team Nutrition. These successful schools conducted the following policy and system change activities:

- *Made more healthful foods available* through various venues in the school, such as school meals, à la carte offerings, and vending machines, based on the fact that increasing the variety of nutritious choices makes it more likely that students will choose nutrient-dense foods and that they will see such foods as the norm.
- *Established nutrition standards* to help schools select the foods to offer outside the national school meals program. Nutrition standards are the criteria that determine which foods and beverages can and cannot be offered on a school campus. These standards resulted in most of the schools adding such healthful items as water, low-fat or nonfat milk, 100% juice, air-popped popcorn, fresh fruit, salads or salad bars, sandwiches, baked chips, and whole-grain breads.
- *Influenced food and beverage contracts* that gave vendors selling rights for up-front cash and noncash benefits to a school or district. Schools canceled them, did not renew them, or negotiated contracts that promoted more healthful eating.
- *Adopted marketing techniques to promote healthful choices.* Schools identified and offered healthful food products that were appealing and met the nutrition standards, placed these healthful products in sites that were easily accessible to students, promoted them so that students would be motivated to try the foods, and set the price at a level that encouraged students to purchase them.
- *Limited students' access to foods that were competitive to the national school meals program.* Most schools removed such less healthful items as sweetened beverages, candy, deep-fried foods, and snack cakes.

Source: Food and Nutrition Service, U.S. Department of Agriculture; Centers for Disease Control and Prevention, U.S. Department of Health and Human Services; and U.S. Department of Education. 2005, January. *Making it happen! School nutrition success stories* (FNS-374). Alexandria, VA: Authors.

---

from local farmers' markets or local farms in farm-to-schools programs. Schools can buy many other farm-fresh foods, such as eggs, meat and beans, or honey. These programs are initiated locally. You may want to consider promoting these options if they are relevant to your program (French & Wechsler, 2004). Farm-to-school programs usually also provide experiential learning opportunities through having farmers visit classrooms, sponsoring educational events at farmers' markets, and making field visits to farms. Children learn about local food and agriculture and are energized to try new foods when they see where their food comes from. Schools can fulfill their mission to provide wholesome, nutritious foods that children want to eat, and farmers have access to a new market. Information on the many activities in different states can be found at the National Farm to School Program website (www.farmtoschool.org) and in Nutrition Education in Action 13-2.

School gardens. Schools are increasingly seeing the relevance and importance of having school gardens in which to grow vegetables. Children learn where food comes from and become more interested in nutrition. You may need to develop coalitions with relevant knowledgeable individuals or groups in order to initiate and maintain such gardens if you do not have the expertise to do so within your own team but deem it an important supportive activity for your program. See www.edibleschoolyard.org for more information. Nutrition Education in Action 13-3 describes an example of the use of school gardens to make changes in schools and in communities.

Policy and Food Environment Activities in Workplaces
Many of the strategies described previously also apply to environmental support activities in workplaces. However, they are usually more difficult to implement because food

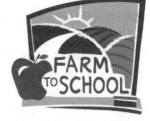

NUTRITION EDUCATION IN ACTION 13-2

Farm-to-School Programs Connect Schools with Local Farms

Farm-to-school programs are programs in which schools buy and feature farm-fresh foods such as fruits and vegetables, eggs, honey, meat, and beans in their menus; provide students experiential learning opportunities through class visits to farms, gardening, and recycling programs; and incorporate nutrition education into their activities. Farm-fresh salad bars are often offered as part of the National School Lunch Program, and local foods are often featured in the cafeteria or in fundraising events. Thus, farmers and schools develop partnerships so that farmers have access to the school market and at the same time participate in programs designed to educate children about local farms and agriculture.

Legislation titled "Access to Local Food and School Gardens" as part of the Child Nutrition and WIC Reauthorization Act of 2004 permits schools to compete for grant funds to help school food service personnel develop procurement relationships with local farmers and equip their kitchen facilities to handle local foods. The program also supports agriculture-based nutrition education, such as school gardens, to teach students where their food comes from. There are over 400 farm-to-cafeteria programs in 23 states that not only feed children fresh, local food, but get them excited about it.

Source: National Farm to School on the Web. http://www.farmtoschool.org.

---

service operations are generally managed by external for-profit companies, which do not necessarily share the interest of the workplace in improved employee health.

If your program will be conducted in a workplace, you can include the following strategies in your plan.

- *Build collaboration and foster buy-in.* Make presentations, meet with, and educate key food service decision makers about the importance of your program's goals. You may need to work with a regional manager of the food service company as well as the site manager.
- *Use a phased approach: start with simple changes first.* With the manager, identify a short list of items currently served that meet your criteria for individual foods that support your program's behavioral goals (e.g., fruits and vegetables). Indicate these with signs and your logo. If these are well received, then using a computer analysis of nutrient content, identify entrées, soups, and other meal items that satisfy your criteria. When it is clear that these changes do not have a negative financial impact, the food service mangers may be ready to make recipe modifications. Here you can provide technical assistance for making changes.
- *Promote employee advisory committees.* Active participation of workplace employees is vital. Depending on the scope of your program, you may help to form a nutrition advisory committee made up of employees as well as management that will provide ongoing feedback and suggestions to food service personnel. Committee members can take over your functions for long-term institutionalization of food service changes.

Policy and Food Environment Activities in the Community

The extent to which you will try to increase environmental supports at the community level for the behavioral targets of your intervention will depend on the scope of your intervention and the resources available. Activities will most likely require collaboration with several to many other groups. Where existing organizations and social structures are in place, your role may first be an educational one, to help them see the importance of the behavioral goal of your program. Your role may then be a partner, providing support and technical assistance as needed. Where community social structures are weak, your role may be to facilitate collective efficacy to accomplish mutually desired goals.

Active participation of community members in all activities is crucial—from planning to implementing to evaluating. Consequently, as described for institutional activities in schools and workplaces, your first activity is to locate decision makers in other organizations—whether these are grocery stores or community gardens—discuss your program with them, and seek strong collaborations. This collaborative group can decide on strategies. The following strategies can be considered, to the degree they are relevant for your program.

- *Provide point-of-purchase information.* You can collaborate with grocery stores relevant to your program and provide posters, brochures, and shelf labels for foods targeted by your intervention (Glanz & Yaroch, 2004). Shelf labels can enhance awareness of the foods and increase use of the information. The strategy of provid-

NUTRITION EDUCATION IN ACTION **13-3**

Food $ense CHANGE: Cultivating Health and Nutrition Through Garden Education

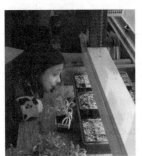

Learning about where food comes from: indoor gardening

Food $ense CHANGE improves the nutrition of limited income children and their families by teaching a nutrition curriculum enhanced by gardening, cooking, and other hands-on activities. In addition to teaching classroom lessons, primarily in elementary schools, CHANGE instructors act as a support system and resource for teachers as they incorporate nutrition education into their daily classroom work. CHANGE instructors also participate in school family nights and other family or adult outreach activities.

CHANGE teaches students how to make good food choices, how to grow food, and how to prepare healthy snacks and meals. Through outdoor garden education, students plant seeds, measure their growth, and harvest fruits and vegetables to eat. They learn where their food comes from and make the connection between what they eat, their health, and the environment.

The goals of CHANGE are:

- Teacher nutrition through gardening and cooking to limited-income youth and their families, resulting in the consumption of more fruits and vegetables and higher quality, nutrient-dense foods.
- Train school teachers to integrate nutrition education into their existing curricula resulting in the delivery of consistent messages about healthy eating.
- Encourage behavior changes in Food $ense schools to create an environment of healthy eating.

The Food $ense CHANGE program in schools includes the following:

- The CHANGE curriculum that teaches nutrition experientially through gardening and cooking.
- The CHANGE curriculum of 40 lessons, taught in four 10-lesson units. There are two units for primary (1–3) grades and two units for intermediate (4–5) grades.
- Enhancement of reading and comprehension skills, teamwork, math skills, science concepts, and creativity while students grow food plants in their classrooms and outdoor gardens and harvest produce for cooking and eating in class.
- Inquiry-based science and nutrition activities.
- Guidance and support for creating school gardens. Each garden meets the needs and environment of each school. Whether gardens are dug in the ground, or grown in large containers, children learn about nutrition by experiencing the excitement of growing, harvesting, and cooking their own food.
- Field trips to local farms, where children have the opportunity to see where their food is grown, talk to the farmers, and learn valuable lessons about nutrition, fresh fruits and vegetables, and caring for the environment.

Results showed that about 75 to 85% of youth reported improved eating practices such as eating breakfasts that includes three food groups and using food labels.

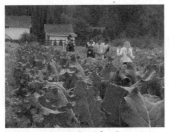

Learning about where food comes from: visiting a farm

Healthy Food in Motion

After learning about food advertising in a CHANGE class, students asked why they don't see any ads for fruits and vegetables. As a result, Food $ense CHANGE decided to place fruits and vegetable advertisements drawn by children in metro buses. Children in 40 elementary school classrooms participated in a contest to draw the advertisements. The 120 colorful expressions of health foods were chosen for the signs, which were accompanied by appropriate messages in multiple languages to reach all bus riders.

Adult Outreach

CHANGE educators use every opportunity to share information about healthy eating directly with parents. Parent newsletters, family nights, and other school and community events involving adults, allow parents to meet and discuss the positive changes that nutrition education can make in the household. Educators provide parents with information to support the behavior changes being attempted by their children and to improve the household's eating habits.

Source: Washington State University King County Extension 2006. Food $ense CHANGE. Funded by Food Stamp Nutrition Education Program. Logo used with permission. http://king.wsu.edu/nutrition/change.htm.

ing point-of-purchase information can also be used in restaurants and other places where food is served.

- *Provide coupons at stores and farmers' markets.* Your program may issue coupons for program participants to use in selected stores that are redeemable for foods relevant to your intervention, such as low-fat milk. Your program would need to pay for these. Government farmers' market coupon programs for various low-income populations have increased shoppers' attendance at farmers' markets and can be used as an environmental support to your program.

- *Work with community food assistance organizations.* Many community organizations are involved in providing food assistance to communities, such as food recovery or food gleaning programs, food banks, and community kitchens or soup kitchens. You may be able to link activities within your educational program to such programs in your community. If your nutrition education is being provided through these organizations, then the foods made available in these settings should be supportive of your program's behavioral goals. You may wish to develop policies as to which kinds of foods the organization is willing to accept for redistribution to those in need to ensure that they are wholesome and nutritious. America's Second Harvest (www.secondharvest.org) is the nation's food bank network of more than 200 regional member food banks and food rescue organizations.

- *Community-supported agriculture (CSA).* You may be able to link individuals in your educational program to community-supported agriculture. CSA helps to support family farms that are struggling to stay in business, while providing city people, particularly those in low-income neighborhoods, with access to high-quality, locally grown, affordable produce. During the winter and spring, the CSA farmer sells shares in his or

her farm's upcoming harvest to individuals, families, or institutions. The share price goes toward the cost of growing and distributing a season's worth of produce and paying the farmer a living wage. Each week, from June through November, the CSA farmer delivers the week's share to a central neighborhood distribution site—usually a community center or house of worship. Members collect their food at their neighborhood sites. Organizations in your community may be able to link your program participants with local CSA farmers.

Multiple-Level Community Nutrition Education

The local- and state-level nutrition education networks and collaborations found in most states, and described in Chapter 6, provide an example of activities at many levels to improve the diets of youth and adults. Many networks are partnerships among a variety of groups, usually with funding from the USDA Food Stamp Program (www.nal.usda.gov/foodstamp) and from state and other sources. These networks provide nutrition education to food stamp recipients and eligible individuals in a variety of settings. The primary partners, with contractual arrangements, are the state Food Stamp agencies and some other agencies such as the state Cooperative Extension Service or department of health, whose task is to organize the networks in their state. The networks are usually relatively informal collaborations. The average network has several dozen public- and private-sector member organizations as partners, such as the Cooperative Extension Service, WIC, welfare agencies, university nutrition or medical departments, professional and voluntary associations (such as the American Cancer Society and the American Diabetes Association), food banks and other food-related organizations, and for-profit organizations (such as supermarkets).

An example of the kinds of activities conducted by state nutrition education networks is provided in Nutrition Education in Action 13-4. The California Nutrition Network for Healthy, Active Families uses a broad-based approach to reach its behavioral objectives, conducting activities at all levels of intervention, from individual- to community-level projects and to environmental and policy change. It funds many local community-based projects throughout the state. Each community-based project is asked to address several levels of prevention at the same time.

Case Study

Our ongoing case study has been with middle school youth, addressing the goal of increasing their intake of fruits and vegetables. A potential program for parents and a program to address the school environment are shown in this chapter. In the parent component we educate parents to be more supportive of the behaviors targeted by the program. We do so by designing theory-based strategies to address potential

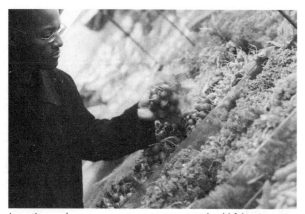

Incentives such as coupons can encourage more healthful eating.

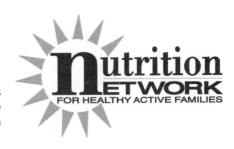

NUTRITION EDUCATION IN ACTION 13-4

California Nutrition Network for Healthy, Active Families

Mission Statement

The mission of the California Nutrition Network for Healthy, Active Families is to create innovative partnerships so that low-income Californians are enabled to adopt healthy eating and physical activity patterns as part of a healthy lifestyle.

Behavioral Objectives

The network seeks to increase Californians' consumption of fruits and vegetables to five or more daily servings, increase daily physical activity to at least 30 minutes for adults and 60 minutes for children, and achieve full participation in federal food assistance programs.

About the Nutrition Network

According to its website, the California Nutrition Network assists local public entities to enhance their nutrition education programs and promotion of physical activity through an ongoing Local Incentive Award (LIA) program. This local assistance program supports nutrition education and physical activity promotion that targets food stamp–eligible and similar low-income consumers throughout the state. These local programs use strategies that will increase the likelihood of low-income consumers making healthy food choices (specifically, eating at least five servings of fruits and vegetables daily) and becoming more physically active and create access to nutrition assistance programs by doing the following:

- Encouraging changes in policy, systems, and the environment. For example, changes in a worksite where low-income consumers work could include changes in cafeterias and vending machine food choices or promoting walking breaks.
- Working for changes in the community such as bringing farmers' markets or even a supermarket to an economically depressed neighborhood, establishing a community garden, and providing safe parks and places to exercise.
- Making changes in organizations and institutions, such as improving school lunch menus and promoting school gardens.
- Facilitating changes at the interpersonal level, which includes promoting healthy lifestyles at places of worship, worksite programs, and grocery store tours.
- Influencing individual lifestyle choices by providing skill-building opportunities in nutrition/cooking classes and food demonstrations and providing community resource information regarding food assistance programs.

Program Description

The network uses a broad-based social marketing approach to meet its behavioral objectives. This includes the following components.

- *Partnership and research development.* The network funds over 100 projects, including LIAs, special projects, California Project LEAN (Leaders Encouraging Activity and Nutrition) regions, 5 A Day–Power Play! regions, and network partners that serve as "ambassadors" in delivering the 5 A Day and physical activity messages.
- *Research and evaluation.* The network conducts statewide surveys focusing exclusively on healthy eating and physical activity. The surveys are used to help set state and local priorities and to raise public awareness. Focus groups, pilot tests, and economic studies are also conducted.
- *Media and retail.* The network and the 5 A Day campaign have conducted media and public relations activities, including the purchase of television and radio airtime; placement of outdoor ads, such as mobile billboards and bus wraps; and regional media tours conducted by trained state and local spokespeople, supported by public relations activities at the community level. The retail merchandising components of the program have included customized point-of-sale materials, ad slicks for print advertisements, in-store recipe booklets and brochures, and a CD-ROM containing advertising copy, graphics, health tips, and nutrition information to be used by retailers.
- *Community interventions/development.* The network and the 5 A Day campaign have facilitated the efforts of a wide range of community-based organizations to promote healthy eating and physical activity by increasing access to tested social marketing interventions, fostering partnerships, stimulating community development initiatives, and

(continued)

Nutrition in Education 13-4 (continued)

encouraging new interventions by LIAs. In a typical year, these efforts include activities in school districts, local health departments, food security organizations, African-American faith organizations, Project LEAN regions, 5 A Day–Power Play! campaign regions, public colleges and universities, healthy cities and communities, tribal organizations, park and recreation departments, city government agencies, and cooperative extension agencies. Cancer research projects also support network interventions.

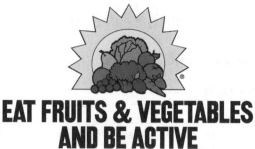

- *Policy, environment, and systems change.* The network asks all its funded projects to change organizational policies and the physical environment and help low-income families eat more fruits and vegetables, be more active, and participate in U.S. Department of Agriculture nutrition assistance programs.
- *Children's nutrition and physical activity.* The network works to facilitate the efforts of a wide range of physicians, health departments, school districts, and community-based organizations to promote healthy eating and physical activity habits in school-aged children and their parents.

Source: State of California. 2004. California Nutrition Network. http://www.dhs.ca.gov/ps/cdic/cpns/network/net_about.htm. Logos used with permission of California Nutrition Network.

mediators of change in the parents' behaviors. These strategies build on the educational objectives that we developed in Step 4 (Chapter 10).

Changing the food environment means educating decision makers and policy makers and then working in partnership with them to create a healthy food environment. This involves designing strategies to address potential environmental mediators at the interpersonal level—social and informational support—and at the institutional level—changes in food accessibility and in food policy. Both the parent and school environment components of the case study are shown at the end of this chapter.

Conclusion

Nutrition education programs can work with partners to promote policy, food environment, and community interventions that increase supports for program participants to engage in the nutrition- and food-related behaviors targeted by the program. Thus the food environments of intervention sites such as schools, Headstart programs, workplaces, and congregate meals sites for older adults can make healthful foods available and accessible as well as encourage and reinforce the behaviors or practices targeted by the program you are designing. In schools, school-wide food-related policies can be developed addressing beverage availability, vending machines, and school stores as well as school cafeteria offerings to provide students the opportunity to have easy access to the healthful food choices being promoted and to see healthful food practices modeled. In workplaces, healthful alternatives can be made available in the cafeteria and in vending machines and can be promoted. In all settings, the nutrition education program can work with decision makers to make healthful choices easier to enact. The active participation of community members and worksite employees as well as leaders through community organization and community building must be incorporated into any intervention. Indeed, community empowerment and collective efficacy are high priorities. Adopting these comprehensive approaches enhances the likelihood of improving the effectiveness of nutrition education interventions.

Questions and Activities

1. Describe how you might make existing social networks more supportive for (a) children and (b) adults.
2. Describe several key features for designing a social support group for your intended audience so that it will likely be effective.
3. Describe three reasons why collaborations and partnerships are important in nutrition education and three reasons why they may be challenging. How might you overcome these challenges?
4. Describe the key steps in developing an effective school or worksite nutrition-related wellness policy. What is the role of the nutrition educator in this process?

CASE STUDY 13-1   **Step 5c: Environmental Support for Action**

Title of program session: The Whys and Whats of Colorful Eating

Component: Parental/family program

Behavioral goal for parents: Parents or family members will make a variety of fruits and vegetables (F&V) available and accessible to their children.

General educational objectives of the parent/family component (from case study Step 4): Parents or family members will

- Demonstrate understanding and valuing of the importance for their children of eating a variety of F&V

- Provide social support to each other

- Develop skills in preparing and making F&V accessible for their children

- Demonstrate commitment to providing F&V for their children

Personal Mediators of Behavior and Educational Strategies*	Specific Educational Objectives for Potential Personal Mediators of Parents (from Step 4)	Learning Experiences or Educational Activities
Motivation-related mediators	*At the end of the session or program, learner will be able to:*	
Outcome expectations *Perceived benefits*	State benefits: energy, important for healthy growth, build strong bones & muscles for athletic performance	Use colorful visuals, striking statistics, short trigger films to emphasize the importance of F&V for their children's health. Bring in a variety of differently colored F&V.
	State the importance of eating a "rainbow of colors"	Provide colorful visuals of nutrients in differently colored F&V.
Parental role *Perceived obligation*	Value importance of providing many opportunities for children to become familiar with different F&V	Learning task to show that children need help to eat more F&V; parents can help.
Social norms/social models	State ways that other parents have made changes at home to support their children; recognize that media personalities support F&V intake	Have parents share their successes in providing F&V to children. Show pictures or film clips; tell stories of media personalities advocating F&V.
		Discuss parents as role models and the importance of talking about nutrition with their child; explain intent of TV advertisements.

Personal Mediators of Behavior and Educational Strategies*	Specific Educational Objectives for Potential Personal Mediators of Parents (from Step 4)	Learning Experiences or Educational Activities
Action-related mediators	At the end of the session or program learner will be able to:	
Barriers	Describe ways to select F&V to lower cost	Talk about and show data that buying in season and storing correctly can reduce costs.
Self-efficacy	Describe how F&V can be used in meals and as snacks	Provide tip sheets and simple recipes.
Social support	Appreciate that other parents share their challenges and successes	Provide family fun nights to meet other parents; share information; newsletters with parents' stories.
Behavioral capability (Food- & nutrition-related knowledge & skills)	Demonstrate skills in quick and easy preparation methods and recipes using F&V	Provide food demonstrations or food preparation tasks for parents to learn new recipes.
	Possess skills to make F&V readily accessible and available to children	Describe ways to cut up vegetables and place in accessible shelf in refrigerator for children to eat; fruit washed and on the counter.
Behavioral intention	State a commitment, in writing, to make F&V readily accessible and available to children	Parents will make an action plan for exactly when, how, and where they will make F&V available to their children.
Reinforcement	Maintain their commitment to support children	Newsletters sent home on a regular schedule to reinforce healthful eating; tips and recipes.

* Theory-based educational strategies are shown in italics in the first column.

Title of program session: The Whys and Whats of Colorful Eating

Component: School environment program

Behavioral goal for youth: Adolescents will increase their intake of a variety of fruits and vegetables (F&V).

General school environmental support objectives to support the program goal behavior(s) from case study Step 4 (Chapter 10):

- The nutrition education program will provide many opportunities for youth to taste F&V.

- The school will provide more F&V in the school meals and through other food venues.

Environmental Mediators (Current status)	Environmental Support Objectives: School	Strategies to Achieve Environmental Support Objectives
Food environment Barriers (Taste, convenience, cost)	School will provide many opportunities for students to taste F&V	Nutrition educators and food service staff will provide taste tests for F&V in the cafeteria
	School food service personnel will increase fruits and vegetables in meals; obtained from local farmers in a farm-to-school program	Meet with food service director to identify changes Provide professional development and manuals for food service personnel; provide information on potential vendors for local produce.
Food policy (No policy about food)	Establish or activate school food policy council to develop guidelines for foods available in school	Presentations for or conversations with school administrators, teachers, parent associations about need for school policies
	School nutrition advisory council will develop food policies	Recruitment to council; school council to be made up of administrators, food service staff, teachers, students, parents, and others
	Develop guidelines of items in vending machines and school store	Provide technical assistance to develop guidelines for vending machine items
	Vending machines will carry healthful F&V items	Vendors will supply healthful items in vending machines; develop system for monitoring compliance
	School stores will carry healthful F&V food items	Develop guidelines of items in school store (e.g., 50% will be healthful items); develop system for monitoring compliance
Decision-makers' awareness and motivation (Administrators have other priorities; funds from vending machines important financially)	Increase school administrators' beliefs in importance of healthful school environment (outcome expectations)	Individual meetings or presentations to staff about importance of healthful eating for learning; discussion of financial impacts, success stories
	Increase awareness of options for school food service personnel to increase students' F&V intake	Professional development, information on success stories; data on healthful options within budgetary constraints; potential vendors
Social support (No support for F&V by school staff and teens; no role models)	Increase social modeling by valued celebrities	Bring in celebrities for school assembly
Information environment (Eating F&V not normative)	Make eating F&V normative; dvelop posters for cafeteria; newsletter to family	Focus group with teens; design posters with teens about eating F&V; post them
		Write and design newsletter to families to make eating F&V normative (include principal and teachers)

REFERENCES

Ammerman, A.S., C.H. Lindquist, K.N. Lohr, and J. Hersey. 2002. The efficacy of behavioral interventions to modify dietary fat and fruit and vegetable intake: A review of the evidence. *Preventive Medicine* 35(1):25–41.

Bogden, J.F. 2000. *Fit, healthy and ready to learn, a school health policy guide. Part I: Physical activity, healthy eating, and tobacco-use prevention.* Alexandria, VA: National Association of State Boards of Education.

Brener, N.D., L. Kann, T. McManus, B. Stevenson, and S.F. Wooley. 2004. The relationship between school health councils and school health policies and programs in US schools. *Journal of School Health* 74:130–135.

Centers for Disease Control and Prevention. 1996. Guidelines for school health programs to promote lifelong healthy eating. *Morbidity and Mortality Weekly Report* 45(RR-9):1–33.

———. 2004a. *School Health Index: A self-assessment and planning guide. Elementary school version.* Atlanta, GA: Author.

———. 2004b. *School Health Index: A self-assessment and planning guide. Middle school/high school version.* Atlanta, GA: Author.

Cho, H., and M.Z. Nadow. 2004. Understanding barriers to implementing quality lunch and nutrition education. *Journal of Community Health* 29:421–435.

Cullen, K.W., J. Eagan, T. Baranowski, E. Owens, and C. deMoor. 2000. Effect of à la carte and snack bar foods at school on children s lunchtime intake of fruits and vegetables. *Journal of the American Dietetic Association* 100:1482–1486.

Cullen, K.W., and I. Zakeri. 2004. Fruits, vegetables, milk, and sweetened beverages consumption and access to à la carte/snack bar meals at school. *American Journal of Public Health* 94:463–467.

French, S.A., and H. Wechsler. 2004. School-based research and initiatives: Fruit and vegetable environment, policy, and pricing workshop. *Preventive Medicine* 39(Suppl. 2): S101–S107.

Glanz, K., and A.L. Yaroch. 2004. Strategies for increasing fruit and vegetable intake in grocery stores and communities: Policy, pricing, and environmental change. *Preventive Medicine* 39(Suppl. 2):S75–S80.

Green, L.W., and M.M. Kreuter. 1999. *Health promotion planning: An educational and ecological approach.* 3rd ed. Mountain View, CA: Mayfield Publishing.

Gregson, J., S.B. Foerster, R. Orr, et al. 2001. System, environmental, and policy changes: Using the social-ecological model as a framework for evaluating nutrition education and social marketing programs with low-income audiences. *Journal of Nutrition Education* 33:S4–S15.

Kramer-Atwood, J.L., J. Dwyer, D.M. Hoelscher, T.A. Nicklas, R.K. Johnson, and G.K. Schulz. 2002. Fostering healthy food consumption in schools: Focusing on the challenges of competitive foods. *Journal of the American Dietetic Association* 102:1228–1233.

Kremers, S.P.J., G. deBruijn, T.L.S. Visscher, W. van Mechelen, N.K. de Vries, and J. Brug. 2006. Environmental influences on energy balance-related behaviors: A dual-process view. *International Journal of Behavioral Nutrition and Physical Activity* 3:9.

Kubik, M.Y., L.A. Lytle, P.J. Hannan, C.L. Perry, and M. Story. 2003. The association of the school environment with dietary behaviors of young adolescents. *American Journal of Public Health* 93:1168–1173.

Kubik, M.Y., L.A. Lytle, and M. Story. 2001. A practical, theory-based approach to establishing school nutrition advisory councils. *Journal of the American Dietetic Association* 101:223–228.

———. 2005. Soft drinks, candy, fast food: What parents and teachers think about the middle school environment. *Journal of the American Dietetic Association* 105:233–239.

McLeroy, K.R., D. Bibeau, A. Steckler, and K. Glanz. 1988. An ecological perspective on health promotion programs. *Health Education Quarterly* 15:351–377.

Medeiros, L.C., S.N. Butkus, H. Chipman, R.H. Cox, L. Jones, and D. Little. 2005. A logic model framework for community nutrition education. *Journal of Nutrition Education and Behavior* 37:197–202.

Michigan Department of Community Health. 2005. *The Healthy School Action Tool (HSAT).* Lansing, MI: Author. http://mihealthtools.org/schools/.

Rosenthal, B.B. 1998. Collaboration for the nutrition field: Synthesis of selected literature. *Journal of Nutrition Education* 30(5):246–267.

United States Department of Agriculture. 2000. *Changing the scene: Improving the school nutrition environment.* Alexandria, VA: Author.

Wechsler, H., N.D. Brener, S. Kuester, and C. Miller. 2001. Food service and foods and beverages available at school: Results from the School Health Policies and Programs Study 2000. *Journal of School Health* 71:313–324.

Step 6: Design the Evaluation for Theory-Based Nutrition Education

· ·

OVERVIEW   This chapter describes key issues in designing and conducting evaluations and how they may be applied to evaluating the outcomes of theory-based nutrition education programs.

OBJECTIVES   At the end of the chapter, you will be able to

- State reasons for conducting evaluations of nutrition education interventions
- Distinguish between the major types of evaluation
- Explain the relationships among educational objectives, mediating variables, and measures of outcome
- Describe types of measures for evaluating mediators and behaviors
- Describe key features to consider in creating evaluation measures
- Judge the appropriateness of different evaluation designs for the given intervention and audience
- Demonstrate skills in designing an evaluation for a nutrition education intervention

· ·

SCENARIO

An American Peace Corps volunteer came to Malawi to work in an under-five's clinic. There he saw many malnourished children and started trying to convince mothers to enrich their babies' food. He finally wrote and recorded a song with the following message: put pounded peanut flour in your baby's maize porridge and feed it to him three times a day if you want your child to weigh a lot. The song was a success; it became number one on the national radio hit parade. Did this very original and apparently successful approach to nutrition education change the mothers' behavior and improve the nutritional status of children in Malawi? Unfortunately, we shall never know.

COMMENT

Reading about nutrition education, one is amazed at the large amounts of dedication, creativity, and resources that have been invested in programs and at how little we know about the effects they have produced.

Introduction

We are now on the last step of the procedural model for designing theory-based nutrition education: designing the evaluation of outcomes. This chapter examines how to evaluate the impact of our sessions or programs as well as the process of how we conducted our programs.

Most nutrition education practitioners enjoy designing group nutrition education sessions and programs and gain great satisfaction by making presentations and conducting the programs they have designed. When it comes to evaluating the effectiveness of these session or programs, however, our eyes tend to glaze over. Much as we agree that evaluation of nutrition education is important, there are many obstacles to carrying it out in any systematic way. When time, energy, and other resources are limited, we are hesitant to take them away from activities that will directly benefit our target audiences and allocate them to something whose value is less obvious. Financial and other resource constraints present a problem. Indeed, both the "befores" (the identification of issues and the analysis of needs and assets) and the "afters" (evaluation) seem like luxuries—much the way appetizers and desserts are for someone eating on a limited budget.

The topic of evaluation can also be an emotional and personally threatening one. It affects our present and our future and gives shape to many memories drawn out of our educational pasts. Many of us fear that the evaluation may point to inadequate performance on our part or be interpreted in a way that is unfavorable to us. It thus affects how we see ourselves and how others see us. Since to us nutrition education programs are "obviously" beneficial to the participants we work with, we tend to resist any evaluation that might threaten our intuitive perception. Moreover, most of us are highly committed to our work and put in much more time than is called for by our job descriptions. We thus fear that we would be very demoralized by an evaluation—usually by the funding agencies or some other outside persons—that we might consider unfair, especially since the effects of education may be subtle or delayed in their expression.

For some programs, political considerations may also influence the evaluation process. The survival of many programs depends on government or other funding sources, and for many working within these programs, it may seem better not to evaluate at all than to obtain evaluation results that fall short of the expectations of these funding sources. On the other hand, some programs may be so inherently politically attractive that no one, from the politicians who initiate the programs to the institutions that develop and implement them, wants to see them evaluated, lest they are shown to be of little value.

Even where there is the desire to evaluate nutrition education programs, the technical or methodological problems are still quite formidable. Although attempts have been made to compile sourcebooks of nutrition education evaluation instruments, there really is no set of ready-made instruments that nutrition educators can simply take and use with a given population in a given situation. Generally we have to design instruments specific to the intervention and test them before use. Other technical problems remain regarding what should be evaluated and when. For short interventions of one or several sessions, what might be appropriate measures of their effectiveness? For longer, more comprehensive programs, what kind of evaluation design should be used? Do quantitative methodologies adequately capture the effects of nutri-

INPUTS: COLLECTING ASSESSMENT DATA		DESIGNING THE OUTPUTS			DESIGNING OUTCOMES EVALUATION
STEP 1 ←→ **Analyze needs and behaviors: Specify the behavior or action focus of the program** • Assess needs and identify audience: select need(s) or issue(s) to address • Identify behaviors of concern that contribute to need(s) or issue(s) • Select core behaviors or practices to address	**STEP 2** ←→ **Identify relevant potential mediators of program behaviors** • Identify potential personal psychosocial mediators • Identify potential environmental mediators	**STEP 3** ←→ **Select theory, philosophy, and components** • Select theory and/or create appropriate model • Articulate educational philosophy • Clarify perspectives on content • Determine program components	**STEP 4** ←→ **State educational objectives for potential mediators** • Select relevant mediators to address • State educational objectives for each selected mediator: —Personal psychosocial mediators —Environmental mediators	**STEP 5** ←→ **Design theory-based educational strategies and activities to address potential mediators** • Design strategies and activities for each selected mediator: —Personal psychosocial mediators —Environmental mediators	**STEP 6** **Design evaluation** • Design evaluation of program's impact on behaviors and mediators • Design process evaluation

tion education? On the other hand, how do we conveniently analyze qualitative data for programs with large numbers of participants? But if we do not ask what worked and what did not and why, we will not learn from our experience. As John Dewey once noted, we do not learn from our experience; we learn from *reflections* on our experience. The evaluation of a program must be planned at the same time as the intervention is being planned; hence it is described here, *before* the next section of the book that focuses on the nuts and bolts of implementation.

Evaluation is a vast topic, with scores of books available on its nature and role in every field of human endeavour. Even in the field of nutrition and health, the literature is substantial. This chapter has space to discuss only the relevant essentials and examine how they can be used to design evaluations for behavior-focused nutrition education programs that are based on theory and evidence. We then apply the information to our ongoing case study. Several reviews in the area of nutrition education can provide further guidance (Thompson & Byers, 1994; Freedman & Perry, 2000; Kohl, Fulton, & Casperson, 2000; McPherson et al., 2000; Gregson et al., 2001; Keenan et al., 2001; McClelland et al., 2001; Medeiros et al., 2001; Contento, Randell, & Basch, 2002).

What Is Evaluation?

With the word *value* embedded in the term *evaluation*, it is not surprising that a simple definition of the term is that evaluation is the process of determining the value or worth of an enterprise. In our everyday lives, we are always making judgments of worth: Is dinner at this restaurant worth the money I will spend? Will this workshop be worth my time and effort to attend? In the case of food and nutrition education, evaluation could mean any or all of the following:

- Did the program achieve the *stated* behavioral goals and objectives? (That is, was it of worth in achieving the objectives?)
- Did it serve some specified larger value goals? For example, did it improve the nutritional well-being of the participants, or their behaviors? Did it enhance their motivations and skills? Did it increase their opportunities for taking action?
- Was it of worth or value to the sponsoring organization or funding source?
- Was the program or educational intervention of worth or value to the participants?

The judgmental nature of such considerations arouses considerable anxiety, and often resistance, among those being evaluated. Many thus prefer a more nonjudgmental definition of evaluation as providing information for decision making. Although this approach helps to ally anxiety among both practitioners and program participants and improve their attitudes toward evaluation, many point out that it is

unrealistic to ignore one of the main features of evaluation—that of judging merit or worth. Indeed, it has been argued that "people who believe that measurement and evaluation are neutral or value free delude themselves" (Green & Lewis, 1985).

These two definitions of evaluation are not mutually exclusive. Certainly evaluation provides information for decision making; however, the information may be used nonjudgmentally or judgmentally, depending on the time at which it is collected and its function. Thus the information may be used to improve the program, especially toward the beginning of program implementation. However, given limited resources, information about the relative effectiveness of nutrition education programs or program components may also be used for allocating these resources appropriately. In this case, the information is still used for decision making, but the decisions, of necessity, carry judgmental overtones.

Why Evaluate?

We have designed our program based on theory and evidence, so why do we need to evaluate it? In general, evaluation can be seen as serving research purposes, program evaluation purposes, or both. For research purposes, we investigate whether and how interventions influence potential mediators and how mediating variables influence nutrition behavior so that we can learn exactly how and why interventions do or do not work. Such understandings can be incorporated into evidence-based theory making to enhance the effectiveness of nutrition education.

In practice settings, practitioners are held accountable for the programs they conduct. In these settings, evaluation can serve many functions, examples of which are given in the following list. These functions vary in their relative importance depending on the nature of the program and the context in which it occurs.

- Determining whether the goals and objectives of the nutrition education intervention we designed have been met
- Judging whether the program has contributed to the improved well-being of the intended audience, or has had impacts on the targeted behaviors or on the mediating variables of the behaviors
- Determining whether the message or content was suitable to the target group
- Providing information on whether the educational strategies and activities (such as format, duration, and frequency) were appropriate for the given group and contributed to the achievement of the goals and objectives
- Determining whether the program was implemented as planned, and if not, why not
- Providing participation of, and feedback to, the intended audience

- Providing evidence to our funding sources that their funding was well spent and achieved their goals or the larger goals of society (such as chronic disease reduction, overweight prevention, or reduction in the loss of small, local farms)

Information such as the above can be used to improve the planning and implementation of the nutrition education program the next time around, as well as to judge its overall worthwhileness. Evaluation can also serve sociopolitical functions. For example, evaluation may be used to improve public relations by demonstrating to the public how good the program is and how worthy of further public- or private-sector funding. An evaluation report released to the various media may also be used to increase the visibility of an organization's work or to apply political pressure for legislative action in the area of nutrition education.

Finally, evaluation may serve psychological functions. Learning that they have been effective can be very motivating for all involved in the nutrition education program, but especially to those actually delivering the programs to the intended audience—whether they are teachers, workplace employees, or community nutrition educators.

Evaluation: What Kinds, for Whom, and by Whom

Evaluation is not the end of the nutrition education process. Rather, it is an ongoing part of the entire process. This section examines the different functions and types of evaluation.

Types of Evaluation

There are four major types of evaluation that you can use to evaluate your program, depending on your needs: formative, summative, outcome, and process.

Formative Evaluation

The function of formative evaluation is to develop or improve an ongoing activity such as programs or educational sessions.

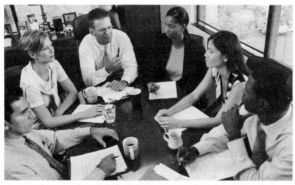

Among the considerations for practitioners as they design programs are goals, objectives, target audience, and appropriate activities.

It is usually used during the early developmental or formative stages of program development. The information collected in this type of evaluation is intended to serve decision making. However, it is important during all phases of the educational enterprise—from the initial identification of needs and assets to the determination of goals, objectives, and activities and their implementation. It helps to shape the features of the intervention prior to implementation.

For example, formative research can determine whether the intended audience understands the messages. Knowing how the program is doing as we go along will help us to improve the program. Also, pilot testing and revising each of the program components will ensure that the program as a whole will be stronger. For example, the lesson plans or curriculum (manual of activities) that you have just designed is based on your identification of issues, concerns, and assets, the research evidence, and theory. You may now want to send this curriculum draft to a sample of teachers or community nutrition educators and ask them to conduct some of the activities to find out whether the goals and objectives are clear, whether the issues included are considered relevant, whether the educational activities are appropriate, interesting, and feasible to carry out, and whether the evaluation procedures are useful. You can now use such information to clarify the objectives and educational strategies of the curriculum. You will also want to test the food-related activities and recipes that are included. Formative evaluation also includes more systematic field tests carried out on the new curriculum or program materials before the final product is published.

Summative Evaluation: Impacts and Outcomes

Summative evaluations are carried out at the end of the program to sum up or provide information on the overall effects of the program or intervention, and are sometimes called *effect evaluations*. These are statements of the results of the program. That is, did the nutrition education program actually accomplish what it was designed to accomplish? This type of evaluation carries the connotation of accountability. A good effect evaluation or summative evaluation, however, should not just report whether the educational intervention was or was not effective, but why or why not and under what conditions. Thus, even effect or summative evaluations may have formative implications.

The terms *impact evaluations* and *outcome evaluations* are used to describe these summative evaluations. Different agencies and researchers use these terms differently. The distinctions are quite arbitrary, and the terms are often used interchangeably. We will use the term *outcome evaluation* as used in the community nutrition education logic model described in Chapters 6 and 13 (Medeiros et al., 2005). Outcome assessments address the question of whether or not anticipated group changes or differences occur in connection with the intervention. By itself, however, measuring outcomes may not provide definitive evidence that the observed outcomes are due to the intervention. In order to definitively conclude that the observed outcomes are a result of the intervention, an *impact evaluation* has to be conducted, whereby a systematic design or plan is used to eliminate alternative explanations for the observed differences. Such a design is called the *impact evaluation design* and is described later in this chapter.

These logic models usually distinguish between short-term, medium-term, and long-term outcomes. Short-term outcomes usually refer to changes in mediating variables; medium-term outcomes refer to changes in behaviors and practices; and long-term outcomes refer to impacts on health, social, environmental, and other outcomes.

In the research literature, a distinction is made between effectiveness and efficacy evaluations. An *efficacy evaluation* is one conducted under optimal conditions (such as when the researchers or program designers themselves deliver the program with outside funding and supports), whereas an *effectiveness evaluation* is evaluation of a program under real-world circumstances (such as conducted by teachers or by practitioner staff as part of their jobs).

Process Evaluation

In process evaluation, you want to know whether the program was delivered to the persons for whom it was intended and whether it was implemented as designed or planned. If so, what worked and what did not? If it did not work, why not? It is especially instructive to probe failures as well as successes. Included in this kind of evaluation are data such as how many people attended, and how participants judged the intervention activities or components (e.g., they liked some but not others).

Summary

Some of the purposes of evaluation are best served by formative evaluations and others by outcome ones. Many evaluation experts prefer the less judgmental, formative aspects of evaluation. And certainly, nutrition educators and administrators in a given program tend to find formative evaluations as well as the process evaluation more useful. However, realistically, when some agency has funded a project, it wants to know whether the funds were effective in bringing about stated or desired goals. It is thus primarily interested in the outcome evaluation. The purposes of an evaluation, then, are very much dependent on the intended recipients of the evaluation information.

The different functions require different methods for gathering data. Hence, you should spell out the functions of evaluation early in the intervention process so that you can include the appropriate evaluation methods in the design and implementation phases of the program.

Evaluation: For Whom?

Who should be served by an evaluation? Clearly, many people are interested in the information generated by an evaluation. The term *stakeholders* is usually used to refer to all those who have some stake in the outcome of an evaluation. Policy makers and program practitioners often have different opinions regarding what should be indicators of effectiveness, and a fair evaluation must take into account the different needs of the various groups involved. It is best to include all stakeholders early in the evaluation design process so that all needs are articulated and considered.

Food and Nutrition Educators

For most food and nutrition educators, from the curriculum developer to the mass media campaign designer, the most important function of evaluation is to provide information about whether the intervention was effective, that is, whether it achieved the stated goals and objectives. It is also important to know what worked, what did not, and why. Other aspects of interest are as follows: Were the learning activities and message content suitable? Was the educational style or approach used appropriate? Were the print, audio, or video materials used effective? Was it easy to implement the program as designed? What facilitated and what hindered implementation? If you are conducting one-shot educational events, this may be the only function of a brief evaluation carried out at the end of a given session. Such information can guide future activities with the same group or similar groups, or provide feedback to the educator that is helpful for the future.

At a personal level, a favorable evaluation may provide a means of increasing a person's status in the organization or even prevent the elimination of his or her job. In some organizations, the evaluation process can be a powerful motivating force to perform well if it is combined carefully and appropriately with some other reward system. For nutrition educators working as independent consultants, a well-conducted evaluation may mean more business. Both formative and outcome evaluations are important to this group.

The Sponsoring Organization

The organization sponsoring the program, whether it is a national or community governmental or private voluntary agency, school system, nonprofit organization, corporate worksite, or fitness center, needs evaluative information to determine whether the goals and objectives of the program are being met and whether the program is being well managed. Information may also be needed to satisfy funding agencies (if other than the sponsoring organization itself) demanding evidence for program effects. Evaluation results are important for decision making about future courses of action. The organization also needs evaluative information to demonstrate to other organizations that it is conducting worthwhile programs and to potential participants or clients that its programs are effective and hence worth their time or money. The sponsoring organization may be more interested in outcome than formative evaluations.

The Funding Agency

The funding agency may be the sponsoring organization itself or may be some other private foundation or public agency. The funding agency is interested in evaluation information because it needs to know about the impact or effectiveness of the nutrition education program. The funding agency is concerned whether its allocation of funds served useful or desirable ends. If effectiveness was not as great as expected, the agency needs to be provided with information as to why not and how changes might be made in the future. The funding agency also needs to know about the efficiency of program operation and to verify that the actual use of funds conforms to that originally agreed upon. It also requires information that it can use to demonstrate the impact of the program in a political context, for example, through press releases or government reports.

Participants

Those participating in the program, such as community members, workplace employees, or school students, have the greatest stake in its outcome or impact. For them, evaluation may provide a sense of accomplishment and sense of self-worth or objective information on whether their eating patterns and health have improved. It also provides information to those participants who are paying directly for the nutrition education service (e.g., a cardiovascular risk reduction group) by which they can judge whether the effect was worth the money they spent. For school students, evaluation provides feedback on whether they have adequately acquired needed health knowledge and skills. For them, the evaluation activities may actually be interesting to do.

Evaluation: By Whom?

Who should conduct the evaluation will depend on the scope of the nutrition education. If you are providing only one or several in-person group sessions, you will probably be the one conducting the evaluation. If the nutrition education is more extensive, who should be involved will depend primarily on two factors: the resources available and the need for objectivity.

Resources include not just time and money but also the technical skills needed to conduct the evaluation. Simple evaluations do not require many resources. Pencils, paper, a duplicating machine of some sort (optional), and knowledge of how to construct and analyze a simple questionnaire are probably all that is needed for a simple but formal quantitative postsession evaluation for a one-time educational event. An informal or qualitative evaluation requires even less in the way of physical resources but probably more technical skills: making verbal inquiries of participants about what they learned. However, evaluating a curriculum in nationwide field tests or evaluating a mass media campaign requires more resources. Such an evaluation will require people with the technical expertise for planning and implementing an evaluation design and analyzing the results. It will also require considerable time and money. Most nutrition education program evaluations are somewhere in between in scope.

Usually, the more resources spent on an evaluation, the higher its quality. However, the choice of how much to spend on the evaluation component of the nutrition education should include careful consideration of the trade-off between the information that will be gained and the resources it will cost. Sometimes the evaluation process can become an end in itself. What you want is the least evaluation that will provide you with the information you need.

For evaluation results to be credible, they need to be obtained in such a way that those reading the results believe that they are objective. Should the evaluation, then, always be conducted by someone who has no stake in the results—for example, some outside person or group? Although the advantage of this approach is that the results will be considered more credible, the outside evaluators may be less familiar with the program, and may be culturally or socially different from those implementing or participating in the program. Their evaluations therefore may not capture important intricacies of the program or the real-world context in which it is occurring. In-house evaluations, on the other hand, have the advantage that those conducting them are more familiar with the program, have access to more information, and are better able to identify problem areas as well as solutions to them. The disadvantage is that if continuation of the program or of individuals within the program depends on evaluation results, obtaining them objectively is very difficult. Even when objectively done, an in-house evaluation may not be believed to be so by outsiders because of the presumed vested interest of those conducting it. In addition, time-consuming evaluations may take away personnel time for program delivery. In many situations, it is possible to use both in-house and outside evaluations, with some aspects (e.g., formative evaluations) primarily done by in-house personnel and others (e.g., outcome evaluations or those involving staff members' jobs) done by an outside person or group.

What Should Be Evaluated?

Evaluations of a nutrition education intervention should involve inquiry into both outcomes and process: inquiry into the program's effectiveness in bringing about the intended results (impact evaluation) and inquiry into the operation of the program, such as how well the program was implemented or managed (process evaluation), to help shed light on why interventions worked well or did not.

Outcome Evaluation

Outcome evaluations are based on the goals and objectives of the nutrition education sessions or program. In behavior-focused, theory-based nutrition education interventions or communications, this generally means that the primary outcomes to be assessed are the behaviors that are targeted by the program; that is, the assessment is of whether the *behavioral goals* of the program have been achieved, such as an increase in consumption of fruits and vegetables, eating more healthful diets, breastfeeding, or using food stamps to shop at a farmers' market. These behavioral outcomes might be considered *medium-term outcomes*.

You will also want to measure whether there have been improvements in the mediators of targeted behaviors, such as perceived threat, perceived benefits and barriers of taking action, preferences for healthful foods, self-efficacy, and intentions, as well as food- and nutrition-related knowledge and skills or goal-setting and self-influence skills. In some cases, movement of participants through the stages of readiness to change may be measured. These may be called *short-term outcomes*. As we have discussed at some length, these mediators are the targets of the general educational objectives of a program. For many nutrition education programs, although demonstration of achievement of specific actions or behaviors is often sought, achievement of these short-term outcomes may be all that can be expected given the duration, intensity, and scope of the program. If the research evidence indicates that there is a strong relationship between these mediating variables and the behavior itself, then changes in these mediators can serve as good indications that the impacts may be translated into action under suitable conditions. For example, in many studies the relationship between self-efficacy and behavior is strong, so that an increase in self-efficacy by program participants may be meaningful. Information about changes in these mediators of behavior will also help to explain how and why the intervention or its component activities worked, or did not.

In some educational interventions, physiological parameters are the desired primary end points, such as changes in serum cholesterol levels or weight. These are *long-term outcomes*, requiring educational interventions of considerable intensity and duration. Choice of outcome may be influenced by the function of the evaluation and funding sources.

At the time of designing the educational intervention, it is best to design ways to evaluate each *behavioral goal* (behavior) and each *general educational objective* (mediator of behavior). You will need to decide whether to evaluate all the *specific* educational objectives and all the environmental support objectives, or only a sample of them. This will depend on the purposes of the evaluation and how detailed or comprehensive the evaluation needs to be.

Program or Process Evaluation

In a program or process evaluation, you want to know answers to the following questions: Did the program reach the intended audience? How many attended? Was the program implemented as designed or planned? If so, what worked and what did not? If it did not work, why not? Were all the activities implemented? To what degree? How did participants judge the intervention activities or component? In terms of environmental support activities, process evaluation questions might include the following: How many coalition partners were involved? How effective was communication among partners? How did the partners feel about the program?

It is just as important to probe failures as successes. Failures may bring to light flaws in the original design and identify breakdowns in the internal operations of the program. Failures also help us understand the limitations of what the program can accomplish.

Designing the Evaluation

Evaluation procedures should be selected at the time the educational intervention is being planned so that they can be incorporated into activities of the program. Even before we have implemented the program, we need to plan for the kinds of information we will need as we go along and at the end of the program, and to design appropriate measurement tools. The logic model we have used as the conceptual framework for nutrition education, as well as our design model, will serve as our framework for evaluation (Figure 14-1).

Since evaluation involves judgment of worth, it requires the development of some way to assess or measure worth. An analogy might clarify the difference between measurement and evaluation. In everyday terms, *measurement* is saying that the temperature in a room is 68°F; *evaluation* is saying I feel cold at this temperature. The measurement instrument (a thermometer, in this instance) has to be accurate and reliable, and my judgment has to be based on ruling out competing explanations for why I might feel cold (I might be sick that day and hence feeling cold). When we say "It's cold today," we are mixing measurement and evaluation. *It* is not cold: it is 68°F (measurement); *I* feel cold (evaluation).

Designing the Process Evaluation

Process evaluation is described first because this is most familiar to us, tends to be done routinely, and is easier to design and carry out. We are participating in a process evaluation when, as students, we complete an end-of-semester evaluation of the course and the instructor, or when, as professionals, we complete an evaluation instrument at the end of a conference or professional meeting asking us our opinions of the learning experience. Banks do it; airlines do it. This section describes the kinds of questions we might want to ask about the program we are designing.

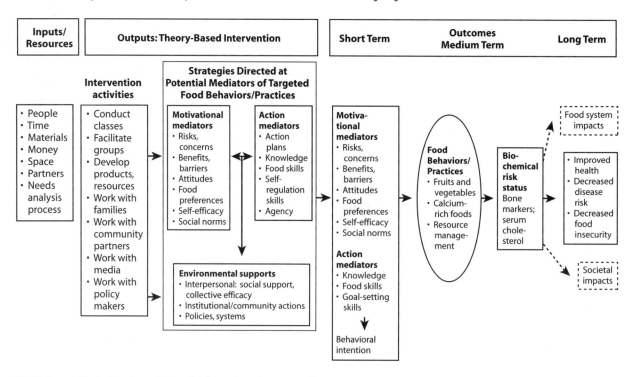

FIGURE 14-1 Designing the evaluation for theory-based nutrition education.

Clarifying the Process Evaluation Questions

In general, process evaluation focuses on the inputs and outputs components of the logic model. Process evaluation questions might be related to program activities and reach, program implementation and fidelity, program design, and program management in some cases. During program implementation and at the end you may want to know the following.

Program Activities and Reach

- What are the components of the program? What are the materials of the program? (Descriptive information on how many and what components, such as classroom plus school environment plus parent component, or groups plus media campaign; how often the sessions are held; what are the handouts, and so forth.)
- Did the program reach the intended target audience? To what extent? (What proportion of the intended audience participated or are participating?) How many participated or are participating?
- What were participants' and practitioners' degree of satisfaction with both the content of materials, learning activities, or media messages and the form in which it was delivered?
- In terms of the coalition component, how many partners or coalition members were or are there? What were or are their roles?

- What activities did coalition partners conduct separately or together?
- What degree of satisfaction did or do the coalition partners express about their participation?

Program Implementation and Fidelity

- How many of the activities designed for the program were actually delivered?
- Was the program implemented, or is it being implemented, as designed? How extensively (part or all)? How frequently?
- If the program was or is not being implemented as designed, why not? What are the obstacles?
- How well did the coalition function or is it functioning? Did coalition partners conduct the activities they committed themselves to do? If not, why not?

Program Design Review

- Are the program behavioral goals and educational objectives that have been designed directed at, or consistent with, the issues identification and needs analysis data collected in Step 1?
- Are educational strategies and learning experiences appropriately designed to achieve stated goals and objectives?

- Are educational strategies and learning experiences appropriately based on nutrition behavior theory and research findings?

Program Management

- How well was the program managed or is it being managed? Did it stay within budget? Was or is the flow of information to those needing it timely and adequate? Was the coalition managed satisfactorily?

Gathering the Process Evaluation Information

How the evaluative data are collected depends on the size of the program and the extent of the resources allocated to the evaluation phase of the program. Collection can involve many different strategies: examining existing documents (e.g., issues identification or needs and assets analysis data, program goal statements, materials and curricula developed), interviewing key individuals, and discussing matters with a group of participants (or the entire target group if it is a small one) and relevant others as the program is being implemented or at the end. Making process evaluation possible requires all the program design materials to be maintained and easily accessible (in binders or in physical or computer files), such as the description of the program, the lesson or education plans used by the nutrition educator or given to participants, and handouts. These materials will provide information on whether the behavioral goals and educational objectives are directed at, or consistent with, the issues identification and needs analysis data and whether the educational strategies are consistent with theory and evidence. Records related to coalition partnerships should also be maintained and available for review—for example, meeting agendas, announcements of accomplishments, program plans, or products developed.

Gathering the evaluative data may also involve the development of appropriate instruments or forms for recording the data. These might include attendance sheets to provide information on number of participants, and instruments to assess fidelity to the program—such as a checklist of activities for each session for the nutrition educator to check off how much of the session content was delivered and note whether other material was added. If ongoing records are to be obtained from the participants, such as three-day food records, you will need to design some way to keep track of whether these records were turned in or are being turned in. You will also want to develop an evaluation form for participants to complete, asking them to rate the usefulness of the nutrition education experience—whether it was one session or a program of several months. More important, it should ask them to state which parts of the program were most useful and which least useful, what topics should have been covered in greater depth or less, and what other topics or activities should have been included.

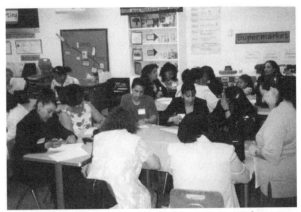

Evaluating the parent component can provide important information for a program.

The data collected can be used in a formative way to decide how to improve participation rates and degree of satisfaction with the program; how to improve the process of delivery, such as better training for personnel, better materials, or more clarity about intervention strategies; or how to improve management. The data collected in a summative evaluation can be used to identify specifically why the program was or was not effective in bringing about desired nutritional goals. In other words, information obtained about program functioning can help to interpret the results obtained from the outcome evaluation about the effectiveness of the program (or lack of it).

Designing the Outcome Evaluation

Figure 14-1 provides the framework for designing the outcome evaluation. As you can see, we can measure short-term, medium-term, or long-term outcomes. Designing the outcome evaluation generally involves the following steps:

1. Clarifying the outcomes that will be evaluated
2. Specifying indicators and measures of outcome effectiveness
3. Selecting, adapting, or designing the instruments for measuring program effectiveness
4. Constructing an appropriate evaluation plan to measure impacts
5. Designing the methods for collecting the evaluation data

Clarifying the Outcomes That Will Be Evaluated

Outcome evaluations are based on the goals and objectives of the nutrition education sessions or program. Hence, at the time of designing the educational intervention, it is best to design ways to evaluate each behavioral goal, general educational objective, and environmental support objective. So in a major way, your evaluation outcomes have already been determined by your statement of objectives. Outcomes of a nutrition education program can thus be evaluated in terms of mediating variables, behaviors or practices, or food intakes, as shown in Figure 14-1.

What you will use as the criterion of effectiveness for a given program needs to be carefully clarified at the outset. Selection of outcomes should be based on the purpose, duration, and power of the intervention. What exactly is meant by "behavior" in this intervention? For example, will achievement of the actual behavior change (such as increased intakes of fruits and vegetables) or engagement in the targeted actions by the intended audience (such as buying at farmers' markets) be used as the criterion of outcome effectiveness? On the other hand, for an intervention of short duration, the behavior change expected can be quite small, such as trying new vegetables when offered. Changes in behaviors, food intakes, or practices are considered to be medium-term outcomes in our logic model shown in Figure 14-1.

Will outcome effectiveness be judged not just on whether participants engaged in the target behaviors but also on whether there were changes in the physiological parameters or risk factors for health problems that result from engagement in the targeted actions, such as change in weight or biochemical markers? These are referred to as long-term outcomes.

On the other hand, is behavior change an appropriate criterion for the particular audience or for the power, duration, or intensity of the intervention? Will behavioral intentions be sufficient? Will improvement in the stages of motivational readiness to change be sufficient? Are changes in mediators of behavior an appropriate measure of the outcome of the given intervention? If you are conducting only one or two sessions, changes in awareness and motivation and in relevant knowledge and skills may be appropriate outcomes. These are referred to as short-term outcomes in our model.

Perhaps the philosophical approach of the program is that participants will choose which changes to make or whether even to make any. What criteria will you use to evaluate effectiveness? How will you report to stakeholders the effect of the program?

Identifying Potential Indicators and Measures of Outcome Effectiveness

In order to evaluate outcomes of your program, you will need to develop some indicators of effectiveness. *Indicators* are the ways to operationalize theoretical constructs, activities, and behaviors in order to identify that change has occurred or that an action has been taken with respect to the desired outcome. *Measures* are the specific tools or instruments that you use to evaluate the change that has occurred. You will need to select the indicators and measures that are appropriate for your program. To evaluate outcomes you will develop tables that have the following columns: Outcomes, Indicators for achievement of outcomes, and Measures for the indicators.

The following subsections discuss some potential indicators and measures in four categories: (1) short-term outcomes: mediators of goal behaviors, (2) medium-term outcomes: goal behaviors, and (3) long-term outcomes: physiological parameters, environmental supports for goal behaviors.

Evaluating impacts on mediators of goal behaviors: short-term outcomes. As we have stated before, general educational objectives are written to address potential mediators of action or behavior change. Thus, impacts on mediators—short-term outcomes—are evaluated on the degree to which these general educational objectives have been achieved. Excerpts from our ongoing case study are shown in Table 14-1 to illustrate. The full set of outcomes, indicators, and measures are shown in the Case Study at the end of the chapter.

You used mediators as the basis of your educational objectives, and you used them as the basis for designing educational strategies to address the educational objectives. Now they will be the basis of your evaluation—which is another reason why the evaluation is designed at the same time as goals, objectives, and strategies. You may not want to measure impacts on all of the potential mediators (or mediating variables)—some may be more important than others for judging the effectiveness of the intervention. Now is the time to specify which mediating variables you will actually measure, then state what will indicate that the program has been effective in changing a given potential mediating variable.

The *indicators* can be as follows:

- Increased awareness of risks or issues of concern
- Increased outcome expectancies or beliefs in the perceived benefits or pros of action
- Decreased sense of the barriers or cons of change
- Increased preferences for or enjoyment of targeted foods or behaviors
- Improved attitudes or feelings toward the targeted behaviors, such as healthy eating
- Increased understanding of the participant's own social norms and skills
- Increased self-efficacy
- Increased understanding of moral or ethical responsibility issues
- Increased food and nutrition knowledge related to the behavioral goals of the program
- Improved skill in selection of targeted/healthful diets
- Increased skill in preparation of targeted/healthful foods
- Improved stage of readiness to take action or to change
- A stated intention to engage in the action or to change
- Improved ability to engage in a goal-setting process for the program goal behaviors

For social marketing or communications campaigns, the following are important indicators:

TABLE 14-1 Evaluating Impacts on Potential Personal-Level Mediators of Goal Behaviors (Case Study)

Potential personal mediator	Outcomes in Relation to the Mediators (Based on General Educational Objectives)	Indicators of Achievement of Outcomes	Measures/Instruments for Indicators
Outcome expectations	Understanding and appreciation of the importance of eating a variety of fruits and vegetables	Increased understanding of benefits of eating more F&V; knowledge of scientific basis for eating F&V Specific indicators: List of specific benefits and understandings	Scale on benefits with responses of 1 to 5, from strongly disagree to strongly agree; knowledge instrument: multiple choice questions on impact of F&V on health and disease risk reduction
Barriers	Decreased barriers to intake of F&V	Decreased perception of barriers on an instrument	Scale with responses of 1 to 5, from strongly disagree to strongly agree
Attitudes	Express positive attitudes toward eating a variety of F&V	Improved attitudes toward F&V and toward self eating specific fruits and vegetables Specific indicators: List of specific attitudes	Scale with responses of 1 to 5, from strongly disagree to strongly agree, on attitudes about specific F&V; and on self eating more F&V (e.g., "I feel I am taking care of myself when I eat F&V")
Self-efficacy	Increased self-efficacy in eating a variety of F&V each day	Increased confidence in being able to eat more F&V Specific indicators: Confidence in various situations, including difficult ones	Scale with responses of 1 to 5 on how confident participant feels about eating F&V (e.g., "If I wanted to, it would be easy to eat more vegetables")
Behavioral capability	Increased knowledge and skills in incorporating F&V into their daily food patterns	Increased food- and nutrition-related knowledge and improved skills Specific indicators: List of specific knowledge and skills	Knowledge and skills instrument: Multiple-choice questions and some open-ended questions related to importance of variety, and serving sizes; ways to add F&V to daily diet

F&V = fruits and vegetables.

- Recall of advertisements or other messages
- Level of exposure to other interventions within the campaign—that is, other classes, workshops, health fairs or festivals, food demonstrations, or materials brought home from school or workplace

Measures. Various ways can be used to measure changes in indicators, although the most usual way is through the use of survey instruments. Theory constructs or mediating variables are operationalized as a series of questions that participants answer or a series of statements to which the participants respond. Many formats can be used. For most mediators, participants are given a series of statements and asked to indicate their opinion on a 5-point agreement scale such as whether they strongly disagree (given a score of 1), disagree (given a score of 2), are neutral (given a score of 3), agree (given a score of 4), or strongly agree (given a score

of 5). Statements might include "I feel that I am helping my body by eating more fruits and vegetables" (perceived benefits), "I feel that fruit is too expensive" (perceived barriers), or "People in my family think that I should eat more fruits and vegetables" (perceived social norms).

A scale might also be stated in terms of amount or frequency. For example, "In your household, how much control do you have in buying/preparing the food you eat?" with a scale ranging from "very little control" to "complete control." Self-efficacy is often measured in terms of how confident individuals are in being able to carry out a given action, such as "How sure are you that you can eat two or more vegetables at dinner?" or "How sure are you that you can add more vegetables to casseroles and stews?" Individuals' readiness to take action can be measured using a series of statements that places them in one of the stages of change: "I am not thinking about eating more fruit" (precontemplation), "I am thinking about eating more fruit" (contemplation), "I am planning to start eating more fruit within 6 months" (contemplation), "I am definitely planning to eat more fruit in the next month" (preparation), "I am trying to eat more fruit now" (action), and "I am already eating two or more servings of fruits a day" (maintenance).

Some examples of instruments are shown in Tables 8-1 and 8-2. These instruments can be given using a pencil-and-paper format (most common). Participants usually complete the instruments on their own. Questions are usually read aloud to young school-aged children or low-literacy audiences, who then complete the questionnaire. The questionnaires should look inviting and be motivational to complete, using pictures, drawings, or other visuals to add interest. Various interactive approaches can also be used. One interactive approach used with school-aged children is to alternate team games to answer some questions with individual responses to questionnaires tapping mediating variables and behavior (Eck, Struempler, & Raby, 2005). Instruments can be read aloud to individuals in an interview setting where literacy is low. They can also be administered through computer or Web-based technologies.

To evaluate whether there have been improvements in the selected mediators of behavior, you calculate changes in scores in these variables. You average the score of all participants for each of the questions in the pretest given at the beginning of the program, and you average the score of all

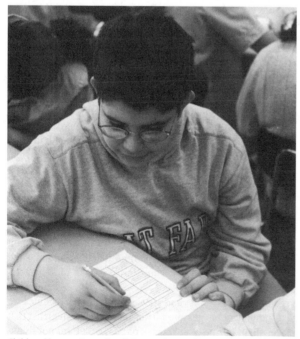

Children like questionnaires if they are interesting.

participants on the same instrument given as a post-test at the end of the program. You then examine whether there has been an improvement in scores and whether this improvement is statistically significant. (You will generally also compare this improvement to that of a group that did not get the program to see if the improvement is due to the program.)

In many programs, the changes in indicators are expressed in terms of percentage of individuals who demonstrate ability to engage in skills that are relevant to the behavioral target of the program, such as the percentage who can adjust menus or prepare foods to achieve the goal behaviors (e.g., reduce fat or increase fruit and vegetable content of menus) or who can set goals, develop action plans, and practice self-regulation skills.

Information on impacts on mediating variables can also be obtained through in-depth interviews, focus groups, and other qualitative methods (Straus & Corbin, 1990). In this case, the interviews are first transcribed and then analyzed for categories and emerging themes. The analysis involves an iterative or repeated process, in which cases are first reviewed and the data grouped into categories or codes that may be based on prior research or program goals. As new cases are reviewed and added to the coding scheme, the categories and themes may change. This is repeated until there is consensus that the codes have captured all the information. The findings may also be shared with the recipients as validation.

Evaluating impacts on the program goal behaviors or practices: medium-term outcomes. In behavior-focused and evidence-based nutrition education, increased engagement in the program goal behaviors is usually the major outcome of interest in an evaluation. This outcome is usually sought by various stakeholders, including participants themselves. Individuals usually give of their time and effort to participate in nutrition education programs because they desire to eat more healthfully or in a way that fosters sustainability of the food system, or for other reasons. The goal behaviors or practices are selected early in the nutrition education design process (Step 1 in our system). You will need to select the indicators and measures that are appropriate for your program. The following are some potential indicators and measures for you to consider.

Indicators of behavioral outcomes can include the following:

- Improved intake of specific foods or increase in behavior targeted by the program. This could include increased intake of certain foods (such as fruits and vegetables or calcium-rich foods), decreased intake of targeted foods (such as sodas or high-fat, high-sugar foods), eating a healthy diet (defined), or increasing physical activity.
- Improved intake of nutrients derived from these foods, such as a decreased percentage of fat in the diet, or an increased amount of carotene or calcium.

- Engagement in the program goal behaviors. These are visible food-related actions that individuals take. The behaviors can be very specific, such as reducing fat in the diet; eating one or more servings of vegetables at lunch and dinner; drinking sweetened beverages; eating breakfast; or eating at a fast food restaurant. Behavioral indicators can also involve practices such as shopping at local farmers' markets or buying organic foods.

Measures. Tools for measuring behaviors depend on the exact indicators of effectiveness chosen, the size of the group, the level of accuracy desired, the purpose of the evaluation, and the resources available. A detailed discussion of these methods is outside the scope of this book: they are usually described in nutritional assessment books. Many of the ones commonly used in nutrition education interventions have been reviewed (Kristal & Beresford, 1994; McPherson et al., 2000; Hersey et al., 2001; Keenan et al., 2001; McClelland et al., 2001; Medeiros et al., 2001; Contento, Randell, & Basch, 2002). They may include the following.

Food Intake

- *Observations of intake.* In school settings, this usually involves observing how much of meals that were served is eaten or thrown away; thus, the method is often called measurement of estimated plate waste. This can be done by preweighing the average serving size of each item served. Students in groups, such as classes sitting together, are observed or asked to leave their trays, and the amount left on each plate is recorded on a predesigned recording sheet or is videotaped and analyzed. This is a very labor-intensive method and requires trained personnel. It is also time-consuming for the participant (called *respondent burden*).
- *Recalls of foods consumed, usually over the previous 24 hours (24-hour dietary recall).* Here program participants are asked to recall all the foods and beverages that they consumed during the previous 24-hour period. This is usually done individually but can also be done as a group, such as a class. The recalled foods can be manually scored for the quantity of intakes of the foods targeted by the program, such as fruits and vegetables or calcium-rich foods, or they can be converted into nutrients of interest to the program, such as percentage of fat in the diet, using a computer diet-analysis program. This is a very labor-intensive method and requires trained personnel; respondent burden is moderate.
- *Food records.* In this instance, participants keep a record of their intakes of food and drinks over a three-day or seven-day period. The records can be analyzed for the targeted foods, such as fruits and vegetables, snacks,

soda, or high-fat foods, or analyzed for nutrients (e.g., percentage of calories as fat, amount of calcium), as for the 24-hour recalls. This too is a very labor-intensive method, requiring trained personnel, and respondent burden is very high.

- *Food frequency questionnaires.* There are standard food frequency questionnaires that you can use that contain fairly long food lists. Individuals indicate how frequently they have eaten foods on this list during the past year or some other time period. The foods on this list can again be scored for the individual foods of interest or can be converted to nutrients, again using a computer program. These standardized questionnaires usually use forms that can be optically scanned. These can be self-administered in a group setting. The respondent burden for participants is moderate, and lower than for the methods listed previously (Willett et al., 1987; Block et al., 1992).
- *Food intake checklists or short food frequency questionnaires.* These are food frequency questionnaires that are usually shorter than the ones described in the last item and may include behaviors as well as intakes of specific foods (e.g., Kristal et al., 1990; Yaroch, Resnicow, & Khan, 2000; Townsend et al., 2003). Examples of validated short food frequency instruments are shown in Table 7-1 and Box 7-2.
- *Brief checklists or screeners.* These are even shorter food frequency questionnaires, involving only a short list of the foods of interest, such as fat intake screeners or fruit and vegetable screeners. Some examples are the Centers for Disease Control and Prevention's Behavioral Risk Factor Surveillance System (BRFSS) (Serdula et al., 1993), the National Cancer Institute's 5 A Day fruit and vegetable screener (NCI, 2000), or the Rapid Screener for Fat and Fruit and Vegetable Intake (Block, 2000).

A note about food frequency questionnaires: The food list must use an appropriate inventory of foods commonly eaten by the audience you are working with, and the names of the foods should be clearly understood by the audience (these often differ by ethnic group). Food frequency questionnaires tend to overestimate intakes and so are best used to compare intakes before and after the nutrition education program rather than to provide estimates of actual intakes. They also ask about intake over a time span of a month to a year, and hence may not be suitable for short-term community programs.

Eating Behaviors or Patterns

- *Food behavior checklists or questionnaires.* These instruments or tools measure specific observable food-related behaviors, such as behaviors related to high-fat diets, eating fruits and vegetables, buying local or organic foods, shopping practices, food safety behaviors, or food insecurity. Excerpts from a widely used instrument for fat- and fiber-related diet behavior are shown in Box 7-2 (Shannon et al., 1997). Here the behaviors related to reducing fat in the diet are categorized as modifying foods to make them lower in fat, avoiding fat as a seasoning or condiment or in cooking, using lower-fat substitutions, or replacement of high-fat foods with fruits and vegetables and other lower-fat foods.. Those related to fiber are categorized as eating cereals and grains, eating fruits and vegetables, and substituting high-fiber for low-fiber foods.

- *Eating patterns.* These tools provide information on specific eating patterns, such as whether the participants are eating breakfast.

Diet Quality

- *Dietary quality indices or questions.* Sometimes a single question can be used, such as "How would you describe the quality of your diet?" Other instruments provide an assessment of the overall quality of the diet. A prime example is the USDA's Healthy Eating Index. For this, however, you will need both food intake information and nutrient (fat) intake information. The index is available online for use by individuals.

Evaluating impacts on Physiological Parameters: Long-term outcomes. In some nutrition education programs, the expected outcomes are reduced risk for chronic disease or improved health. The indicators are improvements in nutritional status (iron deficiency, bone health) or in physiological diseases risk status.

- *Biochemical or physiological measures.* A variety of measures are used. For example, for those with diabetes, maintenance of appropriate blood glucose levels may be the appropriate measure; for a weight gain prevention program with youth, body mass index (BMI) may be the primary outcome measure. For heart disease prevention program, serum cholesterols may be used as the outcome measure.

Evaluating changes in environmental supports. Indicators and measures of program effectiveness in terms of changes made in the environment to make it more supportive of the program goals are very specific to each program. Some examples are shown here, but you will need to develop specific indicators and measures for your program. Figure 14-2 shows a framework for evaluating the multiple levels of intervention that may be addressed by an intervention.

Tables 14-2 and 14-3 describe some examples of indicators and measures that can be used to evaluate the impact of a

program on the social support of children by their parents (Table 14-2) and on the social support provided by family, coworkers, and participant groups in workplaces (Table 14-3). These measures can be assessed before and after the program; changes in scores on these measures are indicative of the impact of the program on these outcomes.

Many changes in environments to make them more supportive of healthful eating require the collaboration and partnership of nutrition educators with various individuals and groups that provide food or services or have decision-making power in that environment, such as school administrators, workplace and institutional managers, community organizations, and food providers, as described in Chapter 13. The role of the nutrition educator is to educate these individuals and institutions about the importance of nutrition, health, or food system issues; to work in collaboration with them; and to provide technical support where appropriate. In schools, the food environment is more controlled than in workplaces. The intervention, and hence the evaluation, can be more formal and systematic. In workplaces, the changes usually involve adding food options to existing menus and making some changes rather than systematic changes. Table 14-4 describes indicators and measures of change for institutional environmental supports. Table 14-5 lists indicators and measures for community food and social environments.

Criteria of effectiveness. For each of the measures you choose to evaluate the program, you will also need to decide the level of change that you will consider as necessary to judge effectiveness. Will a statistically significant change be the demonstration of effectiveness (such as an increase in intake of fruits and vegetables, or an improvement of self-efficacy or perceived benefits)? Or will the change have to reach some criterion level (such as five or more servings of fruits and vegetables per day)? For stages of readiness to change, will any movement be considered acceptable or does the movement have to be from motivation to action (e.g., from precontemplation or contemplation to preparation or action)?

In terms of change objectives directed at environmental supports for the targeted behaviors, what will serve as criteria of effectiveness? All changes made at the 100% level (e.g., all school meals are to be 20% to 35% fat), or an average for the week? Is the criterion whether fresh fruit and vegetables are available every day, or just some days? Should the criterion be the availability of low-fat options in all worksite cafeteria meals or some? By what percentage should food stamp redemptions at farmers' markets increase?

Gathering the Outcome Evaluation Data: Selecting, Adapting, or Designing and Testing the Instruments for Measuring Program Effectiveness

There is no handbook of evaluation tools or instruments for nutrition education from which you can select one that is right

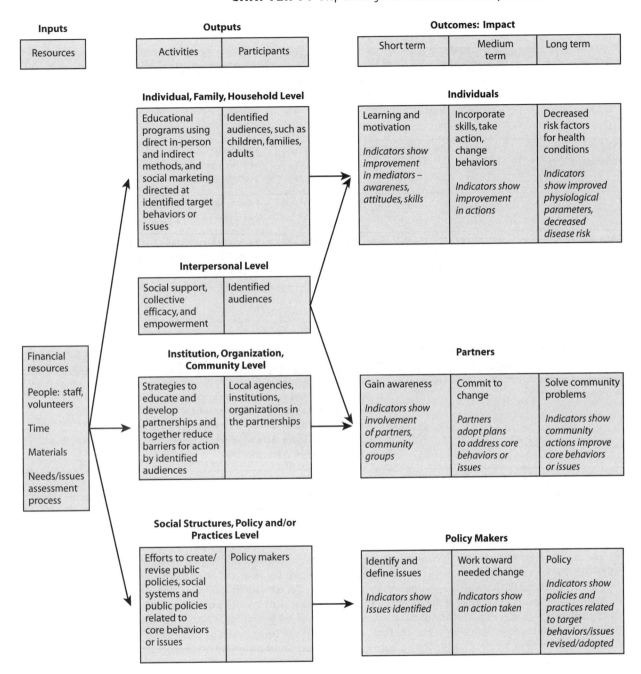

FIGURE 14-2 A logic evaluation model for nutrition education involving multiple levels of intervention. *Source:* Based on the Community Nutrition Education (CNE) Logic Model, Version 2: Overview. January 2006. Helen Chipman, National Coordinator, Food Stamp Nutrition Education, CREES/USDA, and Land Grant University System Partnership. Used with permission.

for you. There are many reasons for this: nutrition education interventions need to be specific to the behavior that has been selected as the focus and to the intended audience. Rarely are two interventions identical. Tools need to be appropriate to the specific intervention, so it is not easy to find one that is exactly appropriate for the intervention you are designing.

TABLE 14-2 Examples of Outcomes, Indicators, and Measures for Evaluating Parental/Household-Level Support of Healthful Behaviors

Outcomes	Indicators of Achievement of Outcomes	Measures (Surveys) for Indicators
Behaviors	Parents/family members demonstrate increased availability and accessibility of healthful foods for their children, as targeted by the program	Parents indicate from a list whether healthful foods targeted by the program are present in the home and offered at meals (e.g., Marsh, Cullen, & Baranowski, 2003).
Outcome expectations: *Perceived benefits*	Increased understanding of the impact of F&V on health.	Knowledge instrument (written or oral) on role of various nutrients in F&V in health and disease (multiple choice).
		Parents report on policies with respect to children's tasting new foods and choosing how much to eat.
Social modeling	Parents/adults in household are serving as role models for their children by increased consumption of healthy foods targeted by the program.	Parents report quantity and frequency of personally eating a list of fruits and vegetables (e.g., Reynolds et al., 2002).

TABLE 14-3 Examples of Indicators and Measures for Evaluating Family, Coworker, and Support Group Support at Workplaces

Indicatorsof Achievement of Outcomes	Measures or Instruments for Indicators
Increased coworker support; increasedfamily/household support	Individuals complete surveys; for example, on whether coworkers, family, or social support group members never, seldom, sometimes, or often • Compliment their attempt to eat healthfully • Bring healthful foods or fruits or vegetables them to try Encourage them to eat more healthful foods (e.g., more fruits and vegetables) (Sorensen, Stoddard, & Macario, 1998)
Increased number of social support groups and high degree of functioning within groups	Observations of support group functioning and checklists Qualitative interviews of group participants and group facilitators

However, research on instrument development is ongoing, and many usable tools are being constantly generated and tested. These can be identified through a search of the literature or government sources. The *Journal of Nutrition Education and Behavior* and *Journal of the American Dietetic Association* are rich sources of potentially useful instruments. There are many other journals as well. For example, some instruments have been validated with low-resource adult audiences in the domain of reducing fat in the diet or increasing fruit and vegetable intake; some have been validated for upper elementary school-aged children, and so forth. When selecting, adapting, or developing a new instrument, you need to consider the following.

Appropriateness. In some types of educational interventions, the educational activities that participants will complete can also serve as evaluations. For example, in school food and nutrition education, activities in community nutrition education, or WIC clinics, many of the evaluations work best as activities that participants will complete as part of the learning units. In this case, some system must be set up to record the results of these evaluation activities.

For educational purposes, it is useful to consider an evaluation activity for *every* specific educational objective. This will let you know whether the educational objectives you set are being achieved. Sometimes this may be quite informal—how many individuals seem to be engaged as assessed by how many are actively participating, or how many are able to carry out a new skill (such as label reading), or how many individuals stated an intention to take action by actually writing a contract for a goal they want to achieve. In our ongoing case study (presented later), we show some of these activities.

In most cases, nutrition educators will use specific instruments administered separately from the educational activities. These should measure achievement of your behavioural goal and general education objectives directed at mediators.

TABLE 14-4 Institutional Environmental Supports: Examples of Outcomes, Indicators, and Measures for Evaluating Supports for Healthful Action

Outcomes	Indicators of Achievement of Outcomes	Measures or Instruments for Indicators
Food environment		
School food service personnel or workplace food vendors will provide healthful meals.	Training conducted for food service personnel Manuals developed for food service personnel	(Process measures: Was training conducted? Were manuals developed?)
	Behaviors: Staff follows recommended food purchasing and preparation methods	Interviews and observations using checklists to identify how many, which, and how often recommended practices are carried out Review of purchase records
	Food quality reflects changes recommended by program	Analysis of planned and actual menus (computer nutrient/food composition programs) Observation of food services on-site
Food service personnel or workplace vendors will conduct food-related activities in the cafeteria.	Increased promotional activities in cafeteria	Checklist completed by staff on number of activities per month Review of quality of foods promoted: checklist or observation
Vending machines will carry healthful items.	Guidelines for healthful vending machine items developed and implemented	Review of guidelines (process measure)
	Increased number/proportion of healthful items in vending machines	Number and/or proportion of healthful items available in the vending machines, using a checklist
School or workplace stores will carry healthful food items.	Guidelines for school stores developed and implemented; increased number/proportion of healthful items in stores	Review of guidelines (process) Count of number and/or proportion of healthful items available in stores
School, workplace, or health care setting catering will use foods from local farms or local processors.	Increased number or proportion of selected foods from local sources	Count of number and/or proportion of foods from local sources being served in cafeteria meals
Grocery stores will highlight items supportive of program's behavioral goal.	Product labeling (and maybe pricing); educational or promotional signage	Degree to which labels are in place; signage in place

continues

Table 14-4 (continued)

Outcomes	Indicators of Achievement of Outcomes	Measures or Instruments for Indicators
Information environment The information environment will be supportive of healthful eating.	Posters: Positive and consistent messages about healthful eating provided throughout the school	Number of posters designed and posted; content consistent with program goals
	Informational materials	Number of brochures, newsletters distributed Survey of students/employees: number read, degree of satisfaction, what learned
Policy environment or organizational climate Good policies are supportive of healthful eating.	Schools: Existence of food (or health) policy council Participation on council by a variety of stakeholders	Review of documents; interviews Review of minutes of meetings; lists of participants; agendas
	Policies for foods available in schools or workplaces encourage healthful eating	Mission statements; annual reports with a description of policies (existing and newly adopted) that have been implemented (number and degree of implementation)
	Worksites: Existence of employee advisory boards	Minutes of meetings; lists of participants; agendas
	Participation on boards; activities	Survey instrument of participatory strategies (e.g., Linnan et al., 1999; Ribisl & Reischl, 1993)
Organizational climate is supportive of healthful eating.	Assessment of organizational and policy climate	Schools: Changes in scores on a school health index or score card, such as the School Health Index for Physical Activity, Healthy Eating, and a Tobacco-Free Lifestyle: A Self-Assessment and Planning Guide (CDC, 2004a, 2004b); or Changing the Scene Healthy School Nutrition Environment Improvement Checklist (USDA, 2000)
		Workplaces: Changes in scores on checklist of workplace policies and environment such as Heart Check (e.g., Golaszewski & Fisher, 2002)

TABLE 14-5 Community Food and Social Environments: Increased Support for Healthful Action

Outcomes	Indicators of Achievement of Outcomes	Measures or Instruments for Indicators
A social environment that is supportive of healthful action	Coalitions and partnerships: number, type, depth, and strength of partnerships	Number of organizations in the coalition or network Scales to describe the depth of the partnerships: Dialogue and information sharing from referrals to common focus and sharing of resources to longer-term commitment to joint action and joint leadership to formal links and decision making; contributions of each partner (Gregson et al., 2001)
	Nature and frequency of media coverage; community events (to enhance social norms for action)	Print media: Number of news articles, inches of column space times circulation Electronic media: Minutes/seconds of airtime and monetary value of that time Pubic relations events: Amount of materials disseminated
Community food environment	Number of grocery stores that now carry or highlight targeted foods	Observations at the sites using checklists; interviews; data maintained by organization
	Number of farmers at farmers' markets who now accept food stamps	

They need to be appropriate for the intended audience. If you need to design your own instruments, remember that designing such instruments is not easy, even for a one-time session or for short interventions. How much time and effort you should spend on such instruments depends on the purpose of evaluation and the degree of measurement accuracy needed or desired.

The most commonly used procedure is to identify those instruments that are close to your intervention in terms of behavioral focus and mediators addressed and to modify or adapt them for use with your specific audience. If you are working with adolescents or a low-resource audience, for example, check whether the instrument you have identified as potentially useful has been developed and validated for that group. Whether you modify or develop your own, you will need to consider the issues related to nutrition education tools or instruments described below.

Validity. *Validity* is a generic term that refers to different kinds of accuracy—the degree to which the instrument adequately or correctly measures the variable or concept under study, whether that variable is in the domain of knowledge or of mediating variables, or is a behavior. The following list provides a brief description of the different types of validity. Check for these when you are reading nutrition education intervention articles, selecting your instrument, or developing your own.

- *Content validity*. Are the items on the test, questionnaire, or inventory reasonably representative of the larger domain or content covered? For dietary intake, are the items on the food frequency questionnaire truly representative of what is typical for this audience? If we are interested in knowledge about fruits and vegetables, are the items representative of that domain?
- *Face validity.* Face validity is an aspect of content validity in which a panel of experts review the instrument to ensure that it measures what it is intended to measure. In addition, are the language, formats, and procedures of the instrument understandable and reasonable from the program participants' point of view?
- *Criterion validity.* Does the score generated by the instrument correlate well with data obtained with a criterion measure? For example, does the fruit and vegetable questionnaire correlate well with seven-day food records or serum carotenoid levels?
- *Construct validity.* Does the instrument clearly measure the construct it is supposed to be measuring, such as self-efficacy?

Reliability. *Reliability* is a measure of the consistency and dependability of the instrument. There are several kinds of reliability.

- *Reproducibility or test-retest reliability:* Consistency or stability over time. It is the degree to which the instrument, used at different times with the same people, will give the same result.
- *Internal consistency:* Consistency within a set of items. Is the instrument internally reliable or consistent? For example, if you have four self-efficacy items, is there consistency among them? For knowledge items, split-half reliability or KR-20 coefficient is usually calculated, whereas for mediating variables, item-total correlations or Cronbach's alpha coefficient (Cronbach et al., 1980) are calculated.
- *Interrater reliability:* Consistency among data collectors. If two or more people will be collecting the information or coding it, has interrater reliability been established? For example, do two nutritionists code the fruit and vegetable intake data from 24-hour recalls in the same way?

Sensitivity to change. *Sensitivity* is the degree to which an instrument can detect changes resulting from an intervention.

Cognitive testing: Readability and understandability. *Readability* is the ease of comprehension of the evaluation tool by the intended audience given its vocabulary, sentence length, writing style, or other factors. Reading-level formulas can help make that determination. *Understandability* goes beyond readability to assess whether the instrument content is understood by the audience the way you intend. This can be judged by having participants tell you what they think each question means or is asking about, a process called *cognitive testing.* Even if you choose to use an existing instrument, you should still test it for understandability with your particular audience.

Qualitative data. Qualitative data, such as information from observations, in-depth interviews, focus groups, or open-ended surveys, are also subject to reliability and validity considerations. In this case, the criteria are dependability, credibility, and trustworthiness. *Dependability* is somewhat like reliability, in that other people need to be able to follow the procedures and decision trail of the original investigator to understand how the findings were obtained; documentation of all steps is thus crucial. The *credibility or trustworthiness* of the findings is indicative of validity. Credibility is increased through engagement with the individuals over a sufficiently long time to understand the phenomenon being studied, through persistent observation, and through the use of several sources and methods to study the same phenomenon, yielding consistent information. This process is called *triangulation.* Often, the findings are shared with the participants for verification, called *peer debriefing.* In addition, the findings need to ring true to readers, in that they can recognize an aspect of human experience is being described, even though they have only read the study.

Pilot testing. Extensive pilot testing of instruments and data collection procedures is absolutely essential. This cannot be emphasized enough. Whether borrowed or developed anew, instruments must be tested with your particular audience.

Selecting an Appropriate Evaluation Plan to Measure Impacts

The purpose of an evaluation plan or design is to ensure that evaluation results are due to the nutrition education program and not to some other confounding factors. Thus, evaluation plans are designed to rule out competing explanations for the results that you get. This allows you to measure the true impact of the program. The nature of the design depends largely on which plan is most feasible given the type of power, duration, or intensity of the educational intervention and the context in which it is occurring and the financial and time resources and expertise available.

The *true experimental design* or *randomized control trial* (RCT) is considered ideal for research purposes. It is routinely used in clinical studies. In this design, individuals, WIC clinics, schools, or worksites are randomly assigned to two groups, one receiving the nutrition education program (intervention condition) and the other receiving the usual education or another unrelated intervention (the control condition). Both groups are given test instruments before and after the intervention. One major advantage of this design is that the randomization process ensures that significant differences in outcomes are attributable to the program. A disadvantage is that randomization is very difficult to do in practice settings.

Quasi-experimental designs are traditionally viewed as more realistic models for field evaluation studies. The most common design within this category is the *comparison-group design with pretest and post-test,* in which one group receives the program and is compared with a second matched comparison group that does not receive the program and is selected from a similar population and matched on various characteristics, such as age, gender, ethnicity, or socioeconomic status. Both groups are given pre- and post-tests. Gain scores are compared between the two groups. In school settings, this means that entire classes may be matched with similar classes in the same school, or entire schools matched with other schools. WIC clinic groups receiving an intervention may be matched with groups from WIC clinics with similar characteristics. Although these designs do not guard against all competing explanations for the results, they do control for various important sources of error while remaining a fairly workable method for most programs in practice settings.

Nonexperimental designs use two common approaches. In the *one-group pretest and post-test design,* scores are compared before and after the program in the same group. There is no comparison group. In the *post-test-only design with non-equivalent comparison groups,* the scores of those who have received the program are compared with a similar group that did not receive the program. These designs make it difficult to rule out other explanations. However, such designs are often the only ones feasible in practice settings and can provide important insights.

In *interrupted time series designs*, a number of observations are made over a period of time as a baseline, and then the program is introduced. A series of observations are then made after the program. If the scores remain constant for a time before the program and then increase after the program and remain constant at that higher level for some time after the program, the increase may be attributable to the program. This conclusion is strengthened if the observations are accompanied by time series observations of a no-treatment comparison group. Again, while many sources of error remain, this design can provide some insight into the effectiveness of the program.

Surveillance studies monitor the status of a population or group on outcomes of interest such as dietary intakes or attitudes toward healthful eating. Such studies can document how a group is doing over time but cannot explain what causes the observed status.

Qualitative evaluation methods can be used as an alternative to quantitative designs. These methods are generally inductive in nature and rely on such strategies as observations, structured and semistructured individual and group interviews, focus groups, historical records, and questionnaires. Qualitative methods can boost the power of quantitative methods by focusing on the dynamics and contexts of change since the latter tend to focus on the outcomes of the interventions. Qualitative methods also enlarge the observational field to capture actual, and often unintended, changes. Qualitative methods can help to develop and delineate program elements, such as current practices, values, and attitudes of participants, leadership styles, staffing patterns, and relationships among program activities

Conducting Evaluations Ethically: Informed Consent

Evaluations should be conducted ethically. This means that you should obtain informed consent from program participants to participate in the evaluation. Participants should not be coerced into completing evaluation activities. Their responses should be anonymous or confidential and should not jeopardize them in any way. Participants should not be denied essential services on the basis of their responses or lack thereof.

Your Turn

As we have noted before, designing nutrition education programs is an iterative process in which we go back and forth between various tasks. The design of evaluation methods goes hand in hand with the design of educational strategies. Thus, at the time that each of the educational objectives and

educational strategies is being designed in Steps 4 and 5, an evaluation method should be considered. Now is the time to finalize the evaluation methods.

Instructions and examples have been given throughout the chapter for how to design evaluations for your program. Because evaluations are so varied and the possibilities are so numerous, no worksheets are given for overall evaluation processes. Worksheet 14-1 is provided to help you think about developing evaluation measures to evaluate the impact of a program on potential mediators of behavior change or action.

Case Study

Our ongoing case study has been with middle school youth, addressing the goal of increasing their intake of fruits and vegetables. The conceptual framework for evaluating the intervention described in our case study uses a logic model and is shown in Figure 14-3. The inputs of the program are the resources invested. The outputs include the activities conducted within the three major components of the program—students, parents, and school environment— and the specific theory-based strategies that are used to address the specific mediators of behavior change: motivational mediators, action mediators, and environmental mediators. As you can see from the model, outcomes can be short, medium, or long term. Given the resources available, the case study intervention will measure short-term and medium-term outcomes. Long-term outcomes are shown and can be measured later in time.

The evaluation in Case Study 14-1 shows the potential methods for evaluating the impact of the intervention on the behavioral goal, the general educational objectives directed at the potential mediators of the behavioral goal, and the specific educational objectives for the two sessions designed in Step 5. For each of these impacts, indicators of achievement of impacts are shown as well as the measures used, as follows.

- *Impact of program on goal behaviors.* The behavioral goal is for adolescents to increase their intake of a variety of fruits and vegetables. The indicator for this impact is fruit and vegetable intake. The measure to be used is a food frequency questionnaire validated for youth.
- *Impacts of educational strategies on mediators of goal behaviors.* Recall that in order to develop theory-based strategies to address specific mediators of behavior, the mediators are first expressed in terms of educational objectives. The case study evaluation lists the educational objectives as well as the mediators of each educational objective (in parentheses). Indicators of each of the mediators are then shown, along with potential measures.

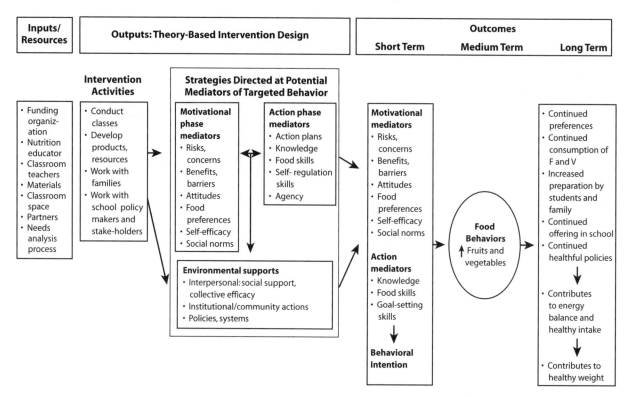

FIGURE 14-3 Conceptual framework for designing the evaluation for The Whys and Whats of Colorful Eating.

Questions and Activities

1. Give three reasons why it is important to evaluate nutrition education, no matter how briefly.
2. Distinguish between formative and summative evaluation and between outcome and process evaluation.
3. In terms of evaluation, describe each of the following terms, indicating the relationships among them and to educational objectives:
   a. Outcomes
   b. Indicators
   c. Measures
   d. Instruments
   e. Evaluation plan
   f. Data collection methods

4. Describe four ways for measuring each of the following:
   a. Behavioral outcomes
   b. Potential mediators of behavioral outcomes
   c. Policy change
   d. Changes in school food environment
5. Distinguish between a true experimental design or randomized control trial (RCT) and quasi-experimental designs.
6. Distinguish between validity and reliability in terms of evaluation instruments. What is the relationship between these two features?

STEP 6 WORKSHEET Design the Evaluation for Theory-Based Nutrition Education

WORKSHEET 14-1 Evaluation Worksheet Example for Developing Measures for Potential Mediators of Behavioral Change

Theory Constructs or Mediating Variables	Outcomes	Indicators of Achievement of Outcome	Measures
Outcome expectations; knowledge of scientific evidence of benefits	Understanding and appreciation of the importance of targeted behavior (e.g., eating a variety of fruits and vegetables (F&V))		
Personal risk assessment	Evaluate their own intake of F&V compared with recommendations; understanding of one's personal risk; recognition of specific enacting target behavior		
Barriers	Identify barriers		
Preference/sensory-affective response to eating F&V	Enjoyment of target behavior (e.g., eating a variety of F&V)		
Attitudes	Positive attitudes toward target behavior		
Behavioral intention	Intention to initiate target behavior increase own F&V intake		
Self-efficacy	Increased self-efficacy for target behavior		
Behavioral capability	Increased knowledge and skills for targeted behavior		
Self-regulation/goal-setting skills	Action plans to increase their consumption of F&V developed and implemented using goal-setting and decision-making skills		

CASE STUDY 14-1   Step 6: Evaluation

Title of program: The Whys and Whats of Colorful Eating

Impact of program on goal behaviors

- *Behavioral outcome*: Adolescents will increase their intake of a variety of fruits and vegetables.

- *General indicator for this outcome:* Increases in fruit and vegetable intake

- *Specific indicator:* Increases in intakes of a specific list of F&V

- *Measure to be used:* A food frequency questionnaire validated for youth

- *Criterion of effectiveness:* A statistically significant increase in intake of fruits and vegetables compared with baseline and compared with the intakes in a matched comparison class of middle school students

Impacts of educational strategies on potential mediators of goal behaviors: Desired outcomes for mediators of behaviors are addressed by general educational objectives.

Outcomes in relation to mediators (General educational objectives): Adolescents will be able to
- Demonstrate understanding and appreciation of the importance of eating a variety of fruits and vegetables (Mediators are outcome expectations and scientific knowledge of benefits.)

- Evaluate their own intake of fruits and vegetables compared with recommendations (Mediator is personal risk assessment.)

- Identify barriers to intake of fruits and vegetables and propose ways to overcome them (Mediator is barriers.)

- Express enjoyment of and positive attitudes toward eating a variety of fruits and vegetables (Mediators are preferences/sensory-affective response to eating fruits and vegetables and positive attitudes.)

- State intention to increase own fruit and vegetable intake (Mediator is behavioral intention.)

- Demonstrate increased self-efficacy in eating a variety of fruits and vegetables each day (Mediator is self-efficacy.)

- Demonstrate increased knowledge and skills in incorporating fruits and vegetables into their daily food patterns (Mediator is behavioral capability.)

- Prepare action plans using goal-setting and decision-making skills to increase their consumption of fruits and vegetables (Mediator is self-regulation/goal-setting skills.)

Table 14-1 listed potential mediators, outcomes in relation to the mediators (based on general objectives), and general indicators of achievement of these outcomes. Table A follows up with a list of *specific* indicators that operationalize the general indicators and specific measures/instruments. Tables B and C describe evaluation measures for specific educational objectives in our case study's pre-action, motivational phase lesson (Table B) and action-phase lesson (Table C). Strategies and measures for evaluating the impacts of the program on promoting environmental supports are shown in Table D.

TABLE A Indicators and Measures of Impact for Potential Mediators of Program Goal Behaviors

Specific Indicators	Measures/Instruments for Indicators
Outcome expectations Increased understanding of benefits of eating more F&V and risks associated with not eating sufficient F&V	Scale with responses of 1 to 5, from strongly disagree to strongly agree. Outcomes might be as follows: have more energy, make me stronger, and help me do well in school, help me maintain a healthy weight, and so forth.
Youth will be able to demonstrate increase in scientific knowledge of a list of specific diet–health relationships & importance of variety	Knowledge instrument: Multiple choice questions on scientific evidence linking F&V and skin health, bone development, disease risk reduction, and importance of variety.
Preference Increased preference for 15 commonly eaten and nutritious F&V	Scale with responses of 1 to 5, from dislike a lot to like a lot
Increased positive attitudes toward themselves eating F&V	Scale with responses of 1 to 5, on attitudes about self-eating more F&V (e.g., "I feel I am taking care of my body when I eat F&V.")
Self-efficacy Confidence in being able to eat more F&V in general, and in specific situations, including difficult ones	Scale with responses of 1 to 5 on how confident learner feels about eating F&V (e.g., "If I wanted to, it would easy to eat more vegetables") Questions would also ask about difficult situations: "If I decided to eat fruit every day, I could still succeed when I did not feel like eating fruit," "when there are other sweets," etc.
Food- and nutrition-related knowledge and skills Youth will be able to demonstrate increase in knowledge of a list of specific ways to add F&V to daily diet	Knowledge and skills instrument: Multiple choice questions and some open-ended questions, scenarios.
Intention to eat more fruits and vegetables	Two items with responses from 1–5 on "I intend to add two or more servings of fruits and vegetables each day" and "It is likely that I will add two or more fruits and vegetables each day to my diet."
Goal-setting skills Youth will demonstrate increased ability to use specific skills in setting goals, making plans	Scenarios with questions about setting goals, planning ahead, and developing strategies to overcome roadblocks; multiple choice questions based on scenarios

F&V = fruits and vegetables.

TABLE B Measures of Specific Educational Objectives: Pre-action, Motivational-Phase Lesson

Potential Mediator of Behavior (*Educational strategies*)	Specific Educational Objectives for Mediator	Learning Experiences, Messages, or Content	Evaluation Measures
	At the end of the session or program, the learner will be able to:	Gain attention by bringing in a variety of F&V of different colors, shapes, & sizes: ask group to guess names & talk about them. Today will focus on the *whys* of eating a rainbow of colors, and next time will focus on the *whats*.	
Outcome expectations *Health benefits/pros of behavior*	State benefits of eating F&V: energy, hair, skin; build strong bones & muscles for athletic performance	Use a worksheet activity, or have group volunteer benefits of eating F&V; list on newsprint. Build on prior knowledge and experience (grounding or anchoring).	Correct answers orally or on a questionnaire at the end of the sessions about F&V contributions to health and other benefits
	State the key reasons for eating a variety of F&V ("a rainbow of colors")	Emphasize the need for variety of intake (a colorful plate). List the five colors: blue/purple, green, white, yellow/orange, and red.	Correct answers orally or on a questionnaire on nutrients in colorful F&V
Personal risk *Self-assessment/ personalizing risk*	Describe risks to health from eating too few F&V	Provide scientific evidence that eating F&V makes for strong bodies; clear up misconceptions.	Correct answers orally or on a questionnaire on nutrients in colorful F&V
	Evaluate personal risk of not eating enough F&V	Checklist, or 24-hour recall, of own intake of F&V and compare with recommendation for number and colors: Is there a rainbow on your plate?	Completion of 24-hour recall and correct identification of how many and which F&V to eat
Barriers and self-efficacy	Identify barriers to eating F&V	Group brainstorms barriers to eating F&V; list on newsprint.	Self-efficacy questions, tapping confidence in being able to eat more F&V
Overcoming barriers	Identify ways to overcome barriers to eating F&V	Group brainstorms ways to overcome barriers.	
	Describe ways in which F&V can be easy to eat	Group discusses ways to make behavior easy to do.	
Social norms *Exposing peer pressure; modeling*	Describe the role of peers in influencing food choices	Students express what peers say when they eat F&V.	Instrument asking about importance of social norms
	Appreciate that vegetables are cool to eat	Provide relevant models (media models, stories) eating F&V, showing it is cool.	
Outcome expectations: taste *Direct experience with food*	Appreciate that fruits and vegetables taste good	Provide a fruit salad or vegetables and dips for tasting.	A preference scale with list of F&V

Potential Mediator of Behavior (*Educational strategies*)	Specific Educational Objectives for Mediator	Learning Experiences, Messages, or Content	Evaluation Measures
Behavioral intention *Values clarification* *Decisional balance*	Evaluate the pros and cons of eating a variety of colors	Group activity: Present value statements, and group discusses. Worksheet for each person to record pros and cons of adding F&V to diet	Questions about attitudes toward F&V and about self eating F&V.
	State an intention to add one fruit or vegetable a day to diet	Make decision about actions to take— individually or share with group.	State an intention to eat more F&V in the next day or week.

F&V = fruits and vegetables.

TABLE C Measures of Specific Educational Objectives: Action-Phase Lesson

Potential Mediator of Behavior Change (Educational strategies)	Specific Educational Objectives for Mediator	Learning Experiences, Messages, or Content	Evaluation Measures
Behavioral capabilities *Food- & nutrition-related knowledge & cognitive skills*	*At the end of the session/ program, the learner will be able to:* State the key reasons for eating a variety of F&V ("a rainbow of colors")	Review reasons for eating a variety of F&V; key nutrients in them, health benefits, and need for variety of intake.	Knowledge instrument: Correct answers about nutrients in colorful F&V, serving sizes, and comparisons between F&V and energy-dense snacks
	Compare the nutrient content of F&V snacks with processed & packaged energy-dense snacks	Show commonly eaten packaged energy-dense snacks; worksheet for students to calculate & compare fat and vitamin C content with F&V.	
	Estimate servings sizes of F&V	Show serving sizes; do engaging group activity for estimating serving sizes (e.g., group contest for correct answers).	
Behavioral skills *Familiarity*	Describe how these F&V can be used in meals and as snacks	Present tips on how to use F&V in meals & snacks.	
	Prepare simple recipes using F&V		
	State satisfaction in trying new F&V	Provide exciting cooking experience if possible; or, teens in groups make different snacks from new fruits and/or vegetables: salads, salsa. Teens eat foods or snacks they prepared.	
Personal action goals *Action plans*	State clear personal action goals to eat more F&V	Teach skills in goal setting & developing action plans to achieve personal action goals; provide contracts.	Review contracts students wrote to ensure appropriate statement of goals
	Make action plan to eat all the colors during a given week	Worksheet for action plan to eat all the colors during the following week.	
Self-regulation skills *Goal setting Self-assessment; action plan; contracting; self-monitoring; rewards*	Appreciate the importance of recognizing hunger and satiety cues during a busy day	Activity to teach students to identify hunger, mood, and cues for food intakes.	Review contracts written and progress toward goals selected
	Develop plan, incorporating F&V, to satisfy hunger when it occurs and follow plan during a busy day	Provide opportunities to plan F&V to eat during a busy day; make contract; monitor progress toward that goal; reward self when goal is achieved. If more than one session, provide opportunities for feedback and rewards.	In instrument, present scenario involving goal setting and obstacles; ask about appropriate goals, ways to overcome obstacles, and ways to reward self

F&V = fruits and vegetables.

TABLE D Impacts of Program on Promoting Environmental Supports

Environmental Determinants (Current status)	Environmental Support Objectives	Strategies to Achieve Environmental Support Objectives	Evaluation Procedures
Food environment Barriers (Taste, convenience, cost)	School will provide many opportunities for students to taste F&V.	Nutrition educators and food service staff will provide taste tests for F&V in the cafeteria.	Document number of events, quality of F&V items served; survey participants about quality and impact
	School food service personnel will provide healthful low-fat, high-vegetable meals.	Meet with food service director to identify changes; professional development & manuals will be provided for food service personnel.	Were manuals developed and training conducted? *Behaviors:* Did staff follow recommended purchasing and preparation practices? • Interviews and observations using checklists to identify how many, which, and how often recommended practices are carried out • Review of purchase records • Analysis of planned and actual menus (computer nutrient/food composition programs) *Impacts:* Has food quality changed? *Students:* Do they notice or like changes?
Policy environment	Establish school food policy council to develop guidelines for foods available in school.	Presentations with school administrators, teachers, and parent associations about need for school policies.	Was policy council established? How many and who on it? (Review of membership list, minutes of meetings)
	School nutrition advisory council will develop food policies.	Recruitment to council: administrators, food service staff, teachers, students, parents, and others.	
	Develop guidelines for items in vending machines and school stores.	Develop guidelines for vending machine items.	Were guidelines developed and implemented?
	Vending machines will carry healthful F&V items.	Vendors will supply healthful items in vending machines.	Number of healthful items available in the vending machines and in stores
	School stores will carry healthful F&V food items.	Develop guidelines for items in school store (e.g., 50% will be healthful items).	
Social support (No role models)	Provide social models.	Bring in celebrities for school assembly.	How many? Issues addressed? Survey students for response
Information environment (Eating F&V not normative)	Develop posters for cafeteria; newsletter for family.	Focus group with teens; design posters with teens about eating F&V; post them.	Number of posters designed and posted
		Write and design student newsletter to make eating F&V normative (include principal and teachers).	Number of newsletters sent; quality of information

REFERENCES

Block, G., F.E. Thompson, A.M. Hartman, F.A. Larkin, and K.E. Guire. 1992. Comparison of two dietary questionnaires validated against multiple dietary records collected during a 1-year period. *Journal of the American Dietetic Association* 92:686–693.

Block, G., C. Gillespie, E.H. Rosenbaum, and C. Jenson. 2000. A rapid screener to assess fat and fruit and vegetable intake. *American Journal of Preventive Medicine* 18:284–288.

Centers for Disease Control and Prevention. 2004a. *School Health Index: A self-assessment and planning guide. Elementary school version.* Atlanta, GA: Author.

———. 2004b. *School Health Index: A self-assessment and planning guide. Middle school/high school version.* Atlanta, GA: Author.

Chang, M.W., S. Nitzke, R.L. Brown, L.C. Bauman, and L. Oakley. 2003. Development and validation of a self-efficacy measure for fat intake behaviors of low-income women. *Journal of Nutrition Education and Behavior* 35:302–307.

Contento, I.R., J.S. Randell, and C.E. Basch. 2002. Review and analysis of evaluation measures used in nutrition education intervention research. *Journal of Nutrition Education and Behavior* 34:2–25.

Cronbach, L.J., et al. 1980. *Toward reform of program evaluation: Aims, methods, and institutional arrangements.* San Francisco: Jossey-Bass.

Eck, S.M., B.J. Struempler, and A.A. Raby. 2005. Once upon a time in America: Interactive nutrition evaluation. *Journal of Nutrition Education and Behavior* 37:46–47.

Freedman, D.S., and G. Perry. 2000. Body composition and health status among children and adolescents. *Preventive Medicine* 31:S34–S53.

Golaszewski, T., and B. Fisher. 2002. Heart Check: The development and evolution of an organizational heart health assessment. *American Journal of Health Promotion* 17:132–153.

Green, L.W., and F.M. Lewis. 1985. *Measurement and evaluation in health education and health promotion.* Palo Alto, CA: Mayfield.

Gregson, J., S.B. Foerster, R. Orr, et al. 2001. System, environmental, and policy changes: Using the social-ecological model as a framework for evaluating nutrition education and social marketing programs with low-income audiences. *Journal of Nutrition Education* 33:S4–S15.

Hersey, J., J. Anliker, C. Miller, et al. 2001. Food shopping practices are associated with dietary quality in low-income households. *Journal of Nutrition Education and Behavior* 33:S16–S26.

Keenan, D.P., C. Olson, J.C. Hersey, and S.M. Parmer. 2001. Measures of food insecurity/security. *Journal of Nutrition Education* 33(Suppl. 1):S49–S58.

Kohl, H.W., J.E. Fulton, and C.J. Casperson. 2000. Assessment of physical activity among children and adolescents: A review and synthesis. *Preventive Medicine* 31: S54–S76.

Kristal, A.R., B.F. Abrams, M.D. Thornquist, et al. 1990. Development and validation of a food use checklist for evaluation of community nutrition interventions. *American Journal of Public Health* 80:1318–1322.

Kristal, A.R., and Beresford, S.A. 1994. Assessing change in diet-intervention research. *American Journal of Clinical Nutrition* 59(Suppl.):185–189S.

Linnan, L.A., J.L. Fava, B. Thompson, et al. 1999. Measuring participatory strategies: Instrument development for worksite populations. *Health Education Research* 14:371–386.

Marsh, T., K.W. Cullen, T. Baranowski. (2003). Validation of a fruit, juice, and vegetable availability questionnaire. *Journal of Nutrition Education and Behavior* 35: 93–97.

McClelland, J.W., D.P. Keenan, J. Lewis, et al. 2001. Review of evaluation tools used to assess the impact of nutrition education on dietary intake and quality, weight management practices, and physical activity of low-income audiences. *Journal of Nutrition Education* 33:S35–S48.

McPherson, R.C., D.M. Hoelscher, M. Alexander, K.S. Scanlon, and M.K. Serdula. 2000. Dietary assessment methods among school-aged children. *Preventive Medicine* 31: S11–S33.

Medeiros, L.C., S.N. Butkus, H. Chipman, R.H. Cox, L. Jones, and D. Little. 2005. A logic model framework for community nutrition education. *Journal of Nutrition Education and Behavior* 37:197–202.

Medeiros, L., V. Hillers, P. Kendall, and A. Mason. 2001. Evaluation of food safety education for consumers. *Journal of Nutrition Education* 33:S27–34.

National Cancer Institute. 2000. *Eating at America's Table Study: Quick food scan.* Bethesda, MD: National Cancer Institute, National Institutes of Health. http://riskfactor. cancer.gov/diet/screeners/fruitveg/allday.pdf.

Reynolds, K.D., A.L. Yaroch, F.A. Franklin, and J. Maloy. 2002. Testing mediating variables in a school-based nutrition intervention program. *Health Psychology* 21:51–60.

Ribisl, K.M., and T.M. Reischl. 1993. Measuring the climate for health at organizations. Development of the worksite health climate scales. *Journal of Occupational Medicine* 35:812–824.

Serdula, M., R. Coates, T. Byers, et al. 1993. Evaluation of a brief telephone questionnaire to estimate fruit and vegetable consumption in diverse study populations. *Epidemiology* 4:455–463.

Shannon, J., A.R. Kristal, S.J. Currry, and S.A. Beresford. 1997. Application of a behavioral approach to measuring dietary change: The fat and fiber-related diet behavior questionnaire. *Cancer Epidemiology, Biomarkers and Prevention* 6:355–361.

Sorensen, G., A. Stoddard, and E. Macario. 1998. Social support and readiness to make dietary changes. *Health Education Behavior* 25:586–598.

Straus, A.L., and J. Corbin. 1990. *Basics of qualitative research: Grounded theory procedures and research.* Newbury Park, CA: Sage.

Thompson, F.E., and T. Byers. 1994. Dietary assessment resource manual. *Journal of Nutrition* 124(11 Suppl.):2245s–2317s.

Townsend, M.S., and L.L. Kaiser. 2005. Development of a tool to assess psychosocial indicators of fruit and vegetables intake for 2 federal programs. *Journal of Nutrition Education and Behavior* 37:170–184.

Townsend, M.S., L.L. Kaiser, L.H. Allen, A. Block Joy, and S.P. Murphy. 2003. Selecting items for a food behavior checklist for a limited-resources audience. *Journal of Nutrition Education and Behavior* 35:69–82.

United States Department of Agriculture. 2000. *Changing the scene: Improving the school nutrition environment.* Alexandria, VA: U.S. Department of Agriculture, Food and Nutrition Service. http://www.fns.usda.gov/tn/Healthy/index.

Willett, W.C., R.D. Reynolds, S. Cottrell-Hoehner, L. Sampson, and M.L. Browne. 1987. Validation of a semi-quantitative food frequency questionnaire: Comparison with a 1-year diet record. *Journal of the American Dietetic Association* 87(1):43–47.

Yaroch, A.L., K. Resnicow, and L.K. Khan. 2000. Validity and reliability of qualitative dietary fat index questionnaires: A review. *Journal of the American Dietetic Association* 100(2):240–244.

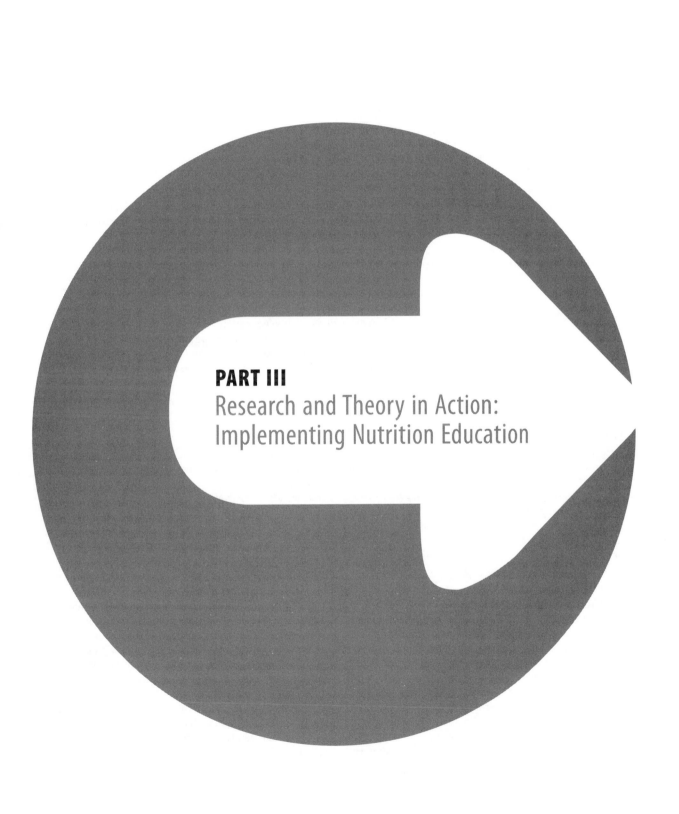

PART III
Research and Theory in Action:
Implementing Nutrition Education

Communicating Effectively in Group Settings

OVERVIEW   This chapter provides an overview of communication principles, learning styles, and group dynamics and how they can inform practical methods for implementing nutrition education with groups.

OBJECTIVES   At the end of the chapter, you will be able to

- Describe basic principles of communication and a communication model for nutrition education
- Apply learning style research in delivering nutrition education
- Use information on group dynamics to more effectively deliver nutrition education
- Describe key features in conducting facilitated group discussions and dialogues
- Apply public speaking principles to making presentations and leading workshops

---

SCENARIO

You have attended a comedy show and laughed all the way through. You want to share the jokes with your friends, so you decide to memorize one of the routines word for word. You present the jokes to your friends and do not get the same laughs. Why not? Because you were not able to *deliver* the jokes in the same way the comedian did. He was effective because of his manner of presentation, his facial expressions, the inflections of his voice, his gestures, and most important, his perfect sense of timing. Likewise, a wonderfully designed nutrition education session can be ruined by poor delivery. This does not mean that wonderful delivery will turn a poorly designed session into an effective one. The issue you want to address must be important and relevant to the group. But having something to say or planning an interesting session is not enough. You must also know how to deliver it.

Introduction: Understanding Communication

You have designed the nutrition education program, including its goals and objectives and theory-based education strategies, and have laid out your evaluation plan. You are ready to do what you like to do most—conduct nutrition education. Now what? How exactly should you proceed in the designated setting? Part III describes exactly how to deliver the intervention in practice through a variety of channels, including group sessions, printed materials, and other media. Conducting group activities and developing other supportive activities requires numerous skills even after the intervention content and activities have been carefully planned. This chapter focuses on working with groups, and the next chapter focuses on implementing nutrition education through a variety of other channels that might accompany group sessions, such as supporting visual media, written materials, grocery tours, health fairs, mass media communication campaigns, social marketing activities, and other venues.

Although the design and delivery of nutrition education are described in different sections of the book, you will probably find that you will go back and forth between these two activities. For example, as you think about how exactly you will deliver what you have designed, you may find that you need to go back to Step 5 of the procedural design model to make changes in your educational plans to make them more in line with your delivery strategies. Because all interactions among people involve communication, communication is at the heart of nutrition education with groups. This chapter begins with a brief description of communication.

Communication is one of those terms we use frequently and yet would have a hard time defining. The word comes from the Latin *communis*, meaning "common." In general it refers to all methods of conveying thought and feeling between individuals. Most definitions have in common the notions that communication is the process of sending and receiving messages and that for a transmission of messages to be successful, a mutual understanding between the communicator and the recipient must occur. Communication refers to what is expressed verbally or nonverbally; it applies to articulated words and to unvocalized feelings. In a broad sense, then, communication includes all methods that can convey thought or feelings and describes interactions between individuals and groups as well as between various media and people.

The term *interpersonal communication* is often used to describe the communication context that involves direct, face-to-face interaction among persons, whether one on one or in small groups. The term *mediated communications* is often used to describe the communication that occurs through some nonpersonal channel such as television or radio, printed materials, telephone, and advertising.

Basic Communication Model

How much time do you spend each day talking with other people? If you are like other adults, you spend about 30% of your waking hours talking with or communicating with others. Thus we are all very familiar with the notion of communication. Communication consists of very complicated processes that are described in numerous books and articles. Here we briefly describe only its chief features. First we describe a model that captures the basic elements of communication, and then we expand on this model for the nutrition education context.

This model states that communication involves the following components arranged in the following sequence:

1. Communication source, or sender
2. Message (sent through one or more channels)
3. Channels
4. Receivers (audience)

In the case of nutrition education, the communication source or sender is the nutrition educator, who sends a message (which can be as simple as "Eat more fruits and vegetables" or much more complex, such as how to get your child to eat healthfully) through channels such as lecturing, making a presentation, leading a group discussion, newsletters, interactive media, or mass media campaigns to receivers, who are groups or individuals, such as mothers of young children, who *attend* to the message, *comprehend* it and *process* it cognitively and affectively, and *act on it*, either by accepting it or rejecting it.

This basic model is clearly unidirectional, with a message being sent by a source to receivers, who receive the message somewhat passively. It does not capture the richness and complexities of interactions *among* individuals in groups that influence message processing. For example, in group discussion, all individuals take turns being the sender and the receiver through the channel of speaking. However, this model can be used to implement some mediated communications through nonpersonal media and in interpersonal settings such as presentations and lectures, where there is very little interaction among group members. After we explore the basic components of this model, we then describe how the communication process is modified by complex interactions in social settings, where much of deliberate nutrition education occurs.

Communication Source Characteristics

We need to begin with the recognition that just as we cannot *not* behave, so too in any situation involving social interaction we cannot *not* communicate. This means that you, as the nutrition educator, are communicating at all times, regardless of whether you are conscious of it or whether the communication is intentional or successful. Communication of the message is more likely to be effective if nutrition educators have the following characteristics.

High credibility. Nutrition educators are more likely to have high credibility if they are perceived by the audience as having competence and trustworthiness. Competence refers to having the skill, knowledge, and judgment relevant to the issue. Credibility can be *extrinsic*, which refers to the audience's perception of the source before the message is delivered (e.g., by virtue of the nutrition educator's position or reputation), or *intrinsic*, which refers to the image of authoritativeness that the nutrition communicator, such as a speaker to a group, creates as a direct result of how the message is delivered.

To increase credibility, then, when you introduce yourself or are introduced you need to let the audience know your professional qualifications and experience. This needs to be done with sensitivity: you cannot be boastful or self-serving, but you should not be overly modest either. The audience needs to know that you are qualified to lead the group. It will help them relax and feel that they are in good hands. How you come across during the session also influences your credibility and trustworthiness. For instance, if your tone is authoritative and you are organized, the audience will be much more convinced than if you sound tentative.

Trustworthiness refers to nutrition educators coming across as having no ulterior motives for the opinions they offer or the actions they advocate. That is, they have "good motives." To ensure an audience's trust, you need to make clear to audience members that you are not using the occasion to sell something to them. If you do represent your own business or practice or a given group, corporation, or industry, you need to clearly indicate this to the audience.

Attractiveness or dynamism. Sources are more effective when they are likable or attractive in the sense of having an attractive and dynamic personality and being seen as healthy. This is especially true when the audience is not initially motivated. Your enthusiasm will go a long way.

Similarity or common ground with the audience. Effectiveness is enhanced if the audience perceives that the nutrition educator has some common ground with the audience or at least a sense of affinity with them. Communication specialists point out that because emotion always influences decisions, the audience must sense that the communicator understands their problems and cares. Empathy, or affinity with the audience, is called for, not sympathy, which can be patronizing. Audiences need to feel that they are respected.

Thus, you are more effective if you establish some common ground by initially expressing some views that are also held by the audience and by demonstrating understanding of the opinions and lives of group members. For example, while discussing the topic of food labels, you may want to acknowledge how confusing and time-consuming reading food labels can be (a personal story can be very powerful here). Then go on to provide the necessary label-reading skills. In discussing parenting practices, you can express understanding and respect for what the (parent) audience members face on a day-to-day basis. Again, a personal story about your own children, or children you have worked with, can be very helpful. It is important to be authentic, however. Using the latest hip language with a group of teenagers, for example, when it is obvious that this is not congruous with who are and how you would normally speak, will only make the teenagers think you are phony.

Message Characteristics

Every communication has a content aspect, which is the manifest or overt information being conveyed. These are the words we speak, the message we are trying to convey, or the illustrations and pictures we present, such as about breastfeeding. Every communication also has an implied or metacommunication aspect, which is information about the information, or a set of rules for interpreting the manifest information, whether this is conveyed consciously or not. In verbal communications it could be our tone of voice or facial expressions. In the case of printed messages, metacommunication could be conveyed through the pictures we use, the layout, and the ordering of content. This meta-level information provides the audience with rules for interpreting the content: it helps the audience judge whether the nutrition educator thinks the information being presented is really important or whether the nutrition educator is being humorous or serious.

Message characteristics to increase processing by audience. Message characteristics have been the focus of this book and are at the heart of Step 5 of the design model, described in Chapters 11 to 13. A health message or nutrition communication is really a set of arguments for a particular behavior or practice or information on how to take action, or both. These arguments are based on the perceived benefits or outcome expectations for the given practice for the intended audience that we have talked about throughout the book. We have referred to these arguments as "why-to" or motivational information. These arguments form the basis of much of your nutrition education content. Such information can be based on the scientific evidence for the desirability of the behavior or practice, such as breastfeeding or eating calcium-rich foods. It can also be based on benefits of a personal nature or can address some emotion related to the practice. An example we have given before is the Pick a Better Snack campaign: here the message about eating fruits and vegetables focuses on overcoming barriers to taking action by showing how easy it is to do. This message thus also addresses an attitudinal or emotional aspect—that is, it is not a bother to eat fruits and vegetables. Messages can also convey information and skills of a "how-to" nature, such as how to read a food label or how to prepare a given food.

The *elaboration likelihood model* of communication reminds us that individuals differ in their ability and motivation to process educational messages, or arguments, thoughtfully (Petty & Cacioppo, 1986). (See Chapters 4 and 11 for more details.) To increase the *ability* of the audience to process messages, make your messages straightforward and clear, repeat or reinforce them, and present them with a minimum of distractions. To increase the *motivation* of the audience to process messages, make the messages unexpected or novel, memorable, culturally appropriate, and, most important, personally relevant. The messages can be expressed in terms of what participants will gain from taking action, as well as what they will lose by not taking action. Messages can involve humor, warmth, or other attributes as found to be appropriate for a given audience. The use of emotion-based messages through materials and activities has been shown to be especially effective (McCarthy, 2005). Use these principles whether you deliver the messages through the mass media, brochures, newsletters, or in a group setting.

Nonverbal communication accompanying the message. When nutrition education is delivered in person, nonverbal communication always accompanies the verbal message and is often more influential than the verbal. Receivers learn to trust their interpretations of the nonverbal messages because they know that these cannot be consciously selected or controlled by the sender. Indeed, communication experts believe that the image the nutrition educator projects may account for over half of the total message conveyed to a group at first meeting. Nonverbal communication includes facial expressions, tone of voice, eye contact, gestures, and touch. Nonverbal cues, particularly facial expressions and tone of voice, can express acceptance and support for group members or judgment and disapproval.

Nonverbal cues can indicate whether you are working *with* the group to state barriers and identify ways to overcome them or manipulating them to come up with the solutions you think are best. We are often judgmental and do not know it; however, the audience is very quick to pick up on it. For example, a nonjudgmental tone is straightforward and sounds provisional instead of dogmatic or defensive. Tone of voice and mannerisms can also express whether you respect the group and consider yourself a member or whether you feel superior. Compare expressions such as "You may not be able to grasp this, but believe me, I have been doing this for 10 years and it works," with "That sounds like a good idea. I have worked with others who found it did not work for them, but you are the one who must be satisfied with the eating pattern. So you can experiment and find whether it works for you. Let us know how it goes." As you work with groups or make a presentation, be very aware of the nonverbal messages that you are transmitting.

Nonverbal communication also accompanies verbal communication through nonpersonal channels, such as videos, media campaigns, websites, posters, or newsletters. The graphics, colors, visual images, and music or sounds used all convey information. Thus all these features must be carefully selected to support the message.

Receiver or Audience Characteristics

Identifying the characteristics of the audience is extremely important in any health communication model. This is done through a process of assessment of audience interests, needs, and characteristics, sometimes called *formative research* or *marketing research*. In our procedural model for designing theory-based nutrition education, the predisposition and interests of receivers are carefully identified in Steps 1 and 2, where we analyze the behaviors and practices of our audience and the potential mediators of these behaviors and practices, such as their stage of emotional readiness to change and which social psychological factors influence their food-related practices. This information formed the basis of your educational design in Step 5 and therefore will not be repeated. The following are a few characteristics that are likely to affect how audience members may attend, comprehend, and react to the message.

Personal motivation to process the message. Audience members are predisposed to react to messages in a particular way by their own experiences, beliefs, attitudes, and habits. Successful communication takes into account these predispositions and the reasons behind them. That is, the message must be personalized or tailored to the predispositions, outcome expectations, attitudes, and needs of the audience, as we have emphasized throughout the book, in order to increase motivation to process the message. As noted earlier, these personalized messages should be meaningful and memorable.

Message-processing skills. Audience members' skills in processing the message also influence the effectiveness of the communication. Receivers must understand, process, and elaborate on a message before it can have an effect on their attitudes or behaviors. Thus receivers' abilities to listen, read, think about, or understand the nutrition concepts you wish to communicate are important considerations when designing and delivering the message. Make the message clear and straightforward for the given audience, but never condescending.

Life situation. Sometimes other things are going on inside receivers that may interfere with their willingness and ability to process messages. As researchers have noted, cognitive information is filtered through our affective states (Achterberg, 1988). Audience members who are sick or in pain or who are anxious and worried will not be able to attend to messages as well as those who are calm and well. This means that the messages or session content and methods used must gain the attention and affect the comprehension of the audience despite such interference.

Learning style. Participants' preferred learning styles influence how much attention they pay to a message. For example, in the context of group sessions, listening to you lecture may be the last thing a group of adolescents will want to do, whereas a cadre of executives may be perfectly comfortable listening to your message; they may indeed prefer this mode of communication. These learning styles are explored in greater detail later in this chapter.

Social roles. The social status roles of the audience also influence response to the message. These roles are behaviors expected of people because of their position in society—for example, the role of "mother," "busy executive," and so forth. Audience members must feel that the message is appropriate for their role in society.

Communications in Social Context

The complexity of food- and nutrition-related behaviors and the social nature of communication has led to a more complex understanding of nutrition communications (Gillespie & Yarbrough, 1984). The social context of communications also affects their reception in various ways.

The receivers' reference groups may influence response to the message. People are socially organized, with formal or informal group memberships or reference groups. These can be peers, family, and others whose opinions are valued by audience members. Research indicates that the response to messages is a social phenomenon that involves not only what the audience members think of the messages but also what trusted others, such as family members, close friends, or coworkers, think of the message. That is, individuals' responses are influenced by what they think others will think of their new opinions or actions. For example, teenagers will be more likely to change beverage choices if they think the change would be acceptable to their peers.

The nutrition educator and receivers both provide inputs into the communication process. Communication is a two-way, not a one-way, street. The nutrition educator designs the sessions, but the audience provides inputs, more formally through the needs analysis process (as in Steps 1 and 2 of our design process), and *always* during the sessions themselves. This is often called *feedback*. As we saw earlier, we cannot *not* communicate. This means the audience in a group setting cannot not communicate to the nutrition educator as well. Even in a very structured situation such as a lecture class, it has been found that when students in one half of the class look bored, pass notes, and start having side conversations and those in the other half are fully alert and interested and asking questions, the instructor will soon direct all his or her attention to the latter half of the class. The audience has thus shaped the behavior of the communicator.

Complex interactions among individuals influence outcome. This interaction may be of two types: between the audience and the communicator, and between audience members and their reference groups or peers. These complex interactions influence acceptance or rejection of the communication. The nutrition educator and the audience communicate with each other verbally or nonverbally, consciously or unconsciously, and these interactions influence outcome, as we have just noted. Others also influence audience members in the group. For example, if the reference group norm for teens is that answering the nutrition educator's questions during question-and-answer periods is not cool, then you will need to find other ways to engage students, such as small group discussions or projects.

Consequently, messages and group sessions are more likely to be effective if interactions between the communicator and the audience and between the audience members and their peers are built into the communication process. For example, women are more likely to adopt breastfeeding if they think this practice will be acceptable in the eyes of their peers. Here a group process whereby women can share their perceptions and feelings with others in the audience would enhance communication. Successes and challenges can be shared, and mutual learning can take place. Indeed, Freire's dialogical method of critical consciousness-raising (Freire & Shor, 1987) or Vella's method of facilitated dialogue (Vella, 2002), in which educators or communicators pose questions and engage in dialogue with the group to facilitate understanding of the causes, consequences, and possible solutions of problems identified by the group, may be very suitable in certain circumstances. We discuss these issues in greater detail later in this chapter.

Implementing nutrition education as designed requires attention to the considerations regarding the characteristics of the communicator, audience, and message just discussed. We now explore in greater detail two characteristics of receivers that influence how they will process our nutrition messages: their styles of learning and their social interactions in group settings.

Understanding Learning Styles

One of the receiver characteristics that we need to keep in mind is that individuals have different learning styles. A given audience may have one predominant learning style, but more likely, the group will include people with different learning styles. Thus, different types of learning activities are needed within each session to accommodate these differences. The various design features we emphasized in Step 5 took learning style into consideration, although we did not state so at the time. Here we first describe the different learning styles and then relate them to the design features in Step 5.

Kolb's Model of Learning Styles and Experiential Learning

Based on his research of the experience of learning, Kolb proposed that individuals differ in the way they understand their experience of, and adapt to, the world, and that these variances can be placed on a continuum of perception (Kolb, 1984). At one end of the continuum are the sensing/feeling individuals who project themselves onto the current reality of each experience by sensing and feeling their way around. Conversely, people on the thinking end of the continuum tend to analyze experiences logically through their intellect. People do move back and forth on the continuum, but most of us have a comfortable "hovering place." Each of these two kinds of perception has strengths and weaknesses. Both are valuable. Learners need both perspectives.

The second way in which people learn differently is in how they process experiences and information. When confronted with learning new things, some people watch and reflect first to filter the experience through their own value system. Other people jump in and act immediately, saving the reflection for later, if at all. Watchers need to internalize; doers need to act. Neither way is better, but rich learning involves both.

When these two kinds of perceiving and processing are looked at together, a four-quadrant learning style model is formed (Figure 15-1).

- *Imaginative learners* process information reflectively and process it by intuiting and feeling. They want the world to be a meaningful place for them and therefore strive to connect personally to the content they are learning. They believe in their own experience and are interested in people and culture.
- *Analytic learners* perceive information abstractly and process it reflectively. They learn by thinking through concepts and pay attention to expert opinions. They

are industrious and thrive in traditional classrooms and nutrition education lecture settings. Verbally skilled and avid readers, analytic learners sometimes see ideas as being more fascinating than people.

- *Commonsense learners* perceive information abstractly and process it actively. They learn by applying theories to practice and are avid problem solvers. They need to know how things work and wonder how (and if) what they learn in a nutrition education session can be of immediate use to them.
- *Dynamic learners* perceive information concretely and process it actively. They learn by trial and error and are enthusiastic about new things. They are at ease with people and enjoy taking risks and wrangling with change. Dynamic learners pursue interests through a variety of avenues, and therefore the structure of formal nutrition education sessions seems limiting to them.

Kolb (1984) suggests that each session or series of sessions include learning activities that address each of these learning styles, in the following sequence: concrete experiences, observations and reflections, formation of abstract concepts and generalizations, and testing the implications of concepts in new situations (Table 15-1).

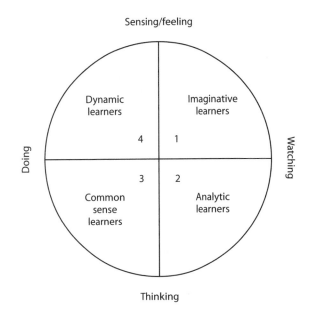

FIGURE 15-1 The four major learning styles. *Source:* Kolb, D.A. 1984. Experiential learning. Englewood Cliffs, NJ: Prentice Hall.

TABLE 15-1 Learning Activities to Address Each Learning Style

What does using the learning style approach look like in terms of instructional activities? Use activities to address all the learning styles by "teaching around the cycle."

Quadrant and Learner Type	Focus	Educational Activities
Quadrant 1: *Imaginative learners*		
Creating a concrete experience	Focus on sensing and feeling. Activate knowledge by making learning meaningful. The focus is on the learners and how they can connect what is being learned to themselves. The aim is motivation of learners.	Trigger films, demonstrations, hook questions, brainstorming, word webbing, puzzles, observations, games
Quadrant 2: *Analytical learners*		
Observing, reflecting, and analyzing experience; integrating reflective analysis into concepts	Focus on watching/reflecting. Assist learners to gain knowledge by introducing needed content. Learners reflect on prior experience from quadrant 1 and develop concepts and skills. The aim is to facilitate ability to take action.	Discussions, mini-debates, journals or logs, thinking questions, analyses of pros and cons, mini-lectures (graphs and charts, pictures or overheads, summaries), readings
Quadrant 3: *Commonsense learners*		
Developing abstract concepts and/ or skills; practicing skills	Focus on thinking. Assist learners to examine how they can apply what they have learned. The aim is to provide opportunities for practice.	Making or completing graphs/charts, drawings, conclusions; case studies; writing activities; "minds-on" worksheets
Quadrant 4: *Dynamic learners*		
Practicing and adding something of oneself; analyzing application for relevance or usefulness	Focus on doing. Encourage creativity and self-expression by asking group members to take what they have learned and practiced and expand on it in their own way. The aim is to challenge the group to incorporate new motivations, learning, and skills in an ongoing way into their lives.	"Hands-on" activities; contracts, commitments, or action plans; developing products or videos, puzzles and/or skits, and simulations; field study; field visits

1. The sessions can begin with asking participants to investigate their own prior knowledge, attitudes, or behaviors through an activity. We called this self-assessment in earlier chapters. There may be other concrete ways to make the session personal and relevant to the participants.
2. The second part of the session or program can address why-to knowledge for the audience to observe and reflect on, such as the latest scientific information about the benefits of taking action. This could be a mini-lecture, incorporating graphs and visuals where appropriate. Together these two sections of the sessions will increase interest and motivation.
3. The next part can focus on activities for the individuals to begin to form their own understandings of the issues related to taking action, such as through needed how-to knowledge and skills.
4. Finally, the group can take steps to apply the knowledge gained by setting goals for specific actions they will take (Beffa-Negrini & Cohen, 1990).

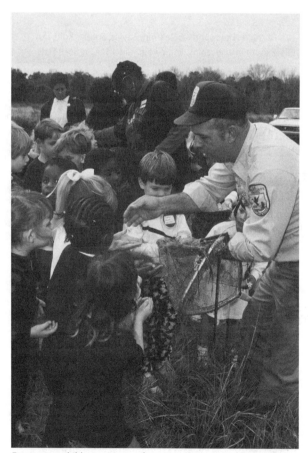

For younger children, a trip to a farm to see how vegetables and fruit are produced may be a great way to create a more hands-on learning experience.

As you can see, these steps reflect the instructional sequence advocated by Gagne (1985) and modified by Kinzie (2005) that we used as the basis of our educational plan or design sequence in Step 5. That sequence of the events of instruction, as you recall, is as follows:

1. Gain attention.
2. Present stimulus or new material, based on the prior knowledge and experience of the audience.
3. Provide guidance.
4. Elicit performance and provide feedback.
5. Enhance retention and transfer.

Learning style research tells us *how* to design activities in each of the events of instruction so as to incorporate different learning styles. Such an approach integrates behavioral nutrition theory, learning styles research, and instructional design principles.

It should be noted that as nutrition educators, we tend to teach according to our own learning style preferences, so we should be aware of what they are and follow this sequence to ensure that we will deliver nutrition education in ways that will reach individuals with different learning styles and enrich their repertoire of ways of learning (and perhaps our own at the same time!). With this information about learning styles in mind, you may need to go back and revise your educational plan or lesson plan and educational strategies to be appropriate for these considerations.

Implementing Learning in Groups

You have already designed learning experiences for nutrition education group sessions in Step 5. The following discussion concerns how to deliver the educational experiences that have been planned.

Methods for Implementing Learning Experiences

The sessions that you have designed may be delivered through many different instructional formats, such as lectures, demonstrations, hands-on learning tasks, or group discussions. These various formats are described in the following subsections.

Lecture

Lecture is still the predominant educational delivery method used today. It is how most of us were taught, and many of us tend to teach as we were taught. During lecturing, group participants play a passive role as learners while the leader assumes the role of expert. As we noted earlier, people remember only 10% of what they hear, so lecturing is not considered the most desirable method for reaching the public. A survey found that a group of mothers in the Women, Infants and Children (WIC) program, struggling with complex issues regarding getting their children to develop healthful eating patterns, gave lectures a very low rating.

The lecture method should not be ruled out entirely, however. It can be useful in classroom settings when presenting new information that students will be required to master later on, or at professional meetings when new information is presented to participants. In addition, lecture may be the preferred style of some types of learners. For example, one study examined the usefulness of social cognitive theory–based strategies such as taste testing, role playing, brainstorming, and goal setting to improve business executives' away-from-home eating behaviors (Olson & Kelley, 1989). The study found that these busy business executives hated the use of hands-on behaviorally based activities. They were already interested in making changes in their eating practices and wanted the necessary how-to information delivered quickly and compactly. Activities just took too long. This affirms the importance of finding out audience learning style preferences in the needs analysis in Step 2.

Generally, lecture works best when it is delivered in short, palatable bites. The average person can listen for no longer than 10 minutes before needing to stop to process the information being taken in. Visuals such as charts, graphs, and pictures enhance the presentation of vital information while helping to accommodate learners who are not keen on the lecture as a viable mode of delivery. Analytic learners may be amenable to a longer lecture, whereas dynamic learners will begin to squirm after the first 5 minutes. Of course, listening to an engaging nutrition educator on an issue of interest will make any lecture seem shorter.

Short mini-lectures can be embedded in an otherwise activity-based session. For example, a mini-lecture is very useful during the part of the session in which scientific evidence of perceived outcomes of behavior, both positive and negative, is presented. Likewise, a mini-lecture may be useful for providing evidence-based information about effective actions for reducing risk or improving health, whether personal, community, or environmental.

Brainstorming

Brainstorming is an effective method for getting groups of participants to generate lists in a creative way. Everyone has a creative streak in them, but as educators we need to get rid of the blocks that keep good ideas pent up. Establishing rules for brainstorming will help participants keep on track and feel safe enough to contribute. Dynamic and imaginative learners will prefer brainstorming over passive learning strategies. Brainstorming can be divided into two phases, for which the rules are as follows.

Phase One

- All critical judgment is ruled out; all ideas count.
- Wild ideas are expected; spontaneity, which comes when judgment is suspended, will flourish. Practical consideration is not important at this phase.

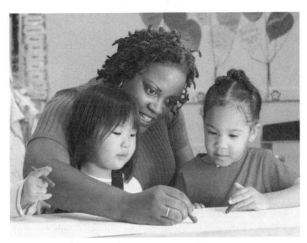

Brainstorming provides an effective, interactive way to involve everyone in a nutrition education lesson.

- Quantity, not quality, counts.
- Pool ideas and build on the ideas of others.

Phase Two

- Apply critical judgment—evaluate proposed ideas for feasibility.
- As a group, decide on the one or two best options if the group is interested in taking action.

Brainstorming can be useful in nutrition education for such purposes as generating a list of barriers to eating healthfully among teenagers, ways to get children to eat more healthfully, or easy meals for working moms to prepare.

Demonstrations, Including Cooking Demonstrations

Demonstrations can serve many functions. They can be used to show how something is done. They can also serve a motivational role and help the group explore ideas and attitudes. Often they serve both functions. For example, cooking demonstrations can teach skills. At the same time, they reduce the barriers to action in the participants watching and thus enhance their motivation and likelihood to take action. Other demonstrations do not specifically teach skills but are designed to enhance motivation. For example, you can spoon out the amount of fat or sugar in some popular fast foods and sweetened beverages. This will mean bringing to the sessions the target foods. We suggest bringing empty wrappers of the demonstration foods because the audience may want to know what you plan to do with the food after you are done. Saying you will throw it away gives the nonverbal message that you are comfortable with wasting food (not an appropriate message for any audience, and especially inappropriate for a low-resources audience). Or they may ask if they can take it home, which of course undermines your latent message.

Conducting demonstrations means that you must have all the materials you need at the site or must bring them with you. It has often been said that a major qualification for a nutrition educator is the willingness to take materials with you to sites, including food or food ingredients. Those with cars often find that their trunks are full. Those in inner cities using public transportation find other means. For example, one nutrition educator uses a suitcase on wheels to bring needed materials to sites: one that is large enough to include a portable butane stove plus a few needed pots and pans, utensils, paper towels, and so forth. She takes it in taxicabs and buses. A second major qualification of a nutrition educator is the willingness to be flexible, that is, to use whatever is available to make the demonstration work. For example, if you want to show how blood vessels can get clogged during a lifetime of eating high-saturated-fat foods, you may not be able to purchase the demonstration materials. But you can buy some clear tubing in a hardware store (to serve as the blood vessel), solid cooking fat, some food coloring, a funnel, and a large bowl. You can place some of the fat in the tubing to block it partially (you do not want to block all of it), dissolve red food dye in water, and pour it through the funnel into the tube, with the large bowl ready to catch the colored water.

It is important to practice demonstrations ahead of time to know that they will work under the circumstances of your session. This is especially important for demonstrating food preparation skills.

Activities and Learning Tasks

Activities and experiences can heighten learning in a way that no passive learning can. Indeed, as we have noted before: "I hear—and forget; I see—and remember; I do—and understand." In addition, we know from earlier in this chapter that active learning not only increases awareness but also enhances motivation. The doers—dynamic and common-

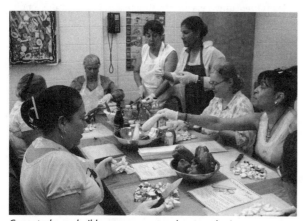

Group tasks can build empowerment and group cohesion.

sense learners—will prefer hands-on learning. These include the many activities and learning tasks that you might design for your participants, such as calculating fat or sugar content in foods, completing checklists, sorting items into categories, completing worksheets comparing foods in terms of cost and nutritional content, or analyzing local restaurant menus for the most healthful meals. If it is feasible, other learning experiences might be taste testing, cooking or simple food preparation, grocery store tours, and visits to farms or farmers' markets. See Table 15-1 for a summary of kinds of activities that can be done, particularly with youth.

Debates

Debates offer a lively vehicle for highlighting the two sides to an issue. There is much controversy in the area of foods and nutrition, as we are all aware. Instead of lecturing about the pros and cons of a given matter, have participants research each side and then go at it in the session. All learners will enjoy a good debate, but the doers—dynamic and common-sense learners—will probably prefer to do the debating, whereas the watchers will be content to sit and absorb the show. Good issues for debate might include whether to take dietary supplements, whether children should drink low-fat milk, and how to introduce healthy foods into the home.

The instructional strategies mentioned here are effective, diverse methods that promote learning across the styles spectrum. Most of them involve active participation in which group participants step beyond the role of passive sponges. Important in each of these approaches is for the nutrition educator to evaluate whether the task involves purely hands-on work or whether there is indeed a thinking, minds-on dimension serving the learning objectives that you have state in your educational plans.

Discussions

Discussions are one of the most constructive strategies for learning. In traditional schooling, a quiet classroom was considered a productive one. We now know that higher-order thinking skills require complex cognition, which is facilitated by verbalizing what we know, do not know, or want to know (Johnson & Johnson, 1991).

As nutrition educators, we can encourage our group participants to talk to each other. For example, we can use the enthusiasm that participants have for each other to promote learning. Passive learning, such as listening to the nutrition educator talk, does not employ the richer cognitive processes that promote memory, elaboration, or attitudinal changes. Imaginative learners will enjoy discussions regarding "what if" questions, analytic learners "why" questions, and commonsense learners "how" questions; dynamic learners will appreciate all three perspectives.

Interesting discussion questions in each category for nutrition education might include the following.

What if . . .

- You could only eat three foods for a whole week—what would they be?
- You lost the ability to taste—would you still enjoy eating?
- We could get all the nutrition we needed from one food—would every one eat that food and only that food?

Why . . .

- Can't we eat just eat ice cream for all our nourishment?
- Do people gain weight?
- Is there not enough food in the world to feed everyone?

How . . .

- Does the food you eat turn into you?
- Come there isn't one perfect food?
- Did the first loaf of bread get baked?

We discuss the use of facilitated group discussions in nutrition education after we have talked a little about the nature of groups and group dynamics.

Creating Environments for Learning

Kurt Lewin, who is considered a leading developer of the field of social psychology and who made profound contributions to our understanding of motivation of behavior, as we noted earlier in the book, is also generally considered to be the founder of modern group dynamics. His work on field dynamics or field theory has had enormous influence on our understanding of human behavior in the context of others.

He emphasized that our individual beliefs, attitudes, and habits are intimately related to those of the groups to which we belong. As humans, who always live in groups, we are constantly involved in dynamic interactions with others. These interactions can be symbolic or can be affective and emotional in nature. In his view, the group is not the sum of its members. It is a structure that emerges from the interaction of behaving individuals who constantly and dynamically adjust to each other to form a "field" (Lewin, 1951). The result of this mutual adaptation is a set of ever more complex patterns of behavior within the group. Neither the individual nor the group structure has an independent existence—they are mutually and dynamically dependent on each other, resulting in a set of group dynamics (Lewin, 1935, 1947).

Since then, investigators have conducted considerable research to try to understand the dynamics of human behavior in groups, including such concerns as the roles of group members, settings and purpose, cohesive and disruptive forces in group behavior, group learning, collective problem solving, and group leadership styles. Such under-

standings have led to applications in psychotherapy, education, the management of organizations, and other settings. Because most learning about food and nutrition is social in nature, these understandings are especially important to us as nutrition educators. There are many kinds of groups, from groups convened to accomplish specific tasks (e.g., committees, teams at work) to those involving formal and nonformal classes. Most of this chapter is devoted to understanding the kinds of dynamics that exist in the nutrition education groups with which we work and the skills required of the group leader.

Lewin always liked to put his ideas to the test and to work out their practical implications. He therefore conducted many studies on "social climates." In one, Lewin and his collaborators set out to investigate the effects on their members of small groups organized along "democratic," "authoritarian," and "laissez-faire" patterns. The study involved task groups of 10-year-old youths in boys' clubs (Lewin, Lippitt, & White, 1939). The studies were experimental in nature and carefully controlled. The setups and results are shown in Table 15-2.

The results suggest that the authoritarian atmosphere impaired initiative and independence and bred hostility and aggression. In some groups the children were apathetic and bodily tensions increased. In the laissez-faire group, there was low morale, poor quality of work, and much frustration. The democratic climate permitted the children to thrive. The same kinds of results were obtained from a controlled experiment with workers in various kinds of work climates (Lewin, 1947, 1948). Workers' resentment toward authoritarian management was found to reduce productivity. When workers could air their views and participate in the decision-making process, their motivation improved and their productivity exceeded previous levels.

These findings led Lewin to a series of experiments on changing people's food beliefs and attitudes (or *values*, as he called them) and food habits, as we discussed in Chapters 3 and 4. During World War II when meat was scarce, he and his collaborators conducted several studies to compare "the relative effectiveness of a lecture method and a method of group decision for changing food habits" (Lewin, 1943). These studies were experimental in nature and carefully controlled for leader effect and socioeconomic and ethnic differences. In one study with housewives, Lewin compared these two ways of encouraging people to eat organ meats (kidneys, sweetbreads/brains, and beef hearts), purposely chosen because they are normally rejected. The lecture used health, status, and patriotic appeals, followed by handouts with recipes. The second method involved a short presentation by the leader, also linking the problem of nutrition to health, status, and the war effort. Then there was ample opportunity for the women to discuss why they rejected these meats and to share experiences with each other. They then identified ways to overcome barriers (with ideas from the leader if needed).

Now the group members were ready to make a decision whether to try one of these meats the following week using the recipes provided. They verbalized their decision to the others. Of the women in the lecture-only setting, only 10% served one of the recommended foods, whereas of those who had an opportunity to discuss and make a group decision, 52% served the recommended foods.

Lewin conducted a similar study with a different audience—college students—emphasizing whole-grain bread. In this case he compared a "request" to the students to eat more whole grain bread instead of white bread, with group decision and obtained similar results (Lewin, 1943). His work suggests, therefore, that group dynamics are important and that a democratic social climate, in which group members have the opportunity to be involved in making decisions for themselves, is more conducive to social change than other social climates. He emphasized that the method was one of *group decision* rather than just group discussion because closure in terms of decision making was considered important to the approach, along with public commitment. Such commitment made in the context of supportive peers was a motivating factor to make good on one's commitment to oneself.

As Lewin noted, no pressure tactics were used; instead, "the group setting gives the incentive for the decision and facilitates and reinforces it" (Lewin, 1943).

Since then, there has been considerable research on group structure and development, group behavior, leadership issues, group learning, and group development in a variety of settings, such as education, worksites, and communities. There have also been numerous professional conversations about the appropriate roles of educators and group members, particularly in work with adults (Rogers, 1969; Brookfield, 1986; Vella, 2002). All, however, agree that creating an emotionally safe learning environment is crucial.

Creating Safe Learning Environments Conducive to Change

Many of the individuals we work with want to make changes in their lives but are also afraid to do so. Food- and nutrition-related behaviors are embedded in so many other aspects of our lives that making a change in this one aspect may involve drastic changes in other aspects. Educators and psychologists (Rogers, 1969; Freire & Shor, 1987; Knowles, 1990; Vella, 2002) have noted that learning environments must be challenging enough to stimulate growth but also safe enough to allow peo-

TABLE 15-2 Group Dynamics: Leadership Patterns and Social Climate in Groups

Authoritarian	Democratic	Laissez-faire
Set-up of social climate		
All policies determined by the leader	All policies a matter of group discussion and decision, assisted by the leader	Complete freedom for group or individual decision, with no participation by leader
Leader dictates the work task and work companions of each person	Work tasks decided by group, and members chose with whom to work	Complete nonparticipation by leader
Leader was "personal" in his praise and criticism; impersonal and aloof, but friendly and nonhostile	Leader was "objective" in his praise and criticism; participated as a group member	No comments unless specifically asked; no participation or interference with course of events
Results		
Greater quantity of work	Slower, but more motivated	Less and poorer quality of work
Greater hostility and competition	Increasingly productive	Greater amount of time on horseplay
Greater aggressiveness (30 times greater than in the democratic climate)	Greater friendliness and teamwork	Talked more about what they should be doing
Greater dependence	Greater satisfaction	More aggressive than democratic, and less than authoritarian
Less originality on tasks	Praised more frequently	Expressed preference for democratic (after experiencing all three)

Sources: Lewin, K., R. Lippitt, and R.K. White. 1939. Patterns of aggressive behavior in experimentally created "social climates." *Journal of Social Psychology* 10:271–299; Lewin, K. 1947. Frontiers in group dynamics. I. Concept, method, reality in social science: Social equilibria and social change. *Human Relations* 1:5–41; and Lewin, K. 1948. *Resolving social conflicts: Selected papers on group dynamics.* New York: Harper.

ple to grow and change in perspectives, knowledge, attitudes, motivation, or action. Cooperative learning is more effective than competitive learning in this context (Johnson & Johnson, 1991). This means respecting that individuals come with a set of fears and defenses. It also means that the design of the sessions, the atmosphere in the room, and your approach to the situation should all signal that this is a safe space and time to learn and change. This feeling is especially important for adult learners in nonformal settings. Group leaders, such as nutrition educators, are often referred to as *facilitators* of such learning groups, rather than teachers or instructors.

Participants in any group bring with them a set of fears. We describe a few of them in the following list. Box 15-1, based on work by Sappington (1984), discusses how we can address these fears to make the learning environment safe for our participants.

- *Outcome fears.* These include participants' fear that they will not get what they want, that the information and activities may not be relevant to their personal needs, that there will not be enough time, and that the session will go over time.

BOX 15-1 Creating a Safe Learning Environment

The following lists present ways to reduce audience fears and create a safe learning environment.

Outcome Fears
- *Provide a welcoming start.* Make sure the room is comfortable in terms of light, heating, and ventilation. Arrange the setting or seating to be appropriate to the learning situation. Conscious decisions need to be made about whether to arrange seating in a circle or half circle (more intimate than rows), around tables, and so forth. Have coffee out if appropriate, and name tags.
- *Greet the group and introduce yourself.* If appropriate to the setting and size of the group, have the group members introduce themselves as well.
- *Set the time frame.* Let the audience know approximately how long the session will last.
- *Make your competence and experience clear,* either through prior material you hand out or through your introduction. This will make the group feel confident in your being able to provide a valuable experience for them.
- *State the objectives of the session clearly and provide a brief overview of the agenda or activities.* This will make the participants feel assured that the material will be relevant to their needs and that the activities are well organized.

Interpersonal Fears
- *State ground rules about how individuals will relate to each other.* Ask the group to contribute so that all are comfortable with the rules. Key ground rules are to respect each other and the facilitator and to listen to each other.
- *Design activities to be done first in dyads and then in small groups,* before having a large group discussion.
- *As the facilitator of the group, provide nonjudgmental responses to individual contributions.* By listening carefully to the feelings behind the questions and comments, you can gauge the fear or safety level in the individual and the group. Model the desired behavior and use warm, accepting humor where appropriate.

Evaluation Fears
- *Validate each response* either verbally or by writing responses on newsprint.
- *Provide nonjudgmental responses.* For example, rather than say that what a group member said was "not quite accurate," thank the person for bringing up that point because it is something that many others also think and then say, "The latest information on that point is . . . ."
- *Provide constructive feedback.*

Internal Fears
- Be respectful of each individual.
- Validate individuals' past experiences.
- Use genuine dialogue as the approach, in which you ask open-ended questions and listen to responses so as to allow for the free-flowing exchange of ideas so that all group members can learn from each other.

- *Interpersonal fears or social concerns.* These are often the greatest barrier to significant learning and change. They include fear of embarrassment, looking stupid or incompetent to peers or to the nutrition educator, criticism by others in the group, being called on when one is not ready, judgment of one's beliefs or positions, feeling vulnerable, unfamiliarity with others in a new group, or competition with others.
- *Evaluation fears.* These include fear of failure at the tasks that have been chosen and fear that participants' verbal responses are not correct.
- *Internal fears.* The deepest fears that group participants often bring are those that challenge their self-concept. Fear of incompetence or inadequacy arises from a genuine fear of not being able to do what is suggested. Changing would suggest that previous beliefs, attitudes, or actions were inferior or bad.

In general, safe environments are created when people feel respected; when their feelings are honored, their self-worth is assured, and their fears are overcome; and when the "delights of growth outweigh the anxieties of growth." Building safe learning environments is a crucial part of facilitated group discussion and dialogue, which is described next.

Facilitated Group Discussion as an Educational Tool: Focus on Adults

The importance of facilitating learning and change through emotionally safe group learning environments has recently been brought to the attention of nutrition educators (or brought *back* to our attention, if we consider that Lewin conducted the first group discussion and group decision work in the food habits area and Rogers focused on this issue in the 1970s). Although an emotionally safe learning environment is important for all age groups, discussions tend to be most useful for adults.

Guided discussions can range considerably in the degree to which the nutrition educator exerts leadership. You may make presentations with added activities; these would not be considered facilitated discussions. Or you may design sessions with open-ended questions and discussion but following a specific lesson plan. Or you may provide mini-lectures interspersed with guided discussion. These approaches are the most widely used and are appropriate for many group settings. There are group learning situations in which the entire session is devoted to a facilitated discussion. These adult group learning settings are described variously as facilitated group discussions, facilitated dialogue, or learner-based education (Abusabha, Peacock, & Achterberg, 1999; Sigman-Grant, 2005; Husing & Elfant, 2005), which vary somewhat in the degree of leadership provided by the nutrition educator. This approach is described in Chapter 17.

No matter whether the entire session is a facilitated group discussion or consists of mini-lectures interspersed with guided discussion, the role of the facilitator is to guide the group unobtrusively and to encourage interaction among members. You can do this by addressing questions posed to you to other group members, by saying things such as "Do you have any reactions to that or suggestions, Maria?" You can also look away from the speaker in the group as he or she attempts to make eye contact with you. The speaker will soon get the idea that he or she should look to others for responses. A good way to increase group interaction, especially at first, is the following technique: tell the group that after a given person speaks, he or she will pick the next person who wishes to speak, who will then pick the next person, and so forth.

The facilitator also needs to know when and how to take control. This depends on the degree of leadership you have decided is appropriate for the given group. Although an authoritarian approach can stifle group discussion, being too uncertain, timid, or laissez-faire can make the group feel unsure of itself and undermine your authority in the group. You can retain your authority while setting up an open, safe, and democratic social climate. When the group goes off track, you can gently bring it back by saying something such as, "Those are important issues, but the issue we are addressing today is *x*."

Understanding Dynamics in Group Nutrition Education Sessions

Even if you have designed engaging activities and wish to incorporate group discussion, you can confront situations that consistently plague instructors and group discussion leaders. If you are not ready to face spontaneous aspects of group dynamics, you may find yourself distracted, frustrated, or even becoming hostile. Defuse the anxiety by considering ahead of time how you will respond in some situations you might face, such as those shown in Box 15-2. These situations can be issues of authority (yours) and power (the audience's). Here we discuss some ways you might handle these situations. In facilitated discussions or dialogues of groups that have met for some time, members of the group may take on many of the following roles.

- *Quiet members.* It is important to respect all individuals in the group in terms of whether they wish to participate in discussions or not. They may be shy, or their quietness may be cultural. However, silence may also be a reflection of boredom, indifference, or a person's sense of superiority, timidity, or insecurity. Thus, it is important for you to figure out why group members are silent. If they are shy or insecure, it is helpful to provide activities such as icebreakers, brainstorming, or working in dyads or small groups. You can also reinforce and praise each attempt they make to speak up in the group. Sometimes quiet members really wish to speak up and will do so if you give them some encouragement, using smiles, nods, and perhaps asking them to respond. If they have blank expressions, it would be unwise to invite them to participate.

- *Dominant or talkative members.* The most common problem facilitators have is what to say to those who are overly dominant and talkative. It is important to handle the situation carefully because what you do will have an impact on all the others in the group. It is crucial to treat individuals with respect and not to humiliate or embarrass them. Being disrespectful is not only hurtful for the individual but also makes others in the group feel unsafe and uncomfortable.

  Several techniques may be effective in dealing with dominant or overly talkative participants. Some people are overly talkative because they are insecure and repeat themselves because they are not sure that the points they are making have been understood. It this is the case, you might interrupt them gently but firmly by thanking them for their response, paraphrase concisely what they have said or reflect their feelings so that they feel they have been understood, and then turn to others for responses. Usually these participants will stop talking because they feel they have been understood. Others are talkative because they enjoy talking or they believe that they can raise their status within the group by sharing information. They will not stop talking even when you or others in the group have paraphrased what they said or reflected their feelings. In this case, you might want to acknowledge their contributions and then say that short comments are easier for others to follow and that lengthy comments tend to lose people. If the pattern persists, you may need to talk with the participant privately. Talkative group members are often unaware of the fact that others may not appreciate their lengthy comments. You can emphasize that you have noticed that others want to talk but cannot because time is always limited in group learning settings.

- *Distractors or disrupters.* These individuals may carry out side conversations or make side comments to the group or frequently get up and leave the room, disrupting the group, whether the nutrition educator is presenting or leading the discussion or others are talking. Generally, you need not embarrass members who are engaged in side conversations if these are brief and intermittent. If the conversations are disrupting, you might stop talking and ask the individuals involved an easy question or ask them to share their thoughts with the group. If the disruptions persist, you should speak with them in private and point out that their behavior distracts and disrupts learning and is disrespectful of others.

BOX 15-2 Give Your Session a Fair Trial: Be Aware of the Effects of Group Dynamics

You know your content. You have designed activities that are based on theory and research and are engaging, interactive, and fun. But you confront situations that have plagued instructors and discussion leaders forever. If you are not ready to face spontaneous aspects of group dynamics, you may find yourself distracted, frustrated, or even hostile. Defuse the anxiety ahead of time. These can be issues of authority (yours) and power (the audience's).

Consider how you would handle each of these chronic instructional problems:

1. Only a few people are on time. When should you begin?
2. People arrive late (missing critical content or instructions).
3. One person dominates the session.
4. People do other work while you are presenting.
5. Some refuse to join the activity.
6. Many tangents are raised.
7. Someone wants to link every issue to a long personal story.
8. A heated argument erupts over a content issue.
9. People leave early or exit the room frequently.
10. Someone thinks he or she should be teaching the session rather than you.
11. Someone nods off.
12. Two people chat continuously at the back of the room or within the circle.
13. Some people are much more informed on the topic than you.
14. You are asked a string of questions you cannot answer.
15. Some people let it be known that the only reason they are there is because they are required to be.

Source: Morin, K. 1998. Presentation at Teachers College, Columbia University, New York.

- *Complainers.* Some participants are always complaining about some aspect of the group or about the physical surroundings. Acknowledge them and thank them for their concern. Ask them for suggestions for alternate approaches. Indicate that you will explore their suggestions and then be firm about staying on track. It the complaining persists, again take the individuals aside and talk with them privately.

- *Digressors.* These group members constantly digress from the main issues of the discussion or activities by talking about matters unrelated to the issues. You can respond by saying, "What you say is interesting, but let's get back to. . . ." Or you can ask, "How does this relate to what we are talking about?" Or again, "This is interesting, but given our time constraints, we can discuss these issues later if we have time."

- *Resistors.* These individuals say that whatever is being proposed by you or the others can't be done, or they just can't do it. This response may stem from fear or insecurity. Acknowledge their feelings and indicate that all change is difficult and that we can take one step at a time. If possible, partner them with someone else in the group who can provide support.

- *Know-it-alls.* Some group members may indicate that they know more than you and keep correcting you. Acknowledge that they seem to know a lot. You might ask them about their sources of information. Even if you believe the source is very questionable, ask them what makes them believe the source. Remain questioning and probing. You might also ask the others in the group to respond. It may be effective for you to place such persons in some leadership role.

- *Wisecrackers.* Some degree of humor may be helpful in the group. However, you will need to determine when the humor stops being helpful in relieving tension and starts interfering with group learning. This usually occurs when more attention is focused on the person who is making the wisecracks than on what is being said. You can say to the person, with a smile and in a tone that suggests that you appreciate what he or she has said, that it is time to get back to the issues. If the wisecracks continue, you may have to say it again, but with a firm tone.

- *Latecomers.* If one or two individuals are late for an ongoing group or learning situation, you may ignore it. However, if they are consistently late, you may need to say something such as "I know it is not always easy to get here on time, given the traffic and your situation, but I do want to remind us all that learning works best when we are all here from the beginning of the group session. It is also respectful of the others who may have made considerable effort to be here on time." If lateness persists for some individuals, you may want to talk with them privately to find out what the issues are for them. If the entire group consistently arrives late, you will need to carefully examine your own hidden messages to the group. Perhaps you do not start or end on time. This may convey the message that the group is not that important and thus not worth being on time for. This will arouse considerable resentment, particularly from those who

make an effort to be on time. It may be interpreted as disrespect for group members' time.

Oral Presentations and Workshops

Leading group discussions is not the only way we implement nutrition education with groups. The session or sessions that you have designed may be delivered as a presentation, a series of presentations, or as workshops. Or you may make a mini-presentation followed by group discussion. The principles of communication described at the beginning of the chapter are particularly useful here.

Preparing and Organizing Oral Presentations

The key to holding the attention of the group in delivering your designed session as an oral presentation is to be well organized, focused, concise, and coherent. When we first begin making presentations, we often have the impulse to tell our audiences everything we know about food and nutrition. Yet listening requires concentration on the part of the audience. By covering too much, we overload our audiences. In describing the use of the procedural model for designing theory-based nutrition education design earlier in the book, we emphasized that it is very important to write clear goals and objectives in designing educational plans or session guides. This is even more important if you are delivering the session through the channel of an oral presentation. Whatever the presentation's length may be, you have a limited time and you should be very clear what you want to accomplish in that time. What kinds of changes do you wish to take place in the audience—greater awareness of an issue, more motivation to consider action, or readiness to take a specific action? The audience should leave the presentation with the ability to state the main goal of the presentation and several supporting arguments or pieces of evidence, or *why-to* information, and a clear understanding of the conclusion or of what they should now do and *how to* do it. Thus, being organized is extremely important.

In addition, being organized throughout enhances the credibility of the nutrition educator. The audience gets only one chance to grasp your ideas and will become impatient if you ramble from one idea to another. The introduction to the session topic, discussion of the objectives of the session, explanations of learning activities, and transitions between activities should flow into each other in an organized fashion. Handouts, flip charts, PowerPoint slides, videos, and other ancillary materials should be ready for use and organized.

The Introduction

Presentations are generally described as having three parts: an introduction, body, and conclusion. Each serves a specific purpose. The functions of the introduction are to establish the speaker's credibility and goodwill, gain the attention and interest of the audience by providing an overview of what the *audience* will gain from the presentation, develop rapport with audience, and preview what the *presenter* intends to cover. The order of the first two functions may differ depending on the situation. If you have been adequately introduced, you may go directly to a way to gain the interest of the audience.

In terms of the first purpose of an introduction, credibility is established if you appear to be competent and trustworthy, as noted at the beginning of the chapter. Thus, when you introduce yourself or are introduced, let the audience know about your credentials and experience—with sensitivity and without bragging, of course—so as to indicate that you are qualified. For example, you can say "In an article I wrote. . ." or "From my work with. . . ." Your credibility does not necessarily depend only on your own accomplishments. You can say, "I have been interested in this issue for some time and have read widely on it." As discussed earlier, your being qualified helps the audience relax and feel reassured that they will get something out of the presentation. Your effectiveness is also enhanced if you can establish some common ground and connections with your particular audience. For example, you can say something like "As those of us who live in this community can attest. . . ," "As a mother of three children myself, I know how difficult it is. . . ," or "I know how hard it is to find out where the food in our grocery stores comes from."

A major function of the introduction is to get the attention and interest of the audience. This is done by focusing on what the audience will gain from the presentation. The design section of this book emphasized the importance of designing activities at the beginning of a session to be motivational, emphasizing "what's in it for me." Here are a few ways to do this in the format of a presentation. They must all be relevant to your topic.

- *Relate the topic or issue to the audience in a way that is personal.* For example, if you are talking to a group of teenagers about world hunger, you might begin with the following: "How many of you barely got to school for your first class today? You jumped out of bed, showered, dressed, and were out the door without breakfast. By ten o'clock you are more aware of your growling stomach than of what the teacher is saying. You say to your classmate, 'I'm starving.' Imagine feeling like that all day, not just for an hour or two before lunch. And day after day. This is what it is like for millions of teenagers around the world."
- *Emphasize the importance of your topic or the issue.* On the issue of eating locally, you might begin with, "Every hour of every day, America is losing *x* acres of farmland, land that produces the food we all need to survive and grow. We want for there to be farmland for our children and our children's children, to produce the food they will need."

- *Make an intriguing statement.* For example, a presentation to teenagers about the importance of bone health and osteoporosis prevention could begin as follows: "Every day our bones are broken down and dissolved, and every day they are rebuilt. We do not see it happening or feel it happening, but it is happening nonetheless. We can't stop the breaking-down process. But what we eat can make a big difference to how well and how much bone is rebuilt."
- *Ask a stimulating question.* The question can be rhetorical or a way to get the audience to think about the topic in a new way. "What is the first word that comes to mind when I use the word *elderly*? The word *adult*? *Older adult*?" This can then lead into a speech about the experience and needs of older adults.
- *Tell a story.* Any story you tell should be clearly relevant to the main goal of the speech. "It happened about a week ago. I was early to a meeting at work, and several of us were chatting. One of my colleagues asked, 'How's your AIDS going?' The room fell silent as the others all looked at me. I then said, 'You mean my speech on AIDS and nutrition. It's going well.' There was palpable relief in the room, but for a moment I understood what it is like for someone to have AIDS in our society."

After gaining the audience's attention, you should devote the final section of the introduction to a clear statement of the main topic of the presentation and a listing of the points you will cover or issues you will address. Preferably your presentation should consist of only three or four main points, which are the three or four objectives of your session. By demonstrating that you are clear and organized, you also increase your credibility. Your credibility is also enhanced when the supporting materials you use are professional looking and clear. We discuss this issue in depth in Chapter 16.

The Body

The body of the presentation consists of the objectives and content that you designed earlier using the procedural model for designing theory-based nutrition education. In translating these objectives and content into the format of an oral presentation, your first task is to identify the main points you want to make. These main points are usually the information on why to consider a food- or nutrition-related action and how to take action. This should be your "educational plan" from Step 5 of the design model. Since these main points are the central focus of your presentation, choose them carefully, phrase them precisely, and arrange them into some kind of strategic order.

From your educational plan, you can develop a speaking outline for use on the day of the presentation. Its aim is to help you remember what you want to say. Label the introduction, body, and conclusion. Make sure your outline is clear and easy to read. It is helpful to use large enough type so you can see the main points just by glancing down. Some people like to put their notes on index cards, large enough so the notes are clearly readable. You may be using slides throughout. These will contain only key ideas; thus, it is important, even in this instance, to have a speaking outline with key information on it. The PowerPoint program provides space to make notes on each slide. Those pages can serve as your speaking outline, with crucial supporting information on them.

It is also useful to write out the first few sentences for the beginning of the presentation—especially the dramatic opening you have planned—and the beginning of each new section so that the transitions will be smooth. Make other notations as needed, such as "pause." Be sure to include important technical information so that you will not forget. You will probably also want to write out your conclusion. Rehearse from this speaking outline. Here are some factors to consider as you plan the body of your presentation.

- *Message vividness versus data summaries.* People tend to give greater weight to vivid and personalized information. Case studies, personal examples, and visual images such as slides are more vivid than recitations of facts, and people can remember and recall them more easily even though they may be less representative of the issues being presented. Statistical data and impersonal information, on the other hand, are less vivid and thus will have less of an impact on attitudes and behavior, even though they may be more accurate. The challenge is to use personal and vivid—but accurate—information if we wish to be effective in increasing awareness, concern, or active contemplation. Statistics can be presented in a vivid way.

- *A single message versus many ideas.* A message or session should provide enough information to be convincing, enhance decision making, or provide new skills, yet it must be manageable in length and complexity. We do not need to tell our audience everything we know about an issue! Too many ideas, especially if they are thrown together haphazardly, create clutter in the receiver's mind so that no single message comes through clearly or sticks. Remember that the audience has only one chance to hear each idea. It is better to have a single message or theme in a given session, supported by a few clearly developed ideas or arguments, than to have too many different ideas. These supporting ideas are the "main points" in your outline. Plan to have only two to five main points because the audience can't keep track of too many of them. Each main point should have one single idea, which should be worded clearly and later spoken with emphasis so that the audience will know which are your main points.

"Less" is definitely better than "more" in this context.

Being focused in your message does not mean that you should be simplistic. You should not underestimate the amount and depth of information that many people want. Indeed, oversimplistic messages may frustrate the audience because they do not provide the information the audience needs and may even lead to misunderstandings. Knowledge of the audience will help you judge the correct level of complexity. This knowledge can be obtained from a needs analysis or from the individuals or organization that invited you to make a presentation.

- *One side versus two sides.* Should you present only one side of a controversial issue or both sides? It is often more effective, and enhances your credibility, to present both sides. It shows that you know and understand more than one viewpoint and have taken a stand in light of these differing viewpoints. It can be quite powerful to present objections or counterarguments to your own message (that breastfeeding is best, for example) and then show how these objections are invalid or do not negate your message.

- *Order of presentation of main points or arguments.* The order of the main points will depend on the purpose of the presentation: we have consistently suggested that focusing on motivational information first followed by how-to information is a good way to organize nutrition education presentations. But other orders are appropriate depending on the audience, issue, and setting.

- *Emotional appeals.* As we have seen, the audience is more likely to consider your message seriously if they believe you are credible and the evidence you present for taking action is strong and persuasive. However, you can deliver the why-to information in a fashion that will have a greater impact if the words you use appeal to people's feelings as well as their reason. We discussed these issues earlier in the book in regard to most learning objectives having an affective as well as a cognitive aspect. Here we will just remind you to use language vividly and clearly to help the audience effectively process your message emotionally as well as cognitively. For example, one way to say to mothers of young children that they should make sure their children gets enough calcium to have good teeth is to say "You have the opportunity to give your child a smile for a lifetime" and show a photo of a child with a great smile (McCarthy, 2005). Vivid examples can also convey feeling (e.g., what it is like to be hungry, or to have AIDS and not be able to cook or shop for oneself), as noted earlier. Most important, it is your sincerity and conviction that the audience will feel and respond to.

The Conclusion

The conclusion of the presentation is extremely important. Its main purpose is to reinforce the audience's understanding of the central idea or their commitment to the main goal of the presentation. The conclusion is what you want the audience to remember, to make a commitment to, or to take action on. You may want to summarize your speech briefly. You have heard the old advice that in a speech one should "tell the audience what you will tell them, tell them, and then tell them what you told them." Your communication will be more effective if the conclusions are explicitly stated than if the conclusions are implied. You might refer back to the introduction to show your progression of ideas and how they led to the conclusion. You might also conclude with some kind of dramatic statement.

Delivering the Oral Presentation

As the presenter, you will be sized up by the audience from the moment you enter the room, so it is important that their impressions of you from the very first are positive. You should arrive early, meet the audience, smile, chat, and look confident whether you feel that way or not. This relaxes the audience or group and makes them want to listen to what you have to say. It also helps establish that you have an attractive personality. Appropriate attire and grooming also contribute to your credibility. After you have been introduced, walk confidently and with poise to where you will speak from, such as the front of the room, behind a podium, or onto a stage. Take a moment to look at the audience, smile, and make eye contact here and there with audience members. This establishes that you are interested in the audience, not just in what you want to say.

It is important to create a safe learning environment by continuing to develop rapport with the audience through looking at them and being comfortable with them. This gives permission for the audience to ask questions and make comments, if appropriate given the size and setting. You will need to decide whether you want audience members to ask questions throughout or at the end.

Room Arrangements

Another reason to arrive early is to check out the physical arrangement and technology in the room. Depending on the size of the group and the physical setup of the room, you may have the opportunity to arrange the seating so as to encourage effective learning in that setting. Decide whether you want to rearrange the seating to be in a circle, around tables, or some other arrangement. If you will be using audiovisual materials, be sure you know how to operate the equipment you will be using. Check out the temperature settings. If you will be using flip charts or newsprint to record group responses, make sure you have the markers you need. Make sure your handouts are ready to distribute.

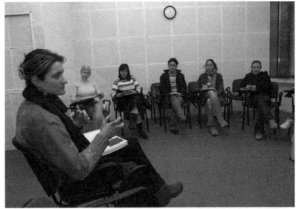

If you arrive early, you can rearrange your teaching area so it encourages communication and learning.

Some speakers like podiums or lecterns. However, these present a barrier between you and the audience, and it is important to create an arrangement that allows you to connect with the audience. Instead, you could use a table on which to place your materials. What, then, to do with your notes? You may be able to see them from the table, or keep them in your hand. You may find it useful to place your notes on cards that you can hold in your hand.

Nervousness and Anxiety

You should never share your internal feelings of nervousness or anxiety. Others cannot see or feel your anxiety unless you bring it to their attention by saying such things as how nervous you are, how intimidating the audience seems, or that you did not have a chance to prepare. Even if asked, do not acknowledge your fright. The group wants to learn and enjoy, and a safe learning environment is established when you seem relaxed and comfortable. When audience members are aware of the leader's fragility or stage fright, they become nervous in sympathy and start worrying for you instead of focusing on your message or the activities you have planned. The best way to reduce nervousness and anxiety is to be well prepared and to rehearse your presentation ahead of time.

Reading the Presentation or Speaking from an Outline

How we write and how we speak are usually very different in terms of language use and sentence structure. When we speak we tend to use simpler words, shorter sentences, and more informal language. Some nutrition educators are able to write speeches in a way that sounds conversational, much as speechwriters do for politicians. Most of us are not good at this kind of speechwriting, however, so that reading from a written text can be extremely dull. A memorized speech can also be dull. In both cases, the presentation becomes a monologue, spontaneity is lost, and the tone can become monotonous. Generally, therefore, the presentation should not be read or memorized. Instead, you should rehearse and deliver the speech from the speaking outline you have developed.

Time Management

Paying attention to how you are doing in terms of your outline and the time available for your presentation is crucial. However, you should find a way to monitor the time without your audience being aware of it. Looking constantly at your watch can give many unintended messages, such as that you can't wait for the presentation to be over or that you are afraid you are going to go over time. Place a timepiece where you can see it unobtrusively.

Language and Diction

The language you use needs to be clear, vivid, and appropriate. The audience members cannot go back to figure out something you said, as they could if they were reading a book. Therefore what you say has to be clear and understandable the first time around. Use familiar words and the active voice instead of passive voice to the extent possible. The language you use should also be appropriate to the occasion (formal or informal) and to the audience. To be effective, the words, idioms, and style of the presentation must be suitable to the group, culturally appropriate, and nonsexist. The language you use should also be appropriate for you. As noted earlier, you have to be authentic to who you are; you can't be someone else—telling jokes or using hip language when these can be seen as forced and inconsistent with your personality and background. You can work out a style that is effective for you.

However, your diction is also important. Your credibility with the audience will be influenced by your diction. When you misarticulate words, such as saying "wanna" for "want to" or "wilya" for "will you," and mispronounce words, such as "revelant" for "relevant" or "nucular" for "nuclear," the audience may develop negative impressions of you. Likewise, the use of *ums* and *ahs* between words can grate on the audience. Listen to yourself speak when you rehearse, and train yourself to speak with clear diction in settings such as these.

Voice, Volume, Pitch, and Rate of Speaking

No matter what kind of voice we were born with, we can learn to make good use of what we have to make effective presentations. Whether you use a microphone or not, adjust your volume to the acoustics of the room. You want the individuals in the last row to hear you, but you do not want to shout. Your natural pitch could be high or low, but your speaking will be livelier when you vary your pitch by going up and down as you emphasize a point or ask a question. By varying your pitch (these variations are called *inflections*), you convey a variety of emotions and come across as

dynamic, as opposed to when you speak in a monotone. Your inflections reveal whether you are being sincere or sarcastic, angry or anxious, and interested or bored. Enthusiasm about what you are saying goes a long way.

Pacing the rate (or speed) at which you speak is also important. If you speak too slowly, you may bore your audience. But if you speak too fast, the audience may not be able to keep up with your ideas. They may also get anxious because they suspect you are anxious. Indeed, people do tend to speed up when they are nervous. So pay attention to your pacing and practice a speed that seems appropriate for the audience. Pause from time to time at the end of a section for a point to sink in or for the audience to catch up with you. Since our minds can go much faster than our speaking, we can scan the group for "feedback" as we speak. Do they appear bored or puzzled? You might adjust what you are saying to fit your feedback.

Provide Signposts and Summarize Periodically

Provide signposts as to where you are in the speech, saying, for example, "first . . . ," "second . . . ," and so on. Use signposts to emphasize important points you want to make as well. You can say things such as "The most important thing to remember about X is . . . " or "Above all, you need to know. . . ." Summarizing periodically is also very helpful. As you begin the second main point, you could summarize in one sentence the key idea of the first point before proceeding.

Nonverbal Communication

As noted previously, nonverbal communication can be as powerful as the verbal communication it accompanies. Your personal appearance, facial expressions, gestures, bodily movement, and eye contact all convey information to the audience, and you want this information to be favorable so that the audience will focus on your message and not on you.

Listeners always see speakers before they hear them. There is evidence that how a speaker dresses and is groomed affects a speaker's credibility and reception considerably. The Madonnas and Einsteins of the world can get away with looking or wearing whatever they wish; the rest of us cannot. The main point is that you want the audience to focus on the message and activities you have designed, not on your personal appearance and grooming. So check out the setting before you go to judge what will be appropriate to the audience and setting and to who you are. Remember that you will also be seen as a representative of the nutrition education profession.

When and how much to move can present a challenge. We can look for opportunities to break the invisible barrier between presenter and audience, so moving toward the audience or moving around a little can be helpful. However, pacing back and forth, fidgeting with your notes or with coins in your pocket, or playing with your hair are signs of nervousness and can be distracting. At the other end of the spectrum, standing rigidly in the same place signals nervousness. Pay attention to what you do, and practice coming across as confident. Saying to yourself "I like the audience and the audience likes me" can be helpful.

What to do with our hands can be problematic. Clasp them behind our backs? Put them in our pockets? Let them hang at our sides? How much should we gesture? There are no rules about this, and we are all comfortable with different ways of holding our bodies and with when and how to gesture. The best way to think about this issue is that whatever you choose to do should appear natural and should not distract from your message.

Eye contact with the group helps you to establish a bond with the group. Look at individuals, not at some space between people, and move your eye contact from person to person around the entire room. Don't focus only on one side of the room or only on those who look most interested. How you look at the audience is also important—pleasantly, personally, and with sincerity. You want to convey that you are pleased to be there, that you have something important to say, and that you want them to believe that the message is important.

Delivering the Conclusion

The audience may be keeping track of your three or more points and may thus know that you are almost finished. However, you should still signal that you are coming to a conclusion by using such phrases as "in conclusion" or "in summary." The conclusion should be quite short; once you say "in summary," do not go on and on, and certainly do not say "in summary" multiple times! Come rapidly to the end.

Co-presenting or Co-leading Group Sessions

Often two people will be involved in making the presentation. This has many advantages: you can prepare together, and each brings special strengths. This is likely to increase the quality of the presentation. When you are co-presenting, you can draw energy from each other. By interacting with each other, you are likely to be more lively and enthusiastic. In addition, many of the tasks described earlier can be shared. Thus, while one person is speaking, the other can be monitoring the audience and keeping track of time and how the content is being covered. Co-presenters can also help each other out if necessary. If one gets off track or goes blank, the other can jump in. Experienced co-presenters have suggested the following formats for how two presenters can work together (Garmston & Bailey, 1988).

- *Tag team.* In the tag-team format, one person presents and then the other does. This method is especially useful for those who do not regularly co-present together or when there is considerable material to cover and it is easier for each person to become an expert for each segment.

- *Speak and add.* In the speak-and-add format, one person is the lead presenter and the other is the support person. The lead is in charge of the content and decides when and how to proceed. The support person adds information when it seems useful or appropriate.

- *Speak and chart.* In the speak-and-chart format, the lead person presents content and elicits responses from the audience, and the support person records the information on newsprint or on an overhead transparency. Both presenters must be clear about their roles, and the support person must be able to record the ideas of the lead or the audience quickly and without comment.

- *Duet.* In the duet format, both presenters are on stage together and each presents content in small chunks of about two minutes each. The presentation thus goes back and forth. The presenters stand five to seven feet apart, but look at the audience and each other to cue each other in. They may move toward each other when they speak and move back when they are not speaking. This works best when the two people are experienced presenters or have rehearsed carefully.

Delivering Nutrition Education Workshops

The term *workshop* is used to describe many different kinds of group sessions. Usually, the term refers to some kind of professional development activity, but this is not always the case. Generally workshops run longer than presentations, but not always. They also usually involve more than one leader—but again, not always. What they *do* have in common is that they involve active participation of the group members. Workshops usually consist of a number of the activities we have described earlier in this chapter: presentations, group discussions, and group activities, which will not be repeated here.

The workshop can be structured somewhat like a presentation in the sense of having an introduction, a body, and a conclusion. The workshop usually begins with a group introductory activity or icebreaker to establish a safe environment and sense of cohesiveness. If the group is small enough, participants can be asked to state what they most want from the experience. This is then followed by an overview of the objectives of the workshop, the main issues to be covered, and expectations.

The main body of the workshop can be delivered using a variety of formats to address all the learning styles discussed earlier. This involves a sequence proposed in the design system described earlier. Thus, there should be concrete hands-on experiences or self-assessments to investigate the audience's own prior knowledge, attitudes, or behaviors;

mini-presentations of needed information; time for work in groups to develop skills; and opportunity to apply the skills in their professional or personal lives.

The conclusion should be carefully planned to bring a sense of closure to the workshop, to summarize what has been accomplished, and to provide an opportunity for the group members to state how they plan to use the information and skills in the future.

Conclusion

Working with groups is at the heart of nutrition education. This chapter has described many ways for nutrition educators to work with groups. Different ways work for different audiences, different situations, and different purposes. The aim in all cases, however, is for the method used to be effec-

tive in communicating the objectives of the messages you designed in such a way that the group becomes motivated to actively contemplate your message and to take action when appropriate. Effective communication involves understanding the communication process and the factors that influence it. Working with groups requires understanding different learning styles and how best to create a safe and challenging learning environment for all. It also requires understanding group dynamics and being able to manage difficult situations. Working with groups is challenging and hard work, in both planning and delivery. However, working with groups can be very rewarding for you, the nutrition educator, and a great experience for participants when the environment is safe and the learning experience is carefully planned and effectively delivered.

Questions and Activities

1. Think back on an occasion in a professional setting when you presented an idea for a group to consider and act on. Analyze your interaction in terms of the purpose of your communication and the effect on your listeners. Were you successful in your communication? Why or why not?

2. On a sheet of paper, create a table with two columns. Label one "Characteristics that make nutrition educators *effective* communicators in a group setting." Label the other one "Characteristics that make nutrition educators *ineffective* communicators in a group setting." In each column, list and briefly describe what you think are the five most important characteristics for that category. Candidly review your current strengths and weaknesses in terms of these characteristics. Pick three you would most like to improve.

3. Describe four learning styles that have been identified by some educators. Which kind of learning style best describes you? What can you do to make a group learning experience effective for different kinds of learners?

4. Compare and contrast the following methods for delivering nutrition education to groups: lectures, demonstrations, debates, and facilitated group discussions.

5. Describe authoritarian, democratic, and laissez-faire social climates in terms of the impact of each on the amount of learning that takes place, work accomplished or productivity, and feelings of the group. Have you experienced each of these kinds of social climate? How did you respond in each case? Which did you prefer? Why?

6. List four things you could do to create a safe learning environment for a group of adults. Would you plan the same way if the same if the group was an after-school program made up of upper elementary school children? Explain.

7. If you were the leader of a group, how would you handle the following kinds of group members? Quiet members, complainers, those who dominate the conversation, digressors, those engaged in side conversations, and those who are consistently late.

8. What are some key features for holding the attention of a group when you are making an oral presentation?

9. Why is the introduction to a presentation or talk so important? What are its key components?

10. Why is it important to have a speaking outline?

11. Compare how you usually deliver oral presentations with five of the recommendations in this chapter. Candidly evaluate how many of these recommendations you have been using. Which of the recommendations do you think you will adopt in the future and why? What would you add to the list of recommendations in this chapter, based on your own experience?

12. Rehearse a presentation you are planning to give in front of the mirror. What do you think you are conveying nonverbally?

13. List all the ways you can enhance your credibility as a nutrition educator when you lead a group or make a presentation.

REFERENCES

Abusabha, R., J. Peacock, and C. Achterberg. 1999. How to make nutrition education more meaningful through facilitated group discussions. *Journal of the American Dietetic Association* 99:72–76.

Achterberg, C. 1988. Factors that influence learner readiness. *Journal of the American Dietetic Association* 88:1426–1428.

Beffa-Negrini, P., and N.L. Cohen. 1990. Use of learning style theory in the development of a nutrition education program to reduce cancer risk. *Journal of Nutrition Education* 22:106A–B.

Brookfield, S. 1986. *Understanding and facilitating adult learning: A comprehensive analysis of principles and effective practices.* San Francisco: Jossey-Bass.

Freire, P., and I. Shor. 1987. *A pedagogy for liberation: Dialogues on transforming education.* New York: Bergin & Garvey.

Gagne, R. 1985. *The conditions of learning and theory of instruction.* 4th ed. New York: Holt, Rinehart, & Winston.

Garmston, R., and S. Bailey. 1988. Paddling together: A co-presenting primer. *Training and Development Journal.* January: 52-56.

Gillespie, A.H., and P. Yarbrough. 1984. A conceptual model for communicating nutrition. *Journal of Nutrition Education* 17:168–172.

Husing, C., and M. Elfant. 2005. Finding the teacher within: A story of learner-centered education in California WIC. *Journal of Nutrition Education and Behavior* 37(Suppl. 1):S22.

Johnson, D., and F. Johnson. 1991. *Joining together: Group theory and group skills.* Englewood Cliffs, NJ: Prentice-Hall.

Kinzie, M.B. 2005. Instructional design strategies for health behavior change. *Patient Education and Counseling* 56:3–15.

Knowles, M.S. 1990. *The adult learner: A neglected species.* 4th ed. Houston, TX: Gulf.

Kolb, D.A. 1984. *Experiential learning.* Englewood Cliffs, NJ: Prentice Hall.

Lewin, K. 1935. *A dynamic theory of personality.* New York: McGraw-Hill.

———. 1943. Forces behind food habits and methods of change. In *The problem of changing food habits* (National Research Council Bulletin 108). Washington, DC: National Academy of Sciences.

———. 1947. Frontiers in group dynamics. I. Concept, method, reality in social science: Social equilibria and social change. *Human Relations* 1:5–41.

———. 1948. *Resolving social conflicts: Selected papers on group dynamics.* New York: Harper.

———. 1951. Field theory in social science. *Selected Theoretical Papers.* New York: Harper.

———. 1958. Group decision and social change. In *Readings in social psychology*, edited by T.M. Newcomb and E.L. Hartley. New York: Holt, Rinehart & Winston.

Lewin, K., R. Lippitt, and R.K. White. 1939. Patterns of aggressive behavior in experimentally created "social climates." *Journal of Social Psychology* 10:271–299.

McCarthy, P. 2005. Touching hearts to impact lives: Harnessing the power of emotion to change behaviors. *Journal of Nutrition Education and Behavior* 37(Suppl. 1):S19.

Olson, C.M., and G.L. Kelly. 1989. The challenge of implementing theory-based intervention research in nutrition education. *Journal of Nutrition Education* 22:280–284.

Petty, R.E., and J.T. Cacioppo. 1986. *Communication and persuasion: Central and peripheral routes to attitude change.* New York: Springer-Verlag.

Rogers, C. 1969. *Freedom to learn.* Columbus, OH: Merrill.

Sappington, T.E. 1984. Creating learning environments conducive to change: The role of fear/safety in the adult learning process. In *Innovative higher education.* New York: Human Services Press.

Sigman-Grant, M. 2004. *Facilitated dialogue basics: A self-study guide for nutrition educators—Let's dance.* University of Nevada, Cooperative Extension, NV.

Vella, J. 2002. *Learning to listen, learning to teach: The power of dialogue in educating adults.* Hoboken, NJ: Jossey-Bass.

CHAPTER 16

Beyond Groups:
Other Channels for Nutrition Education

OVERVIEW This chapter provides an overview of how nutrition education can be delivered through various other channels, such as the use of visuals, printed materials, mass media strategies, and social marketing activities.

OBJECTIVES At the end of the chapter, you will be able to

- Apply design principles for developing supporting visuals for group sessions and oral presentations and state guidelines for their use
- Develop written materials for use in nutrition education
- Describe how to deliver nutrition education through activities such as cooking, supermarket tours, and health fairs
- Understand key principles of health communications and social marketing
- Implement nutrition education social marketing activities
- Recognize that there are many other channels and venues for nutrition education

SCENARIO

A nutrition educator has been asked to speak to a class of teenagers about healthy eating. She begins the session by showing the group a number of food items familiar to this audience: a regular hamburger and a supersized one, and a variety of highly processed packaged snacks. She then shows them a can of solid shortening (fat used in baking) and asks them how many teaspoons of fat are present in each food. She does this as follows. Using a teaspoon, she begins to spoon out the shortening onto a plate until the audience tells her to stop. There are gasps in the group when they see how much fat is present in their favorite foods and snacks.

Introduction

An old saying tells us that one picture is worth a thousand words. People understand what speakers say, find it more interesting, and remember more when visual and other media are used in addition to the verbal message. As noted in an earlier chapter, people remember 20% of what they hear, but 50% of what they both see and hear, and 90% when they are actively involved in talking about it as they do something. Today's audiences grew up in the television and computer age and are used to obtaining information visually as well as orally. About 99% of households have television and adults spend an average of 15–17 hours weekly watching. Some two thirds of households have computers and spend several hours each day on them, particularly young people. People watch videos and see advertising billboards. They are used to being bombarded with information and persuasion from a variety of high-quality media sources. These media affect all age groups.

Using visual aids and written supporting materials with presentations or group discussions is thus important for nutrition education. These supporting media might include slides, overhead transparencies, models, food packages, handouts, or other materials. When the supporting materials are of high quality, they will enhance your credibility, make you seem more prepared, and enhance the effectiveness of your message. Supporting visual media are especially important for low-income groups who have limited reading ability and for those whose first language is not English. When real foods are used and tasted, the addition of other senses, such as sight and touch, as well as smell and taste, enhances the message.

Channels other than group sessions and oral presentations can also be important for delivering nutrition education messages, such as health fairs, church newsletters, billboards, social marketing media campaigns, or Web-based interventions. These channels are becoming increasingly important as people have less and less time to attend group sessions.

This chapter describes the use of visual and written media as supporting aids for group sessions as well as the use of other channels to deliver supporting nutrition education for the group intervention.

Using Supporting Visuals in Group Sessions and Oral Presentations

Humans are visual creatures. When news stories on television about events such as tsunamis, hurricanes, or earthquakes are accompanied by visual images, particularly those showing the suffering of individuals, the impact is dramatic. Often before the news program is over, relief organizations are deluged by calls from viewers wanting to make a donation.

Using supporting visuals or visual aids in nutrition education has many advantages, chief among them being that they make your message clearer and more lively. You can outline the main points and thus help the audience or group follow the key messages you wish to convey. Or you can show real objects or pictures, or present a graph of the statistics that you are quoting. These will make the message more vivid. Using supporting visuals will also stimulate interest. And of course, your audience will be more likely to remember your message. In the scenario at the beginning of the chapter, the teens will be more likely to remember how much fat is in some common foods because of the demonstration, and this may help them in their food choices. The next subsection discusses various visual media that you can use. Consider the following questions as you choose which to use:

- Who is the audience? What kinds of visual media are most appropriate for this audience? For example, a low-literacy audience may need different kinds of visuals from a highly educated audience.
- What will the audience prefer?
- What is the setting? Will you be in the front of a long room in which people in the back will be able to see slides but not real objects such as foods?

- What is the size of the audience? Ten, 25, 50, or 100 or more? Some visuals, such as food models, work well only with a small audience, whereas others, such as slides, can work with larger audiences.
- What equipment is available in the room?
- What length of time do you have? What kinds of visuals will fit into that time? For example, a videotape may take too long, but you could use excerpts.
- How much time do you have to prepare the visuals?
- What skills do you have to develop the visuals that you need? Can someone else assist you?

Types of Supporting Visuals

A variety of visuals can be used to support and reinforce your message, ranging from real foods to slides.

Real Objects: Foods and Packages

Showing real foods or packages can have a dramatic impact and make your objectives clearer. For example, a session on the importance of eating a variety of fruits and vegetables can begin with you bringing in an array of differently colored fruits and vegetables and asking the audience if they can identify them or have tasted them. You can bring in and show low-fat food products for a session on reducing fat in the diet. You can also bring in a variety of packaged food products for a session on label reading or as examples of low-fat snacks. Real objects are especially useful for showing portion sizes of different items, such as sodas or small, medium, and large sizes of movie-theater popcorn.

It is best to bring in *empty* packages and containers (such as soda cans or empty popcorn buckets), particularly for the less healthful items: they are easier to carry, you do not have to worry about the foods perishing, and you do not have to decide what to do when individuals want to take the items home! To avoid distraction for the audience, it is best to keep these kinds of visuals out of sight until you are ready to show them. It is also useful to bring in cups and measuring spoons if you want to show serving sizes of foods.

- *Advantages:* Realistic; dramatic; enhances motivation; improves understanding of the message and increases retention. Objects and packages are portable.
- *Disadvantages:* Some foods are perishable; not suitable for groups larger than 15 to 20 members.

Models of Foods and Other Nutrition-Related Objects

Models of foods are actual-sized, realistic, three-dimensional models made of plastic or rubber. They are especially useful for showing the sizes of servings of foods recommended by dietary guidelines, and for foods that are perishable, such as meats (e.g., hamburgers or chicken). Other kinds of models can also be used, such as models of the heart or of clogged arteries.

- *Advantages:* Food models are realistic, portable, and can show actual portion sizes of foods. Other models can be selected to illustrate complex organs or processes.
- *Disadvantages:* Cannot be seen in groups larger than 15 to 20 members.

Poster Boards

For many settings, poster boards prepared ahead of time can be very effective. Pictures from magazines or empty packages of various kinds of food items can be mounted onto poster boards for display. You may also be able to glue on pockets in which you place various pictures or cards of items that you can pull out to show as you need. You can also display pie charts, bar graphs, or line graphs. You may develop a collection of these poster boards to use for sessions focusing on different behaviors.

How exactly to keep poster boards standing presents a challenge that must be resolved before the occasion. A sturdy grade of poster board or foamcore and a method to keep it standing must be devised.

- *Advantages:* Inexpensive; portable; very helpful when there is not much equipment in the room.
- *Disadvantages:* Fragile when carried; limited amount of information; cannot be used with large groups; can get worn with repeated use.

Flip Charts

A flip chart with a display easel is very useful in a setting without much equipment. Flip charts consist of large pads of newsprint sheets that are fastened or glued together at the top (Figure 16-1). Write on the newsprint with crayon or felt-tip pens that do not bleed through the paper. Use a dark-colored pen, and write large enough for everyone in the

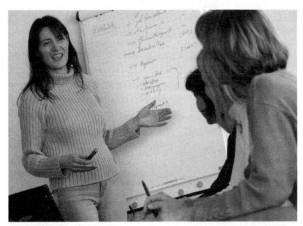

FIGURE 16-1 Flip charts are an inexpensive way to engage your audience.

group to read. You can prepare the sheets ahead of time to contain graphs, pie charts, written outlines, clip art, and so forth. Each sheet is flipped over at the top when you have finished showing the information. Flip charts are particularly useful for group brainstorming activities. The ideas can be recorded and then the sheets torn off and attached to a wall or blackboard for all to see. The sheets can also be taken away after the meeting. Use of different-colored pens can be very helpful.

- *Advantages:* Inexpensive; prepared flip charts can be reused from group to group; appropriate in informal settings such as senior centers or community programs; audience friendly, particularly when information is being collected from the group; information collected during the session can be preserved.
- *Disadvantages:* Cannot be seen in groups larger than 20 to 25 members; inconvenient to carry; requires someone to write clearly and quickly if it is being used to capture ideas of a group; prepared flip charts can get worn with repeated use.

Chalkboard

We often forget that the chalkboard, too, can serve as a visual aid. It can be very useful if you write legibly and large enough for all to see and can spell well. However, it is important not to turn your back to the audience and talk to the board. It also takes time to write on the board, so you need to practice talking and writing at the same time, while facing the audience as much as possible during the process.

- *Advantages:* Inexpensive; easy to use.
- *Disadvantages:* Presenter often talks to the board; takes time to write material; poor handwriting reduces effectiveness.

Overhead Transparencies

Overhead transparencies are sheets of clear acetate, the same size as regular paper, on which you can put type or other visuals and display to an audience with an overhead projector. You can use transparencies to show drawings, graphs, and charts, as well as text (Figure 16-2). Using transparencies permits you to stand facing the audience while you are presenting something visual to illustrate your points. Thus you can maintain eye contact with the audience and maintain attention.

You can use transparencies in one of two ways: the first is to draw or write on them directly using special felt-tip pens designed for transparencies (they come in various colors). You can write the information ahead of time or write as you go along, including writing down ideas from the audience in a brainstorming session. The second way is to prepare the information on a computer and directly print

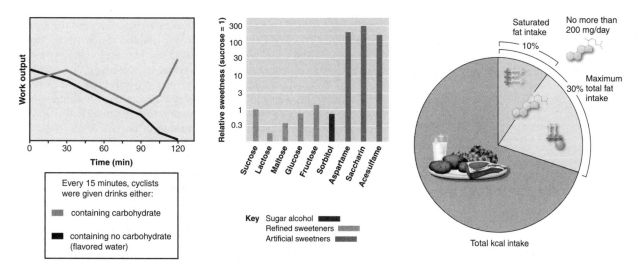

FIGURE 16-2 Example of effective line chart, bar graph, and pie chart presentations. Source: Insel, P., R.E. Turner, D. Ross. 2004. *Nutrition, Second Edition.* Sudbury, MA: Jones and Bartlett Publishers.

the information onto the acetate sheets. You can also print the information onto paper and photocopy it onto acetate sheets using a regular photocopier. If you print directly from the computer, a color printer permits you to produce full-color transparencies. Type should be large enough for your audience to read. The font size will depend on the size of your audience, but should be larger than regular type. For a large audience, a rule of thumb is for the type to be at least a quarter inch high.

Graphs, charts, tables, and cartoons can also be enlarged from other printed sources and photocopied onto transparencies. Photos do not copy well, so you should check whether they are clear to an audience. Make sure all these visuals are large enough for the audience to see or read. In some circumstances you may be standing far away from the projector; in this case, you should have someone else change the transparencies while you talk. Check ahead of time to make sure the projector is working and that you know how to operate it.

- *Advantages:* Transparencies are inexpensive, easy to create, extremely versatile and convenient, and can provide strong visual images. Can be used for medium-sized as well as small groups; can be used with the room lights on. Good way to highlight key points in a presentation. Can maintain sense of connection with the audience.
- *Disadvantages:* Too much text can be unreadable or overwhelming. Visual display is not as sophisticated as PowerPoint or similar slides. In a large, long room, they may be difficult to see from the back.

Slides (PowerPoint, Freelance, Persuasion, Presentation)
Increasingly, those making presentations or working with groups use computer software programs such as Microsoft PowerPoint, Lotus Freelance, Adobe Persuasion, or Corel Presentation to create images involving just about everything from text to graphs, charts, and tables. Photographs can also be scanned in with high fidelity. There are ways to include animation, sound, and video clips, allowing for multimedia presentations. The images are sharp and multicolored and can be made any size you need. The presentation can be printed out on paper and used as a handout at the beginning of the session for the audience to follow along or at the end as reinforcement.

It is best to use colors and graphics on the slides that can be seen without turning off the lights. This helps you maintain contact with the audience. Make the slides visually compelling (Figure 16-3)—use of high technology does not automatically make a presentation interesting. There are now many designs to choose from, and you should exploit these options.

It takes considerable time to learn how to use the software; design the text, graphs, and charts; import images from other sources; and organize all these in a way that is appropriate. So give yourself plenty of time to create the visuals. Arrive early and run through your presentation before the audience or group arrives. In addition, always carry a backup disk or flashdrive. If you have printed out your slides as handouts, you can use the handouts as the basis of your talk if the equipment fails. Finally, be prepared to give your presentation or conduct the group session without the slides if you have to!

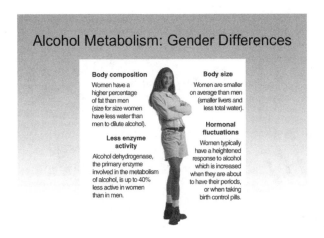

FIGURE 16-3 Example of effective slide presentation. Source: Insel, P., R.E. Turner, D. Ross. 2004. *Nutrition, Second Edition.* Sudbury, MA: Jones and Bartlett Publishers.

- *Advantages:* PowerPoint-type slides provide high-quality lettering, charts, and graphics. Careful use of color and animation can enhance motivation. Your presentation can be saved to a CD or a flashdrive or mini-drive and easily transported from your home or office to the place of presentation. Slides are relatively easy to create once you have learned the program.

- *Disadvantages:* The necessary equipment is expensive and not always available in field settings for nutrition education such as senior centers, after-school settings, or community group education. Use of slides can distance you from the audience, especially when the room is dark and you cannot see the audience. It is easy to put too much information on a slide.

Design Principles for Preparing Supporting Visuals

We have all experienced the presenter who begins a presentation by saying, "I know that you can't read this, but . . . ." You wonder why the presenter even bothered with the supporting visual! Whatever the form of the supporting visuals you are preparing, following certain guidelines will help you make them effective (Smith & Alford, 1989; Knight & Probart, 1992; Raines & Williamson, 1995). Public speaking expert Lucas (2004) provides useful guidelines that have been adapted here for use in nutrition education.

Clear and Simple Supporting Visuals

Supporting visuals should be simple, clear, and directly relevant to your message. They are aids, not the centerpiece. Use only as many real objects and models as are necessary to help visualize what you are talking about. Make slides, flip charts, and overhead transparencies concise; use the fewest words possible, to which you will add as you speak. Thus, the visual will contain much less information than you will actually present: it should not be something that you will read word for word and say nothing else. Each slide or overhead should present only one idea or one set of ideas. It is suggested that the number of words be limited to between 20 and 36. Some have recommended "the rule of six," which is to use no more than six lines of text and no more than six words per line (Raines & Williamson, 1995). This may be overly restrictive, but the principle is not to load the slide with information from margin to margin.

Reproductions of tables and graphs from journal articles or books are rarely effective. Such tables are meant to be studied at the reader's leisure while being held about a foot or so away. They cannot be processed and understood in the few seconds available during a presentation. Unless you are presenting to a professional audience, simplify the tables and graphs and render them boldly so that they can be understood quickly (Figures 16-4 and 16-5). In addition, carefully consider the background you will use. Computer software programs provide numerous different background formats from which to select. However, use simple designs. When you make supporting visuals too busy or complicated or you put too much information on them, you are more likely to confuse your group than enlighten them.

Supporting Visuals Large Enough for the Audience to See

We often have the urge to put a lot of information on the supporting visuals and hence to make the information too small. Remember, though, that if no one can see it, it is not only useless but also may provoke annoyance within the audience. Think about the size of the audience and their distance from you as you select or make your visuals.

For computer-generated slides, use font sizes that can be read from the back of the room when projected. It is recommended that for titles you use font sizes of 36 points; for subtitles, 24 points; and for the text, 18 points. Making fonts bold may increase readability. Capital letters are suitable for short titles of five to six words or fewer, but a combination of capital and lowercase letters is preferable for longer titles. ALL CAPS ARE MORE DIFFICULT TO READ, especially for those of lower literacy (Smith & Alford, 1989). Number lists or use bullets, and underline words for emphasis. Keep paragraphs short.

Choice of Colors

Use of color increases attention. However, it is possible to have too many colors in a supporting visual. Use color sparingly and design it carefully. Use one to three colors at the most, and use them consistently. It is best to decide on the major focus of the visual and select that color first. An effective practice is to select dark lettering or print on a light back-

Older students' (4th - 6th grade) pre-test and post-test scores. Analysis of Variance (ANOVA) comparing the four study conditions on the pre-test and post-test, and post hoc analysis to calculate significant differences between specific groups; unit of analysis is students

	Older students, 4th-6th grade									
	Pre-test					Post-test				
	CS + FEL *4 classes*	CS only *5 classes*	FEL only *4 classes*	Com. *3 classes*		CS + FEL *4 classes*	CS only *5 classes*	FEL only *4 classes*	Com. *3 classes*	
	M±SD (n)	M±SD (n)	M±SD (n)	M±SD (n)	F p^{**}	M±SD (n)	M±SD (n)	M±SD (n)	M±SD (n)	F p
Preferences for plant foods (range 1-5)	2.96±.61 (68)	3.14±.61 (86)	3.20±.64 (65)	3.26±.71 (42)	2.56 *NS*	3.30±.58^{ab} (68)	3.49±.59^a (84)	3.11±.59^b (61)	3.29±.62^{ab} (43)	5.06 *.002*
Attitudes (range 1-4)	2.63±.44^a (68)	2.83±.41^b (83)	3.01±.42^c (63)	2.73±.34^{ab} (42)	10.16 *<.001*	2.78±.43 (67)	2.83±.46 (82)	2.91±.46 (65)	2.76±.42 (39)	1.32 *NS*
Knowledge (range 0-12)	9.68±3.19^a (68)	11.67±3.13^b (86)	11.48±3.42^b (66)	10.26±2.84^{ab} (43)	6.40 *<.001*	16.96±3.72^a (68)	16.19±3.31^{ab} (86)	14.48±3.73^b (66)	11.05±2.81^c (43)	29.77 *<.001*
Self-efficacy in cooking (range 1-4)	3.22±.52 (68)	3.31±.47 (86)	3.26±.41 (66)	3.18±.53 (42)	.85 *NS*	3.31±.43^a (68)	3.50±.33^b (86)	3.28±.49^a (66)	3.27±.54^a (43)	4.51 *.004*
Behavioral Intentions										
Food Intentions Subscale (range 1-4)	2.23±.60 (68)	2.33±.62 (84)	2.38±.49 (65)	2.25±.48 (41)	1.03 *NS*	2.30±.60 (67)	2.40±.60 (85)	2.33±.55 (64)	2.67±.52 (43)	.38 *NS*
Paired Food Choice Subscale (range 0-7)	2.34±1.38 (68)	2.67±1.57 (84)	2.58±1.37 (65)	2.37±1.13 (43)	.89 *NS*	2.92±1.38 (66)	2.95±1.70 (82)	2.95±1.43 (62)	2.59±1.38 (41)	.65 *NS*

CS = Cookshops
FEL = Food & Environment Lessons
Com. = Comparison
Com. = Comparison
higher scores are always "better"

^{abc} different superscripts signify significant differences between those study groups
* n reported for each group was the number of students who took both the pre and post test; actual number of students in the classes was much larger
** ANOVA calculated significant differences among the four groups; to calculate significant differences between specific pairs of groups, Tukey Homogeneous Group Subsets Tests were used

FIGURE 16-4 Example of ineffective presentation of data for general audiences.

Cookshop Results for Older Children (Grades 4–6)

	Cookshop + *lessons*	Cookshop only	*Lessons only*	Control	Pre-post Cookshop *(Lessons)*
Preferences for plant foods (1-5)	3.2	3.4	3.1	2.8	<.001 *(ns)*
Attitudes (1-4)	2.8	2.8	2.9	3.2	ns *(ns)*
Knowledge (0-25)	16.1	16.1	14.1	11.3	<.001 *(<.05)*
Self-efficacy in cooking (1-4)	3.2	3.3	3.0	3.0	<.05 *(ns)*
Plate waste (%)	74	78	91	97	<.10 *(ns)*

FIGURE 16-5 Example of good presentation of data for general audiences.

ground. Some argue for using a dark background, particularly dark blue. In this case the graphics and lettering should be larger and white, or some strongly contrasting, bright color such as yellow. Do not use black on blue. The biggest danger in using a dark background is that the lettering and graphics may not be bright enough to see. In addition, a dark background usually requires that the room lights be dimmed, which means you lose touch with your audience.

Appropriate Fonts

Most computers come with dozens if not hundreds of different fonts or typefaces that you can use. It is best to choose those that are simple and easy to read. Also, limit the number of different fonts you will use in any given presentation. For example, use a squarer font in capitals for the title and a rounder font for the text. The rounder fonts are usually called *serif*, because they have little feet. The squarer typefaces are called *sans* (from the French meaning "without") *serif,* or without feet. A third style is called the *decorative* and includes all those that do not belong in the other two categories. The following list presents some common fonts and their appropriateness.

More Effective	Less Effective
Courier (serif)	*Apple Chancery*
Times or Times New Roman (serif)	*Lucinda Handwriting*
Arial (sans serif)	Harrington
Helvetica (sans serif)	**Textile**

Guidelines for Using Supporting Visuals

Having selected or designed your supporting visuals with care, you need to give careful consideration to how you will use them when you are with your group. You will want to ensure that you use them effectively so as to get your message across.

Ensure That Your Audience Will Be Able to See Your Visuals

When you plan on using visuals such as poster boards, be sure to arrive early so as to identify where you will place them so that all can see. Will you have access to easels? If not, where can you place them so that they will not fall over? If you are using objects, where will you place them so that all those in the audience can see? If you are using slides or overheads, do not stand in front of them and block the vision of the audience.

Show Your Supporting Visuals at the Appropriate Time

If you are using real objects such as food, food models, or food packages, do not show them to the audience until you are talking about them with the group. Leave them in cardboard boxes or bags until you are ready, or cover them up if you need to place them on a table in front of the audience. The same is true of poster boards or flip charts. Ensure that a blank sheet or a sheet with the title of the session is facing the audience as they come in. Likewise, for slides and transparencies, use a title slide as the audience or group enters, and introduce a blank (for slides) or cover up a transparency when you are not using the visuals. When you are finished, cover them up or put them away so as not to distract the audience.

Maintain Contact with Your Audience at All Times

When you are using overhead transparencies, slides, or poster boards, you will often find yourself facing the visuals and not your audience. Be sure you only glance at the visuals and continue talking to your audience so as to maintain eye contact with them.

Use Handouts and Materials Appropriately

You may have only one visual, such as a photo or object, that you want to pass around while you speak. However, doing so will cause you to lose the attention of those who currently have it in hand and are looking at it and distract all the others who are wondering about it. At professional meetings you may hand out copies of your PowerPoint presentation for the audience to follow along and take notes. Do so at the beginning or place them on the chairs before the audience comes in. But in most other settings, it is best to pass out materials such as handouts at the end. If you make handouts for everyone and wish to hand them out at various times, do so at the strategic times and allow time for all individuals to receive them before proceeding. Recognize, however, that these actions may be distracting.

Developing and Using Written Materials

Written materials in this context refers to short printed pieces such as handouts, flyers, brochures, tip sheets, booklets, and recipes that will be used with some intended nutrition education audience. Printed materials have many advantages compared with the other media described so far. Printed materials can be kept. Whereas messages in the visual media fly by, people can read and digest printed information at their own pace and refer to it over time. Printed media can provide information that can be read in private. Many individuals may be reluctant to ask questions in a group setting or to discuss issues they have. But they may be eager for the information provided in handouts or brochures that they can take home. And of course, printed materials can reinforce information discussed in a group setting or provided in a presentation.

The design of written materials should involve similar considerations to that of the six-step model used to design the group intervention itself. Many of the guidelines described earlier for designing supporting visuals apply to supporting printed pieces as well. This section highlights guidelines that may be useful for nutrition educators who are developing simple supportive materials. The advent of desktop publishing makes it possible for most of us to develop and design a variety of materials that are pleasing to the eye and of good quality. However, the services of a graphic designer, professional writer, or editor may be necessary to ensure high quality in the design and readability of written materials.

Planning the Printed Piece

The effectiveness of printed materials is improved if you have clear answers for the following questions for each printed piece:

- *What is the primary purpose for each printed piece?* If you could accomplish just one goal, what would it be? Is this a promotional piece designed to generate interest in the group program or is it an information piece that will be used in conjunction with the program? You should be able to say "The primary purpose of this flyer is to get people to come to the group nutrition education session" or "The purpose of this poster is to make eating a variety of colors of fruits and vegetables seem cool to teens." In other words, is the purpose to enhance motivation to take action and activate decision making (why-to information), or is the material to be used to reinforce the session by providing food and nutrition information that facilitates skills acquisition (how-to information), or some combination of both? What theoretical framework is being used? Which personal mediators of behavior change are addressed? In the example just given with teens, the purpose is to enhance motivation by addressing social norms (why to take action)—a primary theory construct in both social cognitive theory and theory of planned behavior.

- *What are the secondary purposes?* A printed piece usually has more than one goal. However, when you try to accomplish several goals, you risk not accomplishing any of them very well. So think carefully about which goal is your primary purpose and which goals are secondary. Perhaps the primary goal of your poster is to increase motivation, but you also want the poster to have information about eating five to nine servings of fruit and vegetables a day (how-to information). If this is your secondary purpose, you will want to consider a format that makes this clear—perhaps by using smaller lettering or positioning it lower on the page. Remember that there are also unstated purposes, which are the impressions people get from reading your printed piece. In the previously mentioned case of posters for teens, if the posters are hung up or placed in the cafeteria, the unstated purpose may be that the school is concerned about teens' health and welfare. A common

unstated purpose is for the reader to see you as professional and credible, or to see your organization or agency as a leader in the field.

- *What actions or behaviors do you want the audience to take?* What do you want individuals to do as a result of reading your piece? Individuals are more likely to take action if you lay out specific suggestions for what actions they can take. For example, in a brochure on cancer risk prevention, what specific actions are you aiming for? Do you want the individuals to go to a medical facility to get screened? Then spell out how to do so. Do you want them to eat more fruits and vegetables? Then say so and tell them how to do so. Is it a policy document about actions a school can take to ensure a healthy school food environment? Then spell out what a school can do. What would you like the audience to do with the printed piece itself? Pass it on? Then say so. Put on the refrigerator door or on a bulletin board? Say so.

- *How will the printed piece be used?* Will the piece be used only in conjunction with the group intervention? Will it be used during the session and/or taken home? Or should it be able to stand alone?

- *Who is the intended audience?* What is their background in terms of cultural or religious traditions? What are their attitudes and values in relation to the issue or behavior you wish to address? What is most likely to get their attention? Here you should go back to Step 2 of the procedural model for designing nutrition education (Chapter 8) for details on conducting an audience analysis.

  What are the characteristics of the audience, such as age, sex, cultural group, or educational level, that might influence the nature and design of the piece? For example, individuals with low literacy skills will require different approaches than those with high levels of education. What does the intended audience prefer in terms of types of content and layout? A good needs analysis is extremely important here.

- *What length do you need?* Our common urge is to want to tell the audience everything in one printed piece. But it is important to be selective. Do you have enough to say to require a booklet, or will a brochure do? Will a flyer do instead of a poster? If you have too much information for one printed piece, consider breaking up the information into several different handouts, flyers, or brochures.

- *What resources are available for this project?* The most frequently required resources are time, energy, and money. Needing a piece of printed material by a certain date will influence the nature of what you will be able to generate and produce. Likewise, our energy is limited. So think through carefully what you are able to do given your time. Perhaps someone else can work on it or at least help you with it. Finally, most of us work with limited budgets. This calls for creativity and careful thinking. Perhaps instead of a poster, a flyer will do. Or a lighter paper will do. Or printing with several shades of one color will work as well as several colors.

- *How will you evaluate the effectiveness of these materials?* It is important to obtain feedback on the materials, if not from written evaluation forms then from asking the recipients of the materials. You may also discuss with other members of your team such questions as the following: Did the printed pieces fulfill their purpose? What did the readers learn from them? How much time, effort, and money did it take to produce them? Was it worth it? How can they be improved?

Making Your Printed Materials Motivating and Effective

You want your printed pieces to be effective with your audience. Some suggestions follow.

Tailor the Piece to Your Audience

Your audience will be more interested in your printed materials if they can immediately see that the information is relevant to them. This means you need to know your audience well. A careful analysis as outlined in Steps 1 and 2 of the procedural model for designing nutrition education (described in Chapters 7 and 8) can provide you the information you need. In particular, you will need to know the audience's food- and nutrition-related knowledge, their attitudes and values in relation to the issue in your printed material, their living situation, what magazines they read and what visual media they watch, and what their tastes are in terms of written materials.

Make the Writing Motivational and Reader-Friendly

It is important to gain and hold the attention of your readers just as you plan to do when designing lesson plans or presentations for an audience. Several ways to do this are by beginning your printed piece with one of the following:

- *An interesting anecdote or personal story,* preferably of someone similar to the audience and involving a situation familiar to them. "As a group of teens entered the school cafeteria last week, they were surprised to discover it had had a complete makeover and looked very cool."
- *A surprising fact or startling statistic.* "The rate of obesity is increasing. At current rates, all individuals in the US will be overweight by the year *x*."
- *An intriguing question.* "Did you know that it has been estimated that one of three children today will develop diabetes during their lifetime?"

- *A checklist.* Create a checklist of foods or food-related behaviors addressed by the printed piece, such as a list of high-fat foods and fruits and vegetables, and ask readers to check off whether they eat them on most days. Come up with a score and tell them to read the rest of the printed material to learn how to eat a healthier diet.
- *A quiz.* Beginning with "Can you name five vegetables that are red or purple in color?" is likely to engage your readers.

Motivate the reader. We are very interested in food, nutrition, and health, but we can't assume that the reader shares our enthusiasm! Describe the importance of the issue you are addressing, such as eating school meals. List the benefits of the actions you are writing about, such as eating breakfast or calcium-rich foods. Make clear to readers what is in this for them. Again, your needs analysis information from Step 2 will be important here.

Put important information first. Assume that the reader will read just the first sentence, the first paragraph, or the first page. So place the most important information first rather than bury it in the middle of the document. Avoid lengthy introductions and long explanations at the beginning.

Be simple and direct. You are not writing a novel or poem. You are trying to communicate with the reader about important food- and nutrition-related information. So write simply and directly. To do this, consider the following tips:

- *Keep the words simple.* The field of nutrition is full of technical terms, and we often use them when simple ones will do. Often the simplest words have the fewest syllables. Thus, use *better* instead of *more advantageous,* and *use* instead of *utilize.*
- *Use the active voice rather than passive voice.* Active voice makes the writing more personal and lively. For example, instead of "The program participants will be provided with handouts," say "The nutrition educator will provide program participants with handouts."
- *Write strong sentences.* Vary the length of sentences, but generally keep them short. Varying the length of sentences changes the pace for readers and makes the writing more interesting. But express only one idea per sentence. Long and complex sentences are difficult to understand and may discourage people from reading, particularly those with low literacy. Aim for about 9 to 10 sentences per 100 words.
- *Keep paragraphs focused.* Begin sentences with the main topic. For example, say "Watching your weight is very important when you have diabetes," rather than "When you learn that you have diabetes, it is important for you to watch your weight." Begin each paragraph with the topic sentence and keep the paragraph to one key idea or theme.

- *Aim for the right reading level.* Determine the appropriate reading level for your audience. It is often said that the eighth-grade reading level is best for most general printed pieces, and the fifth-grade level for low-literacy audiences. Computer programs will now give you information on the reading level or readability scores for the document you are writing. You can also calculate the SMOG (simple measure of gobbledygook) score as follows: take 10 sentences each from the beginning, middle, and last paragraphs of the document. Count how many words in these 30 sentences have three or more syllables (polysyllabic words) and look up the approximate grade level in Table 16-1. Readability is also influenced by concept density, so keep each paragraph to only one concept or message.
- *Be professional and accurate.* Writing can take on many different styles, from humorous to chatty to serious. Regardless of style, use a professional tone in your writing. Being concise, clear, and readable will increase your credibility. Make sure your information is accurate.
- *Use a positive tone.* This does not mean you should be a Pollyanna. We know only too well that the news in the area of foods and nutrition is often dire. It means speaking to your readers in a respectful and positive manner. Being negative or condescending does not help you communicate your message.
- *Be consistent in your vocabulary*, particularly for technical information. For example, use *hypertension* or *high blood pressure*, but not both interchangeably.

Design Considerations

Make the written material look easy to read. The following tips can help:

- *Keep the document as short as you can.* We often try to say too much in our printed materials. The piece ends up looking crowded and difficult to read—and so it is not read.
- *Use more headings and keep them simple.* Break up the piece with more headlines and make them vivid and informative. This way the reader who only skims the piece will get something out of it. Rather than "Introduction," use "An Overview of the Senior Program." Instead of "Picky Eaters," use "Ways to Handle Picky Eaters."
- *Use more paragraphs and make them shorter.* Short paragraphs make for easier reading, especially in brochures and flyers. Long paragraphs make the page look dense and may discourage readers.
- *Include adequate white (empty) space.* Many of us think of empty or white space between paragraphs or in large margins as wasted space, waiting to be filled.

TABLE 16-1 Calculating Reading Levels: SMOG Conversion Table

Total Polysyllabic Word Counts	Approximate Grade Level (± 1.5 grades)
0–2	4
3–6	5
7–12	6
13–20	7
21–30	8
31–42	9
43–56	10
57–72	11
73–90	12
91–110	13
111–132	14
133–156	15
157–182	16
183–210	17
211–240	18

Source: McLaughlin, G.H. 1969. SMOG grading: A new readability formula. *Journal of Reading* 12:639–646.

However, it has been found that having adequate white space makes a piece easier to read. It is better to sacrifice some text than to have no white space.

- *Divide wide columns of text into two narrower columns for easier reading.* Lines that are too long strain the eye and make you lose track of the content, whereas lines that are too short cause the eye to jump back and forth. A line length of 50 to 70 characters is best because it is less tiring to the eye.
- *Make text left justified with a ragged right margin.* Left-justified text with a ragged right margin is easier to read because the ragged right profile helps the eye distinguish one line from the next. Full justification (lines that go to the same left and right margins) is difficult to read because it is hard to distinguish the lines and the eye has to adjust to different spacing between letters. Indenting the paragraphs is also important.
- *Use a simple font, especially with low-literacy audiences.* As emphasized earlier for designing visuals, using simple fonts and adequate font sizes can help the reader, particularly low-literacy audiences. Remember also that all caps are more difficult to read.
- *Use bullets where appropriate.* Bullets are useful when the information lends itself to a list. Tips, procedures, and things to do can all be listed with bullets. Bulleted lists break up the text and make brochures, handouts, and tip sheets easier to read.

Examples of print materials from the Pick a Better Snack campaign are shown in Figures 16-6 and 16-7. Figure 16-6 shows an article about eating apples to be printed in a newspaper, and Figure 16-7 shows text that can be used for a flyer, poster, or print ad in a magazine or newspaper. You can see that these materials exemplify all the tips we described earlier.

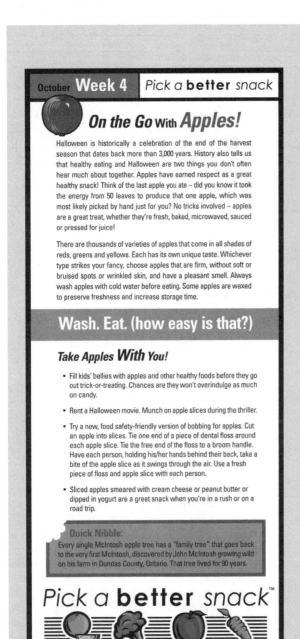

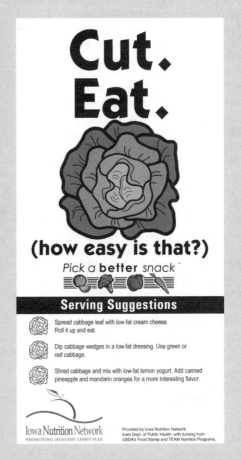

FIGURE 16-6 (Left) Example of good printed material: Printed newspaper story using a template. Source: Iowa Pick a Better Snack Social Marketing Campaign, www.idph.state.ia.us/picka-bettersnack/default.asp. Used with permission of Iowa Nutrition Network, Iowa Department of Public Health and Iowa Department of Education.

FIGURE 16-7 (Above) Text that can be used for a flyer, poster, or print ad in a magazine or newspaper. Source: Iowa Pick a Better Snack Social Marketing Campaign, www.idph.state.ia.us/pickabettersnack/default.asp. Used with permission of Iowa Nutrition Network, Iowa Department of Public Health and Iowa Department of Education.

A Caution

We may think that anything that is hands-on and innovative will be appreciated by our audiences. However, that may not always be the case. A survey of mothers in Head Start and Expanded Food and Nutrition Education Programs once found that participants did not judge all program activities to be equally enjoyable or effective. Their evaluations led to the tips found in Box 16-1.

> ### BOX 16-1 Helping Low-Income Consumers Achieve the 5 A Day Goal: Tips for Nutrition Educators
>
> Focus group interviews and surveys with low-income women found that the following were effective and enjoyable ways to promote fruit and vegetable consumption.
>
> **Taste Testing**
> - Provide tasters with the recipe and demonstrate the preparation steps.
> - Offer ways to prepare "old favorites" (broccoli, carrots, apples).
> - Offer the opportunity to taste new and unusual fruits and vegetables.
>
> **Recipe Booklets**
> - Limit number of ingredients (no more than five).
> - Ingredients should be low cost and on hand.
> - Limit number of steps; they should be quick and easy to do.
> - Do not include steps that use lots of dishes.
> - Do not use terms that people might not understand.
> - Include nutrition information about fat and calories.
> - Include a picture of how it should turn out.
> - Include tips for how to get the best buys when shopping for fruits and vegetables.
>
> **Take-Home Items (Freebies) with Useful Information or Reminders**
> - Calendars (with reminders to eat fruits and vegetables; recipes; health information)
> - Refrigerator magnets
> - Magnetized shopping lists
> - Tote bags
> - Coffee mugs, or juice cups for kids
> - Coloring books with recipes for kids
> - Fruits and veggies (to make the recipes they tasted at home)
>
> The methods listed below were least popular. Participants made the following suggestions for incorporating these elements if you decide to use them.
>
> **Videos**
> - Show videos for no more than 10 to 15 minutes at a time.
> - Select only videos that have "good actors" and "good music."
> - Use food demonstrations and taste testing, or other hands-on activities, in conjunction with the video.
>
> **Handouts or Brochures**
> - Discuss them with the group (don't just give to clients to take home).
> - Make them colorful/appealing.
> - Keep them simple, to the point, and useful to the clients.
>
> **Lecture-Style Presentation**
> - Be an enthusiastic speaker with a positive attitude.
> - Have personal experience with the topic.
> - Avoid use of technical terms (but also do not talk down to the group).
>
> *Source:* Based on focus group interviews conducted in March, 1996, with Expanded Food and Nutrition Education Program groups and Head Start and WIC moms ($n = 61$). Participants graded each of 20 methods using a scale ranging from A+ (12) to E (0). These methods included videos, group discussions, presentations, posters, refrigerator magnets, handouts, storybooks, coloring books and songs for children, recipes, mugs, and tote bags. The tips were generated from these scores. (Michigan Public Health Institute and Michigan Department of Community Health, presentation at the annual meeting of the Society for Nutrition Education, 1997.)

Educational Activities Using Other Channels

Nutrition educators engage in many activities in addition to conducting discussion groups, making presentations, and developing supporting written and visual materials. These include such activities as organizing health fairs and grocery store tours and conducting cooking classes. For all of these activities, plan ahead using the same six-step procedural model for designing nutrition education described in Part II of this book.

Planning the Activity

The effectiveness of your activity is improved if you are clear about the following:

- *What is the specific purpose of the activity?* The objectives of the activity should be clear. You should be able to say "The primary purpose of this activity is to get people to come to the group nutrition education session" or "The purpose of this activity is to teach skills in food selection (or in cooking) so that the audience is able to follow the recommendations of the program." In other words, is the purpose to enhance motivation to take action and activate decision making (why-to information) or is it to provide food and nutrition information and facilitate skills acquisition for those already motivated (how-to information), or some combination of both? What theoretical framework is being used? Which personal mediators of behavior change will be addressed?
- *What actions or behaviors do you want the audience to take?* Do you want the behavioral outcome of the activity, such as a health fair, to be that participants will attend the full program you are offering? Is it a freestanding activity with specific behavioral goals? For example, you may organize a health fair at which participants can be screened physiologically for a condition, such as blood pressure, or screened using a behavioral checklist, such as for their intake of fruits and vegetables. This may be followed by handouts about what to do. Thus, spell out clearly what you wish the action outcomes to be for the activity.

Guidelines for Nutrition Education Through Other Channels

Channels such as cooking experiences, health fairs, or grocery store tours are useful for conveying food- and nutrition-related information. The following guidelines can help.

Cooking or Food Preparation as Nutrition Education

Just about everyone is interested in food, and participating in preparing it can be motivating. There is also evidence that cooking can be effective as a means of nutrition education beyond other hands-on activity-based nutrition education

(Liquori et al., 1998; Brown & Hermann, 2005). Consequently, nutrition education programs often include a session, or part of a session, in which the participants cook or prepare some items that they then all eat together. Below are some tips for conducting such activities.

Getting started. Consider the following:

- *What are your objectives?* Be clear about the purpose or objectives of the food preparation activities. Do you wish to enhance motivation through the activity? For example, do you want to encourage the group members to try new foods? Is it an application of other material learned? Or is it primarily a skills-building activity for those already motivated? Do you want to assist participants to learn new ways of making familiar recipes more healthful?
- *What is the time frame?* What is the time frame that you have available for this activity? Is this a one-time session? How long? Or will this be a series of cooking sessions with a consistent group? These differences will influence your selection of objectives, recipes, and activities.
- *Who is your audience?* Do they come from a variety of ethnic groups with different cultural backgrounds, or are they somewhat homogeneous? Are they low income? These considerations will influence your recipe development.
- *What is the group's cooking skills level?* For example, are you working with teens with few skills or experienced older women with many skills? In all cases, make clear to the group the relationship of this activity to the rest of the nutrition education session or set of sessions.
- *What are the facilities?* Is there a stove in the setting or will you have to bring a butane stove or hot plate? Are there any utensils? Thus, you must check out the facilities ahead of time. If there are no cooking facilities and it is not possible for you to bring a heat source, you can still develop recipes that involve active food preparation such as making a salad. These factors will all influence the recipes you choose.
- *How large will the group be?* Will all the group members participate in the same food preparation or will you have several cooking stations preparing different recipes?
- *What ingredients and materials will you need?* Materials include all the utensils you will need as well as all the food items you will need. When bringing perishable foods, you need to consider issues of food safety, such as travel time in terms of keeping items cold and leaving food out at room temperature for any length of time. You may need to consider a cooler or ice packs. If you will have several stations, you may need several sets of utensils. If you have a lot of food materials, you will need sturdy boxes or suitcases on wheels.

Making the cooking experience motivating and effective. The following guidelines can help.

- *Tailor the experience to your audience.* Your audience will be more interested in food preparation if they can immediately see that the items being prepared are relevant to them, such as healthy and convenient snacks for teens or modifications of recipes for older adults. This means you need to know your audience well.

- *Make the cooking experience culturally appropriate.* One of the most visible and interesting ways in which people express their cultural and ethnic identity is through the food they will or will not eat. Hence it is very important that the recipes chosen and the practices recommended and taught take into consideration cultural differences between groups.

- *Test the recipes carefully ahead of time so that you know that they will work—no matter how simple they seem to be.* Test that they can be prepared in the setting in which the group will prepare them.

- *Always show respect for all participants.* Some may not like the recipes or have different levels of cooking skills, willingness to engage, and adventuresomeness in trying new foods. After all, preferences in food and eating are very personal. All participants bring valuable insights and past experiences to the table, and these should be honored.

- *Divide tasks into small group "assignments."* Each group may make a separate recipe or components of the same recipe.

- *Assemble all ingredients, materials, and utensils needed for each group ahead of time.* Place the ingredients for each group at a designated station or in a bag or box until you are ready to use them.

- *Review the recipes with the entire group.* Write the recipes on flip charts. If the group speaks English as a second language, record the recipe in their language of origin as well as in English. You may need to read the recipe, depending on the literacy level of the group.

- *Select the appropriate time within the session to do the food preparation activity.* You may lead a group discussion plus mini-lecture session first and conclude with the food activity as a skills development activity. Or you may have planned a series of cooking sessions for a group using food preparation as a primary form of nutrition education. In this case, interweave discussion of nutrition content with cooking, and provide motivational, why-to information as well as how-to food- and nutrition-related information. It is best not to talk too long before getting the group members started on the food preparation; provide information as you go along.

- *Review responsible cooking practices with the group.* These practices include the following:

  - Wash your hands before you begin, and wash them again if you cough, sneeze, or touch or hair or face.
  - Be careful with knives—even plastic knives.
  - Treat everyone with respect.
  - Cooking is most fun when everyone cooperates.
  - Listen carefully to the instructions and ask questions if you don't understand.
  - If you don't want to eat something, politely say "No, thank you." Do not say it is gross or nasty—someone else may love the taste.

Conclude with eating together if that is possible or appropriate. Make the ambience pleasant. Some nutrition educators bring paper tablecloths, and even vases of flowers, so that the eating experience is enjoyable.

Nutrition Education in Action 16-1 provides information on CookShop as an example of a program that uses cooking in the classroom as a means of nutrition education (Liquori et al., 1998; Wadsworth, 2005).

Conducting Grocery Store and Farmers' Market Tours

Tours of grocery stores or farmers' markets can be a wonderful experience for all ages. As we have noted before, all of us love food! Such tours can be conducted in a variety of markets, ranging from small to large, and can serve many purposes.

Getting started. Consider the following:

- *What are your objectives?* Be clear about the purpose or objectives of the supermarket or farmers' market tour. Do you wish to enhance motivation through the activity? Is it an application of other material learned? Or is it primarily a skills-building activity for those already motivated? It is generally best to be focused. For example, will you focus on how to identify low-fat foods, or will you introduce people to the large variety of fruits and vegetables available? These objectives should have been determined in Step 4 of the procedural design model (Chapter 10).

- *Who is your audience?* Are they children or adults? This will make a difference in how the experience is structured. Are they of a particular ethnic or cultural group? Are they low in resources? Your audience assessment in Step 2 of the procedural design model can provide you with this information (Chapter 8).

Planning the tour. Get approval if the tour is to take place in a grocery store, especially if you are bringing a group of children. This usually involves the manager. The 5 A Day program encourages grocery stores to provide tours to children, and grocery stores are often happy to conduct them, seeing it as a good opportunity to encourage families to eat more fruits and vegetables and to generate positive community relations and media publicity. You will need to schedule a time that is convenient for the store as well as for your group. Approvals are not usually needed at most farmers' markets.

Develop an educational plan for the tour. This should be designed as part of Step 4 of the design model. Determine the specific educational objectives of the tour and design several activities to achieve them. For children and adults, develop activity sheets that they can complete while at the store or market. These may include a scavenger hunt of some sort to find specific foods, such as low-fat items or specific fruits and vegetables. Or make the participants food detectives. Make the activities humorous or brain-twisters so as to provide interest and challenge.

Map out how you will proceed inside the store or market. Make arrangements for where your group can congregate while you give them the information, and determine to what extent grocery store personnel will be involved.

Making the experience motivating and effective. Make the tour a physically and mentally active experience. Do not just go from aisle to aisle talking about foods! In the store, carry out some verbal activities first. For example, a tour on fruits and vegetable can begin with questions such as "What colors do you see when you look at all these fruits and vegetables?" "Can you name a red fruit that you see? A green one?" and so forth (Dole Food Company, 2001).

Provide clipboards, or the equivalent, so that participants can complete written activities. Perhaps you could have them complete some kind of self-assessment relevant to the foods of focus. Then send them on a food investigation tour with a series of questions in their activity sheets. Assign points for completing various activities. The store may be willing to provide taste testing of some fruits and vegetables or of

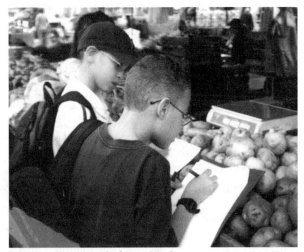
Nutrition education at the farmers' market.

recipes made from them. This would result in a tour that challenges all the senses.

Make the tour informative and relevant to your audience. With adults in particular, the tour should teach skills as well as enhance motivation. Perhaps you can teach preparation methods for various vegetables and supply recipes, point out lower-fat versions of food products, introduce them to whole grains of various kinds, and so forth.

Clearly, there are many options for what you can do, limited only by what your group is interested in and your creativity.

Health Fairs
Many nutrition education programs find that holding a health fair is a useful activity, particularly in worksites, colleges, and community centers. As is the case for the activities described earlier, you need to start with a clear understanding of the specific purpose of the activity and of the actions or behaviors you want the participants to take as a result of participating in the health fair. Health fairs take some effort and planning, so you will have to start early. Develop a time line based on the following considerations.

Getting started. Be clear about the purpose or objectives of the health fair. Do you want the fair to attract attention as a kickoff event to motivate people to attend other activities of the program, such as group education or physical activity sessions? Or is it a standalone event where you want to motivate individuals to take a certain action and provide some skills on how to do it?

Planning the health fair. Consider the following:

- *Site.* Select or find a location. This may depend on how many people you think will attend and hence the space you will need. Will you have break-out activities? Can all of these be done in the same space, or will you need additional rooms?
- *Other potential participants.* Will program staff conduct all the activities or will you invite other similar agencies or groups to participate? For example, if the focus of the health fair is to increase fruit and vegetable consumption, you may want to ask personnel from a nearby hospital to conduct blood pressure screenings as motivation. Or you may want someone from a local gym to demonstrate activities people can do in the home. This will help you decide how many tables you will need.
- *Raffles.* If you will use raffles as a motivator to attend the health fair, early on you will need to seek out local vendors who can provide items to raffle off, such as membership to a gym. This will require letters and/or phone calls.
- *Activities.* Brainstorm the topics or issues you will focus on. Limit them depending on the scope of your fair. For

each, decide on the central message. Each message or topic should have a table or booth, on which you will display posters using a foamcore stand. You will need to develop quizzes, activities, and handouts. These need to be motivating and informative, using theory-based strategies as appropriate.

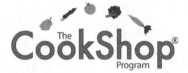

NUTRITION EDUCATION IN ACTION 16-1

CookShop

CookShop Classroom is a nutrition education curriculum designed to increase early elementary school students' consumption of whole and minimally processed plant foods through hands-on exploration and cooking activities. CookShop Classroom began implementation in New York City public schools in 1995. At this time, it was called the CookShop Program and included a cafeteria component. Since then, it has evolved to accommodate changing school and classroom environments to become a year-long, standards-focused, classroom curriculum.

CookShop Classroom strives to increase students' acceptance and consumption of plant foods and foster an understanding of where food comes from. To meet these goals, the curriculum, specifically designed for kindergarten and second grade classrooms, capitalizes upon students' natural curiosity and excitement about cooking and how things grow.

The curriculum consists of twenty-two lessons divided into eleven units: two introductory units and nine plant units. The introductory units familiarize students with the skills used throughout the curriculum. The plant units introduce the students to regionally available plant foods through pictorial letters from local farmers, sensory food explorations, cooking activities, and shared eating experiences in the classroom. Each plant unit consists of two lessons: explorer and chef. During the explorer lesson, students directly explore a plant and learn about how it grows. In the chef lesson, students become chefs, cooking and eating a recipe that focuses on the food explored the previous lesson. This structure provides students with multiple meaningful exposures to the foods they have learned about, and creates stronger academic and behavioral change opportunities.

Experience and research demonstrate that the greatest impacts on student dietary change outcomes come from classroom lessons that provide cooking and eating experiences and that are complemented by related experiences outside the classroom (Liquori et al., 1998; Wadsworth, 2005). With this in mind, two other school-based programs have been created to complement CookShop Classroom and to establish links with the cafeteria and parent components of the school community. SchoolFood Plus Cafeteria (originally part of the CookShop Program) provides exposures to the same plant foods the students learn about in the classroom through incorporation onto the school lunch menus in many of the same New York City elementary schools. In addition, SchoolFood Plus Cafeteria provides cafeteria-based activities and marketing that further promote these plant foods and reinforce classroom learning. CookShop for Adults, the community-based adult counterpart to CookShop Classroom, has been incorporated into some of New York City's elementary schools via parent connections to provide parents with the knowledge, skills, and resources to further students' learning and exposure to plant-based foods at home.

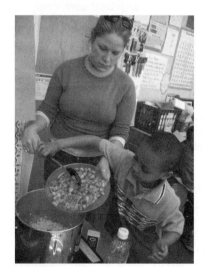

CookShop Classroom

CookShop Classroom and CookShop for Adults are curricula developed at and implemented through FoodChange, a New York City–based nonprofit organization. SchoolFood Plus Cafeteria is a program of the SchoolFood Plus Initiative that involves many partners. More information about the program, its partners, and funding sources can be found on the FoodChange website, www.foodchange.org.

CookShop logo courtesy of CookShop Program, FoodChange, New York City.

Sources: Liquori, T., P.D. Koch, I.R. Contento, and J. Castle. 1998. The CookShop program: Outcome evaluation of a nutrition education program linking lunchroom food experiences with classroom cooking experiences. *Journal of Nutrition Education* 30:302–313; Wadsworth, K. 2005. "From farm to table: The making of a classroom chef," presented at the Society for Nutrition Education Annual Conference, Orlando, Florida.

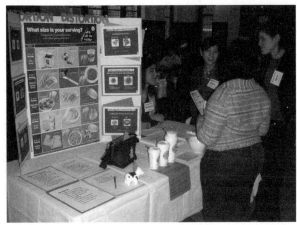

Nutrition education through worksite health fairs.

- *Promotion and advertising.* You can promote the fair using a variety of approaches, such as posters displayed around the institution, postcards sent to various departments or to community groups, email messages sent to selected audiences, or a story in the institution's newsletter or local newspaper.

Making the experience motivating and effective. Staff or volunteers should have on name tags and be ready to greet attendees. Staff should be assigned to meet other vendors or participants and help them set up. The displays should look professional, attractive, and welcoming. The raffle products should be displayed all on one table so that attendees can see what they might get if they complete quizzes or other activities. Have someone take pictures so that they can be used as follow-up motivators if posted, for writeups about the event, and for evaluation or documentation purposes.

Mass Media and Social Marketing Activities

A brief discussion of social marketing and mass media activities is included here because a mass media campaign or social marketing component often accompanies in-person, in-institution activities as part of a larger program. Activities often described as social marketing are really mass media nutrition communication campaigns. Nutrition mass media campaigns involve communication strategies to disseminate messages to targeted audiences through a variety of mass channels such as newspaper articles, radio public service announcements (PSAs), or paid advertising. Social marketing, on the other hand, is a complex enterprise that often includes mass media campaigns, but may not, and involves the larger enterprise of marketing. It is described only briefly here in terms of its use in nutrition education. Whether designing mass media campaigns or developing social marketing activities, nutrition educators usually work in collaboration with mass media or social marketing experts.

Nutrition Mass Media Communication Campaigns

A mass media communication campaign is usually described as an intervention that "intends to generate specific outcomes of effects, in a relatively large number of individuals, usually within a specified period of time, and through an organized set of communication activities" (Rogers & Storey, 1988; Institute of Medicine [IOM], 2002). Such campaigns are designed to reach large audiences, using multiple channels. They usually require substantial resources in terms of money and effort. Campaigns seek to "influence the adoption of recommended health behaviors by influencing what the public knows about the behavior and/or by influencing actual and/or perceived social norms, and/or by changing actual skills and confidence in skills (self-efficacy), all of which are assumed to influence behavior" (IOM, 2002). They are often part of social marketing programs. Such campaigns are sometimes conducted along with efforts to change the environment using a multiple-level, ecological model of health promotion.

The process of developing such campaigns involves consideration of the communication principles described in the last chapter and engagement in a process somewhat similar to that described in the six-step nutrition education design model used in this book, as follows: selecting the intended audience and specific behavioral outcomes, conducting extensive formative research (needs analysis) with the audience, choosing the message strategy and how the messages will be worded and executed, selecting the channels and settings for dissemination, and conducting ongoing monitoring and evaluation. Detailed instructions on how exactly to design and implement health communications can be found in documents such as *Making Health Communication Programs Work,* published by the National Cancer Institute (2004), and *Speaking of Health,* from the Institute of Medicine (2002).

Social Marketing

The term *social marketing* is defined in many different ways. Kotler and Zaltman (1971) first proposed that marketing principles could be applied to socially relevant programs, ideas or behaviors. They saw social marketing as the design, implementation, and control of programs seeking to increase the acceptability of a social idea or practice of a target group. The term often refers to a systematic planning process that focuses on consumer behavior (understanding the target group's values, attitudes, barriers, and incentives to change), developing clear messages, designing interventions, implementing them, and evaluating results on a continual basis. It also refers to a particular conceptual framework about how to bring about behavior change. The definitions have in common the notion that social marketing is a set of systematic procedures to promote personal and societal welfare. Here we first describe the conceptual framework and then the social marketing process.

Conceptual Framework

Social marketing is based on the following set of considerations (Kotler and Zaltman, 1971, Lefebvre & Flora, 1988, Kotler & Roberto, 1989, Andreasen, 1995, Rothschild, 1999, Alcalay & Bell, 2000):

- Social marketing is applied to causes that are considered to be beneficial to both individuals and society.
- It seeks to promote the voluntary behavior of intended audiences so as to reduce risk or enhance health, not simply to increase awareness or alter attitudes.
- It does so by offering intended audience members reinforcing incentives and/or consequences in an environment that invites voluntary change or exchange (see below).
- Social marketing is tailored to the unique perspectives, needs, and experiences of the intended audience with input from representatives of that audience.
- Social marketing strives to create conditions in the social structure that facilitates the behavioral changes promoted.
- Social marketing uses the processes and concepts of marketing.

Here we focus on some central ideas and practices that are useful for nutrition education.

Self-interest

Individuals are assumed to act in their own self-interest. Although there are many determinants of behavior beyond self-interest (Mansbridge, 1990), it has been proposed that self-interest plays some role in most contexts of human interaction. Self-interest can be seen as similar to the concept of outcome expectations (or anticipated outcomes) from social psychological theory– outcomes people can expect from engaging in healthy behaviors such as health or decreased risk of disease. The anticipated outcomes are often long-term rather than immediate as in the example of urging people to increase their intake of calcium-rich foods to reduce risk of osteoporosis. Indeed, these long-term outcomes may be in conflict with more immediate outcomes based on self-interest. For example, people choose to eat the unhealthy foods they do or not to be physically active because they have evaluated their life situations and have made their decisions based on their current judgment of their self-interest. Social marketing thus seeks to promote change by offering benefits that the intended audience perceives to be in their self-interest, as identified through thorough market research or needs analyses. That is, it offers "the benefits they (intended audience members) want, reducing the barriers they are concerned about, and using persuasion to participate in program activity" (Kotler & Roberto, 1989).

Self-Interest

Exchange Theory

Central to social marketing is the notion of voluntary exchange of resources: one party gives up something in exchange for getting something from another party. In the case of nutrition education, this means that participants give up time, effort, convenience, or money in exchange for the benefits of enhanced physical health, improved psychological well-being, or a healthful, wholesome food system (Rothschild, 1999; Alcay & Bell, 2000). Our job as nutrition educators is to demonstrate that the benefits outweigh the costs of taking action. In the design of strategies for enhancing benefits and encouraging action, social marketing uses other theories as tools, such as the theories described in Part I of this book: the health belief model, the theory of planned behavior, social cognitive theory, or the transtheoretical model.

Focus on Intended Audience Members' Wants and Needs

The design of social marketing activities is based on what individuals or consumers want or need. Although evidence from research studies is important and best practices can be very useful, social marketing adds a strong focus on what specific audience members in a given community want and need. Hence it invests heavily in *market research*, which is similar to the needs analysis process described in Chapter 8, to find out about the specific perspectives, values, attitudes, interests, and needs of a given audience. Social marketing also emphasizes pretesting potential materials, messages, and themes with the intended audience so as to refine the message based on their suggestions. If audience members influence the development of the program, it is more likely the intervention will be effective.

Segmentation of the Audience

In order to be able to design messages and activities that are highly specific, social marketers try to segment or subdivide any broad category of individuals into more homogeneous subgroups using demographic criteria such as age, sex, income, and ethnicity; geographic criteria such as urban, suburban, and rural settings; psychological criteria such as motivations, readiness to change, or skill levels; and behavioral criteria such as the degree to which the group already practices the behavior of concern. Selection of which segment or subgroup to focus on can be based on various criteria, such as which group has the greatest need based on the size of the group and the incidence and severity of food- or nutrition-related conditions, which group is most ready to change, or which group has the most influence on others.

Tipping the Scales

Whereas education can increase awareness, promote active contemplation, enhance motivation, and teach food- and nutrition-related behavioral skills and self-regulation skills, social marketing goes beyond education by attempting to modify the relative attractiveness of the specific behavior. This is accomplished through the use of incentives and other benefits that positively reinforce the behavior and through the reduction of barriers or costs associated with the behavior, thereby tipping the scales in favor of the behavior, according to Rothschild (1999). Social marketing focuses on providing direct, immediate, and tangible benefits that are reinforcing. It also attempts to reduce both personal barriers, such as beliefs and expectations, and external barriers by making the environment favorable for the appropriate behavior. In the case of an intervention to increase the consumption of more fruits and vegetables, social marketers not only provide educational messages but also reduce barriers by such activities as increasing the availability of fruits and vegetables in schools, working with grocery stores to lower prices, or providing coupons that participants can redeem at stores.

Key Elements in Planning Social Marketing

The social marketing planning process systematically addresses the five Ps of the "marketing mix" considered by commercial marketers (Alcay & Bell, 2000; Maibech, Rothschild, & Novelli, 2002),

Product. *Product* refers to what is exchanged with the intended audience for a price. The product may not be a tangible item but a service, practice, or intangible idea such as health. For the product to be "buyable," people must first perceive that they have a problem and that the product being offered is a good solution. Here formative research is important to unveil consumers' perceptions about the problem and how strongly they feel that they can do something to solve the problem. Thus, products are desired behaviors, benefits of these behaviors, and any tangible objects and services offered to support the behaviors.

The core product can be a health idea or behavior that is of benefit to individuals. For example, the idea can be improved health, or the action can be eating five to nine servings of fruits and vegetables daily. Supporting products can be material items, such as coupons for fruits and vegetables at farmers' markets, or a service such as a WIC clinic or nutrition education classes (but not the materials used in the classes—which are described later in this chapter in a different category). In designing a program, you have to be very clear about what exactly is your product. If it is a behavior, you need to find out from the intended audience what behaviors they see as realistic, effective, practical, or easy to do. You should also be specific: Is the product the behavior of eating *more* fruits and vegetables, or eating a specific amount such as 2.5 cups a day or more?

Price. *Price* refers to the barriers or costs to the consumer associated with obtaining the product, such as adopting the desired behavior, and any monetary and nonmonetary incentives, recognition, and rewards used to reduce the costs. Costs can include the economic costs of eating more fruits and vegetables as well as the inconvenience and increased time involved in the preparation of healthful foods, or perhaps the psychological costs of learning new ways of eating. Social marketing recognizes that decisions to act are based on considerations of both benefits and costs. Individuals ask themselves, "What will I gain if I engage in this behavior, and what will it cost me?" Often individuals fail to take action not because they do not recognize the benefits, but because the costs are too high.

Social marketing thus seeks to increase the benefits and decrease the price or barriers of engaging in the behavior of concern (Andreasen, 1995; Rothschild, 1999). It does this by addressing the internal determinants of behavior that we have discussed earlier in the book, such as perceived risk, beliefs about outcomes of taking action, knowledge, social norms, and self-confidence or self-efficacy. Social marketing also addresses external barriers such as policy, access, skills, and cultural trends by attempting to create conditions in the social structure and environment to facilitate the actions being promoted. More simply said, it attempts to make the more healthful behavior the easy behavior.

In the case of promoting fruits and vegetables to low-income mothers of young children, the benefits might be the good health of their children or wanting to enhance their children's educational opportunities and performance. Internal barriers might be lack of time and cooking skills or confusion about portion sizes for their children. External barriers might include the high cost of healthful foods such as fruits and vegetables. Food stamps and coupons for farmers' markets would be ways to reduce external barriers.

Place. *Place* refers to where and when the product will reach the consumer. In the case of intangible products, it is the place where the audience will receive the information. This may mean researching which media channels are most effective for reaching the intended audience. It may mean grocery stores, doctors' offices, community centers, WIC clinics, or food stamp offices. Place can also refer to where you might offer program activities (such as classes) so that they are convenient to the intended audience. Social marketing seeks to increase the places where the product may be found, at the right times, and at the points at which audience members make their decisions. Behaviors must be easy to carry out; hence, placement must encourage the behavior. If increasing consumption of fruits and vegetables is the behavior, then the placement strategy might be to have information and messages conveniently located in the grocery store, workplace, or school lunchroom.

Promotion. The targeted audience members can be expected to voluntarily exchange their time, effort, and other resources if they are aware that the product, such as eating fruits and vegetables, offers them attractive benefits at a reasonable cost and can be practiced at convenient locations. The role of *promotion* is to create this awareness. For example, the 5 A Day campaign complemented its efforts by placing the product (messages about fruits and vegetables) in the right places via a promotional campaign in the news media and point-of-purchase materials such as messages on grocery store bags. Promotion requires considerations such as the following:

- *What channels to use to reach the intended audience.* For fruit and vegetable consumption among low-income mothers of young children, the channels might be grocery stores, day-care centers, WIC clinics, food stamp offices, community centers, newspapers, or TV.
- *What types of messages might be effective.* The content of the messages will be based on your audience analysis or needs assessment, as described in Chapter 8. The nature of the message, such as whether to use humor, emotion, or logical reasoning, should again be based on your audience analysis. The tone of the messages should be positive, such as "We know it is hard, but we know that you want to make a change." It should also be respectful, fun, and personal.

Positioning. The product can be positioned in such a way as to maximize benefits and minimize costs. *Positioning* is a psychological construct that involves the location of the product relative to products with which it competes. Positioning is difficult in nutrition education because it means having your product (message) outweigh the competitors. For example, it is very challenging to get teenagers to eat more fresh fruits and vegetables when they feel that the alternative products, such as high-fat snacks, taste much better. However, physical activity can be repositioned as a form of relaxation rather than as exercise (which some may view negatively). Serving fruits and vegetables can be positioned as taking care of yourself, and serving healthful meals to your family can be positioned as an act of love.

Designing Social Marketing Activities

As we have seen, social marketing programs are tailored to the unique perspectives, needs, and experiences of the target audience and also seek to create conditions in the social structure and environment that facilitate the actions being promoted (Andreasen, 1999; Alcay & Bell, 2000). The set of procedures for designing social marketing is similar to that described in models of health communication and the six-step nutrition education design model used in this book. In social marketing these steps are usually referred to as formative research and planning, strategy design, implementation, and evaluation. To develop the social marketing campaign or activities, nutrition educators usually work in collaboration with health communication and social marketing experts. These experts are especially important in the formative

research, message development, and planning stages. Hence the design phase is only summarized briefly here.

Formative research and planning involve setting goals, selecting the audience segment or subgroup to work with, and identifying the focus of the intervention. The focus may be change in individual attitudes or behaviors, community norms, policies, or all three. The various channels are selected at this time, such as posters, classes, community events, changes in availability of the foods in the stores, or policies in schools and workplaces. An environmental analysis is conducted and community participation sought. Formative research seeks to understand the motivations, attitudes, and behaviors of the intended audience, as well as the audience's perceptions of the benefits and costs of taking the recommended action.

Strategy design includes designing the campaign message based on the formative research, and pretesting the message using focus groups and surveys. The marketing mix, or five Ps, is selected at this time.

Implementation usually involves considerable collaboration with individuals and organizations in the community. This is described in greater detail in the next subsection. Funding and changes in social structures are sought so that the programs can be maintained over the long term.

Evaluation is important. There are many approaches, the simplest of which is to see whether the audience can recall campaign messages. Another measure is extent of exposure—the number of activities that audience members have attended, such as classes or workshops, live food demonstrations, or health fairs, or the amount of materials they have taken home. Other measures are surveys of mediator of behavior/change such as knowledge, beliefs, attitudes, behavioral intent, or stage of change. Behaviors can be self-reported through a survey or using monitoring data such as the increase in sales of fruits and vegetables in grocery stores or increased attendance at fitness classes and gyms.

Implementing Social Marketing Involving Mass Media and Related Activities

Social marketing often involves the mass media, but not always. Here we describe the use of social marketing in a program that involves the mass media as a primary channel—the Pick a Better Snack campaign—and in a program that did not—the Food Friends program.

Social marketing that uses mass media as the primary channel usually requires the collaboration of many individuals and organizations. Such campaigns can be local, community-wide, statewide, or national. Some potential practical methods for implementing social marketing are summarized below, based on the literature and best practices of those who have been involved. These methods are useful to nutrition educators who are interested in incorporating mass media and community support components into their programs.

The following suggestions are based on the experience of the Pick a Better Snack campaign in Iowa (Iowa Department of Public Health, n.d.).

Media Activities

1. *Develop media partnerships.* Prior to the initiation of the campaign, actively solicit print, outdoor, and broadcast media partnerships to extend the reach of the campaign to audiences that would otherwise be out of the program's reach for financial reasons.

   ▶ Meet with local television and radio station public service directors, station promotional managers, and print advertising managers to identify opportunities for partnerships.

   ▶ Draw up a simple joint agreement that outlines how each partner will be identified in collaborative efforts, such as whose logos will be on media events. Such agreements avoid misunderstandings later on and engender trust.

2. *Introduce the campaign to the community.* You have only one shot to introduce your campaign. The challenge here is to make as big a splash as you can with a few simple messages and to get media coverage.

   ▶ Plan a kickoff event such as a press conference. Select a site with a compelling visual element for broadcast media where a story can be told, such as at a farmers' market, grocery store, or after-school program.

   ▶ Carefully develop two to four key messages to serve as the focus of the news conference or event.

3. *Sustain ongoing media relationships.* Work with local media to develop periodic articles or special features on the importance of your message, as did the Pick a Better Snack campaign.

   ▶ Identify a few key reporters and news editors who are responsible for covering food or health issues and work on building a good working relation-

ship with them. Contact them from time to time by phone or email with news about campaign events or article ideas. Follow up with information to support your story ideas. Or send them a draft of a potential article for them to modify.

   ▶ Offer to serve as a resource for them on other food and nutrition issues.

4. *Plan an outdoor campaign if feasible.* Place your messages on billboards, bus benches, buses, or bus shelters. These can be paid for or placed as PSAs.

   ▶ Work with outdoor media companies to identify the best locations for your intended audience and obtain cost estimates.

   ▶ Outdoor media companies will frequently run billboards with as PSAs at no charge for the space. These may not be placed in prime locations, so negotiate with them about placement and duration.

Community Outreach

1. *Develop a newsletter.* Develop a simple, inexpensive newsletter to keep key partners and targeted segments of the campaign's audience informed about your activities and progress.

   ▶ The frequency of the newsletter will depend on your ability to develop a simple system for its regular development and distribution, but should be at least quarterly.

   ▶ Because it will go to a variety of stakeholders, the newsletter should also include information relevant to the campaign, such as recipes and actionable ideas for taking the action promoted by the campaign.

2. *Collaborate with community organizations.* Collaborate with community organizations regarding events that would bring benefit to your program and the organization, such as farmers' markets, local food drives, broadcast media, and health fairs.

   ▶ Work with a local farmers' market to organize an event that would both bring people to the farmers' market and bring awareness to the campaign messages. Demonstrate simple recipes reflecting the campaign action (such as eating more fruits and vegetables), decorate with campaign posters, and wear campaign-related tee-shirts.

   ▶ Work with other organizations at special events they may sponsor, such as community health fairs sponsored by local radio or TV stations.

3. *Place campaign literature in strategic locations.* Distribute program literature to the public in several health- and medical services–related settings throughout the community.

   ▶ Work with your local medical society leadership to encourage them to recommend to their members that they participate by being willing to serve as dis-

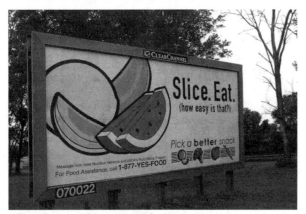

Billboards are another way to get the message out.

tribution points for your campaign literature (such as posters, recipes, or bookmarks) to their clients.

▶ Distribute your written PSAs to county medical groups for inclusion in their regular member newsletters.

Working with Schools

1. *Work with school food service staff.* Provide a campaign promotional package to food service directors for use in school cafeterias, suggests the Pick a Better Snack campaign.
    ▶ In this package include several posters and selected samples of point-of-sale materials to allow them to dress up the lunch line.
    ▶ Encourage food service directors to periodically focus on the campaign for a week, such as to promote fruits and vegetables or low-fat milk that week.
2. *Coordinate with parent–teacher organization (PTO) open houses and school events.* Solicit local schools' PTOs to promote your goal behavior at their social events and fundraising sales.
    ▶ Have a booth at the PTO/school open house to raise awareness that the school is focusing on the campaign goal through its curriculum. Outline what parents can do at home to support the campaign's target goal.
    ▶ Hand out samples of foods promoted by your campaign, as well as recipes, postcards, book markers, and so forth.
    ▶ Seek PTO volunteers to promote imaginative after-school snacks, foods for sporting events, and school fundraisers (in place of bake sales) that support the campaign goals.

Grocery Store Activities

1. *Conduct in-store or farmers' market demonstrations.* Volunteer to conduct in-store food demonstrations in a local grocery store. (See Dole Food Company [2001] for tips on how to conduct one with students.)
    ▶ Work with the store manager to get approval to do a demonstration.
    ▶ Demonstrate only one or two very simple ideas for the promoted foods; hand out recipes and other campaign material.
2. *Use incentive cards to persuade individuals to try promoted foods.* The campaign may develop incentives for children to eat certain foods, such as fruits and vegetables, by handing out cards (through schools, WIC clinics, or other food-related settings) with activities printed on them for the whole family to do. In the Pick a Better Snack campaign, when the family verified that the activity had been completed, they took the card to a participating grocery store or returned it to the school to redeem it

for an incentive. Focus group research in several locations has shown that "unfamiliarity" and fear of wasting food are frequently barriers to trying new foods. Incentives thus can be free samples of campaign-related food items to help families overcome the barrier of fearing to purchase foods that their children will not eat.
    ▶ Develop a system for distribution of the educational incentive items.
    ▶ Work with store managers to develop a redemption procedure.
3. *Provide in-store signage.* Develop signs to identify the foods promoted by the campaign.
    ▶ Set up criteria for classifying food items as qualifying as target foods. For example, if low-fat foods are a focus, define what you mean by *low-fat*. Come with a list of foods that qualify.
    ▶ Work out with the store manager who will place the signs, who will monitor them, and who will change them as needed.

Implementing Social Marketing Involving Other Channels

Social marketing principles can be used to design and implement programs that do not involve the mass media. For example, social marketing has been used to design a variety of community-based and even school-based programs. The key approaches in design are to conduct extensive formative research to identify the potential audiences, the important nutritional issues, and the key channels to use with an intended audience.

Food Friends

The program called Food Friends provides an example of the social marketing process (Young et al., 2004). This program was directed at promoting healthful food choices among low-income families.

Formative Research. Focus groups are a major method of collecting formative research data in social marketing. They can be used to identify the audience segment with which you can work. In this example, focus groups were conducted with low-income elderly individuals and with low-income parents with children. Results from these focus groups usually help you narrow the target population. In the example of Food Friends, families with young children aged 3 to 7 were selected. Next you conduct focus groups with the selected audience. Here you can be more specific, for example, asking about the target group's eating practices, barriers to healthful eating, and preferred communication channels. Through this process, the audience identified in the Food Friends program was preschoolers, the behavior chosen was "trying new foods," and the site for delivery of the message was Head Start centers. Novel foods to include in the program were identified from a food frequency questionnaire.

Campaign Strategy. Formative research provides the basis of campaign strategy. In the case of Food Friends, it led to the selection of an intervention involving education and marketing strategies to be distributed through Head Start programs (not through the mass media). They included nutrition activities, novel foods offered during afternoon snack time, and parental involvement through the publication of articles in the monthly Head Start newsletter. Food Friends is described in Nutrition Education in Action 16-2.

WIC Social Marketing Program

Table 16-2 presents a case example of the use of social marketing to plan strategies to reduce barriers for WIC participants to shop at farmers' markets. The five Ps provide the planning framework.

Comparing Social Marketing and Nutrition Education

Many years ago, an early social marketer, Richard Manoff (1985), who had achieved considerable success in improving nutrition in several developing countries, quipped at a Society for Nutrition Education meeting that "anything that works is social marketing; anything that does not is nutrition education." Others, on the other hand, criticize social marketing as too simplistic, not promoting the critical thinking and reflection that are needed in making informed choices in a complex food system (Van Den Heede & Pelican, 1995). The debate continues even as many nutrition education programs incorporate social marketing activities as a component. Here we compare the two endeavors on three features considered to be central to social marketing: it tailors messages and strategies to the unique perspectives, needs, and experiences of the

---

NUTRITION EDUCATION IN ACTION 16-2

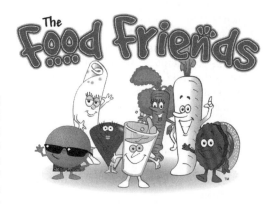

Food Friends: A Nutrition Education Initiative for Preschool Children Using Social Marketing Principles

The Food Friends program was directed at promoting healthful food choices among low-income families in Colorado. It used social marketing as a framework for developing the program, including extensive formative research to identify key behaviors or practices that would promote health. Included in the formative research were focus groups, an extensive food frequency questionnaire to identify foods that preschoolers eat, and concept pretesting. Through this process, the audience identified was preschoolers, the behavior chosen was "trying new foods," and the selected site for delivery of the message was Head Start centers. Children are served meals and snacks in this setting, permitting the program to provide children with the opportunity to taste and become familiar with new foods.

The 12-week program included a blend of education and marketing strategies and used social cognitive theory to support developmental learning skills such as fine and gross motor control, listening and language skills, sensory evaluations, and problem solving. Activities included the following:

- "Food Friend Memory Card game," a memory activity
- "Edible Food Faces," a tasting party
- "Fruit and Vegetable Mystery Bags"
- Reading of storybooks with a "trying new foods" theme
- New foods offered three times per week during afternoon snack time
- Parental involvement: four articles in the monthly Head Start newsletter

The social marketing process and attention to the 4 Ps—product, price, place, and promotion—were helpful in developing a program specifically tailored to preschoolers and their families.

Food Friends logo used courtesy of Department of Food Science and Nutrition, Colorado State University. www.foodfriends.org.

Source: Young, L., J. Anderson, L. Beckstrom, L. Bellows, and S.L. Johnson. 2004. Using social marketing principles to guide the development of a nutrition education initiative for preschool-aged children. *Journal of Nutrition Education and Behavior* 36:250–257.

TABLE 16-2 Social Marketing Case Study Example: Farmers' Market Coupons for WIC Clients

Barriers	Using the Four Ps to Overcome Barriers			
	Product	**Price**	**Place**	**Promotion**
I don't know where to park at the market.	Print places to park on map on new coupon folder.			Have staff visit the market so they can describe where to park.
I'm embarrassed around other shoppers when using coupons, and vendors seem a little irritated with the coupons.	Use mystery shoppers (even WIC staff) to evaluate service.	Consider feasibility of a "scanning" card rather than coupons.		
It's difficult to find signs that qualify farmers for WIC coupons. Sometimes they are below the tables and can't be seen.			Provide "poles" for farmers to use to display a sign that can be seen above the crowds.	Have WIC signs be the 5 A Day sign instead of the "WIC coupons accepted here" sign.
I'm concerned about not getting change back from $2 coupons. It's such a waste.		Reduce size of coupons to $1 versus $2.		
I lose the checks or forget where I put them.	Create a folder for checks, as opposed to loose, similar to an airline ticket folder.			
I'm afraid of what WIC counselors will think if I decline the coupons.		Offer clients with hesitation or barriers "a half pack" of coupons.		
I don't know what some of the fruits and vegetables are that I saw the last time (e.g., kohlrabi).				Use dedicated whiteboard in clinic to describe what's in season.
I don't know how to cook some of the fruits and vegetables.	Offer cooking classes and provide recipes.			
I don't have transportation.			Organize car pools from the clinic office.	
I don't really like vegetables.	Offer cooking classes and recipes.	Offer "half pack" of coupons to see if individual can find things to like.		
I don't know where the market is.	Print places to park on new coupon folder.			Have staff visit the market so they can describe where to park.
I work and can't get there during the week, and on weekends I'm too busy.			Recruit interested farmers to deliver select items to the clinic.	

(continues)

TABLE 16-2 Social Marketing Case Study Example: Farmers' Market Coupons for WIC Clients *(continued)*

	Using the Four Ps to Overcome Barriers			
Barriers	**Product**	**Price**	**Place**	**Promotion**
I don't know what's in season, so I don't know what I'll find at the market.				Use dedicated whiteboard in clinic to describe what's in season.
I'm concerned about returning checks that I didn't use, but I feel bad just keeping them when someone else could use them.		Allow return of unused checks, with no questions asked.		
I can't use all these checks in one visit, and then it takes too much to get back to the market.		Allow return of unused checks, with no questions asked.	Recruit interested farmers to deliver select items to clinic.	

WIC = Women's, Infant, and Children program.

Source: The Association of State Nutrition Network Administrators, Society for Nutrition Education, Division of Social Marketing. 2003. Using the 4Ps to overcome barriers to behavior change. Available at http://www.sne.org/specialinterest.htm.

target audience; it is a systematic consumer-based planning process; and it goes beyond nutrition education by aiming to create conditions in the social structure and environment that reduce barriers and facilitate the actions being promoted.

Social marketing's consumer focus and emphasis on thorough formative research or audience analysis as a first step is similar to the needs assessment or audience analysis process that constitutes the first step in designing theory-based nutrition education. The contrast is in the level of importance given to this step. Social marketing spends considerable time and effort on this step in order to understand its audience and tailor its messages, whereas nutrition education programs often spend little time on this step. However, theory-based nutrition education also requires that a thorough needs analysis be conducted to identify the many mediators of behavior change, including motivators and reinforcers of action and barriers to change. Two chapters in this book are devoted to such assessments. In addition, social marketers also spend considerable resources in pretesting messages with potential audience members. Pilot testing is also always considered an important part of nutrition education. Still, social marketing does provide a good reminder about the importance of understanding our intended audiences.

As we examine the *process* of consumer-based social marketing, we see that it is not very different from the systematic process used in designing good health education or nutrition education. The steps in social marketing of formative research and planning, including a clear statement of objectives; strategy design, including strategy formation, and message and material development; pretesting; implementation; and evaluation and feedback are very similar to the steps of

any systematic educational planning process, including the procedural model for designing theory-based nutrition education used in this book. The use of the five Ps provides an interesting way to think of the strategy design process. Yet a careful examination shows that these five Ps overlap many theory variables. Social marketers do remind nutrition educators, however, to be more systematic in their planning process.

Finally, social marketing is described as going beyond education by attempting to modify the relative attractiveness of the specific behavior. It does so through providing direct and immediate benefits that are reinforcing and through reducing both personal barriers, such as beliefs and expectations, and external barriers by making the environment favorable for the appropriate behavior. Theory-based nutrition education also seeks to increase the perception of benefits and decrease internal barriers, as has been described in great detail in this book. Nutrition education increasingly incorporates environmental supports for action—including policy and system modification—as part of its programming. The use of the social ecological approach, described earlier in the book, is an example of this trend. The two enterprises of social marketing and nutrition education thus share many characteristics.

Social marketing contributes to nutrition education a reminder to involve consumers or the public intensely in developing the program, to value their input, and to offer a sense of participant empowerment. Its set of planning ideas or tools, such as the five Ps, can also be very useful to nutrition education. The channels favored by social marketing, such as the mass media, offer the potential to reach a large portion of the population and to change the informational and normative environment. (Remember, though, that social marketing is not the same as a mass media campaign.)

On the other hand, nutrition education, when conducted with groups, goes beyond social marketing by providing a set of learning opportunities for the intended audience to develop and practice food- and nutrition-related cognitive skills, including critical thinking skills, as well as affective and behavior-specific skills that can assist individuals to make choices and take action on complex behaviors and issues. Venues such as facilitated group discussion also provide for social support and reinforcement of learning. Social marketing can thus be used as a component of a multicomponent nutrition education or health promotion program.

Nontraditional Channels

Many other channels for nutrition education have been explored. A few are briefly summarized here.

Individually Tailored Messages

Individually tailored messages can enhance the effectiveness of communications through nonpersonal media such as letters, newsletters, and computers. In this approach, a targeted group—such as employees at a worksite or clients of a physician—is sent a questionnaire that asks them about their current practices with respect to the target behavior, as well as their beliefs, attitudes, social norms, perceived barriers, or state of change. They are then sent computer-generated letters that specifically address their own particular set of beliefs and practices. The tailored communication can also be a newsletter or a magazine. Evidence shows that such a tailored approach improves communication attention and satisfaction. That is, instead of reading a general mailing or newsletter containing information that may not be relevant, the person reads only information that is specifically relevant to his or her beliefs or stage in the dietary change process. Thus this approach addresses issues that are personally relevant to the target audience and the choices they have to make. Evidence suggests that such an approach may enhance effectiveness compared with general communications (Brug, Campbell, & Van Assema, 1999). Tailoring can also be based on the core cultural values of a given cultural group in addition to behavioral theory constructs and has been found to enhance effectiveness (Kreuter et al., 2003, 2005).

Computer-tailored personal letters, newsletters, and magazines have been used with a variety of audiences: general practitioners' clients, healthy employees, healthy volunteers, retirees, members of health maintenance organizations, and church members. Another channel that can be used is an interactive computer approach: one study was designed to motivate and assist people to eat more fiber by using a very specific food choice strategy; another used touch-screen computers accompanied by in-person counseling and follow-up

telephone counseling (Brinberg, Axelson, & Price, 2000; Stevens et al., 2002). Web-based tailored messages can also be used (Oenema, Brug, & Lechner, 2001).

Other Promising Nontraditional Channels

Besides computer-tailored letters and newsletters, other nontraditional channels have been explored and show promise. Motivational interviewing over the telephone has shown some effectiveness. People calling in for cancer-related information to the national Cancer Information Service received a brief proactive education intervention over the telephone involving motivational and educational messages tailored to the caller's stage of readiness for eating at least five servings of fruits and vegetables daily (Marcus et al., 2001). Though brief, this interaction resulted in significant increase in fruit and vegetable consumption. Members of black churches were also reached with telephone motivational interviewing with some success (Resnicow et al., 2001). A multimedia approach using tailored soap opera and interactive infomercials that provided individualized feedback, knowledge, and strategies for lowering fat based on stage of change was effective (Campbell et al., 1999).

Computers in kiosks in supermarkets used tailored information and self-regulation activities, resulting in improved consumption of fat, fiber, and fruits and vegetables (Anderson et al., 2001). Nutrition public service announcements in grocery stores rotated every 30 minutes, along with two 1-hour videotapes given to individuals, increased fruit and vegetable intake (Connell, Goldberg, & Folta, 2001). Working with Boy Scouts was another avenue explored. A 5 A Day achievement badge program provided opportunities to develop asking skills to increase fruit and vegetable consumption at home and training in making fast and fun foods for home and camping trips. These were accompanied by comic books and newsletters sent home that included recipes (Baranowski et al., 2002). A multimedia, psychoeducational game involving 10 sessions delivered in schools over a five-week period was found to be highly effective in increasing the consumption of fruits, juice, and vegetables in fourth grade children (Baranowski et al., 2003). Given the difficulties of reaching people with nutrition messages, such nontraditional channels can be further explored.

Conclusion

Nutrition education for the public can be delivered through a variety of venues. This chapter has described some of the main channels and media you can use. It is important that you carefully determine your objectives when you use each of the channels and supporting materials. Sessions with groups are enhanced with the use of visuals, which can range from real foods and food packages to flip charts and PowerPoint slide presentations. Visuals should be interesting but simple. They should be clearly visible and appropriate in size so that you never have to say, "I know you can't read this, but. . . ." Written materials such as brochures, flyers, and handouts are also widely used. If they are to be effective, however, you should carefully tailor each piece to your intended audience and make the writing motivational and reader-friendly. Written materials should be designed to look interesting and be easy to read. Other supporting channels include cooking or food preparation activities, conducting grocery tours, and planning health fairs.

This chapter also described how nutrition educators can be involved in mass media communication campaigns as well as social marketing activities. Delivering nutrition education through these channels usually involves working with experts in these fields and within coalitions and collaborations. The principles of social marketing were described as well as many of the kinds of activities that nutrition educators can participate in as part of social marketing campaigns. Several other nontraditional channels were also described. Table 16-3 summarizes various channels and their advantages and disadvantages. It should be clear that there are numerous channels that you can use with any audience. This chapter had the space to describe only some of them. There are many more venues through which nutrition education can be delivered, limited only by your imagination!

TABLE 16-3 Communication Channels and Activities: Pros and Cons

Type of Channel	Activities	Pros	Cons
Interpersonal channels	• Nutrition education with groups • Facilitated group discussion • Workshops • Patient counseling	• Permit two-way, personal discussion • More effective in increasing motivations; influential, supportive • Most effective for teaching nutrition-related and self-regulation skills, helping/caring	• Can be expensive • Can be time-consuming • Can have limited reach for intended audience • Can be difficult to link into interpersonal channels
Organizational and community channels	• Community meetings and other events • Organizational meetings and conferences • Workplace campaigns	• May be familiar to audience, trusted, and influential • May provide more motivation and/or support than media alone • Can sometimes be inexpensive • Can offer shared experiences • Can reach larger intended audience in one place	• Can be costly, time-consuming to establish • May not provide personalized attention • Organizational constraints may require message approval • May lose control of message if adapted to fit organizational needs
Mass media channels Newspapers	• Ads • Inserted sections on a health topic (paid) • News • Feature stories • Letters to the editor • Op-ed pieces	• Can reach broad intended audiences rapidly • Can convey health news and breakthroughs more thoroughly than TV or radio and faster than magazines • Intended audience has chance to clip, reread, contemplate, and pass along material	• Coverage demands a newsworthy item • Larger-circulation papers may take only paid ads and inserts • Exposure usually limited to one day • Article placement requires contracts and may be time-consuming
Radio	• Ads (paid or public service placement) • News • Public affairs/talk shows • Dramatic programming (entertainment, education)	• Range of formats available to reach intended audiences with known listening preferences • Paid ads or specific programming can reach intended audience when they are most receptive • Paid ads can be relatively inexpensive • Ad production costs are low relative to TV	• Reaches smaller intended audiences than TV • PSAs run infrequently and at low listening times • Many stations have limited formats that may not be conducive to health messages • Difficult for intended audiences to retain or pass on material

TABLE 16-3 Communication Channels and Activities: Pros and Cons *(continued)*

Type of Channel	Activities	Pros	Cons
Television	• Ads (paid or PSAs) • News • Public affairs/talk shows • Dramatic programming (entertainment, education)	• Reaches potentially the largest and widest range of intended audiences • Visual combined with audio good for emotional appeals and demonstrating behaviors • Can reach low-income intended audiences • Paid ads or specific programming can reach intended audience when most receptive • Ads allow message and its execution to be controlled	• Ads are expensive to produce • Paid advertising is expensive • PSAs run infrequently and at low viewing times • Message may be obscured by commercial clutter • Can be difficult for intended audiences to retain or pass on material
Internet	• Websites • Email mailing lists • Chat rooms • Newsgroups • Ads (paid or public service placement)	• Can reach large numbers of people rapidly • Can instantaneously update and disseminate information • Can control information provided • Can tailor information specifically for intended audiences • Can be interactive • Can provide health information in a graphically appealing way • Can combine the audiovisual benefits of TV or radio with the self-paced benefits of print media	• Can be expensive • Many intended audiences do not have access to Internet • Intended audience must be proactive—must search or sign up for information • Newsgroups and chat rooms may require monitoring • Can require maintenance over time

PSA = public service announcement.

Source: Modified from National Cancer Institute. 2004. *Making health communication programs work* (NIH Publication No. 04-5145). Bethesda, MD: National Cancer Institute, U.S. Department of Health and Human Services.

Questions and Activities

1. What are the major advantages of using supporting visuals when working with groups?
2. What kinds of visuals might you use when working with groups? Describe how your choice might differ depending on your audience, such as teens in an after-school program, older adults at a senior citizen center, or a professional group at a conference.
3. List the design principles you would use to avoid having to say to a group "I know that you cannot read this, but . . . ."
4. Prepare a poster (or PowerPoint slide) for use with a group that depicts one idea or theme. Write a description of your objectives for the visual and your intended audience. Write an analysis of your visual explaining how you used art and design principles to enhance quality.
5. You have prepared well for your session, your visuals are in place, and you are now in front of the group. Describe five guidelines for presenting the visuals in an effective manner.
6. Many nutrition educators use printed materials. What purposes might they serve? Describe them.

7. Think of the last time you developed a printed piece. What objectives did you expect it to serve? Do you think it achieved your objectives? Why or why not?
8. How would you ensure that your printed materials are motivating and effective? Describe three specific ways of doing so.
9. You have decided that you will use cooking or food preparation as part of your nutrition education intervention. Based on what you have read, describe three guidelines to ensure a successful learning experience for your participants.
10. What purposes might be served by organizing nutrition education events at health fairs? Describe three tips to ensure that your purposes are met.
11. A central concept in social marketing is the concept of the "exchange." Describe this concept carefully.
12. Compare nutrition education and social marketing. How do they relate to each other?
13. Design social marketing for one of the following situations. Indicate what exactly is the exchange in this setting and how you used the five Ps in your design.

REFERENCES

Alcay, R., and R.A. Bell. 2000. *Promoting nutrition and physical activity through social marketing: Current practices and recommendations*. Davis, CA: Center of Advanced Studies in Nutrition and Social Marketing, University of California.

Anderson, E.S., R.A. Winett, J.R. Wojcik, S.G. Winett, and T. Bowden. 2001. A computerized social cognitive intervention for nutrition behavior: Direct and mediated effects on fat, fiber, fruits, and vegetables, self-efficacy, and outcome expectations among food shoppers. *Annals of Behavioral Medicine* 23:88–100.

Andreasen, A.R. 1995. *Marketing social change: Changing behavior to promote health, social development, and the environment*. San Francisco: Jossey-Bass.

Baranowski, T., J. Baranowski, K.W. Cullen, et al. 2002. 5 a Day achievement badge for African-American Boy Scouts: Pilot outcome results. *Preventive Medicine* 34:353–363.

Baranowski, T., J. Baranowski, K.W. Cullen, et al. 2003. Squirrel's Quest: Dietary outcome evaluation of a multimedia game. *American Journal of Preventive Medicine* 24:52–61.

Brinberg, D., M.L. Axelson, and S. Price. 2000. Changing food knowledge, food choice, and dietary fiber consumption by using tailored messages. *Appetite* 35:35–43.

Brown, B.J., and B.J. Hermann. 2005. Cooking classes increase fruit and vegetables intake and food safety behaviors in youth and adults. *Journal of Nutrition Education and Behavior* 37:1004–1005.

Brug, J., M. Campbell, and P. Van Assema. 1999. The application and impact of computer-generated personalized nutrition education: A review of the literature. *Patient Education and Counseling* 36:145–156.

Campbell, M.K., L. Honess-Morreale, D. Farrell, E. Carbone, and M. Brasure. 1999. A tailored multimedia nutrition education pilot program for low-income women receiving food assistance. *Health Education Research* 14:257–267.

Connell, D., J.P. Goldberg, and S.C. Folta. 2001. An intervention to increase fruit and vegetable consumption using audio communications: In-store public service announcements and audiotapes. *Journal of Health Communication* 6:31–43.

Dole Food Company, Inc. 2001. *5 A Day supermarket tours: A guide for retailers*. Oakland, CA: Dole Food Company, Nutrition and Health Program. www.dole5aday.com/Retailers/pdfs/5TourRetailerGuide.pdf.

Frederisksen, L.W., L.J. Solomon, and K.A. Brehony, ed. 1984. *Marketing health behavior: principles, techniques, and applications*. New York: Plenum Press.

Institute of Medicine. 2002. *Speaking of health: Assessing health communication strategies for diverse populations*. Washington, DC: National Academy Press.

Iowa Department of Public Health. n.d. Pick a better snack. http://www.idph.state.ia.us/Pickabettersnack/default.asp.

Knight, S., and C. Probart. 1992. How to avoid saying "I know you can't read this but . . ." *Journal of Nutrition Education* 24:94B.

Kotler, P., and E.L. Roberto. 1989. *Social marketing: Strategies for changing public behavior*. New York: The Free Press.

Kotter, P., and G. Zaltman. 1971. Social marketing: An approach to planned social change. *Journal of Marketing* July, 3–12.

Kreuter, M.W., S.N. Kukwago, D.C. Bucholtz, E.M. Clark, and V. Sanders-Thompson. 2003. Achieving cultural appropriateness in health promotion programs: Targeted and tailored approaches. *Health Education and Behavior* 30:133–146.

Kreuter, M.W., C. Sugg-Skinner, C.L. Holt, et al. 2005. Cultural tailoring for mammography and fruit and vegetables intake among low-income African-American women in urban public health centers. *Preventive Medicine* 41:53–62.

Liquori, T., P.D. Koch, I.R. Contento, and J. Castle. 1998. The CookShop program: Outcome evaluation of a nutrition education program linking lunchroom food experiences with classroom cooking experiences. *Journal of Nutrition Education* 30:302–313.

Lucas, S.E. 2004. *The art of public speaking*. 8th ed. New York: McGraw-Hill.

Maibech, E.W., M.L. Rothschild, and W.D. Novelli. 2002. Social marketing. In *Health behavior and health education: Theory, research and practice*, edited by K. Glanz, B.K. Rimer, and F.M. Lewis. San Francisco: Jossey-Bass.

Manoff, R.K. 1985. *Social marketing*. New York: Praeger.

Mansbridge, J.J. 1990. *Beyond self-interest*. Chicago: University of Chicago Press.

Marcus, A.C., J. Heimendinger, P. Wolfe, et al. 2001. A randomized trial of a brief intervention to increase fruit and vegetable intake: A replication study among callers to the CIS. *Preventive Medicine* 33:204–216.

National Cancer Institute. 2004. *Making health communication programs work* (NIH Publication No. 04-5145). Bethesda, MD: National Cancer Institute, U.S. Department of Health and Human Services.

Oenema, A., J. Brug, and L. Lechner. 2001. Web-based tailored nutrition education: Results of a randomized control trial. *Health Education Research* 16:647–660.

Raines, C., and L. Williamson. 1995. *Using visual aids: The effective use of type, color, and graphics*. Revised ed. Menlo Park, CA: Crisp Learning.

Resnicow, K., A. Jackson, T. Wang, et al. 2001. A motivational interviewing intervention to increase fruit and vegetable intake through black churches: Results of the Eat for Life trial. *American Journal of Public Health* 91:1686–1693.

Rogers, E.M., and J.D. Storey. 1988. Communications campaigns. In C.R. Berger and S.H. Chaffee (eds). *Handbook of communication science.* Newbury Park, CA: Sage.

Rothschild, M.L. 1999. Carrots, sticks, and promises: A conceptual framework for the management of public health and social issue behaviors. *Journal of Marketing* 63:24–37.

Smith, S.B., and B.J. Alford. 1989. Literate and semi-literate audiences: Tips for effective teaching. *Journal of Nutrition Education* 20:238C–D.

Stevens, V.J., R.E. Glasgow, D.J. Toobert, N. Karanja, and K.S. Smith. 2002. Randomized trial of a brief dietary intervention to decrease consumption of fat and increase consumption of fruits and vegetables. *American Journal of Health Promotion* 16:129–134.

Van Den Heede, F.A, and S. Pelican. 1995. Reflections on marketing as an inappropriate model for nutrition education. *Journal of Nutrition Education* 27:141–145.

Young, L., J. Anderson, L. Beckstrom, L. Bellows, and S.L. Johnson. 2004. Using social marketing principles to guide the development of a nutrition education initiative for preschool-aged children. *Journal of Nutrition Education and Behavior* 36:250–257.

Working With Different Population Groups

OVERVIEW   This chapter provides an overview of strategies to use to deliver nutrition education to various age and population groups.

OBJECTIVES   At the end of the chapter, you will be able to

- Describe key features of the cognitive and emotional development of children and adolescents
- Demonstrate understanding of ways to deliver nutrition education activities that are appropriate to the developmental level of youth
- Demonstrate understanding of ways to conduct nutrition education activities that are based on adult education principles
- Describe key features of cultural competence, cultural sensitivity, and cultural appropriateness in the nutrition education context
- Demonstrate understanding of ways to deliver nutrition education activities that are culturally appropriate
- Demonstrate understanding of ways to deliver nutrition education activities that are appropriate for low-literacy audiences
- Apply design principles for written and visual materials for use in nutrition education for low-literacy audiences

SCENARIO

At a nutrition education session, a group of mothers of young children sit in a circle around a room, sharing their experiences of trying to provide healthful meals for their young children. They are animated and fully engaged with each other for an hour as they share challenges and successes. The educator facilitates the discussion unobtrusively and helps the group to come to closure about what they will do about this issue during the coming week.

Introduction

Try to imagine a group of preschoolers sitting in a circle and having a similar discussion for an hour, with little guidance from a nutrition educator. Totally impossible, of course! Clearly, the way nutrition education is delivered must be tailored to the group with which you are working. It is thus important to understand the differing characteristics of different population groups. Nutrition educators work in numerous settings, as we saw in Chapter 1: communities, health care settings, schools, food- and food-system-related community and advocacy organizations, and workplaces. In addition, we work with many diverse audiences, differing by age, sex, ethnicity, developmental stages, socioeconomic status, geographic location, and so forth. We also work with many groups that have specific food- or nutrition-related issues, such as diabetics, pregnant and lactating women, and those who are overweight, to name a few.

This chapter focuses on audiences at different ages and stages of life, from different cultural backgrounds, and with different literacy levels. It provides some background information on each audience and makes suggestions regarding nutrition education delivery methods that are appropriate for each (Contento et al., 1995). Some of these differences in appropriate deliver methods should be considered at the time you are designing your educational plan or lesson plan.

Developmental Level Appropriateness

Children are not little adults. Children are undergoing rapid physical, cognitive, and socioemotional development. Hence they have their own particular set of concerns and ways of viewing the world, and these change from the preschool years through adolescence. They are in the process of developing various cognitive structures and abilities, understandings of the world, motor skills, social skills, and emotional coping strategies that most adults take for granted. They develop these through their explorations of the world (Piaget & Inhelder, 1969) and through social interaction with skilled individuals embedded in a sociocultural backdrop (Vygotsky, 1962; Bronfenbrenner, 1979). Understanding how children develop and how they learn about food and eating is crucial for nutrition education.

The Preschool Child

The way young children view and experience the world is qualitatively different from that of adults. Child development research provides evidence that the cognitive world of preschool children is creative, fanciful, and free. However, they are becoming less dependent on their direct sensorimotor actions for direction of behavior and are increasingly able to function in a symbolic-conceptual mode in their thinking, for example, using scribbled designs to represent people, cars, houses, and other objects. They have some causal reasoning ability, but it does not lead to abstract generalizations or formation of logical concepts, as in older children or adults. Their attention span is short and they cannot distinguish between their perspective and that of another person. It is not surprising, then, that children younger than 4 years cannot consistently discern between television advertising and the informational content of programs. Children between 4 and 8 years can distinguish between television advertising and program content but do not effectively understand that the intent of television advertising is to persuade them.

Preschool children learn by manipulating the environment rather than by passive listening—that is, they learn by exploring, questioning, comparing, and labeling. Physical manipulation skills are being developed when children touch, feel, look, mix up, turn over, and throw things. Emotionally, exploration and the need to test independence are important during this time. They take on more initiative and are more purposeful. They are eager to learn, usually from

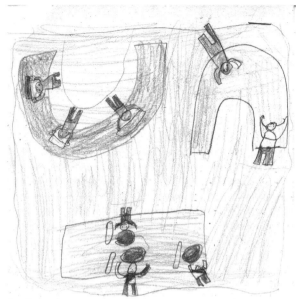

Family meals.

other people: they observe parents, teachers, and other children, they role play, and they start to accumulate and process information.

Young Children's Thinking About Food and Nutrition

Research on preschool children suggests that whereas 2-year-olds are only able to name or identify objects, 3- to 5-year-olds can begin to place them into categories such as size, color, and shape. In the food area, they can easily identify foods and are beginning to classify them. However, they classify foods based on observable qualities such as shape and color and on function rather than by nutrient content (Michela & Contento, 1984; Matheson, Spranger, & Saxe, 2002). They are beginning to be able to relate foods to health (Singleton et al., 1992), but they do not really know what happens to food in the body to bring about its effects on health (Contento, 1981).

When preschool children playing in toy kitchens were asked to make a meal for a research assistant, they demonstrated that they already had some knowledge of meal planning, food preparation, table preparation, food serving, eating, and cleaning up (Matheson, Spranger, & Saxe, 2002). They also had notions about eating rules such as "You must eat a little bit of everything," "Eat it—it is good for you," and "This is mine and that's yours; you can eat whatever you want." These observations suggest that nutrition education should not focus on food group information but should instead emphasize active methods and play activities.

Children are not born with the natural ability to choose a nutritious diet: they have to learn to do so. The accumulating evidence from research suggests that early experience with food and eating has an impact on the development of food preferences and on the regulation of amount of food eaten in several ways.

- *Familiarity with the food.* Very young children show a neophobic response, or reluctance to taste new or unfamiliar foods, a natural and protective mechanism that is one of the most common reasons for food rejection. However, repeated exposures increase children's preference for a food or beverage (Birch, 1999). A longitudinal study found that a large percentage of children's food preferences were formed as early as age 2 to 3 years and did not change over the five-year period of the study, at which point the children were aged 8 (Skinner et al., 2002). Other studies have shown that dislike of foods can be transformed into liking when children are repeatedly exposed to foods through tasting and eating (Wardle et al., 2003a, 2003b).

- *Association of foods with the physiological consequences of eating.* Very young children seem to be able to regulate the amount they eat based almost solely on their physiological reactions to foods (i.e., feeling full) (Birch, 1987, 1999). As they get older, however, children eat substantially more when larger portions are offered, suggesting that the ability to respond solely to internal physiological cues decreases with age as external factors become more influential (Rolls, 2000; Orlet Fisher, Rolls, & Birch, 2003; Rolls, Engell, & Birch, 2002). Indeed they often eat in the absence of hunger (Fisher & Birch, 2002).

- *Association of foods with the emotional tone of the social interactions that surround feeding.* Children come to prefer foods that are eaten in a positive emotional atmosphere (Birch et al., 1987) as well as foods eaten by their peers. A survey of Head Start parents showed that their own positive nutrition-related attitudes were related to more pleasant family mealtimes, fewer negative mealtime practices, and less troublesome child eating behaviors (Gable & Lutz, 2001). Head Start program mealtime environments and practices can thus contribute importantly to young children coming to like healthful foods.

- *Learning and self-regulation.* As children develop the ability to identify which food cues are relevant in beginning, continuing, and ending eating, learning and self-regulation become extremely important. As noted previously, very young children seem to be able to regulate the amount they eat based primarily on their physiological reactions to foods, but as they get older, external factors, including parenting practices, become influential as well. For example, there is some evidence suggesting that in mainstream culture parents who have eating issues of their own or who

impose strong control over their children's intake may interfere with their children's ability to regulate their intake on their own (Faith et al., 2004). The role of parental control may be more complex in children of diverse ethnic and socioeconomic backgrounds (Robinson et al., 2001; Contento, Zybert, & Williams, 2005) because parents' control and restriction may be interpreted as love and responsibility in some cultures (Lin & Liang, 2005). However, the studies do all support the recommended practice that it is the responsibility of the adults in families, day-care centers, and schools to provide healthful foods, and it is the responsibility of the child to choose how much of these foods to eat (Satter, 1999).

From consistent practice in making choices from an array of healthful foods, children learn healthful eating patterns and develop the ability to regulate how much of these foods to eat.

Methods for Delivering Nutrition Education Appropriately to Preschool Children

What practical methods can we use, then, to increase the effectiveness of nutrition education for young children? Based on the information just discussed and on the research literature, the following methods of delivering nutrition education are likely to be useful.

Use food-based activities. Food-based activities such as tasting parties, food preparation, and activities designed to engage the five senses with food are useful. Provide daily exposure to healthful meals and snacks to increase children's preferences for these foods. Nutrition educators note that meals and snacks provided at child-care centers should be seen as the centerpiece of nutrition education and should be offered in a positive eating atmosphere.

Create developmentally appropriate learning experiences. Child development theory and research suggest that no amount of "teaching" will make young children learn concepts that are beyond the capability of their cognitive structures to understand. On the other hand, preschoolers should not just be entertained because they are assumed to be unable to understand (Hertzler & DeBord, 1994). Young children have certain cognitive skills that can be used in nutrition education. Programs need to be tailored to children's level of emotional and motor developmental levels as well. Design activities that take into account the observations that 2- to 3-year-olds can name foods eaten at home or seen in the store and describe the tastes and textures of foods, whereas older preschoolers can classify foods by color and function, identify foods seen on TV, and learn reading skills by reading food-themed story books. In terms of the link between food and health, 2- to 3-year-olds can name body parts and tell the location of organs, such as eyes, and what they do.

Older preschoolers can compare breathing and pulse rate when doing different activities, and can state general connections between food and the body, for example, that carrots are good for your eyes.

Apply activity- and play-based teaching methods. Design activity-based teaching methods and play-based curricula that build on children's naturalistic environments and interests. Studies show that where interventions had an impact on knowledge and eating practices, active participation by children in a nonthreatening environment was most conducive to success. Employ activities such as art projects, songs, jingles, role playing, stories, puppets, and puzzles. Curricula can focus on play. Toy kitchens or grocery stores provide opportunities for nutrition education. In addition, children can role play trying new foods or practicing food safety behaviors in these contexts (Matheson, Spranger, & Saxe, 2002). Children can work in school gardens, learning about how food grows.

Focus on behaviors. Identify specific children's behaviors to focus on, such as trying new foods, eating vegetables, or eating healthful snacks. Then work with parents and preschool staff to model eating healthful meals and snacks, offer foods to children in a positive social environment, and use rewards appropriately. For example, "trying new foods" was the behavior addressed in a social marketing campaign directed at preschoolers, called Food Friends (discussed in Nutrition Education in Action 16-2). It used many of the kinds of activities described earlier: sensory activities that included "fruit and vegetable mystery bags," storybooks, opportunities to try new foods, and parental involvement (Young et al., 2004).

Encourage self-regulation. Parents and preschools can encourage the child's ability to self-regulate. It is the responsibility of families and preschools to provide children with healthful foods in appropriate settings and at appropriate times, but children should be able to choose how much to eat from among these foods. From this practice children will learn to self-regulate the appropriate amounts of food to eat to satisfy hunger. These self-regulation skills will become increasingly cognitive, as well as biological, in nature as children develop cognitively and are exposed to, and have to make conscious choices from, an increasing array of foods, many of which are very attractive in a variety of nonhealthful ways. Children can be encouraged to pay attention to their hunger cues and to eat when they are hungry and to stop when they are full. These are cognitive activities, requiring conscious decisions.

Involve parents and families. Involving families either as major recipients of the program or in conjunction with the program offered to the preschool child is crucial for nutrition education of children this age. Parents and teachers working together can make more of an impact through mutual reinforcement than either can alone. Studies with Head Start

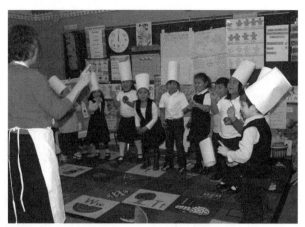

All together now! Let's sing our song about apples!

found that educating and encouraging parents were effective in increasing children's knowledge and reported consumption of more nutritious foods. The Food Friends program incorporated a parent component, as discussed in Nutrition Education in Action 16-2.

Middle Childhood and Adolescence

Children grow and change rapidly during the school years. Middle childhood (ages 6–11) is a time of major cognitive development and mastery of cognitive, physical, and social skills. Children at this age are eager to understand people and the world around them. They like being physically active as their bodies grow steadily in muscle mass and strength and as they grow taller. They progress from dependence on their parents to increasing independence, with an increasing interest in developing friendships with others.

During adolescence (ages 12–19), growth accelerates, leading to dramatic physical, developmental, and social changes that can affect eating patterns. Diet quality declines as children move from childhood through adolescence. Their eating patterns put them at risk for current and future health problems, as shown in Box 17-1. They have considerable spending power, and they often have considerable autonomy in food choices as well. A number of these factors influence the choice of methods for delivering nutrition education.

Cognitive Development

Cognitive maturity influences what children can learn from nutrition education. The child comes to school with a host of ideas about the physical and natural world, and these are different from those of adults. We need to understand these differences to communicate well with them. Children are motivated to learn and acquire knowledge and are full of curiosity. In the early school years, children move beyond intuitive thinking to be able to think causally, although rea-

BOX 17-1 Typical Eating Patterns of Adolescents in the United States and Their Implications

Patterns
- Chaotic eating patterns
- Eat rapidly and away from home
- Spend their own money
- Exposed to more than eight hours per day of various media (TV, computer, radio, magazines)
- Reliance on fast food and convenience food
- Begin to buy and prepare more food for themselves
- Influence parents' buying; do some of the family shopping
- Replacement of milk with soft drinks and other sweetened beverages

Statistics
- Less than 25% of adolescents, grades 9–12, eat at least five servings of fruits and vegetables per day.
- The average teen visits a fast food restaurant just over two times a week and spends $5 a visit, for a total of $13 billion each year in fast food restaurants.
- Teens spend $9.6 billion in food and snack stores each year.
- They spend $736 million each year on vending machines.

Why Are These Patterns a Problem?
- Fast foods tend to be high in fat, sugar, and/or salt.
- Sweetened beverages are high in calories.
- Fast foods tend to be low in iron, calcium, riboflavin, vitamin A, folic acid, and vitamin C.
- Inadequate intake of calcium in adolescence can set the stage for osteoporosis later on.
- The rate of type 2 diabetes is increasing among adolescents.

cessing capacity also increases during the school years, but they use behavioral, concrete, and specific cues to define health, and the criteria for their food choices are specific and immediate (such as taste or cost).

Adolescents begin to think more abstractly and more logically and are able to formulate hypotheses to explain occurrences and imagine alternative explanations for what is observed. They are thus capable of more abstract concepts linking food and health. They begin to develop the ability to grasp the deeper meanings of problems and to think reflectively and critically, keeping an open mind. Becoming more idealistic, they begin to think about idealistic characteristics for themselves and others and to compare themselves and others to ideal standards. They are intrigued by social, political, and moral issues and are willing to speak out on them. In the food area, many become vegetarians or become involved in important food- and nutrition-related causes.

Emotional and Social Development

The emotional and social development of children and youth are important to consider when delivering nutrition education. During middle and late childhood, children spend an increasing amount of time with their peers. Friendships are important because they provide stimulation in the form of interesting information and excitement, a familiar playmate, support, encouragement and feedback, intimacy, affection, and a trusting relationship where aspects of the self can be shared. Friendship also provides a means of social comparison, whereby the child can find out where she or he stands with respect to others. During this period, children begin to understand the perspective of another person and develop greater self-understanding. Development of self-esteem or sense of self-worth is important and can be fostered by providing emotional support and approval and opportunities to develop real skills and a sense of achievement. Self-esteem can also be enhanced by learning to cope with problems realistically rather than avoid them.

During adolescence, pubertal changes occur, resulting in rapid growth and sexual maturation. Adolescents also become intensely interested in their body image. They worry about their sexual appearance. They also develop a special kind of egocentrism. Whereas preschoolers' egocentrism derives from the inability to distinguish between their own perspective and that of someone else, adolescent egocentrism is distinguished by belief in an imaginary audience and in a personal fable (Elkind, 1978). In terms of imaginary audience, adolescents are very aware of other people and believe that others are as preoccupied with them as they are with themselves. They feel they are on stage and the rest of the world is their audience. This leads to the desire to be noticed and visible. At the same time this leads to great concerns. For example, the young woman is sure that everyone will notice and comment on the small, almost invisible spot on her

soning is likely to be limited to concrete objects and specific experiences. They tend to think like scientists, asking many "why" questions. They like to do experiments and can theorize. However, they often maintain their old theories regardless of the evidence and are more likely to be influenced by happenstance events than by overall patterns. They think of food in functional terms. One study found they classified on the basis of sweet versus nonsweet foods; meals versus more versatile foods and drinks; whole, fresh foods versus more highly processed foods; and plants versus animal foods (Michela and Contento, 1984). Children's information-pro-

BOX 17-2 Cognitive and Emotional Development of Children and Adolescents: Implications for Nutrition Education

Middle Childhood
Characteristics
- Have ideas or theories of how the natural world works that are different from those of adults
- Black-and-white thinkers: causal thinking is more developed, but reasoning still limited to concrete objects and specific experiences
- Criteria for food choice are specific and immediate
- Curious and motivated to learn: they particularly like to do experiments
- Trust and respect adults
- Playmates and peer friendships are increasingly important
- Beginning to desire autonomy

Implications for Nutrition Education
- Use fantasy characters and stories in nutrition education
- Address benefits related to having more energy and/or improved performance in sports
- Use active methods
- Focus on the functional meanings of food
- Include handouts with bright pictures and direct messages
- Foster self-esteem
- Use simple goal-setting activities and foster cognitive self-regulation

Early Adolescence
Characteristics
- Causal reasoning becoming more developed
- Criteria for food choice are specific and immediate
- Relationships between food and health are becoming of interest
- Trust and respect adults
- Anxious about peer relationships
- Ambivalent about autonomy
- Preoccupied with the body and body image, and uncomfortable with the physical changes of puberty
- Willing to do or say anything that makes them look or feel better about their body image
- Interested in immediate results

Implications for Nutrition Education
- Address benefits related to looking healthy, having more energy, and/or performance in sports
- Focus on short-term goals
- Include simplified instructions, handouts with bright pictures, and direct messages
- Use active methods

Middle Adolescence
Characteristics
- Abstract thinking skills developing
- Criteria for food choice are becoming more complex, with increased reasoning about consequences
- Greatly influenced by peers
- Mistrustful of adults; recurrently challenging adult authority
- Listen to peers more than adults
- Consider independence to be very important and experience significant cognitive development
- More in charge of the food they eat
- Temporary rejection of family dietary patterns

(continues)

⬤ **BOX 17-2 Cognitive and Emotional Development of Children and Adolescents: Implications for Nutrition Education** (continued)

Implications for Nutrition Education
- Design activities to analyze social influences such as television advertising, the media, what's available in neighborhood stores or stores around their schools, and what their friends eat, and their own response to these influences
- Focus on how to make healthful choices when eating out
- Use food demonstrations and taste tests
- Use simplified problem-identification techniques, role playing, and "what if" scenarios
- Guided goal setting is possible
- Foster teenagers' increasing independence while maintaining a caring, yet authoritative role

Late Adolescence
Characteristics
- Abstract thinking more developed; with experience, teens become more skilled at problem solving and decision making
- Criteria for food choice are becoming more complex: understand the notion of making trade-offs
- More established body image
- Orientation toward the future and making plans
- Becoming increasingly independent; less challenging of adult authority
- More consistent in their values and beliefs
- Developing intimacy and permanent relationships
- Begin to think of long term and about improving their overall health
- Still want to make their own decisions, but are more open to information provided by health care providers

Implications for Nutrition Education
- Build educational experiences around motivations that are particularly meaningful to this age group
- Present dietary recommendations and give the rationales behind them
- Focus on behaviors that adolescents have control over
- Discussions of complex issues are now possible, and homework-type assignments are appropriate
- Foster cognitive self-regulation involving goal-setting and action plans
- Teach skills to address long-term goals
- Provide food preparation experiences if possible
- Respect their independence and encourage their decision-making skills

sweater, or the young man imagines that all eyes will be on the tiny blemish on his face. In terms of personal fable, adolescents believe in their personal uniqueness, which results in believing that no one else can understand how they really feel. To foster this uniqueness, adolescents create stories about themselves that are filled with fantasy. They believe that what is really important is what is going on with their particular circle of friends and events at school.

As they grow older, adolescents become more independent, trying to establish themselves as unique individuals. They also start developing a better understanding of their own strengths and weaknesses and think about the future. They struggle with how they should relate to their friends and family in terms of how to be close to them yet maintain their own independence.

Adolescents' Thinking, Concerns, and Behaviors with Respect to Food, Nutrition, and Health

Adolescents' eating behaviors are influenced by factors at many levels: *individual factors,* both psychological and biological; *social environmental factors* such as family and peers; *community settings* such as schools or fast food outlets; and *societal factors* such as mass media, marketing, and sociocultural norms (Story, Neumark-Sztainer, & French, 2002). Factors influencing food choices include hunger and food cravings, time, convenience, cost and availability of foods, perceived benefits, mood, body image, and habit. Major barriers to healthy eating include a lack of sense of urgency about personal health in relation to other more pressing concerns, and preferring the taste of other foods (Neumark-Sztainer et al., 1999). Box 17-2 notes the implications for nutrition education of the cognitive and social development characteristics of adolescents.

Focus group research has found that adolescents have a significant amount of knowledge about healthful foods and believe that healthful eating involves balance, moderation, and variety. However, they find it difficult to eat healthfully because of their perceived lack of time, the limited availability of healthful options in school, and a general lack of concern about following recommendations (Neumark-Sztainer et al., 1997; Croll, Neumark-Sztainer, & Story, 2001).

The weight and body image concerns of adolescents have been of particular interest to nutrition educators. Studies have found that adolescents often attempt to make their weights conform to societal ideals by practicing many weight control behaviors. Most adolescents practice healthy weight control behaviors (85% of girls and 70% of boys in one survey). Some adolescents, particularly those who are overweight, practice some unhealthy weight control behaviors or even behaviors that are extreme (Neumark-Sztainer et al., 2002). However, those who use moderate methods of weight control have more healthful eating and exercise patterns than those who are extreme dieters or nondieters, suggesting that they might be practicing some degree of self-monitoring and self-regulation (Story et al., 1998).

Cognitive-motivational processes and self-regulation. The fact that children and adolescents are not concerned about health and nutrition issues to any major extent when they are making food choices is not surprising, given that they do not perceive any urgency to change and that the future seems so distant (Story & Resnick, 1986; Newmark-Sztainer et al., 1999). In addition it has been found that nutrition knowledge alone does not ensure that children and adolescents (or adults, for that matter) will adopt healthful behaviors (Gibson and Wardle, 1998).

However, studies show that cognitive-motivational processes do become increasingly important influences on food choice as children become older and more developed cognitively. That is, older children and adolescents become more able to link cause and effect and to perceive the consequences of their actions (Contento & Michela, 1998). Thus, they can make food choices in light of their perceptions of anticipated consequences from eating particular foods. Adolescents can make trade-offs among their desired consequences. For example, dieting adolescents in one study were willing to forego taste and convenience to some degree in order to obtain less-fattening food (Contento, Michela, & Williams, 1995). In another study, adolescents were willing to balance less nutritious items with more nutritious items within a meal, and to balance less healthful lunches with more healthful dinners (Contento et al., 2006).

We need to remember that adolescents are not monolithic in their food choice motivations. One study found they could be divided into several subgroups with distinct orientations to food, ranging from the hedonistic group, for whom taste and convenience were paramount; to the socially controlled group, for whom friends were most important; and to the health-oriented subgroups, who were concerned about personal health (Contento, Michela, & Goldberg, 1988). Those in the health-oriented groups had better diets than those in the hedonistic and socially controlled groups. Other studies have reported similar findings that those concerned about health had better diets (Gibson et al., 1998; Cusatis & Shannon, 1996). It should be noted that health outcomes that have meaning for this group are still short-term outcomes (e.g., that they will have more energy, better athletic performance, or better-looking skin), which should thus be emphasized in nutrition education.

From a social psychological perspective, the picture that emerges from research is that older children and adolescents want particular consequences from the food they eat and become increasingly able to align their food choice behaviors with their goals. They integrate motivations and cognitions in a process of *cognitive self-regulation* (Contento & Michela, 1998). This ability makes it possible for nutrition educators to incorporate the teaching of skills in goal-setting, self-monitoring, and other self-regulatory processes to this age group.

Family influences. What the family serves is still important. Children aged 6 to 11 obtained 76% of their calories at home, and even adolescents obtained 65% (Guthrie, Lin, & Frazao, 2002). Although adolescents are increasingly independent, making food choices in an ever-widening circle of settings, most still eat some meals at home. Several surveys suggest that about a quarter of teens in the United States eat seven or more meals with their family, about 40% eat three to six meals a week with them, and 20% eat about one to two meals a week, with only about 15% never eating with their families (Neumark-Sztainer et al., 2003). Increasing frequency of eating family meals among children and adolescents is associated with more healthful dietary patterns (Gillman et al., 2000; Videon & Manning, 2003; Neumark-Sztainer et al., 2003).

Most adolescents in one survey reported that they enjoyed eating meals with the family and that it is a time to bring everybody together and to talk with each other (Neumark-Sztainer et al., 2000a). Major reasons for not eating together were teen schedules, a desire for autonomy, and not liking the foods served or the family atmosphere (Neumark-Sztainer et al., 2000b). Another study found that many adolescents resolved these meal-related conflicting desires by negotiating with others in the family about what to serve at home (Contento et al., 2006). This means that nutrition education can teach youth to more effectively negotiate with their families and to use what they eat at home to balance what they eat elsewhere.

Methods for Delivering Nutrition Education Appropriately to Children and Youth

Based on the background information just discussed and on the research literature, the following are suggestions for methods of delivering nutrition education that are likely to enhance effectiveness.

Focus on behaviors or practices over which youth have some control. We have seen that a behaviorally focused approach to nutrition education improves effectiveness. In the case of older children and adolescents, choose behaviors for the intervention that are of nutritional concern but are also those over which youth have some control. Examples are eating fruits and vegetables, lower-fat snacks and lunches, regular breakfasts, and calcium-rich foods.

Address motivations that are meaningful and important to youth. Link information about why to engage in healthful behaviors to motivations that are important to youth, such as having energy, being able to perform well both physically and cognitively, being strong, or having healthy-looking hair or skin. Focus on benefits such as convenience, taste, cost, and other attributes of foods and eating patterns that are relevant to them. Explore barriers. Take into account that some are still growing and that satisfying hunger at low cost is a major motivator, whereas others, particularly girls, have made the transition through puberty and have stabilized in terms of growth.

Thus, make the case for healthful eating in terms that are meaningful for youth. For example, you can help them calculate the costs of the beverages and snacks they currently consume and show how more healthful alternatives can cost the same or less. Or show how convenient it is to prepare fruits and vegetables as snacks. This does not mean you cannot increase a sense of concern about healthful eating. You

can. But rather than focusing on their own personal risk for disease, ask youth about whether they have family members who have various chronic diseases such as diabetes and how that makes them feel. This can be a useful way to address the issue of food-related disease risk.

Incorporate self-evaluation and self-assessment. Youth like self-assessments that are interesting and fun and provide a picture of themselves. A possible activity is to have the class as a group write down what they ate and drank the day before and then analyze these lists in terms of the behavior of focus for your sessions, such as eating breakfast, eating fruits and vegetables, or eating at fast food restaurants. Or you could design a checklist of actions that the group could potentially engage in and come up with a composite score to indicate how well they are doing.

Use active methods. Although their attention spans are now longer than those of young children, getting and holding the attention of youth still require active methods of nutrition education, perhaps alternating with mini-lectures. Food preparation or food-related demonstrations with participation of volunteers from the group can be very effective. Provide small group activities to explore issues. Be clear to yourself regarding the purpose of each activity and how it relates to your session objectives. As we have said many times, activities need to be minds-on as well as hands-on so as not to turn into busywork. Carefully structure such activities, with clear instructions on how to conduct the activity and accompanying worksheets or activity sheets. Grocery store or farmers' market tours, for example, are appealing to upper elementary school children. Prepare the students ahead of time and prepare activity sheets for what they will do once there.

Deliver content appropriately in terms of cognitive developmental level. For elementary and middle school-aged children, health outcomes are in the distant future, and hence food and nutrition content needs to be provided in formats that fit their cognitive levels. Children may respond to food and nutrition activities if they involve some kind of intrinsic reward or element of fun (Matheson & Spranger, 2001). Puzzles, fantasy play, contests, quizzes, games, or computer games are engaging because they provide children with a challenge, the level of which can be set by the age of the child or group. These activities also stimulate children's curiosity if there is a meaningful objective that is part of the game or contest. Thus, fantasy, challenge, and curiosity can build on children's interest in investigations and stimulate intrinsic motivation. Nutrition content can be part of the plot or the problem to be solved by the characters involved in the fantasies and stories. One program created characters from another planet—named Hearty Heart, Dynamite Diet, Salt Sleuth, and Flash Fitness—who came to Earth to work with children and help them learn and practice health-promoting eating and exercise patterns (Leupker et al., 1996). A computer curriculum based on stories about invaders of a king-

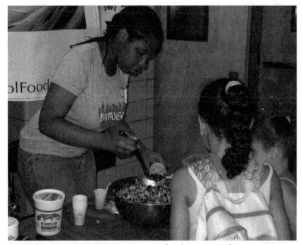

Peer education: Eatwise teens prepare food taste tests for younger children.

dom asked children to become squires to help the king and queen. The squires faced many challenges in their quest. The story included wizards, robots, and other fantasy creatures (Baranowski et al., 2003).

For high school students, hunger and food cravings, time, convenience, cost and availability of foods, perceived benefits, mood, body image, and habit are pressing food choice motivations, as we have seen. However, many issues in the field are controversial, from weight control diets, sales of sweetened beverages in schools, organic foods, and causes of world hunger to local versus global food systems. Stimulate thought and critical thinking through presentation of surprising data, interesting content, and case examples. Given that adolescents like to be challenged, design activities, such as debates or position papers, where they have an opportunity to grapple with these issues. Provide opportunities for students to propose novel or imaginative ideas to solve problems, understand and appreciate different viewpoints, and develop plans to address issues and solve problems.

Address social norms and peer influences. Help youth recognize the power of social environmental influences on their eating patterns by having them analyze television advertising, food marketing techniques, and what's available in neighborhood stores or stores around their schools. Make healthful eating desirable or cool by providing role models of importance to older children and youth. Peer educators can also be incorporated into the program, who can model healthful behaviors and address the participants' concerns.

Remember the importance of the affective domain. Teens' food choices and eating practices are strongly influenced by affective and emotional factors (as is true for all of us). Nutrition education can appeal to their growing sense of independence and ability to make choices for themselves as opposed to being dependent on the opinion of others. They can be encouraged to take charge of their lives. Because self-esteem is very important, activities should be respectful, build self-esteem, and never embarrass children and teens in front of others. Address body image and appearance concerns with sensitivity, being respectful of persons of all sizes.

Conduct food-based activities when possible. All of us are interested in food, and youth are no exception. These activities can enhance motivation, overcome barriers, and provide skill development. Develop simple recipes for food preparation, particularly ones that do not require heating or complicated utensils for where facilities are limited. Be sure to test these recipes first for ease of preparation, taste, and appearance, as well as ease in transporting ingredients and utensils to the site. Unless it is designated as a cooking session, the procedures should be quick in order to maintain attention and motivation. The activity should also engage all the teens, so that you do not have volunteers and onlookers. Set up several food preparation stations with the ingredients already measured out at each station.

Foster cognitive self-regulation. Given the increasing pressure of external forces on the food choices of older children and adolescents, ranging from peer pressure, food marketing practices, and the school environment to busy schedules and time constraints that leave little time to eat healthfully, nutrition education can foster cognitive self-regulation processes that focus on mindful eating through goal setting, planning ahead, and self-monitoring. These processes are described in detail in Chapter 12 of this book. Setting specific and actionable goals is not always easy, even for adults. It is important to take the time to teach goal-setting skills, using a process of guided goal setting, which seems to works best for this age group. Guided goal setting means that you can set the *major goals* for youth to achieve through your sessions or program, such as "eating healthful snacks," and youth can set their own specific and highly individualized *action goals* to achieve these major goals, such as by stating they will "eat fruit for snacks two days next week." Help them to balance meals eaten with peers that may not be so healthful with other, more healthful meals, such as those eaten at home. They can also negotiate within the family for healthful foods they like.

The Adult Learner

Adult learners can't be threatened, coerced, or tricked into learning something new; they must want to know (Brookfield, 1986; Knowles, 1990; Tennant & Pogson, 1995; Vella, 2002). Nutrition educators thus need to focus on behaviors, practices, or issues of immediate relevance to the group.

Characteristics of Adult Learners

Adults need to know why they need to learn something before undertaking to learn it. Much of adult learning is self-initiated and conducted on their own. However, adults also often find themselves participating in learning experiences because of the requirements of workplaces or food assistance programs (such as WIC or senior meal programs), referrals by their doctors and other medical care professionals, or for other reasons. Individuals need to see the immediate usefulness of the new skills, knowledge, or attitudes they are working to acquire. Learning is a means, not an end. Most adults do not have time to waste. They may even have to arrange for child care in order to attend a session, so that the session costs them money as well as time. Not surprisingly, they like to be convinced that the experience will be worth their time and effort.

Orientation to learning. Adults are generally task-oriented, problem-oriented, or life-centered. Thus they are less interested in, or enthralled by, a survey of nutrition such as provided by an overview of the food pyramid. They would rather learn about one or two key ideas and how they can be applied to a problem of relevance to them. However, there may be large differences in their preference for teaching style based on their own learning styles (see Chapter 15). For example, analytic learners may prefer that the needed information be presented to them in a straightforward but interesting presentation, whereas sociable or dynamic learners enjoy discussions. There is some agreement among adult educators that discussion is an ideal format for adult learning: it permits learners to share their own challenges and successes and to learn from the experiences of others. It reinforces their sense of self-worth and fosters their ability to make decisions. Discussions are especially useful for developing critical thinking and for creating new meaning systems out of shared experiences and collaborative interpretations of them (Brookfield, 1986; Knowles, 1990; Abusabha, Peacock, & Achterberg, 1999; Vella, 2002).

Readiness to learn. Adults are ready to learn those things that will help them to cope effectively with their real-life situations. Thus, pregnant women and mothers of young children may become interested in nutrition education because they want to have healthy children. Other life-changing events may also increase the readiness to learn, such as beginning to live on one's own, having teenagers whose eating patterns are of concern, or being diagnosed with some health condition. They seek out a learning experience because they have a use for the knowledge or skill being sought.

Learners' past experience. Adults have a great quantity of prior experience with food and eating. These experiences are unique to individuals, and the differences between individuals are large. We may be the experts on the content, but they are the experts on their own lives. These experiences must be honored and can greatly enrich sessions if they are built into the design of the sessions. You can find out about these past experiences through a careful and thorough needs and resources analysis. Indeed, many adults have greater experience with cooking or child-rearing than the nutrition educator. Others in the group, including the nutrition educator, can benefit from this wealth of knowledge if it is shared.

Learners as decision makers. Adults have a self-concept of being responsible for their own decisions and for their own lives. Healthy adults thus want respect for themselves as decision makers and resist being treated as objects and being told what to do. Indeed, quality of life increases as people are more capable of making decisions that affect their lives. Participants in nutrition education want the information we provide and are grateful for the sharing of experiences and tips from others, but they want to choose whether and how they will apply the information. This makes it imperative that sessions with adults be built on mutual respect and dialogue.

Motivation. Internal or intrinsic motivations to learn and change are more important than extrinsic motivations. Internal motivations include increased self-esteem, quality of life, job satisfaction, and health and avoidance of disease. Extrinsic motivations may include the advice of physicians or the urging of family.

Stage of Life and Roles

Adulthood is not some static state at which individuals arrive when they finish high school or get their first job. Instead, development is lifelong. Individuals grow and change throughout life. As they do, their needs, values, roles, and expectations change. These all have implications for nutrition education.

Life stage influences. Researchers have identified several adult life stages from in-depth interviews of individuals over time (Neugarten, Havighurst, & Tobin, 1968; Gould, 1978; Levinson, 1978, 1996). They suggest that adults experience several main stages: leaving the family between the ages of 15 to 25; with a transition between ages 25 and 30 to becoming an adult, entering a career, and starting a family; leading to settling down and becoming one's own person between the ages of 30 and 40. At this stage, careers are usually set and individuals now have families of their own. In the middle 40s to early 50s, children have left home, and individuals begin to see that time is finite and question life's meaning. Neugarten and colleagues (1968) proposed that until about this time, individuals see life in terms of "time since birth." The future stretches forth and there is time to do and see everything. The orientation is toward achievement, and death is an abstraction. After this period, individuals see life as "time left to live," where time is finite and there is time enough only to finish a few important things. Sponsoring others becomes important, and death becomes more personal. Some experience this midlife transition as destabilizing (the so-called midlife crisis), but most do not. This is then followed by restabilization in the 50s, where there is a renewed interest in friends and reliance on spouse or partner. This process is well illustrated in the nutrition area by the description of one woman about her changing perspective:

> When you're in your twenties you think you're not vulnerable to anything. When you're in your thirties you think you still have time. When you're in your forties you see things begin to creep up on you that have never affected you before . . . so you begin to seriously consider some of the things you've been reading about. [In your fifties] you make more conscious efforts to stick with foods and diets and meal planning that conform to better health standards. (Devine & Olson, 1991)

Women's motives for preventive dietary behaviors have been found to vary with life stage because of altered perceptions of health status, body weight, and family roles and responsibilities (Devine & Olson, 1991). Women with young children at home were more likely to be concerned for their children's health, resulting in a positive impact on their own diets because they prepared balanced family meals and sought to set a good example. For mothers of teenagers, there was tension between their desire to make healthful changes for their own health and the lack of acceptance of these changes by the family. The departure of grown children from the home allowed older women to make dietary changes for their own personal health, and many expressed that this stage was very satisfying.

There are also cohort effects (Neugarten, Havighurst, & Tobin,1968): those who grew up in the idealistic 1960s, for example, have different values, attitudes, expectations, and behaviors than those who grew up in the baby boomer or "me" generation (see Box 17-3). This has been found in the nutrition area as well: those growing up between 1944 and 1954 differed from those born two decades before in their perspectives on food and gender roles in the household and the ways in which differing kinds and degrees of public information about food and nutrition affected family meals growing up (Devine & Olson, 1991). The perspectives of today's generations X and Y and younger on food and nutrition issues likewise differ from those of the baby boomers. We need to be mindful of these cohort effects as we deliver nutrition education.

Life-course perspective on food choice. A central concept of a life-course perspective on food choice is that the development of individual food choices takes the form of stable trajectories or pathways over a person's life course. A food choice *trajectory* is a person's persistent thoughts, feelings, strategies, and actions with food and eating developed over a life course in a social and historical context (Devine et al., 1998; Devine, 2005). Embedded in trajectories are transitions and turning points. *Transitions*, such as changes in roles or in health conditions, can help to shape trajectories but do not necessarily change the direction of those pathways, whereas *turning points* are salient transitions, situations, or events that create long-term redirections in individuals' pathways (Devine, 2005).

In the nutrition arena, these pathways are the accumulation of experiences from food upbringing, roles, ethnic traditions and identities, location, and personal health and physical well-being. Research in food choice suggests that individuals make adjustments to accommodate life-course transitions such as motherhood, menopause, midlife, and older age, but relatively few adults report major turning points (Edstrom & Devine, 2001; Devine, 2005). Nutrition education activities should take into account how these past experiences may influence current beliefs, attitudes, and expectations.

Methods for Delivering Educational Strategies Appropriately to Adults: Making Learning Meaningful
What are the best ways, then, to conduct nutrition education to specifically take into consideration the special educational preferences and experiences of adults? Based on the background just discussed and on the research literature, the following methods of delivering nutrition education are likely to be effective (Contento et al., 1995; Vella, 2002; Sahyoun, Pratt, & Anderson, 2004).

Provide immediately useful information. At the beginning of a session, you can explain the purpose of the session and reassure participants that the session will be of immediate use to them. Provide adults with what they want and need to know—directly, clearly, and in a straightforward manner. Focus on only one or two key messages or specific behaviors, such as how to increase milk consumption or provide healthful snacks to their children. Provide realistic, not idealistic, information. Making the session relevant to any particular group of participants means that you must conduct a good assessment of the past experiences, needs, and desires of the group. If the group is ongoing, tell participants they will have an opportunity at the end of the session to suggest issues and topics to be addressed in future sessions.

Create a safe learning environment. To encourage learning, ensure that the room is physically comfortable and establish ground rules about respecting the time frame of the session; confidentiality; mutual trust, respect, and helpfulness; freedom of expression; and acceptance of differences. How to create such an environment is described in great detail in Chapter 15.

Develop respectful relationships. Adult educator Vella (2002) emphasizes the importance of respectful relationships between the group leader and learners and among learners. Relationships of the nutrition educator to the group can involve power-over or power-with. *Power* in this context refers to providing knowledge, decision-making control, and the right to ask questions (Abusabha, Peacock, & Achterberg, 1999). *Power-over* is when the professional provides all the information and gives advice, expecting the group members merely to comply. Although studies show that such a means for transfer of information can result in knowledge gains, it is less likely to lead to improved problem-solving skills, reflective thinking, attitude change, or changes in behavior. In the *power-with* approach, power is shared by the expert and the participants in an active partnership. In this approach, you listen actively to what each participant is saying, you do not talk down to participants but treat them as equals, you accept them exactly as they are, and you are warm, caring, trusting, and flexible. Even where individuals may prefer presentations as a way to receive information (Olson & Kelly, 1989), the attitude of respect for group participants is still crucially important.

Recognize that adult learners are decision makers. Respect adult learners as decision makers in their lives. Also respect that they should have some say in the content of the sessions. You can achieve this in many ways. For example, when new content is introduced, the nutrition educator can first describe in outline what can be included in this section, and then ask the group what they feel they need or want to learn about the topic. Learners can thus decide what occurs for them in the learning event. This involves their taking responsibility for their own learning and not being pas-

▶ **BOX 17-3 Characteristics of Different Age Cohorts**

The GI Generation, or Greatest Generation

Born between 1901 and 1924, today they are aged mid-80s and up. At 60 million strong, they were molded by the Great Depression and World War II. They won World War II and provided the nation with seven presidents. Members tend to be conservative; as a whole, they constitute the most satisfied generation.

Tips for Working with Them

- Emphasize realistic strengths, not weaknesses.
- Don't tell them they are old; just provide larger type.
- Make access easy.

The Silent Generation and Idealistic Generation

Born between 1925 and 1942, today their ages range from the late-60s to the early 80s. About 49 million strong, they were influenced by the GI generation before them. The older members of the cohort were silent in their youth, and the younger were idealistic and activist. This generation produced every major figure in the 20th-century civil rights movement, from Martin Luther King to Caesar Chavez. The Peace Corps was important to them. Members of this generation tend to be compassionate problem-solvers who find strength in human relations. They are healthy and active.

Tips for Working with Them

- Emphasize expertise.
- Provide statistics and information (they are readers).
- Stress wellness.
- Emphasize willingness to help others.

Baby Boomers, or the "Me" Generation

Born between 1943 and 1964, baby boomers are now in their mid-40s to mid-60s. About 79 million strong, they were born after World War II. Many are beginning to retire. This generation tends to be focused on the individual: the "inner world," consumption, and self-gratification. They want jobs that involve individual creativity. Denial is not in their dictionary. Emphasis is on youth: a longer life means extended middle life, not old age. Nostalgia is important.

Tips for Working with Them

- Promote quickness and convenience.
- Emphasize what is in it for them to eat healthfully.

Generation X

Born between 1965 and 1981, today they are in their mid-20s to early 40s. Almost 93 million strong, they are creating new families. This generation is very group oriented. Friends have taken the place of absent parents and relatives. Group dates are common. Members are often great shoppers: going to the mall is part of their social life. The generation is diverse and entrepreneurial. Because of job insecurity, they want to control their lives. They are wired, with email addresses, laptops, and cell phones. Members tend to be interested in environmental issues.

Tips for Working with Them

- Be visual, musical, and dynamic.
- Emphasize price value.
- Stress balance in life and the impact of food behaviors on the environment.

Generation Y

Born between 1982 and 1998, today they range in age from 10 to mid-20s. About 60 million strong, they are the children of baby boomers. This generation is practical and pragmatic. Members often grew up in dual-income and single-parent families, and are very involved in family purchases. They are technologically savvy: computers and other gadgets are like pens and pencils to them, and they grew up with the Web. They expect multiple options and think of time in seconds. They tend to be action oriented and socially and ecologically aware.

Tips for Working with Them

- Be visual, musical, and dynamic, but also use technologically sophisticated formats, such as CDs and PowerPoint presentations.
- Emphasize quickness and convenience.

Source: Adapted from "Who are your customers? What do they want?" *On-Site Magazine*, May 1999, pp. 21–42.

sive listeners. There will no doubt be different viewpoints on any particular issue. The group should feel secure that their opinions will matter and that they will not be criticized. After all viewpoints have been expressed, they can then be sorted out and evaluated for their scientific merit. The role of the facilitator is crucial in keeping the group on track and ensuring that the conclusions being drawn are scientifically accurate and based on evidence. Where there are misconceptions, the nutrition educator can correct them with respect, such as saying, "I am glad it worked for you, but research suggest that . . ."

Engage learners. Design activities that will actively engage learners. For example, design active learning tasks that can be carried out in small groups or dyads. Where appropriate, the outcome of these tasks should be open-ended and based on what the group or dyad comes up with. Provide for the opportunity to reflect on the task. These learning tasks should build on the past experience of the learners. Facilitated dialogue is another format in which all group members are fully engaged: they actively participate in learning by listening to each other and sharing with each other. Facilitated dialogue is described later in this section.

Build on learners' past experience and knowledge. Adults need to be able to integrate new ideas with what they already know if they are going to keep—and use—new information and skills. Information that conflicts sharply with what is already held to be true, and thus forces a reevaluation of the old beliefs and attitudes, should not, of course, be avoided, but recognize that it is integrated more slowly. Likewise, information that has little conceptual overlap with what is already known is acquired more slowly. So learn about the current perceptions, beliefs, or attitudes of your audience toward the issue at hand in order to build on what is known.

Sequence the learning experiences and reinforce them. If new how-to food and nutrition information is to be provided or new skills are to be taught, such as new food preparation methods, sequence the learning tasks from simple to complex and provide plenty of opportunities for observation and practice. Reinforce information, skills, and attitudes by repetition in diverse, engaging, and interesting ways until the knowledge and skills are learned. In group discussion, frequently summarize the key points of the discussion.

Come to closure with solutions. After a group of adult learners grapples with the issues that are the focus of the session and shares challenges and successes, the nutrition educator can summarize the discussion and facilitate the group coming up with common solutions. Good solutions come from full participation of the group and the shared understandings and meaning that evolve through discussion. The group feels more commitment to the solutions adopted by the group because they shared in the responsibility of arriving at final decisions about what actions to take.

Support cognitive self-regulation. As with older children and adolescents, adults also have busy schedules and experience time constraints that leave little time to eat healthfully. When group participants decide individually or collectively to take action, we can support their cognitive self-regulation processes through teaching skills of goal setting, planning ahead, and self-monitoring. These processes are described in detail in Chapter 12 of this book. Setting specific and actionable goals is important.

Example of Nutrition Education Program Based on Adult Education Principles

Choosing Healthy Options In Cooking and Eating, or the CHOICE project, was a program directed at older women that incorporated the features just discussed. The project is described in Nutrition Education in Action 17-1.

Facilitated Group Dialogue as an Educational Tool

Facilitated dialogue is an example of an effective tool for working with adults that incorporates all the previous strategies (Abusabha, Peacock, & Achterberg, 1999; Vella, 2002; Sigman-Grant, 2005). The word *facilitate* is derived from the Latin word meaning "to enable, to make easy." The *facilitator* is thus a person who makes it easier for people to understand (Sigman-Grant, 2005). The facilitator's job is to make the group atmosphere comfortable for discussion by incorporating the actions described previously to address each of the types of learner's fears (Abusabha, Peacock, & Achterberg, 1999). The facilitator's role is also to move the discussion along without dominating it. The facilitator assists group members to express their ideas, helps them to think critically about issues, encourages them to talk to and listen to each other, and assists them to come to conclusions based on group input. The aim is for active participation by all of the group members and shared understandings. Use of this approach has resulted in sessions that are lively and in which group participants feel motivated and empowered (Reid & Gerstein, 2005).

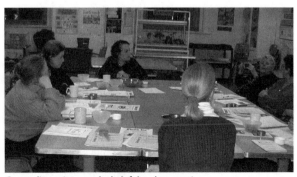

Group discussions can be helpful and supportive.

NUTRITION EDUCATION IN ACTION 17-1

Choosing Healthy Options in Cooking and Eating (The CHOICE Project)

The Program

The major causes of death and disability among American women today include cardiovascular disease, cancer, and osteoporosis, and there is consensus that diet is related to these conditions. This program was designed to help non–at-risk, healthy older women in a free-living setting to develop eating patterns that would reduce the risk of these conditions. They were randomized into three conditions:

- A moderate fat diet, operationalized as the American Heart Association (AHA) eating plan
- The addition of flaxseed (a good source of phytoestrogens) to the AHA eating plan, provided as a dietary supplement
- A diet high in plant foods and low in animal foods, in the form of a macrobiotic-style eating plan

During the course of 12 months, participants met for 24 nutrition education and behavioral change sessions: weekly for 14 weeks, biweekly for the next 10 weeks, and monthly for the remaining six months. The behavioral intervention strategies used to maintain subject participation and dietary adherence included:

- Seven cooking classes with hands-on experience alternating with behavioral sessions during the first 14 weeks; information provided on how to eat according to the assigned eating plan
- Cooking demonstrations with tastings at all other sessions
- Individual goal-setting and development of action plans each session
- Regular feedback and encouragement based on three-day food records completed monthly by the women
- Monthly telephone calls on a random day to collect 24-hour dietary recalls, as an incentive for adherence
- Group bonding through icebreakers at start of sessions, sharing of addresses and phone numbers, facilitated discussion
- Chef's knife, apron, mug and tote bag with CHOICE logo
- Monthly newsletter to participants during six months of monthly sessions

Evaluation Results

Results showed that women on the macrobiotic-style eating plan were able to achieve significant changes in diet, in the desired direction, for many key categories of foods targeted in the intervention. They tripled their whole grain intakes, tripled their intake of beans and legumes, and doubled their intake of fish. They decreased their intakes of refined grain products; cut their meat, poultry and eggs, and whole milk products intake; and reduced their consumption of high-fat sweets compared to baseline values. They made these changes within the first three months and maintained them for most of the 12 months. The women in the other two eating plans, based on the AHA moderate fat diet, made changes in their diet but these were not significant, largely because the women were already eating diets moderately low in fat.

Source: Contento I.R., A. Persaud, E. Solomon, et al. 2004. Changes in food patterns during an intervention with women placed on eating plans with varying amounts and types of phytoestrogens. Presentation at International Society for Behavioral Nutrition and Physical Activity Annual Meeting, Washington D.C.

In the context of nutrition education, what is the role of the facilitator? What does group facilitation mean? How exactly does one function as a nutrition educator to make a group session a democratic and valuable group learning experience? How does one find the right balance between being authoritarian as a facilitator and being laissez-faire?

Some believe that the facilitator is just another member of the group, who should not direct the activities of the group. Brookfield (1986) notes that because much of adult learning is concerned with such issues as the resolution of moral difficulties, development of self-insight, reflection on experi-

ence, and reinforcement of self-worth rather than technical knowledge, there are those who argue that discussion cannot be directed, for to attempt to do so would be to close people's consciousness to alternative interpretations of the issue under discussion before these alternatives were even stated (Peterson, 1970).

The facilitated dialogue reflects this approach to some extent: it is described as a method of group teaching that involves the active participation of all group members and the leader. Learners and facilitators are equal partners in the learning experience (Sigman-Grant, 2005). The group sits in a circle, and the leader sits alongside the group members in the circle. Ideally, the group members do all the talking and in essence conduct the session. The leader talks very little as group members share with each other and learn from each other. Although the nutrition educator may be the expert on food and nutrition issues, the group members are experts on their own lives and how and whether they can incorporate the provided information into their own situations. Those who use a learner-centered approach state that "the most central point of learner-centered education is that the learner is a decision-maker. They choose *if* they learn and *if* they will change their behavior. We cannot decide for them. The learning is in the *doing* and *deciding*" (Husing & Elfant, 2005).

However, it is acknowledged that open discussions about whatever topic comes to the minds of group members in laissez-faire fashion without much input from the nutrition educator are not fruitful either. Group members often express frustration with a lack of sense of progress toward any clear learning objective. In addition, as nutrition educators working in specific programs that have specific missions, we are accountable for certain outcomes that involve addressing specific behaviors, such as recommended infant feeding practices or eating more fruits and vegetables (Sigmund-Grant, 2005).

In general, the sessions based on facilitated discussion are planned ahead of time, involving the preparation of an educational plan. Norris (2003) and Sigmund-Grant (2005) suggest that the sequence of activities during the session can follow four "A"s as follows:

- *Anchoring:* Introduction and/or review
- *Add:* Active learning and facilitated dialogue; introduction of new concepts and new information
- *Apply*: Providing an opportunity through an interactive exercise for all participants to consider ways to use the new material and the points made within the discussion to their own lives
- *Away:* Summarizing, bringing to closure, and selection of action plans

As can be seen, the four As procedure is very similar to the sequencing of learning described in chapter 11, which is: gain attention, present new material by building on prior learning, provide guidance, elicit performance and feedback, and enhance retention and transfer. An example of a specific sequence of activities for how such facilitated discussion can be carried out in the Women, Infants and Children (WIC) program is shown in Box 17-4.

Facilitating a group does not mean that the group should not be challenged. Indeed, we are charged as educators to assist group members to analyze assumptions, challenge previously accepted and internalized beliefs and values, and contemplate the validity of alternative behaviors or other ways of doing things (Brookfield, 1986; Abusabha, Peacock, & Achterberg, 1999). All these acts can at times be uncomfortable

and may even contradict the stated needs of the group. Thus the job of the facilitator is to create learning environments that are both emotionally safe *and* challenging. In addition, in nutrition education groups, there is often much nutrition science–based motivational why-to information and how-to information and skills that need to be addressed. Thus the educator has a role, and the group members have a role.

It can be seen, then, that facilitating groups requires considerable skill and practice to find the right balance of acceptance and challenge, of leading and being a member of the group. The nature of the facilitator's role and the degree of guidance and control will depend on the food and nutrition issue being addressed and the nature of the group.

Working with Different Cultural Groups

The United States is becoming increasingly multicultural, with people living in it who come from diverse ancestries and who have become part of the mainstream to varying degrees. New York City has over 170 distinct ethnic communities. More than 130 languages and dialects are spoken by students in the Washington, D.C., school system. Los Angeles has more people of Mexican descent than any city in the world except Mexico City. Even states such as Iowa and Alabama are getting used to people speaking Spanish in their midst. Some are recent immigrants, and others have been in the country for several generations. Whereas in the past all became a part of a general "melting pot," in recent decades racial/ethnic groups have shown a wish to be acknowledged, honored, and respected for their unique heritage and contributions, resulting in more of a mosaic. Although often referred to as minorities, such subsets of the population are often a majority of the population in certain locations, and hence such a term is inaccurate and inappropriate in these cases (Bronner, 1994). We thus face the challenge of providing nutrition education to a variety of people who come from a variety of cultures that are different from our own. This requires us to better understand our own culture and those of others.

Culture has been described as a set of beliefs, knowledge, traditions, values, and behavioral patterns that are developed, learned, shared, and transmitted by members of a group. It is a worldview that a group shares and hence influences perceptions about food, nutrition, and health (Sanjur, 1982). Knowledge and beliefs include accepted understandings, opinions, and faith about the world. Beliefs help determine which foods are edible, appropriate preparation methods, or the meaning of a food. Traditions are customs about which foods are eaten on what occasions (e.g., weddings, birthdays), what will be eaten for health or to cure illness, or religious traditions about fasting and feasting. Values are widely held beliefs about what is worthwhile, desirable, or important for well-being. Values considered desirable in one culture may not be considered so in another culture, and these differences in value systems can influence food and nutrition practices.

▶ **BOX 17-4 Specific Guidelines and Techniques for Facilitated Group Discussions in the Special Supplemental Nutrition Program for Women, Infants, and Children**

Build the Group from Within
- Assure members that the group will be structured to fit their needs and concerns.

Establish Ground Rules
- Set the time, agenda, and length of the session.
- Set rules of respecting confidentiality, sharing group responsibilities, and respecting and listening to opinions of other group members.

Begin with an Icebreaker Exercise
- Ask each group member to make a brief statement about herself, her child's needs, and anything new that happened to her during the past month.

Ask Open-Ended Questions
- Ask questions that cannot be answered by "yes" or "no."
- Involve group members in describing their own experiences.

Guide the Discussion
- Encourage others to speak.
- Keep discussion on track.
- Gently bring topics to a conclusion.

Encourage Full Participation
- Encourage quiet members to voice their ideas.
- Listen intently to each member.
- Repeat members' comments when necessary.
- Give a positive feedback verbally or physically (e.g., nodding head, smiling).

Focus the Conversation
- Clarify different views.
- Restate the objectives of the session when necessary.
- Summarize the important points of the discussion.

Correct Misconceptions Artfully
- Avoid turning into the "lecturer."
- Emphasize the worth of the member's experience.
- Use responses such as "I am glad this worked for you, but other people have found . . ."
- Ask what other group members think about the statement.

Create an Atmosphere of Acceptance
- Accept people and respect each member's feelings even when you disagree with her viewpoint.
- Do not hurt members' feeling by abruptly negating or putting down their ideas and experiences.

Summarize the Discussion
- Bring ideas together and repeat relevant information.
- Strive to make the summary the result of the members' discussion, not your own analysis.
- Repeat and clarify the solution to the nutrition problem that members agreed on.

Be Patient
- Remember, it takes time for a group to grow and develop trust.

Have Fun
- Keep a smile and enjoy sharing with and learning from the group.

Source: Abusabha, R., J. Peacock, and C. Achterberg. 1999. Facilitated group discussion. *Journal of the American Dietetic Association* 99:72–76. Used with permission of the American Dietetic Association.

Culture, then, is a learned experience, not a biologically determined one (Sanjur, 1982). It is the product of interaction among generations, always being modified over time. Consequently, it can also be unlearned. Cultures are constantly changing. Thus we can view food habits as a dynamic process, always changing. However, every culture also resists change by self-generated mechanisms to perpetuate its cultural traits and to maintain its boundaries.

All societies have a dominant set of beliefs, values, and traditions that are shared by the majority of people. In the United States, the norms have been described as an emphasis on education, a work ethic, materialism, religion, physical appearance, cleanliness, high technology, punctuality, independence, and free enterprise. Those cultural groups whose beliefs, values, and traditions are different may not always be treated with understanding and respect (Bronner 1994).

Understanding Cultural Sensitivity and Cultural Competence

Working with a variety of cultures requires that the nutrition educator become culturally competent. This may involve several steps, according to Bronner (1994). *Cultural knowledge* is the process of learning about the worldviews of other cultures. This can be accomplished by reading books, attending workshops, watching audiovisual presentations, perusing government documents, and so forth. We can learn about the food habits and beliefs of various ethnic groups through these means. *Cultural awareness* is the process of becoming aware of our own learned biases and prejudices toward other cultures through self-assessment, while becoming aware of the beliefs, values, practices, lifestyles, and problem-solving strategies of other groups. This leads to *cultural sensitivity*, which is the awareness of our own cultural beliefs, assumptions, customs, and values as well as those of other cultural groups. We recognize that cultural differences as well as similarities exist, without assigning values to these differences as good or bad, right or wrong.

Cultural competence is a set of knowledge and interpersonal skills that allows individuals to increase their understanding and appreciation of cultural differences and similarities within, among, and between groups and to work effectively in cross-cultural situations (Bronner, 1994). Being competent in cross-cultural functioning means learning new patterns of behavior and effectively applying them in the appropriate settings. Knowledge about a culture does not equal cultural competence. In fact, "book" knowledge of a culture may lead to inappropriate generalizations, such as stereotyping. Through frequent cultural encounters and engagement, nutrition educators can become aware of the heterogeneity within cultural groups. For example, although individuals from a given culture may have similar beliefs, attitudes, and practices in terms of food and nutrition, there are also many variations due to differences in education,

age, religion, socioeconomic status, geographic location, and length of time in the country.

The goal for nutrition educators is to accompany knowledge of the culture with awareness, respect, and acceptance of the group's cultural beliefs and practices, and willingness and ability to work within the values, traditions, and customs of the participants' community (Bronner, 1994).

Not only individuals but also organizations need to exhibit cultural competence. Thus cultural competence has been defined as "a set of congruent behaviors, attitudes, and policies that come together in a system, agency, or among professionals and enables that system, agency, or those professionals to work effectively in cross-cultural situations. Operationally defined, cultural competence is the integration and transformation of knowledge about individuals and groups of people into specific standards, policies, practices, and attitudes used in appropriate cultural settings to increase the quality of services, thereby producing better outcomes" (King, Sims, & Osher, 2006).

Consequently, systems and agencies, such as health systems, food and nutrition agencies, and nutrition education programs, need to become more culturally competent. Five elements have been identified as essential for contributing to a system's ability to become more culturally competent (Cross et al., 1989; Isaacs & Benjamin, 1991; King, Sims, & Osher, 2006).The system should (1) value diversity, (2) have the capacity for cultural self-assessment, (3) be conscious of the "dynamics" inherent when cultures interact, (4) institutionalize cultural knowledge, and (5) develop adaptations to service delivery reflecting an understanding of diversity between and within cultures (King, Sims, & Osher, 2006). Further, these five elements must be manifested in every level of the service delivery system. They should be reflected in attitudes, structures, policies, and services.

Appropriate Delivery Methods for Nutrition Education for Culturally Diverse Audiences

What, then, are the implications for how nutrition education can be delivered to culturally diverse audiences? It should be noted that the psychosocial theories and models that we have used throughout the book can provide a framework for designing the program for various cultural groups (Liou & Contento, 2001). However, the theory constructs need to be operationalized to be culturally appropriate. There may also be culturally specific constructs that are important to consider in delivering nutrition education. In applying the concepts related to cultural sensitivity to health promotion and nutrition education, Resnicow and colleagues (1999) suggest that is it helpful to consider the following distinctions.

Cultural sensitivity or *cultural appropriateness* is the extent to which the design, delivery, and evaluation of nutrition education and health promotion programs incorporate the ethnic or cultural experiences, beliefs, traditions, and behaviors of a given group as well as relevant historical, social, and environmental forces. *Cultural competence,* as we have seen, is the capacity of individuals and organizations to exercise interpersonal cultural sensitivity. Thus, cultural competence refers to practitioners and agencies, whereas cultural sensitivity or appropriateness refers to the intervention messages and program materials. *Multicultural* refers to incorporating and appreciating the perspectives of multiple racial or ethnic groups without assumptions of superiority or inferiority. Thus, culturally sensitive programs are implicitly multicultural.

Cultural targeting is the process of creating culturally sensitive interventions. This often involves adapting existing materials and programs for racial/ethnic subgroups. *Culturally based* programs and messages are those that combine the culture, history, and core values of a subgroup as a medium to motivate behavior change. For example, nutrition education programs for indigenous Americans can focus on traditional foods and spiritual systems.

Surface Structure and Deep Structure

Programs and materials can focus on a *surface structure* dimension, whereby materials and messages are matched to the observable social and behavioral characteristics of given cultural groups by using people, places, language, music, clothing, or food familiar to, or preferred by, the target audience (Resnicow et al., 2005). You might also use media channels that are most watched or settings uniquely used by the group to deliver the nutrition education, such as churches or ethnic community centers. Ideally you would want to match staff ethnically to the participants. Surface structure indicates how well the intervention fits within the culture, experience, and behavioral patterns of the audience.

Programs and materials that focus on *deep structure* are culturally based by building on general core values and historical, cultural, social, and environmental factors that may influence the food and nutrition behavior of the target audience (Resnicow et al., 1999). Core values that have been considered when working among some Asian groups, for example, are the importance of family, respect for older people, and the importance of maintaining balance for health, including the use of hot and cold foods to address hot and cold health conditions. Programs with African Americans have been built on the core values of commitment to family, communalism, connections to history and ancestors, and a unique sense of time, rhythm, or communication style (Resnicow et al., 1999, 2002, 2005). For the Latino culture, core values include importance of family, respect for elders, fatalism, and the importance of positive social interactions that can be the foundation for nutrition education (Bronner, 1994). You need to understand and value the core values of the different groups with which you work as you deliver your program. In particular, there are differences in body image

issues, such as what is an appropriate weight in the eyes of a given cultural group (Kumanyika & Morssink, 1997).

In terms of food choice specifically, one qualitative study with three ethnic groups (African American, Latino, and white) found that ideals, identities, and roles interacted reciprocally and dynamically with each other and with food choices and influences on food consumption (Devine et al., 1998). *Ideals,* or deeply held beliefs about food and eating, came from multiple sources, of which ethnicity was one. For some individuals, ethnicity was dominant; for others, age or religion or other interests, such as health and fitness, were also important. *Identity* is the way people think of their own distinguishing characteristics and self-image. Ethnic identities in this study existed along with others, such as regional or family background and travel experiences, which sometimes overrode ethnic identities. Ethnic identities were most often expressed in holidays and family celebrations. Individuals also have multiple *roles,* some of which influence food choice. Women in all three cultural groups were usually the family food managers. Some African American and white men were the primary cooks for the family. *Contexts* enhanced or constrained all food choices and influenced the ability to enact cultural ideals and roles.

It is essential to remember that there are wide variations within groups in terms of ethnic/racial identity, which may be defined as the extent to which individuals identify and gravitate toward their racial/ethnic group psychologically and socially (Resnicow et al., 1999). Ethnic identity includes individuals' extent of acculturation; the degree to which they have affinity for in-group culture such as food, media, or clothes; racial/ethnic pride; attitudes toward maintaining one's culture; and involvement with those within the group and those outside the group.

Appropriate Language

There are many differences in communication styles between cultures, such as whether to speak loudly or softly; to look at the person who is speaking or avert one's gaze; to smile, nod, or interject when someone is speaking to acknowledge understanding of what the speaker says or to show little expression; and whether to rarely ask questions and provide yes/no responses or to use a direct approach and ask direct questions (Sue & Sue, 1999). Rather than ask whether the group understands—which is likely to yield a yes answer in some cultures, say "Tell me which things are not clear to you." In some cultures, it is impossible to say no to a request, so individuals may respond with "maybe" about whether the time for the session is a good time or whether they will come to the next session. In some cultures, it is acceptable to make a commitment and then to decide later to make changes to it or to decline altogether. It is assumed that one cannot predict events in one's life that may occur in the meantime. It is thus very important to learn about the specific culturally appropriate communication styles of the groups with which you will be working.

Strategies for Enhancing Cultural Appropriateness

Several strategies for making health promotion programs and materials more culturally appropriate have been proposed (Kavanagh & Kennedy, 1992; Kumanyika & Morssink, 1997; Resnicow et al., 1999; Kreuter et al., 2003). Those proposed by Kreuter and colleagues (2003) are briefly described in the following list. These strategies are not mutually exclusive, and most nutrition educators use several when planning programs and materials.

- *Peripheral strategies* use preferred colors, images, fonts, or pictures of group members to convey relevance to the group and to enhance acceptance. That is, the strategies match materials to the surface structure characteristics described previously. These strategies are called peripheral because they appeal to the peripheral route to attitude change identified by Petty and Cacioppo (1986) and described earlier in the book.

- *Evidential strategies* seek to enhance the perceived relevance of the health issue for the particular group by providing scientific or epidemiological evidence for the impact of the issue on the group. For example, you can provide evidence that the group has a high incidence of heart disease or hypertension, thus raising perceived risk.

- *Linguistic strategies* strive to make the programs or materials more accessible by using the language of the group. Sometimes this just involves translating the materials into another language, or using an interpreter when you are leading groups. In some situations the interpretation may be into more than one language if the audience is multicultural.

- *Audience-involving strategies* draw directly on the experience of the intended audience by using staff members, paid or volunteer, who are drawn from the same cultural group and by involving lay community members in planning and decision making for the programs.

- *Sociocultural strategies* focus on the cultural beliefs, traditions, and behaviors, or deep structure characteristics, of the intended audience. Such strategies build upon and reinforce the group's core values in order to provide context and meaning for the programs and messages.

All these strategies can be used in one program (Kreuter et al., 2003). For example, a program for Latina women could use the kinds of bright colors that appeal to the women (peripheral strategy), address the increased incidence of a health condition such as diabetes experienced by Latinas compared with other groups (evidential strategy), present group sessions using straightforward words and phrases in Spanish (linguistic strategy), include stories and testimonials of other women from the community (strategy of involving the audience community), and address the belief in fatalism (sociocultural strategy).

Process for Developing Culturally Appropriate Programs and Materials

Given the wide diversity between cultural groups, it is essential that the materials and programs are appropriate to a given specific cultural group. You can do so through use of focus groups and extensive pretesting.

Focus groups. Use focus groups to provide the basis for developing your message content and format. Using this format, you can identify both surface and deep structure elements by exploring the thoughts, feelings, language, assumptions, and practices of the group, including food preferences, shopping and cooking habits, and perceived benefits and barriers. You can also explore cultural differences by using "ethnic mapping" (Resnicow et al., 1999). Here you can ask the group whether certain foods they eat or behaviors they engage in are "mostly an ethnic thing," "equally an ethnic and white thing," or "mostly a white/American thing." Such focus groups should include individuals representing the heterogeneity within the cultural group.

Pretesting. After you have designed a draft of your materials (e.g., videos, printed materials) or program content, it is essential that you show them to a sample from your target audience for their feedback on format and content, reflecting both surface and deep structure characteristics. Some groups may like the images to portray individuals from their same racial/ethnic group, but others may not, for example. Test the concepts being addressed and the language being used. Find out whether the group perceives any of the features to be stereotyping or insensitive.

Examples of Effective Interventions

An intervention conducted with black women illustrates how a program can be made more culturally sensitive by appropriate targeting (Kreuter et al. 2003, 2005). The study, designed to increase mammography and fruits and vegetable consumption, was based on four potentially important cultural characteristics that had been identified as being salient because they were found to be prevalent among African Americans, were associated with health-related beliefs and practices, and could be measured:

- *Religiosity,* represented by church attendance, prayer, spirituality, and beliefs about God as a causal agent in health. A message might be as follows: "The Lord has given us a powerful tool for helping find cancer before it is too late. Getting a mammogram, together with the power of prayer, will give you the best chance to live a long and healthy life" (Kreuter et al., 2003, p. 140).

- *Collectivism*, which is the belief that the basic unit of society is the community or family, not the individual, and that collective survival is a high priority. Hence, important values were cooperation, concern and responsibility for others, forgiveness, family security, friendship, and respect for tradition. A message might be as follows: "As black women, we have many important jobs. We keep our families together. We help build our communities. We work inside and outside the home. But our most important job may be to keep ourselves healthy. If we don't take care of ourselves, it is harder to take care of others" (Kreuter et al., 2003, p. 140).

- *Racial pride*. Individuals vary in a continuum in terms of the degree to which they remain immersed in their own cultural traditions, adopt the mainstream white culture, or participate in the traditions of both their own and mainstream culture. Racial pride is manifested in interest and involvement in traditional practices, preferences for African American media, belief in the importance of promoting black art and literature, or degree of practice of traditional eating practices and preferences, such as fried food. A message might be as follows: "Did you know that most cancers affect blacks more than whites? Only about 10% of blacks in our community eat five fruits and vegetables as recommended by health professionals. But you can reverse this trend by . . . " (Kreuter et al., 2003, p. 141).

- *Perception of time*. The notion of time is socially constructed, as we noted in Chapter 2. The traditional white perception of time is that it has a past, present, and future and can be divided into discrete units, which, like money or other goods, can be saved, spent, wasted, or even bought, as in "buying time" (Kreuter et al., 2003). Time well spent now can lead to a better future. People with such a future orientation are thus more likely to engage in health-promoting behaviors. In the health area, it has been found that African Americans are more present-oriented. Hence a message can be "It is hard to think about the future when you are feeling fine today. But sometimes you can take steps today to make life better tomorrow. Getting a mammogram is another step you can take today to make life better tomorrow, since finding cancer early increases the chances of successful treatment" (Kreuter et al., 2003, p. 142).

Another study, the Healthy Body/Healthy Spirit trial, examined the effect of a culturally sensitive, multicomponent self-help intervention on fruit and vegetable intake and on the physical activity of members of a set of socioeconomically diverse black churches (see Nutrition Education in Action 17-2).

Low-Literacy Audiences

In the United States, the average reading level is at the eighth grade, with about one in five reading at the fifth-grade level, and for those older than 65 and for many cultural subgroups, about two in five reading below the fifth-grade level. This means that about 20% of the population are functionally illiterate—they can't read newspapers or physician instructions for medications. Another 30% have marginal reading skills (Doak, Doak, & Root, 1996). Those with low literacy skills may not be able to read the handouts or booklets we give them or the written food and nutrition instructions we provide them.

Doak and colleagues (1996) point out that we cannot identify low-literacy individuals by their appearance or by conversation with them. They are often very good in other forms of communication and have learned to compensate, so that their lack of literacy skills is not obvious. They can be poor or affluent, immigrant or native born. Sometimes those who have low literacy in English are highly literate in the language of their country of origin; others, born in this country, just never developed the skills. Low in literacy skills does not mean low in intelligence. Our nutrition education can be effective if we find the appropriate format.

Poor readers, compared with skilled readers, read slowly, often one or two words at a time, so that they lose the meaning of the whole sentence. They think in terms of individual items of information rather than in categories or groups with common characteristics. They often do not understand information if it is implied; how the information is to be used must be spelled out clearly (Figure 17-1). Thus, they often have difficulty with analysis and synthesis of information as well as with literacy.

Comprehension is about grasping the meaning of instruction or materials and is an important aspect of literacy. Comprehension, whether verbal, written, or visual, requires that we pay attention to information and remember it for when we need it. Gaining the attention of the intended audience at the beginning of a session or a piece of printed material is important for activating the memory system. As we have noted many times in this book, this can be done by vivid stories, striking visuals, or dramatic data. Getting the information into our audience's short-term memory requires us to be aware that this form of memory has a limited capacity and a short storage time. We can usually store only up to seven independent items at a time. Any more than that may mean that we will not remember *any* of the items. For those of low literacy, the number is more like three to five. Transfer from short-term to long-term memory, and storage in long-term memory, requires that the new information links to what the audience already knows, is repeated often, and actively involves the audience.

NUTRITION EDUCATION IN ACTION 17-2

Healthy Body/Healthy Spirit: A Church-Based Nutrition and Physical Activity Intervention

The Program

The Healthy Body/Healthy Spirit program was a culturally targeted self-help intervention to increase consumption of fruits and vegetables and levels of physical activity. It was based on addressing both dimensions of *surface structure*, in which materials and messages are matched to observable social and behavioral characteristics of the intended audience, and *deep structure,* in which the intervention is based on cultural, historical, and psychological factors that are unique to the racial/ethnic identity of the audience.

The intervention built on surface structure involving food preferences, cooking practices, and exercise patterns of the audience. It also addressed deep structure issues, which included unique attitudes to body image, safety concerns, lack of time for exercise, effect of exercise on hair, religious themes, and interest in improving the health of the community (as opposed to personal health).

The study was conducted in 16 socioeconomically diverse black churches in the Atlanta area. Church members were randomized into three groups. One group received standard educational materials. The second group received culturally sensitive self-help materials, and the third received self-help materials plus motivational interviewing. The materials provided to the intervention group participants were as follows:

- *Forgotten Miracles:* An 18-minute video that centered around two families, one that tended to eat healthfully and the other that did not. Key messages were conveyed with biblical themes, such as the story of Daniel, who rejects the "kings' diet" for his own "natural diet" high in fruit and vegetables, and messages about the body being "God's temple." These culturally sensitive messages conveyed information about the health benefits of eating fruits and vegetables, analysis of costs, recipes, and cooking tips.
- *Eat for Life cookbook:* A cookbook containing recipes submitted by church members that met specified criteria. The recipes were first tested by staff.
- *Healthy Body/Healthy Spirit exercise video:* A 20-minute video hosted by African American celebrities from the Atlanta area and based on footage taped in church members' homes so as to provide real-world role models.
- *Healthy Body/Healthy Spirit guide:* A 37-page, four-color manual to accompany the video.
- *Audiocassette:* A cassette with gospel music to match a three-phase workout: warm-up, aerobic activity, and cool-down. Biblical quotes and brief excerpts from the pastors' sermons were interspersed with the music.

Evaluation Results

Slightly over a thousand individuals were recruited from the 16 churches, of whom 906 were assessed at the end of one year. A subset of the individuals also received four culturally sensitive telephone counseling calls based on motivational interviewing techniques. Results showed that those who received the culturally sensitive intervention significantly increased their fruit and vegetable intakes and their physical activity levels compared with those who received standard educational materials.

Sources: Resnicow, K., A. Jackson, R. Braithwaite, et al. 2002. Healthy Body/Healthy Spirit: A church-based nutrition and physical activity intervention. *Health Education Research* 17:562–573; and Resnicow, K., A. Jackson, D. Blisset, et al. 2005. Results of the Healthy Body Healthy Spirit trial. *Health Psychology* 24:339–348.

Appropriate Delivery Methods for Low-Literacy Audiences

How shall we apply these considerations to delivering nutrition education to low-literacy audiences? Many have written about this problem (e.g., Doak, Doak, & Root, 1996), and some key strategies are described briefly here.

General Strategies

The following strategies are applicable to all components of nutrition education.

- *Know your audience.* Assess the needs and preferences of the intended audience thoroughly before designing your program, using the procedures described in Steps 1 and 2 earlier in this book. What is the group's literacy level and its readiness to learn? Focus groups, personal interviews, or interviews with those who work closely with this audience, such as agency personnel, are all valuable means for gaining this information.
- *Pretest all materials through cognitive testing.* Use focus groups to guide you as you design your sessions. How

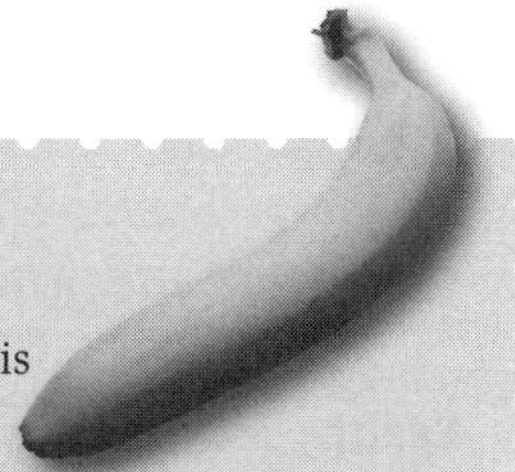

Fiber is fantastic!

There are two kinds of fiber, and they are both very good for your health. One kind of fiber is called <u>soluble</u>. The other kind of fiber is called <u>insoluble</u>.

Think of <u>soluble fiber</u> as a sponge—it soaks up water, and slows down anything going through your intestines. It also helps lower cholesterol. You can find it in fruits like bananas and apples, or vegetables like carrots and peas.

Think of <u>insoluble fiber</u> as a bristle-brush that helps clean out your tube-like intestines. It keeps things moving, which helps keep you regular! You can find it in the skins of fruits, like when you eat whole grapes or whole cherries. You can also find insoluble fiber in the skins of vegetables, like when you eat potato skins, or corn on the cob. Either way, fiber is good news for your health!

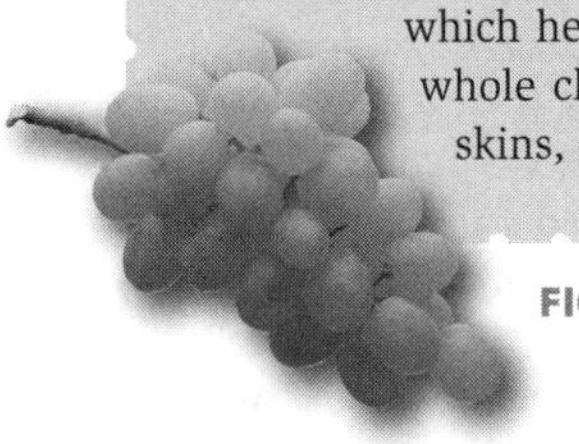

FIGURE 17-1 Low-literacy material: short words and sentences and underline instead of bold.

should the issues be framed for this audience? What educational strategies do they prefer? After you have designed a draft of your sessions, pretest your message with your intended audience to determine whether the message to be delivered through educational sessions or written materials conveys the meaning you intend. This is referred to as *cognitive testing* (Alaimo, Olson, & Frongillo, 1999). In particular, cognitively test any evaluation instruments that you intend to use, such as food frequency checklists or attitude items. Here, individual interviews are most helpful. Present individuals with the materials and have them complete the assignments, such as worksheets or evaluation instruments. Then use read-aloud procedures to ask them to explain to you what they think each item means. This will force you to use the language of the intended audience in your materials.

- *Limit your educational objectives.* Limit the number of educational objectives for group sessions or written materials. These objectives should state exactly what actions or behaviors the audience will be able to accomplish as a result of the educational intervention. Present the smallest amount of information possible to accomplish your goals. Three or four items of instruction are enough at any one time. This translates into one major concept—your behavioral goal—two or three motivation-related concepts on why to take action, such as perceived benefits and barriers, plus two or three examples of how to take action. Teach only "need-to-know" rather than the "nice-to-know" information.
- *Focus the content on behaviors or actions rather than on facts and principles to facilitate the ability to take action.* This entire book is based on this premise, but it is especially important for low-literacy audiences. The

nutrition science information and principles we present may imply what the behaviors should be. But for a low-literacy audience, the behaviors must be spelled out clearly, not just implied. In addition, this audience usually does not need all the underlying nutrition science information in order to engage in the behavior.

- *Present information using a variety of ways to enhance learning.* For example, use mini-lectures, discussions, small group activities, and visuals, as well as appropriate printed materials.
- *Use familiar examples and a conversational style.* Build on what they already know, and use familiar examples from their lives. For all audiences, but particularly if your audience is also a low-resource audience, refer to foods or dietary practices familiar to the audience rather than to exotic foods and national data. This will help to anchor your message in memory. Talk to them the way you would a friend.
- *Actively engage your audience.* During educational sessions, encourage people to ask questions and to share information and experiences through discussion and dialogue. Allow time for individuals to commit themselves to doing something before the next session. Then in the next session allow time for them to report what they did on their commitment. In printed materials, engage the readers in some activity—checklists to check off, completing the blanks, circling items, and so forth.
- *Frequently repeat and review.* If the individuals are experiencing the sessions primarily through oral means, key concepts need to be repeated often so that information can move from short-term memory into long-term memory. Allow time to process information, and at the appropriate points, review what has been said or accomplished through activities. Bring the session to closure with clear conclusions. If you use hand-

outs that require the audience to write something, be sure to have pencils ready and to allow plenty of time for them to complete the activity. For older audiences, you may need to allow time for them to find their reading glasses.

- *Treat people with respect and dignity regardless of their literacy level, and of course, regardless of socioeconomic status, race/ethnicity, religion, or country of origin.* If your audience is also a low-resources audience, note that disadvantaged groups often mistrust authority figures, so you must to willing to initiate trusting relationships. Show the group that you believe in them.

Tips for Written Materials

Many strategies for writing effective written materials are described in Chapter 16. They apply to low-literacy audiences as well. Here we emphasize those features that are additionally, or particularly, important for low-literacy audiences.

- *Write the way you speak: use the active voice.* Literacy experts such as Doak, Doak, and Root (1996) note that when you do this, your written materials become easier to read because the readability index automatically drops. They become more interesting to read. They will be easier to understand. The extra words we use when we speak help the reader to process the information.
- *Use common words.* These are words you would use when talking with a friend who was not familiar with nutrition concepts. Common words are usually short and simple words, but not always. *Doctor* is more common than *physician*, but many people are very familiar with the term *medication* even if it is a four-syllable word. If you use uncommon words, such as *hydration*, explain them. Some words are short but conceptually difficult, such as a *variety* of foods or a *balanced* diet. What exactly do we mean by *variety* or *balanced*? Explain such conceptual words.
- *Use short sentences.* Short sentences of under 10 to 15 words are easier to understand. However, you should not sacrifice conversational style. If it is more natural to say something in a longer sentence, then do so.
- *Put the key information first.* The first part of a message is remembered best (newspapers know this). So put the behavior or information that is key to your message up front, in the position most likely to be remembered. Assume that the reader will read just the first sentence, the first paragraph, or the first page. So put the most important information first. For example, say "eating lots of fruits and vegetables [the behavioral goal of your program] each day can help lower your risk of heart disease," and then go into greater detail about the many benefits of why to eat more fruits and vegetables and how to do so.

- *Create headings, subheadings, and summaries.* Use headings to serve as guideposts or road signs. Headings and subheadings make the text look less formidable. They alert readers as to what is coming up next and help them focus on the intended message. Keep the headings simple, using perhaps three to five words, and locate them right before the text that they introduce. This process also allows for delivering the written information in chunks that can be remembered.
- *Use layout and typography that makes the text easier to read.* As noted in the last chapter, use short paragraphs and plenty of white space, simple fonts such as sans serif fonts, and adequate font sizes. Use short lines of 30 to 50 characters and spaces, and use bullets where appropriate, such as for lists of tips, procedures, or things to do. Highlight important information with circles, arrows, or underlining rather than all capital letters. Remember that all caps are more difficult to read. Make the page look as though it can be read in a few minutes.

Tips for Visuals

The following tips apply to the use of illustrations, charts, lists, tables, and graphs with low-literacy audiences.

- *Use visuals to enhance learning.* We all remember information better when we see the message, not just hear it, as we have noted in earlier chapters. Visuals make information vivid and real. As Doak and colleagues note (1996), most poor readers rely on visuals and the spoken word. Visuals with a minimum of text help them to understand instructions without having to struggle with the text. Visuals, appropriately designed, can help the low-literacy reader follow step-by-step instructions for complex procedures. Visuals can also provide emotional impact that is more memorable. The written message saying that "when a mother drinks alcohol, the baby drinks alcohol" can be converted into a line drawing showing a baby inside the mother drinking from a cup when the mother does so. This can carry a more powerful and memorable message than the written word (Doak, Doak, & Root, 1996).
- *Use visuals to enhance motivation.* Make the cover of a booklet or the beginning of a brochure or handout appealing while clearly conveying the key message of the material. Because reading is not easy for low-literacy individuals, an appealing cover or introduction can provide the impetus to open the page or read the material. The style of artwork or the photograph needs to be appropriate to the culture so that readers can easily recognize it as familiar and can visualize themselves in the situation. Realistic line drawings are recommended over stylized or abstract images, which are often not

understood. Test the style of the artwork or photograph with the intended audience for its appropriateness and motivational power.

- *Include visuals to clarify the text, but use visuals carefully.* Place the visual near the text to which it refers so that the readers' eyes do not have to go elsewhere to find the written text to understand the message. Break the information into small chunks and provide one visual for each chunk to make it easier to follow. For example, if you want to encourage walking and stair climbing, show separate drawings for walking and stair climbing. Use a simple action caption for each drawing. Or if you use a table to provide a list of foods high in fat, break up the foods into groups with a heading over each. To engage the learner, you can provide a checklist with boxes to check as a means of self-assessment. Doak and colleagues (1996) provide many examples on how to develop effective visuals.

- *Use simple and clear illustrations.* Illustrations should include enough detail to emphasize the message but should not be so detailed as to become complex and distracting. Line drawings of people should look as real as possible and therefore should include eyes, mouth, nose, ears, and facial expressions (Doak, Doak, & Root, 1996). If you want to illustrate a procedure with many steps, number each of them. Photographs are also effective if they are uncluttered and the message is clearly depicted.

- *Use color appropriately.* Color can attract and hold attention and is almost expected today given the high quality of the visual media by which we are all surrounded. The preference for colors varies considerably by age, gender, socioeconomic status, and ethnicity. It is thus very important to test your color choices with the intended audience to find out whether they will convey the meanings and message you intend.

Conclusion

Although the key principles in designing nutrition education described in Part II of this book apply to all groups—that is, a focus on enhancing motivation and facilitating the ability to take action—the methods for delivering the educational plan for the intervention in actual practice will need to differ depending on the audience. Working with different population groups requires ensuring that your educational delivery methods are appropriate for the particular group.

In this chapter we learned that children are not little adults—they are experiencing various stages of physical, cognitive, emotional, and social development. At each stage, they have different needs and abilities and different ways of thinking about themselves and the world that must inform the educational design and activities. Preschool children need repeated experience with tasty and healthful foods to become familiar with them, and play-based activities. As children develop, they can process more information, and cognitive motivational processes become more important. Goal-setting and cognitive self-regulation skills become more developed. At the same time emotional and social forces are important. Nutrition education needs to identify motivations that are meaningful to youth and provide opportunity to practice goal-setting and cognitive self-regulation skills.

Adults tend to engage in learning only when they see that the learning is of immediate use to them. Adults differ in life stage and roles. Nutrition education for them should build on previous experience, respect them as decision makers, and engage them actively in their own learning. Facilitated discussion or dialogue is a useful educational tool.

Given the cultural diversity in the United States, groups often differ in cultural background, which should influence how nutrition education strategies are delivered. Nutrition educators should aim to become culturally competent, which means possessing a set of knowledge and interpersonal skills that allows them to increase their understanding and appreciation of cultural differences and similarities within, among, and between groups and to work effectively in cross-cultural situations. Nutrition education programs should seek to be culturally appropriate to their intended audience. Likewise, nutrition education programs should be mindful of the literacy level of their audiences and develop oral, visual, and written communications that are appropriate to their level.

Questions and Activities

1. You have been asked to provide suggestions to a Head Start center regarding their nutrition education program for their youngsters. From what you have learned, what advice would you give?

2. You are looking over a nutrition education curriculum for grades 4 and 5. Based on what you have read in this chapter, list three features the curriculum should have that would make you conclude that the curriculum is at the appropriate developmental level.

3. You will be providing two after-school nutrition education sessions to a group of teens aged 13 to 15. Describe three educational formats you will be sure to use to gain their attention and provide skill development.

4. You plan to facilitate a group discussion and dialogue session to implement your educational plan with a group of mothers of young children. What do you see as your role as a facilitator? What challenges do you anticipate? How will you know that you are being an effective facilitator?

5. Pick a cultural group that you would like to learn about. Read about the culture of the group or talk with people from that group. For this group, what are two key nutritional concerns? Go to a grocery store that stocks foods for this cultural group. Pick two foods and learn more about them. Then identify a nutrition education material, such as a handout, pamphlet, poster, video, or healthy cookbook, that you might use with this group. In what ways is it culturally sensitive? Describe how it uses surface structure or deep structure features or both. Be specific.

REFERENCES

Abusabha, R., J. Peacock, and C. Achterberg. 1999. How to make nutrition education more meaningful through facilitated group discussions. *Journal of the American Dietetic Association* 99:72–76.

Alaimo, K., C.M. Olson, and E.A. Frongillo. 1999. Importance of cognitive testing for survey items: An example from food security questionnaires. *Journal of Nutrition Education* 31:269–275.

Baranowski, T., J. Baranowski, K.W. Cullen, et al. 2003. Squire's Quest! Dietary outcome evaluation of a multimedia game. *American Journal of Preventive Medicine* 24:52–61.

Birch, L.L. 1999. Development of food preferences. *Annual Review of Nutrition* 19:41–62.

Birch, L.L. 1987. The role of experience in children's food acceptance patterns. *Journal of the American Dietetic Association* 87(suppl):S36–S40.

Bronfenbrenner, U. 1979. *The ecology of human development*. Boston: Harvard University Press.

Bronner, Y. 1994. Cultural sensitivity and nutrition counseling. *Topics in Clinical Nutrition* 9:13–19.

Brookfield, S. 1986. *Understanding and facilitating adult learning: A comprehensive analysis of principles and effective practices*. San Francisco: Jossey-Bass.

Contento, I.R. 1981. Children's thinking about food and eating: A Piagetian-based study. *Journal of Nutrition Education* 13(suppl):S86–S90.

Contento, I.R., G.I. Balch, Y.L. Bronner, et al. 1995. The effectiveness of nutrition education and implications for nutrition education policy, programs and research. A review of research. *Journal of Nutrition Education* 27:279–418.

Contento, I.R., J.W. Michela, and C.J. Goldberg. 1988. Food choice among adolescents: Population segmentation by motivation. *Journal of Nutrition Education* 20:289–298.

Contento, I.R., J.W. Michela, and S.S. Williams. 1995. Adolescent food choice: Role of weight and dieting status. *Appetite* 25:51–76.

Contento, I.R., J.W. Michela. 1998. Nutrition and food choice behavior among children and adolescents. In Goreczny and Hensen, eds. *Handbook of pediatric and adolescent health psychology*, p. 249–273. Allyn & Bacon: Boston.

Contento, I.R., S.S. Williams, J.L. Michela, and A.B. Franklin. 2006. Understanding the food choice process of adolescents in the context of family and friends. *Journal of Adolescent Health* 38(5):575–582.

Contento, I.R., P.A. Zybert, and S.S. Williams. 2005. Relationship of cognitive restraint of eating and disinhibition to the quality of food choices of Latina women and their young children. *Preventive Medicine* 40:326–336.

Croll, J.K., D. Neumark-Sztainer, and M. Story. 2001. Healthy eating: What does it mean to adolescents? *Journal of Nutrition Education* 33:193–198.

Cross, T., B. Bazron, K. Dennis, and M. Isaacs. 1989. *Towards a culturally competent system of care*. Vol. 1. Washington, DC: Georgetown University Child Development Center, CASSP Technical Assistance Center.

Cusatis, D.C., and B.M. Shannon. 1996. Influences on adolescent eating behavior. *Journal of Adolescent Health* 18:27–34.

Devine, C.M. 2005. A life course perspective: Understanding food choices in time, social location, and history. *Journal of Nutrition Education and Behavior* 37:121–128.

Devine, C.M., M. Connors, C.A. Bisogni, and J. Sobal. 1998. Life-course influences on fruit and vegetables trajectories: Qualitative analysis of food choices. *Journal of Nutrition Education* 30:361–370.

Devine, C.M., and C.M. Olson. 1991. Women's dietary prevention motives: Life stage influences. *Journal of Nutrition Education* 23:269–274.

Doak, C.C., L.G. Doak, and J.H. Root. 1996. *Teaching patients with low literacy skills, Second Edition*. Philadelphia: Lippincott.

Edstrom, K.M., and C.M. Devine. 2001. Consistency in women's orientations to food and nutrition in midlife and older age: A 10-year qualitative follow-up. *Journal of Nutrition Education* 33:215–223.

Elkind, D. 1978. Understanding the young adolescent. *Adolescence* 13:127–134.

Faith, M.S., K.S. Scanlon, L.L. Birch, L.A. Francis, and B. Sherry. 2004. Parent–child feeding strategies and their relationships to child eating and weight status. *Obesity Research* 12:1711–1722.

Fisher, J.O., and L.L. Birch. 2002. Eating in the absence of hunger and overweight in girls from 5 to 7 years of age. *American Journal of Clinical Nutrition* 76:226–231.

Gable, S., and S. Lutz. 2001. Nutrition socialization experiences of children in the Head Start program. *Journal of the American Dietetic Association* 101:572–527.

Gibson, E.L., and J. Wardle. 1998. Fruit and vegetable consumption, nutritional knowledge, and beliefs in mothers and children. *Appetite* 31:205–228.

Gillman, M.W., S.L. Rifas-Shiman, A.L. Frazier, et al. 2000. Family dinner and diet quality among older children and adolescents. *Archives of Family Medicine* 9:235–240.

Gould, R.L. 1978. *Transformations: Growth and change in adult life*. New York: Simon & Schuster.

Guthrie, J.F., B.H. Lin, and E. Frazao. 2002. Role of food prepared away from home in the American diet, 1977–1978 versus 1994–1996: Changes and consequences. *Journal of Nutrition Education and Behavior* 34:140–150.

Hertzler, A.A., and K. DeBord. 1994. Preschoolers' developmentally appropriate food and nutrition skills. *Journal of Nutrition Education* 26:166B–C.

Husing, C., and M. Elfant. 2005. Finding the teacher within: A story of learner-centered education in California WIC. *Journal of Nutrition Education and Behavior* 37(Suppl. 1):S22.

Isaacs, M., and M. Benjamin. 1991. *Towards a culturally competent system of care*. Vol. 2: *Programs which utilize culturally competent principles*. Washington, DC: Georgetown University Child Development Center, CASSP Technical Assistance Center.

Kavanagh, K.H., and P.H. Kennedy. 1992. *Promoting cultural diversity: Strategies for health professionals*. Newbury Park, CA: Sage.

King, M.A., A. Sims, and D. Osher. 2006 How is cultural competence integrated in education? Center for Effective Collaboration and Practice, American Institutes of Research. http://cecp.air.org.

Knowles, M.S. 1990. *The adult learner: A neglected species.* 4th ed. Houston, TX: Gulf.

Kreuter, M.W., S.N. Lukwago, R.D. Bucholtz, E.M. Clark, and V. Sanders-Thompson. 2003. Achieving cultural appropriateness in health promotion programs: Targeted and tailored approaches. *Health Education and Behavior* 30(2):133–146.

Kreuter, M.W., C. Sugg-Skinner, C.L. Holt, et al. 2005. Cultural tailoring for mammography and fruit and vegetables intake among low-income African-American women in urban public health centers. *Preventive Medicine* 41:53–62.

Kumanyika, S.K., and C.B. Morssink. 1997. Cultural appropriateness of weight management programs. In *Overweight and weight management: The health professional's guide to understanding and practice*, edited by S. Dalton. Gaithersburg, MD: Aspen.

Leupker, R.V., C.L. Perry, S.M. McKinlay, et al. 1996. Outcomes of a field trial to improve children's dietary patterns and physical activity. *Journal of the American Medical Association* 275:768–776.

Levinson, D.J. 1978. *The seasons of a man's life*. New York: Knopf.

———. 1996. *The seasons of a woman's life*. New York: Knopf.

Lin, W., and I.S. Liang. 2005. Family dining environment, parenting practices and preschoolers' food acceptance. *Journal of Nutrition Education and Behavior* 37(Suppl. 1):47.

Liou, D., and I.R. Contento. 2001. Usefulness of psychosocial theory variables in explaining fat-related dietary behavior in Chinese Americans: Association with degree of acculturation. *Journal of Nutrition Education* 33:322–331.

Matheson, D., and K. Spranger. 2001. Content analysis of the use of fantasy, challenge, and curiosity in school-based nutrition education programs. *Journal of Nutrition Education* 33:10–16.

Matheson, D., K. Spranger, and A. Saxe. 2002. Preschool children's perceptions of food and their food experiences. *Journal of Nutrition Education and Behavior* 34:85–92.

Michela, J.L., and I.R. Contento. 1984. Spontaneous classification of foods by elementary school-aged children. *Health Education Quarterly* 11:57–76.

Neugarten, B.L., R.J. Havighurst, and S.S. Tobin. 1968. Personality and patterns of aging. In *Middle age and aging*, edited by B.L. Neugarten. Chicago: University of Chicago Press.

Neumark-Sztainer, D., P.J. Hannan, M. Story, J. Croll, and C. Perry. 2003. Family meal patterns: Associations with sociodemographic characteristics and improved dietary intake among adolescents. *Journal of the American Dietetic Association* 102:317–322.

Neumark-Sztainer, D., M. Story, D. Ackard, J. Moe, and C. Perry. 2000a. The "family meal": View of adolescents. *Journal of Nutrition Education* 32:329–334.

———. 2000b. Family meals among adolescents: Findings from a pilot study. *Journal of Nutrition Education* 32:335–340.

Neumark-Sztainer, D., M. Story, P.J. Hannan, C.L. Perry, and L.M. Irving. 2002. Weight-related concerns and behaviors among overweight and nonoverweight adolescents: Implication for preventing weight-related disorders. *Archives of Pediatric Adolescent Medicine* 156:171–178.

Neumark-Sztainer, D., M. Story, C. Perry, and M.A. Casey. 1999. Factors influencing food choices of adolescents: Findings from focus-group discussions with adolescents. *Journal of the American Dietetic Association* 99:929–937.

Neumark-Sztainer, D., M. Story, E. Toporoff, J.H. Himes, M.D. Resnick, and R.W. Blum. 1997. Covariations of eating behaviors with other health-related behaviors among adolescents. *Journal of Adolescent Health* 20:450–458.

Norris, J. 2003. *From telling to teaching*. North Myrtle Beach, SC: Learning by Dialogue.

Olson, C.M., and G.L. Kelley. 1989. The challenge of implementing theory-based nutrition education. *Journal of Nutrition Education* 22:280–284.

Orlet Fisher, J., B.J. Rolls, and L.L. Birch. 2003. Children's bite size and intake of an entrée are greater with larger portions than with age-appropriate or self-selected portions. *American Journal of Clinical Nutrition* 77:1164–1170.

Petty, R.E., and J.T. Cacioppo. 1986. *Communication and persuasion: Central and peripheral routes to attitude change.* New York: Springer-Verlag.

Piaget, J., and B. Inhelder. 1969. *The psychology of the child.* New York: Basic Books.

Resnicow, K., T. Baranowski, J.S. Ahluwalia, and R.L. Braithwaite. 1999. Cultural sensitivity in public health: Defined and demystified. *Ethnicity and Disease* 9:10–21.

Resnicow, K., A. Jackson, D. Blisset, et al. 2005. Results of the Healthy Body Healthy Spirit trial. *Health Physiology* 24:339–348.

Resnicow, K., A. Jackson, R. Braithwaite, et al. 2002. Healthy Body/Healthy Spirit: A church-based nutrition and physical activity intervention. *Health Education Research* 17:562–573.

Robinson, T.N., M. Kiernan, D.M. Matheson, and K.D. Haydel. 2001. Is parental control over children's eating associated with childhood obesity? Results from a population-based sample of third graders. *Obesity Research* 9:306–312.

Rolls, B.J., D. Engell, and L.L. Birch. 2000. Serving portion size influences 5-year-old but not 3-year-old children's food intakes. *Journal of the American Dietetic Association* 180:232–234.

Sahyoun, N.R., C.A. Pratt, and A. Anderson. 2004. Evaluation of nutrition education for older adults: A proposed framework. *Journal of the American Dietetic Association* 104:58–69.

Sanjur, D. 1982. Social and cultural perspectives in nutrition. Englewood Cliffs, NJ: Prentice-Hall.

Satter, E. 1999. *Secrets of feeding a healthy family*. Madison, WI: Kelcy Press.

Sigman-Grant, M. 2004. *Facilitated dialogue basics: A self-study guide for nutrition educators. Let's dance.* University of Nevada, Cooperative Extension.

Singleton, J.C., C.L. Achterberg, and B.M. Shannon. 1992. Role of food and nutrition: The health perceptions of young children. *Journal of the American Dietetic Association* 92:67–70.

Skinner, J.D., B.R. Carruth, B. Wendy, and P.J. Ziegler. 2002. Children's food preferences: A longitudinal analysis. *Journal of the American Dietetic Association* 102:1638–1647.

Story, M., and M.D. Resnick. 1986. Adolescents' views on food and nutrition. *Journal of Nutrition Education* 18:188–192.

Story, M., D. Neumark-Sztainer, and S.I. French. 2002. Individual and environmental influences on adolescent eating behaviors. *Journal of the American Dietetic Association* 2:S40–S51.

Story, M., D. Neumark-Sztainer, N. Sherwood, J. Stang, and D. Murray. 1998. Dieting status and its relationship to eating and physical activity behaviors in a representative sample of US adolescents. *Journal of the American Dietetic Association* 98:1127–1135, 1255.

Sue, D.W., and D. Sue. 1999. *Counseling the culturally different: Theory and practice*. 3rd ed. New York: Wiley.

Tennant, M., and P. Pogson. 1995. Learning and change in the adult years: A developmental perspective. San Francisco: Jossey-Bass.

Vella, J. 2002. *Learning to listen, learning to teach: The power of dialogue in educating adults*. Revised ed. San Francisco: Jossey-Bass.

Videon, T.M., and C.K. Manning. 2003. Influences on adolescent eating patterns: The importance of family meals. *Journal of Adolescent Health* 32:365–373.

Vygotsky, L.S. 1962. *Thought and language*. Cambridge, MA: MIT Press.

Wardle, J., L.J. Cooke, E.L. Gibson, M. Sapochnik, A. Sheiham, and M. Lawson. 2003a. Increasing children's acceptance of vegetables: A randomized trial of parent-led exposure. *Appetite* 40:55–162.

Wardle, J., M.L. Herrera, L.J. Cooke, and E.L. Gibson. 2003b. Modifying children's food preferences: The effects of exposure and rewards on acceptance of an unfamiliar vegetable. *European Journal of Clinical Nutrition* 57:341–348.

Young, L., J.J. Anderson, L. Beckstrom, L. Bellows, and S.L. Johnson. 2004. Using social marketing principles to guide the development of a nutrition education initiative for preschool-aged children. *Journal of Nutrition Education and Behavior* 36:250–257.

CHAPTER

18

Nutrition Educators as Change Agents in the Environment

OVERVIEW This chapter describes ways in which nutrition educators can help to shape the profession and to act as change agents in the larger environment by working with others to shape legislation about nutrition education and by educating policy makers in government.

OBJECTIVES At the end of the chapter, you will be able to

- State reasons why it is important to participate in professional associations relevant to nutrition education
- Identity ways you can help to shape the profession
- Understand the importance of policies regarding outside sponsorship of nutrition education professional activities and conflicts of interest
- Describe ways you can affect the larger environment by participating in community networks and coalitions
- Appreciate the importance of educating policy makers in government, such as elected officials

SCENARIO

You attend your first professional meeting of dietitians, extension nutritionists, nutrition educators, and others. You are amazed to see so many activities going on and are both excited and overwhelmed. At sessions, you hear about various programs and projects that people are involved in. They spark ideas for you to use in your professional work.

You learn new information from research. You hear about committees and task force reports. You learn about government policies at the state and national level that might affect your work and you wonder, Should I get involved? If so, how do I do that?

Introduction

Providing nutrition education directly to the public is our major role as nutrition educators. We do this through direct in-person activities with groups, indirect activities such as printed materials and media campaigns, and policy and systems change activities to foster environments supportive of the program's targeted behaviors and practices. We also have the opportunity to develop and grow as nutrition educators by networking with others and being involved in professional organizations. We can make our voices heard in the organizations of which we are members and even help to shape their

policies and practices by our participation and actions. We also have the opportunity to make a difference in the world by advocating for nutrition education policies and programs in the larger environment. This chapter describes some ways in which you can be involved in the nutrition education professional community.

Keeping Up with Nutrition Education Research and Best Practices

We began this book by saying that this is a great time for nutrition education. It is needed now more than ever, and research

467

and evidence for best practices is providing us with the tools we need to assist the public to achieve health and well-being. We have seen that nutrition education is more likely to be effective when it focuses on behaviors and practices, uses theory and research evidence from behavioral nutrition and nutrition education to guide the strategies it uses, and addresses multiple sources of influence. Effective nutrition education is not short-term work; it takes time to facilitate the progress of individuals and communities through various stages of change: from awareness and active contemplation, through various levels of motivational readiness to change, through how-to activities to enable change, to maintenance of change. Consequently, the motivators and reinforcers of change and the environmental supports of change need to be multifaceted, continually updated, and maintained.

Research in this area is active and ongoing. New understandings of how to facilitate change and new tools are being generated. Keeping up to date on nutrition education research is important to maintain your effectiveness as a nutrition educator. You can do this by reading the relevant journals and by attending nutrition education and behavioral nutrition (not just nutrition science) workshops, meetings, and conferences. Box 18-1 lists some of the professional organizations particularly relevant to nutrition educators.

Helping to Shape the Profession

As nutrition educators we also have the opportunity to participate in and shape our profession. There are many ways to do this. One way is to join one or more professional associations. For example, there are local and state dietetic associations to which you can belong, as well as national associations such as the Society for Nutrition Education and the American Dietetic Association. Through these organizations you will

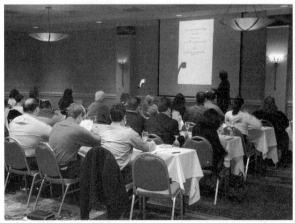

Becoming a member of a professional organization is a great way to become involved in your profession, and the level of participation is up to you.

meet others just like you—individuals who are excited to be in the nutrition education profession and helping the public eat well and who are dealing with the same dilemmas and constraints. These organizations provide a forum for you to network with others and share ideas, learn about best practices, receive updates on information that may be important in your work, and learn about regulations and policy actions that affect the profession or the public at large.

You also have the opportunity to make your opinions heard. Professional associations are member organizations, made up of others just like you. Although state and national organizations may have some paid staff, all are dependent on members' volunteer participation to operate. These associations thus become whatever we as members want them to be. If you are a student member, many organizations have student rates that extend to the first year of "professional enrollment" or "new professionals." Many organizations have what are called sections, divisions, or affiliates. These provide opportunities to network with colleagues who have like interests or are related geographically.

Who They Are

What are some associations where you might find a professional home? For nutrition educators, some of the most relevant ones include the Society for Nutrition Education (SNE), American Dietetic Association (ADA), School Nutrition Association (SNA), American Public Health Association, International Society for Behavioral Nutrition and Physical Activity, American Association of Family and Consumer Sciences, American Diabetes Association, American Association for Nutritional Sciences, and the Society for Behavioral Medicine. Information on some of these is provided in Box 18-1. Of course, many of us belong to several professional associations.

Getting to Know Them and Vice Versa

Getting involved in an organization is key to getting to know it. Reading the organization's journal by itself will not bring about opportunities to participate fully or shape the profession. As you get to know the organization, the organization will get to know you. As you offer to serve on committees and task forces and hold offices, over time the organization will come to you asking for your involvement.

A key way to get started in the process of knowing and getting known is to attend the organization's annual meeting. Annual meetings provide opportunities for more than learning from experts. They are opportunities for meeting your colleagues, expressing your thoughts, and supporting your position in the various units that run the organization and professions. The divisions, special interest units, caucuses, and affiliates all provide opportunities for input. Although these units may meet during the year and have electronic mailing lists and bulletin boards, it is at the annual meetings

BOX 18-1 Professional Associations of Particular Relevance to Nutrition Educators

Society for Nutrition Education (SNE)

Mission: The Society for Nutrition Education advances the food and nutrition education profession to impact healthful food choices and lifestyle behaviors at the individual, community, and policy levels. SNE offers opportunities for members to share best practices, evidence-based knowledge, and diverse perspectives.

Identity statement: SNE represents the unique professional interests of nutrition educators in the United States and worldwide. SNE is dedicated to promoting healthy, sustainable food choices and has a vision of healthy people in healthy communities. SNE provides forums for sharing innovative strategies for nutrition education, expressing a range of views on important issues, and disseminating research findings. Members of SNE educate individuals, families, fellow professionals, and students, and influence policy makers about nutrition, food, and health.

   Special interest units known as divisions include Nutrition Education for Aging Americans, Children, Communications, Food and Nutrition Extension, Higher Education, International, Industry, Public Health, Social Marketing, Sustainable Food Systems, and Weight Realities. SNE also has some regional affiliates and an Advisory Committee on Public Policy that helps provide focus on national issues of importance to society members.

Website: http://www.sne.org

American Dietetic Association (ADA)

Mission: Leading the future of dietetics.

Identity statement: American Dietetic Association is the nation's largest organization of food and nutrition professionals. ADA serves the public by promoting optimal nutrition, health, and well-being. ADA members are the nation's food and nutrition experts, translating the science of nutrition into practical solutions for healthy living.

   Dietetic Practice Groups (DPGs) and state affiliates provide opportunities for networking based on area of practice, interest, and geography. DPGs include groups based on area of practice (e.g., Gerontological Nutritionists DPG) as well as areas of interest (e.g., the Hunger and Environmental Nutrition DPG)

Website: http://www.eatright.org

School Nutrition Association (SNA) (Formerly the American School Food Service Association, ASFSA)

Mission: To advance good nutrition for all children. The association works to ensure all children have access to healthful school meals and nutrition education by

- Providing members with education and training
- Setting standards through certification and credentialing
- Gathering and transmitting regulatory, legislative, industry, nutritional, and other types of information related to school nutrition
- Representing the nutritional interests of all children

Identity statement: SNA is dedicated solely to the support and well-being of school nutrition professionals in advancing good nutrition for all children. Since 1946, SNA has been advancing the availability and quality of school nutrition programs as an integral part of a student's education. SNA has 52 state affiliates and hundreds of local chapters.

Website: http://www.schoolnutrition.org

American Association of Family and Consumer Sciences (AAFCS)

Mission: Members focus on an integrative approach to the reciprocal relationships among individuals, families, and communities, as well as the environments in which they function. The association supports the profession as it provides leadership in

- Improving individual, family, and community well-being
- Impacting the development, delivery, and evaluation of consumer goods and services
- Influencing the creation of public policy
- Shaping social change

Identity statement: AAFCS strives to improve the quality and standards of individual and family life by providing educational programs, influencing public policy, and through communication. Members work to empower individuals, strengthen families, and enable communities.

(continued)

▶ **BOX 18-1   Professional Associations of Particular Relevance to Nutrition Educators** *(continued)*

Through divisions, members provide guidance and practical knowledge about the things of everyday life, including human growth and development, personal behavior, housing and environment, food and nutrition, apparel and textiles, and resource management, so that students and consumers can make sound decisions and enjoy a healthy, productive, and more fulfilling life. Professional sections and state affiliates offer other opportunities for networking.
Website: http://www.aafcs.org

International Society for Behavioral Nutrition and Physical Activity (ISBNPA)

Mission: ISBNPA was formed in 2000 to address the professional interests of researchers from multiple disciplines engaged in investigating behavioral issues in nutrition and physical activity. Its purposes are as follows:

- Conduct scientific meetings, congresses, and symposia in which current research on behavioral issues in nutrition and physical activity will be discussed by researchers in related fields
- Disseminate information on research being done in behavioral issues in nutrition and physical activity through newsletters and other communications
- Provide information to and encourage continued support by public and private bodies that support research in behavioral issues in nutrition and physical activity
- Promote and facilitate the dissemination of knowledge of behavioral issues in nutrition and physical activity to the public and to educators, scholars, and health professionals through any lawful means
- Promote and assist communication between researchers on issues of behavioral nutrition and physical activity and members of scientific and scholarly organizations whose members do research in other related health and medical fields through joint meetings, shared membership lists, joint publications, and any other lawful means

Identity statement: ISBNPA has an international presence, with nearly 400 members representing 29 countries. Its members come together from more than 40 government agencies and industry and professional organizations, as well as close to 150 academic and medical institutions. Members bring to this organization a diversity of experience and expertise.
Website: http://www.isbnpa.org

Association for the Study of Food and Society (ASFS)

Mission: The Association for the Study of Food and Society is a multidisciplinary international organization dedicated to exploring the complex relationships among food, culture, and society.

Identity statement: The ASFS's members, who approach the study of food from numerous disciplines in the humanities, social sciences, and sciences, as well as in the world of food beyond the academy, draw on a wide range of theoretical and practical approaches and seek to promote discussions about food that transgress traditional boundaries. The association holds annual meetings with the Agriculture, Food, and Human Values Society and publishes the journal *Food, Culture & Society*.
Website: http://www.food-culture.org

Society for Behavioral Medicine (SBM)

Mission: The Society of Behavioral Medicine is a multidisciplinary organization of clinicians, educators, and scientists dedicated to promoting the study of the interactions of behavior with biology and the environment, and the application of that knowledge to improve the health and well-being of individuals, families, communities, and populations.

Identity statement: Better health through behavior change. The SBM's goals are to

- Enhance the value of SBM as a base for networking, professional growth, and information exchange
- Establish SBM as a visible and influential champion of behavioral medicine
- Develop the capacity to secure resources to achieve SBM's goals and mission

Website: http://www.sbm.org

that we all come together to discuss, plan, and strategize. This also applies to meetings of state or local affiliates, which often focus on more regional professional issues; membership or town meetings; and gatherings to discuss specific issues.

Finding Where You Fit

Finding your home in the profession involves finding not only the organization but also the specialty units within it that are right for you. Initially it may be the specialty units, defined as divisions, sections, or practice groups, and local, state, and regional affiliates that are of more interest to you than the organization itself. They are smaller and therefore more manageable. They also provide a common ground of interest in specific issues or approaches that may feel comfortable to you. Many of us belong to more than one such unit. Over time you may change your focus or move on, but you will often find that the relationships you have developed keep you involved and, through networking, offer opportunities in other groups and locations.

Attend the business meetings of the specialty unit or division to find out the main issues facing the organization or unit, the activities completed or contemplated, and the financial situation of the organization as well as the sources of funding for the organization.

Determining your fit is based often on your relationships with the people in the unit or organization and the ability to work synergistically to have an impact, discuss common interests, and share war stories. You can join communication forums, such as listservs. Find out if there is a mentoring program. There may be a specific student unit, and often the governing boards have student representatives. Even as a student you have an opportunity to affect the profession.

Join a Subcommittee or Task Force

Professional associations are always seeking interested members to participate. You do not have to wait to be asked! Look for notices seeking participation and input. This, too, is a way to shape the profession. If you don't feel comfortable sitting on a committee or being part of a task force, respond when the organization asks for member input or opinions. Let leadership know you're interested in an issue. Over time, as your name is recognized as an involved member, leadership will come to you. In fact, managing your time so as not to become overextended may become the more important consideration!

Write

You can participate by helping to write for, or edit, the newsletter for your specialty unit or division. You can help to write background papers or participate with others in writing position papers on some issue that is a passion of yours. You can write letters to the editor or write articles. All these actions provide opportunities to be involved and have an impact.

Participate in Program Planning Activities

Organizations and the specialty units within them always need to plan future conferences or meetings. Attend the open planning sessions and provide your suggestions for sessions, topics, or speakers. Join the planning committee if you can. Help shape the agenda for the meetings.

Participate in Member-Initiated Resolutions or Issues Management Processes

Many professional associations have a process whereby an individual, a group of members, or a division or committee can write up and submit resolutions or statements for the membership to vote on, which then go to the association for action. In most cases the resolutions advocate that the association take a position or action on some issue, or advocate that the association establish a policy. The American Dietetic Association uses an issues management process as the communication process whereby members can convey their concerns about contemporary issues to the leadership (ADA, 2001). The Society for Nutrition Education uses a member-initiated resolutions process (SNE, 2006). Such a process is a very effective way to influence the professional association as well as the larger policy environment. Past resolutions of the Society for Nutrition Education are found on its website (www.sne.org). These provide some interesting insights into membership interests and concerns. These resolutions are conveyed to the agencies and groups designated in the resolutions where they often have important impacts on food- and nutrition-related policy. The resolutions of the American Dietetic Association are also available from that organization (www.eatright.org).

Run for Office

Making the commitment to be a part of the process may very well lead you to run for an office. You may be nominated or you may decide to nominate yourself. Don't be shy. If you want to have an impact and be involved, let others know. This applies to running for offices at the specialty unit or division level as well as at the organizational level.

Volunteer

Whatever you do, find some way to be involved. The connections you make can be very important for you over the long term. In the process of volunteering, you get to know others, they get to know you, and the profession becomes stronger because of all the participatory voices. Also keep in mind that professional organizations cannot run on the dues they raise alone or the funds they may acquire through foundation grants. They need volunteers. Some active members have used a rule of thumb of volunteering an hour a week and found it to be very rewarding, both personally and professionally.

Ethics in Nutrition Education: Maintaining Credibility

We said earlier in the book that one of the most cherished assets we have as nutrition educators is our credibility—to our clients and program participants, to the professional community, to government, and to the public at large. When we lose our credibility, we lose our effectiveness. This same principle applies to the professional associations to which we belong, and indeed to the profession as a whole. Our professional associations, and indeed our profession, must be seen as credible sources of information and recommendations.

What does this mean? It means that just as is the case for individuals, so also the recommendations made by the professional associations must be seen as being based on sound science. The professional associations must not stand to gain financially, or *seem* to gain financially, from their recommendations. In recent years, professional associations, as well as private voluntary organizations, research programs using public funds, and all government and quasi-government committees, have developed sponsorship policies that apply to potential sponsors of activities of the organization, and conflict of interest policies that apply to individuals. Much of the impetus for this development came from the concern of members of organizations and of the public about undue commercial influence that might affect the credibility of the organization.

Sponsorship of Nutrition Education Programs and Professional Activities

Professional associations and organizations that provide nutrition education are always in need of funds. Membership dues, government or foundation grants, or grants from academic institutions do not always generate enough funds for these organizations to do what they need or want to do. It would appear natural to turn to the food industry for such funding. Organizations may go to individual corporations or to commodity groups. Funding can be sought for individual activities, such as a specific one-time professional meeting or a specific session or social event at the annual meeting, or for the annual meeting of an organization as a whole. Funds can also be sought for a particular fact sheet or position paper, or for a specific project or particular community outreach activity. The food industry may also contribute to the professional organization as a whole.

Members in several professional associations raised concerns about undue influence, potentially biased positions, conflict of interest, and the appearance of conflict of interest. They were concerned that corporate need for profits and nutrition professionals' interests in the health of the public may at times come into conflict (Nestle, 2002). These concerns were often raised through the resolutions process or issues management process. In response to membership concerns, many professional organizations have developed

guidelines so that sponsorship by, and collaborations with, the food industry can be conducted in an ethical and mutually beneficial manner.

Guiding principles usually include the following (SNE, 2002):

- The organization should secure sponsorship arrangements that further the organization's mission and vision, retain the organization's independence, maintain objectivity, promote trust, avoid conflicts of interest, and guard its professional values.
- The sponsorship should be consistent with the organization's commitment to the free exchange of ideas, opinions, research findings, and other information related to members' interests and activities.
- There should be transparency about relationships, clearly specified expectations, understanding of the value of the sponsor's contribution, and methods of accountability.
- Protection of the reputation of the organization is of utmost importance, along with full disclosure, information that is science based, and avoidance of the appearance of endorsement.

Conflicts of Interest

Members in several professional organizations were also instrumental in initiating policies about conflict of interest and disclosure. Members were concerned that speakers (whether members or invited guests) were not disclosing professional and corporate relationships they had when they spoke at conferences or sat on an organization's boards, committees, and task forces. Members felt it was important to know that a given speaker or board member, whatever his or her primary professional designations, also had paid consulting or other relationships with the food industry or some other relevant group. Because professional associations are member-run organizations, members' voices are important and are heard. The outcome has been that many organizations have developed new policies and procedures that address these concerns of membership.

The American Dietetic Association, for example, has a policy that requires all persons speaking or making presentations at ADA programs to disclose any dualities of interest (conflict of interest) that might be perceived as affecting or influencing their presentations; such disclosures are made known to the attendees and audience for such programs (ADA, n.d.).

Most professional associations or societies now also require all those who are on the governing board, committees, policy bodies, or task forces, and those who are officers at the division or specialty unit level, to complete an annual conflict of interest form. Some associations also require that at the beginning of each committee or task force meeting, the agenda items be reviewed and an opportunity provided for members of the committee to disclose if they have a conflict of interest on any given item. If they do, they may be asked to recuse themselves altogether from that item or to participate in the discussion but not vote (SNE, 2005). All would agree that transparency is good for everyone.

Notice that these policy changes were frequently initiated by members asking for change. This is another example of how you can make a difference in the profession by your actions.

Such self-disclosures of conflict of interest have become routine for all government and quasi-government committees, task forces, and other bodies. They are also required now for all government research and other grant recipients.

Tests for Conflict of Interest
How do you test yourself to determine if you have a conflict of interest? Ask yourself, Would others trust my comments, decisions, actions, or votes if they knew about my relationships with other organizations and/or my situation? How would I feel if the roles were reversed—would I feel misled or betrayed?

Conflicts of interest involve the abuse, actual or potential, of the trust people have in professionals. Conflicts of interest thus not only injure particular clients and employers but also damage the whole profession by reducing the trust people have in professionals in general (McDonald, 2004). Perception is a critical component here. If your colleagues or the public find out information after the fact and perceive a conflict of interest, the perception can do as much damage as the reality. Disclosure and transparency are key ways to address a conflict of interest, allowing others to weigh what you say. It may be appropriate not to participate in a given activity, a determination that can only occur if public acknowledgment of possible conflict is made.

Participating in Community Coalitions

Earlier we discussed ways in which nutrition education intervention programs can include environmental components in order to promote opportunities for participants to take the actions that are advocated by the program (see Chapters 6 and 13). Even if your program does not have an environmental change component, you can, as a nutrition education professional, participate in a number of activities in the community where you can be a change agent in the larger environment.

We need to help others understand that nutrition education professionals are much more than people who offer lectures and workshops. For the public to understand what we do, we need to be out there working with the community. Here are some examples of volunteer opportunities with community coalitions, networks, or other community groups.

Food Policy Councils

A Food Policy Council (FPC) consists of stakeholders from various segments of a state or local food system. Councils can be officially sanctioned through a government action such as an Executive Order, or can be a grassroots effort. The primary goal of many food policy councils is to examine the operation of a local food system and provide ideas or recommendations for how it can be improved (Desjardin et al., 2005).

Who better to be part of the process than the nutrition educator? It makes sense for nutrition educators to play a key role in food policy councils. Desjardin et al. (2005) point out that we contribute food and nutrition knowledge and provide 'legitimacy' as health professionals. Having nutrition professionals on board can broaden the scope of food policy councils, where members may be more concerned with emergency food assistance or agriculture policy in the most traditional sense. It also means a food policy council can get in-house help with proposal and report writing, research and evaluation, and media communication. Nutrition educators can also offer essential organizational and planning skills.

Local Wellness Policy

The Child Nutrition and WIC Reauthorization Act of 2004 (Section 204) required every local school district to develop and implement a local wellness policy (Fox, 2005). The mandate provides that nutrition guidelines must

- Be developed for all foods available on the school campus during the school day
- Include goals for nutrition education, physical activity, and other school-based activities to promote student wellness
- Have a plan for measuring implementation
- Involve parents, students, school food representatives, school board members, administrators, and the public in development

Strong nutrition components will make strong wellness policies, and the nutrition educator can be a facilitator of this process and/or serve as a resource. As is the case with food policy councils, school wellness councils are multidisciplinary, and assessment is important. Examples of self-assessment and planning tools include the School Health Index (SHI) from the Centers for Disease Control and Prevention (CDC, 2005), and Changing the Scene from the Team Nutrition Program of the U.S. Department of Agriculture (USDA, 2000). In New York State, nutritionists are encouraged to participate through the Schools and Professionals in Nutrition Program (SPIN), using the CDC School Health Index. Other states use the USDA Changing the Scene tool, and still others have developed their own. As a nutrition educator, you bring your skills in assessment and in facilitation of dialogue to the table; these are critical to a functional wellness policy. Wellness policies must be evaluated, and you can provide useful skills in this task as well.

Nutrition Education Networks

Nutrition education networks came into being in the mid-1990s when the Food and Nutrition Service (FNS) of the USDA approved cooperative agreements to establish nutrition education networks in 22 states (Association of State Network Administrators, 2004). The funding objective was to create self-sustaining statewide networks to implement nutrition education for food stamp eligible adults and children, building on existing efforts, developing public-private partnerships, and using social marketing. It was envisioned that the networks would be the catalyst to integrate nutrition education messages across the food assistance programs and public-private programs (Association of State Network Administrators, 2004). This networking process would be designed to

- Maximize public and private resources
- Identify specific client needs and relevant ways to address these needs
- Recruit and leverage community organizations to deliver appropriate messages

Such networks continue to exist in many states, using funding from a variety of sources. You should check whether there is one in your state or city. They provide considerable opportunities to network and coordinate nutrition education activities in your local area.

Community Coalitions

There are no doubt many other local or national coalitions of food and nutrition professionals concerned with a variety of issues that would welcome your participation. Issues might include food security, concerns about the sustainability of food systems, urban gardens, farmers' markets, special populations such as those with HIV/AIDS or diabetes, or childhood overweight prevention. Your insights and expertise as a nutrition educator can be very important to the effective functioning of these coalitions.

Advocating for Nutrition and Nutrition Education

You can be a change agent in the larger environment through advocacy activities. These include written communications, providing testimony to governmental and quasi-governmental groups, and helping to shape legislation that affects the nutritional well-being of the public and the support of nutrition education.

Written Communications

Written communications take many forms. The most notable, of course, are letters: you can make your voice heard through writing to newspapers, to legislators, and others. You can also write articles. However, you can also write other documents that can have a tremendous impact on the decision making of individuals, organizations, and government. These can include position papers, policy papers, issue fact sheets, and background papers. Although "key expert members" may write the initial background documents and subsequent

papers, you usually have an opportunity to provide input into these documents if you wish and let your wish be known.

Testimony, Hearings, and Forums

Governmental bodies often seek information from professionals about a specific issue, using a variety of formats. Testimony and hearings usually come about in response to an invitation or public announcement to provide evidence to a session or committee of Congress, or to other governmental or quasi-governmental bodies, such as committees of the National Academy of Sciences. Hearings are usually open to the public and are designed for committees to obtain information and opinions from professionals or the public on proposed legislation, an investigation, or other activities of government. Hearings may also be purely exploratory in nature, a forum for professionals and the public to provide testimony and data about topics of current interest.

Forums or listening sessions provide opportunities for sharing comments in person or in writing. If you feel passionate about a particular issue, you can seek to testify. Sometimes you can do this on your own, on the basis of being a professional in the field. Or you may testify through your professional group, in which case you must make sure the leadership knows you are interested in presenting testimony.

Helping to Shape Legislation

Some legislation, once passed, is permanent. However, some legislation is written so that it must be renewed after some stated period of time or it will expire. This happens typically in five-year increments, but the time period may be longer or shorter. Key examples of federal legislation that impact nutrition education include the following:

- The Child Nutrition and WIC Reauthorization Act
- The Farm Bill
- The Ryan White Act
- The Older Americans Act

See Box 18-2 for more information.

You can help shape such legislation by becoming actively involved in the process of making recommendations. For example, the Child Nutrition and WIC Reauthorization Act was due to expire in 2004. In 2002, concerned organizations began to meet to discuss what they would advocate for at renewal time. A one-day meeting was held, sponsored by the National Alliance for Nutrition and Activity, an umbrella organization with more than 30 member organizations, and the Society for Nutrition Education. The meeting was called "The Future of Nutrition Education: Child Nutrition Reauthorization Opportunities." The purpose of this meeting was to bring together stakeholders to discuss the current state of child nutrition education, develop ideas for strengthening child nutrition education, and aid member organizations in developing policy recommendations regarding child nutrition education.

> **BOX 18-2 Legislation That Affects Nutrition Education Programs**

Child Nutrition Reauthorization

Child Nutrition Reauthorization includes legislation that covers the primary government food programs outside of the Food Stamp Program, and related education components. Programs include the following:

- National School Lunch Program (NSLP)
- School Breakfast Program (SBP)
- Child and Adult Care Food Program (CACFP)
- Summer Food Service Program (SFSP)
- Special Milk Program (SMP)
- Women, Infants and Children (WIC), which includes the WIC Farmers Market Nutrition Program (FMNP)
- Fruit and Vegetable Snack Program
- Team Nutrition Program and language for the Team Nutrition Network
- School Wellness Policy legislation
- Language for access to local foods and school gardens

The Farm Bill

The Farm Bill is a series of ten titles; four in particular relate directly to nutrition education. These cover international and national nutrition education and related programs, research, and "miscellaneous" components (respectively, Titles III, IV, VII, and X). This act is also a key source of nutrition education funding and research.

- Title III, the Trade Title, includes the McGovern-Dole International Food for Education and Nutrition Program.
- Title IV, known as the Nutrition Title, covers the Food Stamp Program (FSP), Food Stamp Nutrition Education (FNSE), and Community Food Project Grants (CFPG); commodity distribution programs that are often associated with nutrition outreach, such as the Emergency Food Assistance Program (TEFAP), the Commodity Supplemental Food Program (CSFP), and the Department of Defense Fresh Program (DoD Fresh); funds for child nutrition programs such as commodities for school meals; primary funding for Senior FMNP and additional funding for the WIC FMNP program; the Nutrition Information and Awareness Pilot Program; and startup grants for some institutions participating in the national school lunch, and school breakfast programs that purchase locally produced foods (the latter two have never received funding).
- Title VII, known as Research and Related Matters, includes the Education and Administration of Land Grant institutions, with programs such as the Cooperative State Education and Extension Service (CSREES), which includes the Community Food Projects (CFP), the Expanded Food and Nutrition Education Program (EFNEP), and Sustainable Agriculture Research and Education Grants (SARE). The title also includes the Organic Agriculture Research and Extension Initiative.
- Title X is for miscellaneous programs such as country-of-origin labeling, irradiated food/pasteurization, and biotechnology education.

The Ryan White Comprehensive AIDS Resources Emergency (CARE) Act

The Ryan White Act is federal legislation that addresses the unmet health needs of persons living with human immunodeficiency virus (HIV) disease by funding primary health care and support services. The CARE Act was named after Ryan White, an Indiana teenager whose courageous struggle with HIV/AIDS and against AIDS-related discrimination helped educate the nation.

Older Americans Act

The Older Americans Act was originally signed into law by President Lyndon B. Johnson. In addition to creating the Administration on Aging, it authorized grants to states for community planning and services programs, as well as for research, demonstration, and training projects in the field of aging. Later amendments to the act added grants to Area Agencies on Aging for local needs identification, planning, and funding of services, including but not limited to nutrition programs in the community as well as for those who are homebound; programs that serve Native American elders; services targeted at low-income minority elders; health promotion and disease prevention activities; in-home services for frail elders; and those services that protect the rights of older persons, such as the long-term care ombudsman program.

Sources: Administration on Aging, U.S. Department of Health and Human Services. *Older Americans Act.* http://www.aoa.gov/about/legbudg/oaa/legbudg_oaa.asp; Health Resources and Services Administration, U.S. Department of Health and Human Services. HIV/AIDS Bureau. http://hab.hrsa.gov/history.htm; National Campaign for Sustainable Agriculture. 2006, January. What's in a farm bill? http://www.sustainableagriculture.net/primer.php; U.S. Congress, House of Representatives. 2002, May. *Farm Security and Rural Investment Act of 2002 conference report to accompany HR 2646.* 107th Congress, 2nd session. Report 107-424. Washington, DC: Government Printing Office. http://www.nrcs.usda.gov/about/legislative/pdf/2002FarmBillConferenceReport.pdf; and U.S Department of Agriculture. 2002. Farm Bill 2002. http://www.usda.gov/farmbill2002/.

The group was made up of nearly 30 participants representing a variety of food and nutrition professional organizations and advocacy groups interested in strengthening child nutrition education. Over the course of the day and through numerous other activities over the course of the ensuing months, the group developed program recommendations such as the following (American Public Health Association, n.d.):

- Allocate adequate funding to reflect nutrition education as a priority.
- Develop and implement evaluation and reporting components.
- Create key nutrition coordinators at the federal, state, and local levels and identify clear roles and responsibilities.
- Provide funding for new and existing staff.

These recommendations became the basis of a white paper on child nutrition education and of other activities that were designed to influence the shape of the legislation. Nutrition educators volunteered their time to participate in these activities. Out of this process came the mandate to set up local wellness committees in school districts to develop policy regarding food and health in schools (see Chapter 13). You can make an important contribution by adding your voice to those of other nutrition educators in activities such as these so as to make a difference in the larger environment.

A number of organizations serve as advocates of food and nutrition policy and legislation at the local, state, and federal level. They monitor the various food and nutrition programs, alert the profession about new initiatives and changes that are being contemplated, and advocate for programs that benefit the public. One such organization is the Food Research and Action Center (FRAC). Located in Washington, D.C., it is a leading national organization working to improve public policies to eradicate hunger and undernutrition in the United States. FRAC describes itself as "a nonprofit and nonpartisan research and public policy center that serves as the hub of an anti-hunger network of thousands of individuals and agencies across the country" (www.frac.org). Its staff includes a variety of professionals, dominated by lawyers. However, nutritionists have an important role to play in organizations such as FRAC at the local, state, or national level. The experience of one such nutrition educator is described in Nutrition Education in Action 18-1.

NUTRITION EDUCATION IN ACTION 18-1

The Nutritionist as Food and Nutrition Advocate

After her undergraduate degree in anthropology, Lynn Parker went to South America to work on various development projects. While there, she became aware that many issues related to development were related to poverty and access to food. She came back to the United States and studied for a graduate degree in nutrition, after which she sought to work on policy issues related to access to food for all.

She now works at the Food Research and Action Center (FRAC). According to its website, "FRAC seeks to harness our nation's resources on behalf of those in our country who are least able to provide for themselves. Hunger reduces a child's ability to learn, decreases a worker's productive energy, weakens an elderly person's resistance to disease. Hunger prevents our nation from reaching its full productive potential." FRAC engages in a variety of activities at the national, state, and local levels to form a comprehensive strategy for reducing hunger in this country. To accomplish these goals, FRAC's activities include the following:

- *Research:* Conducts research to document the extent of hunger, its impact, and effective solutions.
- *Public policy:* Seeks improved public policies that will reduce hunger and undernutrition.
- *Monitoring function:* Monitors the implementation of laws, regulations, and policies affecting the poor.
- *Program support:* Provides coordination and support to a nationwide antihunger network of advocates, food banks, program administrators and participants, policy makers, and others, especially those concerned with the School Breakfast Program, the Summer Food Service Program for Children, and the WIC program.
- *Public information:* Develops media and public information campaigns to help promote changes in public attitudes and policies, and acts as an authoritative source of information on hunger for the news media and public officials.

The organization is staffed predominantly by lawyers. In her role as a nutritionist in the organization, Lynn Parker is involved in many of the listed activities. In particular, she helps the group understand the nutritional impacts of legislative action related to food, attends policy meetings to bring in the perspective of the nutrition profession, and keeps food and nutrition professional associations apprised of legislative action.

Many other nutrition educators work in various food policy and advocacy organizations at the community, state, and federal levels.

Source: Food Research and Action Center. www.frac.org.

Educating Policy Makers in Government

Chapter 13 talked about the importance of educating and working with policy makers and decision makers so as to promote environments that are conducive to food and nutrition behaviors. These policy makers were school principals, community leaders, worksite management, local agencies, and others. Here we discuss educating policy makers in government—our elected officials.

Why Educate Elected Government Officials?

Elected government officials are the ones who will vote on legislation and make policy on issues that are of concern to you as a nutrition educator, such as funding for nutrition and for nutrition education through a variety of programs. Legislators are always sensitive to their constituents, so you, as an individual, *can* have an impact on them.

Who Are Your Elected Officials?

There are policy makers at many levels—local, city, county, state, and federal—and those who participate in nutrition education policy work say that it is important for you to know each one by name. Finding out who represents you should not be difficult in this age of technology. Go to the Web-based page of your local or state government; there will most likely be a tool there that will assist you in identifying your representative. Or try the Government Guide (http://votenote.aol. com/mygov/dbq/officials/). This site provides information on representatives at all levels and keeps you up to date on the activities of your legislators. At the federal level, you can also use www.senate.gov for senators and www.house.gov for members of the House of Representatives.

Get to Know Them and Let Them Get to Know You

Once you know who your elected representatives are, the next step is to find out about them. Go to their websites and find out the following:

- Their interests
- Legislation they support
- Committees they sit on

You put them there through your vote, and now you can help them work *for* you. You may think voting is not important, but it is. When you vote, you are designating the person who is ultimately going to work on your behalf. You need to let them know what you want and why it is important. If there is no funding for nutrition education at the federal level, many members of the public will not get the nutrition education they need, especially those in greatest need, such as those with few resources and those who live in low-income neighborhoods. Many issues of great importance will never be addressed, and many nutrition education jobs will not exist. You can use a variety of tools alone or in combination, but it is imperative to take action. Some methods are listed here.

- *Phone calls.* You can call your local office or, if the legislator travels between home and the state or national capitol, call that office. Either way, the legislator will get your message.
- *Meet legislators and meet with their staff.* It is great for them to know you by face; again, it can be in the district office, at the seat of government, or at both locations. Often you will not be able to meet with the legislator but can meet with the staff. The administrative assistant (AA) often acts as chief of staff and is involved in policy decisions. The legislative director (LD) is in charge of the work of the legislative aides (LAs), who focus on a specific issue, such as health, transportation, or education. In fact, asking to meet and work with the legislative aide who works on your area of interest in the case of federal representatives can be most productive. They are the ones who do the research, provide the recommendations, and often write the legislation that is very important to nutrition education.

  When it comes to making an appointment, do not wait until the last minute. Be sure you are registered to vote. Be prepared to tell the scheduler (an actual position) what you intend to talk about. In fact, it is very likely you will be asked to put your request in writing before it will even be considered. Faxing and email are common since the terrorist events of 2001, but each office is different, so you need to determine what works best for the particular office. Confirm your appointment the day before.

  Prepare in advance, know your key points, and bring your business card. Stay on topic. You are paying them, but be realistic and expect the meeting to last only 15 minutes. Come with a brief handout, and if there is a visual to share, bring it. A picture can say volumes, as can a graph. If you are asked a question and don't know the answer, don't guess. Tell them you will find out the answer and be sure to follow up with whatever you promise and with a thank you note.

  Inviting your legislator to your place of work or your local agency can also be a great opportunity for you and for the legislator. Make the offer and be sincere. Although they might not take you up on it, knowing you want them there can help. Photo ops are very important for them in the communication age.
- *Letters.* Letters can be sent to express your perspective, offer your help on an issue, ask for a meeting, or as a thank you note. Today letters are not as easy a way to communicate with many government offices, especially in Washington, D.C., so you can use email. If you

do use e-mail, stay formal in your letter composition. A resource for writing a letter is the Government Guide (http://votenote.aol.com).

- *Contribute to them.* Although legislators work for you, they still need funds to support their campaigns. There are a number of options, and finding the one that works for you is important. You can give them money directly, go through a political action committee (PAC), attend functions they have, or a combination of these. Contributions do have value and are recognized.
- *Stay in touch with them.* Meeting with legislators is not a one-shot deal. You want to know them, and they need to know you and the nutrition education issues you are most concerned about. If you stay in touch, they will be more ready to meet with you when you want their support for some policy or legislation that is important to you and the nutrition education community.
- *Become a legislative aide yourself.* A great way to influence food and nutrition policy through the legislative process is to become a legislative aide yourself.

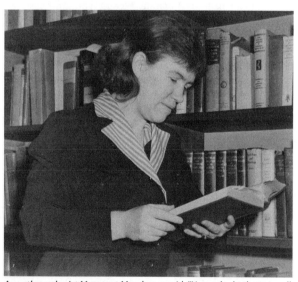

As anthropologist Margaret Mead once said, "Never doubt that a small group of thoughtful committed people can change the world. Indeed, it is the only thing that ever has."

Several nutritionists or nutrition educators have gone to work on the staffs of elected officials. They add expertise to the office, advocate for food and nutrition policy, and help legislators write policy that is needed and sound. One such person is described in Nutrition Education in Action 18-2. Some nutritionists and dietitians have even run for office themselves.

You Can't Do Everything, but You Can Do Something

This book has sought to provide you with the motivation, conceptual understanding, and skills for you to develop, implement, and evaluate nutrition education that is behavior focused and evidence based and that links theory, research, and practice. This final chapter has sought to stimulate you to become actively involved in the profession of nutrition education and to participate in actions that will have an impact on the larger environment. These actions can increase the ability of the nutrition education profession to advance the health of the nation's citizens.

As we have seen, you have many opportunities to make a difference in the world. Although you don't need to do everything, you can do something. Pick one action that you feel you can do:

- Involvement in the profession
- Helping the profession remain ethical and credible
- Participation in community coalitions
- Advocating for nutrition education to governmental and other bodies
- Educating policy makers in government about nutrition education issues

Postscript

Now that you have completed this book, go back to the list you generated in Chapters 1 and 2 of the qualities you stated as important to being a good nutrition educator. You also stated areas in which you felt you needed more work. Reflect on your understandings and skills now.

- How do you see yourself now as a nutrition educator? What knowledge and skills have you gained?
- Where would you like to be a year from now? Five years from now? Describe ways that will help you get from here to there.

NUTRITION EDUCATION IN ACTION 18-2

A Nutritionist Working in Legislation

After he completed his undergraduate degree in psychology, Robert Stern realized that he was interested in community food issues and wanted to make a difference in the world. He returned to school and received a master⊠s degree in nutrition education. While working in a community health center near the capitol of New York, Albany, he had occasion to interact with regional organizations concerned with food issues that worked with the state legislature. He also worked on the campaign of a friend who was elected to state office. When his federally funded job ended, he sent his resumé to his elected friend, who thought he was a good match with the New York State Assembly Task Force on Food, Farm, and Nutrition Policy. The task force had an opening, and he got the job. Over the years he worked his way up to program manager for the task force.

Mission of the Task Force
- To develop programs, legislation, and budget initiatives that mutually benefit New York consumers, producers, and marketers of food in urban, suburban, and rural communities
- To provide oversight of implementation of state and federal food, nutrition, and agricultural programs
- To provide information and support concerning food policy issues to the task force chair, Speaker, assembly, and the public

Task Force Issue Areas
- Federal, state, and local food assistance programs (e.g., food stamps, WIC, school meals, senior meals, emergency food programs)
- Improving the marketing of New York farm and food products (e.g., government, school, and institutional purchasing; sales in supermarkets; farmers' market expansion; small-scale food processing; farm product distribution)
- Nutrition and health; nutrition education (e.g., childhood obesity prevention, concern for foods of minimal nutritional value, and increased fresh fruits and vegetables in schools); food allergies; insurance coverage for nutrition therapy
- Consumer concerns (e.g., labeling of food, contamination of food, genetic engineering, effectiveness of herbal supplements)
- Food-related community and economic development (e.g., farmers' markets, kitchen incubators, food entrepreneurs, restaurants featuring local products)
- Environmental and community impact of farming and food production (e.g., farmland protection, watersheds and farming, farm labor)
- Food policy councils

As program manager, Stern manages the legislative work related to these activities: he responds to and translates policy issues into legislation and budget recommendations; he initiates, develops, and manages public hearings and meetings around the state as needed; he negotiates; and he writes letters, newsletters, and press releases. The work changes over time and is always dependent on the direction the chair of the task force wants to take. Although the politicians make the final decision, he is pleased that he has the opportunity to help shape legislation on issues that are of concern to nutritionists and the public.

Questions and Activities

1. Identify two professional associations, local or national, that you think will be a good home for your interests as a nutrition educator. List their addresses and membership criteria. Make a plan to join.

2. List some of the strengths that you bring to the profession. Based on these, describe two ways in which you can help shape the profession.

3. Why is it important for nutrition education professional organizations to maintain or increase their credibility? Describe policy actions they can take to ensure ethical practices.

4. Define what is meant by "conflict of interest." Why is it important for individuals and organizations to disclose potential conflicts of interest?

5. Describe at least two ways in which member-initiated actions have had an impact on professional association policy changes.

6. In what ways can nutrition educators help to shape legislation that will have an impact on nutrition education?

7. Do you know who your legislators are at the federal, state, and local level? Complete the following table. For each of your elected officials, list his or her address or email address and phone number. Make a date to contact these officials.

Your Elected Official to	Contact Information: Address, email, Phone	Committee That Person Is On; Special Interests	Date You Contacted or Will Contact Person
City/town council			
State senate			
State assembly			
U.S. Senate			
U.S. House of Representatives			

REFERENCES

American Dietetics Association. n.d. *HOD backgrounder: Dietetics professionals and ADA organizational units relations with industry.* http://www.eatright.org/ada/files/Industrybackgrounder.doc.

———. 2001. The issues management process: An evolving process, focused on member value. http://www.eatright.org/cps/rde/xchg/ada/hs.xsl/home_531_ENU_HTML.htm.

American Public Health Association. n.d. National Alliance for Nutrition and Activity: Child Nutrition Program reauthorization recommendations. http://www.apha.org/legislative/factsheets/ChildNutrition.pdf.

Association of State Network Administrators. 2004. *Food Stamp Nutrition Education Networks: Partners for better health.* http://www.ces-fsne.org/pdfs/04ASNNAsummary.pdf.

Centers for Disease Control and Prevention. 2005. *Welcome to the School Health Index (SHI): A self-assessment and planning guide.* http://apps.nccd.cdc.gov/shi/default.aspx.

Desjardin, E., L. Drake, F. Estrow, and S. Roberts. 2005, July. Food policy councils and the role nutritionists play. Presented at the annual conference of the Society for Nutrition Education, Orlando, FL.

Food Research and Action Center (FRAC). 2006. www.frac.org.

Fox, T. 2005, July. Local wellness policies. PowerPoint presentation at the annual conference of the Society for Nutrition Education, Orlando, FL.

McDonald, M. 2004. Ethics and conflict of interest. Vancouver, BC: The W. Maurice Young Centre for Applied Ethics. http://www.ethics.ubc.ca/people/mcdonald/conflict.htm.

Nestle, M. 2002. *Food politics: How the food industry influences nutrition and health.* Berkeley: University of California Press.

———. 2002, January. *Society for Nutrition Education sponsorship guidelines.* http://www.sne.org/sponsorship-guidelines.pdf.

Society for Nutrition Education. 2005. Conflict of interest. In *Society for Nutrition Education policies and procedures manual*, Section 6.9. Approved by the SNE Board April 11, 2005.

———. 2006. *Society for Nutrition Education resolutions process.* http://www.sne.org/documents/FinalResolution-process51305amendedJuly2006.doc.

United States Department of Agriculture. 2000. *Changing the scene: Improving the school nutrition environment.* Alexandria, VA: U.S. Department of Agriculture, Food and Nutrition Service. http://www.fns.usda.gov/tn/Healthy/changing.html.

Photo Credits

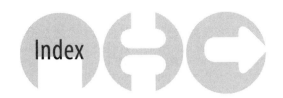

Index